AT QUI CONSILIUM FUTURI
EX PRAETERITO VENIT

(The council for the future
results from the past)

Seneca ep. 83,2
(about 63 A.D.)

History of Dentistry

by

Walter Hoffmann-Axthelm

Professor Dr. med. Dr. med. dent.

Freiburg im Breisgau, Germany

Translated by H. M. Koehler
Chicago, USA

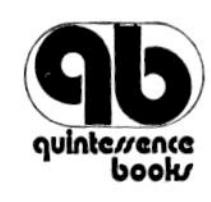

Quintessence Publishing Co., Inc. 1981
Chicago, Berlin, Rio de Janeiro and Tokyo

Dedicated to my wife,
Dr. Irmtraut Hoffmann-Axthelm

Title of the German Edition: Die Geschichte der Zahnheilkunde

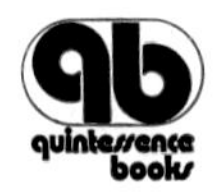

Process engraving: Meisenbach Riffarth & Co., Berlin
Composition and presswork: Kupijai & Prochnow, Berlin
Binding: J. Godry, Berlin
Printed in Germany

ISBN 3 87652 161 0

Preface

"History indeed is the witness of the times, the light of the truth"
Cicero (De Oratore)

The ascendancy of the healing art of the oral structures to the profession of dentistry is the end of a long journey from the roots of civilization to the atomic age of molecular biology. The odd, frustratingly slow, often chilling, often inspiring history in which dentistry only yesterday reached the legal status of an independant branch of the healing profession can be retraced parallel to that of medicine as the issue of the following consecutive epochs: First there is paleontologic evidence of the suffering of our human ancestors from oral ills and the first attempts of treatments by healers and sorcerers. Documents and artifacts then bear witness of a rising recognition of the pathologic conditions at the dawn of a medical science by the "asu" in Akkadian Mesopotamia (3000 B. C.), the Egyptian "sinu" like Hesy Re (2600 B. C.), then the Greek "iatros" like Hippocrates (400 B. C.) and the Roman "medicus" like Galenus (170 A. C.). Then, there followed the dark period of the quackery-pharmacologic and technical, tool making revolution that lasted, short of a few exceptions of scientific pioneering up to the 18th century; charms and salves, pernicious nonsense of anatomical ignorance but also masterpieces of technically ingenious instruments are the mixed legacy of this period of a prevalent charlatanic craftmanship of the dental art. Its ultimate reraise to the free academic profession—as it has been in the antiquity already certified by Hammurapi's code of Babylonian surgery (1700 B. C.)—is due to the scientific acquisitions of prestigious physiologists. This start of the era of oral biology was first heralded in France, then Germany and Great Britain to be accomplished in the United States and Canada. The creation of dental faculties is the cornerstone of this reelevation of dentistry to a free academic profession, a process which in old world countries (Portugal, f. i.) as well as in the developing nations is still under way.

To have put for the first time this universal human struggle toward understanding, treating and preventing oral conditions into a sequential perfectly documented "History of Dentistry" is the merit of Professor Walter Hoffmann-Axthelm. With an encyclopedic knowledge —reflected by his Dental Lexicon*, a rare zest for historic truth, documented by a unique list of exact references, and a detective's eye for pertinent original documents—Professor Hoffmann-Axthelm has pieced together into fluent reading the fascinating tale of man's attempts over millenaries to conquer and prevent oral pain and disease. By abstaining from the usual emphasis on the bizarre and by scrutinizing the painful step by step advancement of scientific discoveries the author has created a text of reference of great scientific importance. Professor Hoffmann-Axthelm's formidable account of the historic past of the art and science of dentistry is indeed a source of enlightment in the never ending pursuit of the provision of dental care to everybody by an ever competent dental profession.

Geneva, September 1980

Louis J. Baume
President FDI

* HOFFMANN-AXTHELM, W.: Lexikon der Zahnmedizin. Buch- und Zeitschriften-Verlag "Die Quintessenz", Berlin, 1978.

Foreword to the German Edition

The last important work on history of the discipline in German language came out more than 45 years ago with the second edition of Karl Sudhoff's "History of Dentistry." This was followed by the 1935 and 1945 description of the 18th and 19th century by the Danish dentist Stroemgren. Still earlier there was the work of Geist-Jacobi in 1896, and several older communications. Worth noting among Anglo-Saxon writings is the "History of Dentistry" of 1909 by the Italian, Guerini, and, among newer contributions, there are several editions of Lufkin and Bremner published since 1938 as well as Weinberger's two-volume opus of 1948. Volume II, however, has a strictly national character.

With the exception of those by Geist-Jacobi and Stroemgren the German books do not consider the decisive development of dentistry during the 1900's. Therefore as the author assumed his functions at the Institute for the History of Medicine at the Free University of Berlin in 1964, he set himself to the task of closing the gap as Sudhoff in 1924 had suggested. As a short introductory history of the important dates of earlier developments was compiled, many new facts came to light regarding the hundred years divided in half by Sudhoff. From this over a period of 8 years an entire chronicle was developed, almost unwillingly, on the history of the discipline until the 1900's. The scope of the work was somewhat frightening, even to the writer.

Yet, several seemingly important procedures and names were missing, for information concerning professional problems, especially for the 1900's, has been treated conscientiously on the side. Until the present time development in individual countries has been so varied that it can only be described without difficulty by national representatives. Although the periods of headings are not always adhered to strictly and the boundaries between history and history of our time disappear, the breakthrough of indispensable framework classification of transitory passages may be accepted by the unbiased reader as well as criticized by historians. In the whole, the author (following the precepts of the great historian in the 19th century, Leopold von Ranke) has attempted to write history "as it actually happened." This may seem to be old-fashioned, but it appeared to the writer to be appropriate to the subject.

With few exceptions original sources were traced and reproductions or reprints were evaluated simultaneously. The footnotes after each chapter refer to these and to secondary reports that were used. The references were not intended to represent a complete bibliography, but merely the portions of texts used. Philological aid received by the author from true helpers was a particularly happy circumstance. This aid is recorded at the close of the corresponding chapters. Only in this manner was it possible to reach the actual source. The cooperation received is responsible in many instances for the first texts translated from the original language.

Collegial support in other countries was given the author by R. A. Cohen in Warwick, Charles Coury in Paris, J. A. Donaldson in London, Åke B. Loefgren in Goeteborg, F. E. R. de Maar at the Hague and Donald Washburn in Chicago. To them belong heartfelt thanks as well as to the late custodians of the Research Institute for Dental History of the German Dental Association in Cologne, F. H. Witt and R. Venter, who made the treasures of their library available for many years.

Special thanks are due to the co-workers at the Institute for the History of Medicine at the Free University of Berlin who, each in his own way, made this comprehensive project possible. Among these many years of aid given by Mrs. Christa Riedel-Hartwich deserves special mention.

The author owes thanks to the publisher, Dr. h. c. W. Haase, who gave him a free hand regarding range and photographic material and to R. Klein for his typical care in preparation.

Berlin, March 1973

Walter Hoffmann-Axthelm

Foreword to the English Edition

This English-language edition of the "Geschichte der Zahnheilkunde," published in 1973, is not a simple translation. Rather, at least in the sections devoted to the nineteenth and early twentieth centuries, it is almost a different book. Results of recent research as well as extensive correspondence elicited by the publication of original, but also new insights, for instance, such as those gained from review of the published chapter about Old Egypt, have made necessary a rather comprehensive revision. The results of that process are presented here after an eight-year interval. They are also the base of a Japanese edition of this book.

For all that the author thoroughly recognizes the problems associated with such a translation; there will never be an absolutely objective writing of history. No author can detach himself from the spirit of the present time or the time in which he grew and matured. Inevitably, despite all the efforts made to attain objectivity, the historian's nationality, contemporary social structures, his own status in society, his religion, or some other factors will be reflected in what he writes. He assumes responsibility for interpreting development—even in dentistry—from external and internal circumstances of the time, in which the particular event occurred. To complicate matters he will usually have an abundance of events from which to choose, and the choosing itself is a subjective process. In the triad that comprises the writing of history today —finding, evaluating, and interpreting source material—the individuality of the author unavoidably is reflected in his writings. The ways and means in which this occurs are decisive in the determination of the quality of his works, even—and especially—for his foreign language readers.

In addition to those whose help has been acknowledged in the earlier foreword and at the end of some chapters the author thanks the translator in Chicago, Mr. Henry M. Koehler, who often had to fight with very delicate texts. Good support in collecting older English literature the author found in the libraries of the British Dental Association and of the Wellcome Institute of the History of Medicine, both in London. Mrs. Aletha Kowitz, librarian of the American Dental Association, assisted with dates and literature of her country. Mr. Bernd-M. Seyffarth performed conscientiously the production and earned great merit by managing all the transoceanic communications.

Very special recognition is offered here to the publisher, Mr. H.W. Haase. Books such as this one, directed to the circle of those interested in history, entail a high degree of publishing risk, especially when—as is the case here—production is undertaken without support from any official source. It deserves express mention that here material interests were subordinated to service to science in the best traditions of publishing.

Freiburg im Breisgau, January 1981

Walter Hoffmann-Axthelm

Contents

Part 1

Dentistry from the Beginnings to becoming Independent in the 18th Century

Part 2

Dentistry in the Industrial Age

Part 1

Dentistry from the Beginnings to becoming Independent in the 18th Century

Introduction

Dentistry first assumed its position as a profession with a certain independence in literature of the eighteenth century, during the Baroque period, a time of absolutism. Thus the actual history of the profession starts during this period. Of course, written traditions and hand-made products of dental procedures have existed for four to five thousand years. These matters may only be attributed in rare instances to actual dental therapists. The overwhelming majority are examples of work done by priests and physicians, magicians and charlatans on the periphery of their practical healing arts, or as the many-faceted remains of prosthetic efforts of skilled artisans. Only the more pressing requirements for control of toothaches, fastening of periodontally loosened teeth and closure of cosmetically unattractive anterior spaces are considered as the first dental procedures.

As disease is as old as life on earth, it is possible to determine the pathological conditions of the teeth and jaws for the corresponding interval to the saurian age, a period of 70 or more million years. Excavated jaw bones from the Glacial Age showed signs of periodontal disease even among pre-Neanderthals and Neanderthals. This condition plagued mankind for over 100 thousand years, as described by the anatomist Hans Virchow, son of the renowned pathologist, regarding the Ehringsdorf jaw, and by Choquet regarding the skull of La Chapelle-aux-Saints. The opposing point of view, that the signs indicate presence of senile atrophy, was rejected by Virchow on the basis of the fissures between the alveolar margin and the root[1] (Fig. 1).

Carious processes, however, were as rare among these obscure paleolithic races as in the much older completely dentulous Heidelberg mandible of the first interglacial period (about 500,000). They were also rare during the post-glacial period, in the Middle Stone Age which was about 8,000 B. C. Ferrier found only 3 % caries among 2,000 teeth from 7,000- to 8,000-year-old skeletons[2]. Mummery saw 2 teeth (2.94 % of those existing) with carious defects in 68 British skulls[3]. Not until the early Stone Age did the incidence of caries increase. A more frequently occuring tooth destroying factor was the severe abrasion caused by coarse food mixed with sand, gravel and—later—milling remnants of primitive grain mills. A contributing factor probably was the prevalent edge-to-edge bite of that period[4] (Fig. 2). Stress of this type did not contribute to the durability of either enamel or dentin or even of the secondary dentin which formed as a result of the abrasion. The result was extreme pain, loss of pulp vitality, and pulp necrosis with the corresponding consequences to the jaw bones and—no longer demonstrable today—the soft tissue[5] (Figs. 3 and 7). In the earlier Iron Age (750—450), findings of this sort could be substantiated in the cemetery of Hallstatt[6]. The marked abrasion could be the reason for the significant predominance of approximal caries over fissure caries[7]. Traces of operative therapy are no more ascertained from these early times than in those of the historically ancient cultures of Asia and Africa. People sought help in the way of conjuring and magic. The first attempts for rational dentistry were limited to medical and physical measures. The oldest recorded procedures of this kind are found in Egyptian papyrus scrolls and on Babylonian-Assyrian clay tablets.

1 H. Virchow (a); (b) p. 66 f.; Choquet (specific literature references can be found at the end of each chapter)
2 Ferrier (a)
3 Mummery
4 Bouvet
5 Gorjanovič-Kramberger
6 Morton et al.
7 Praeger

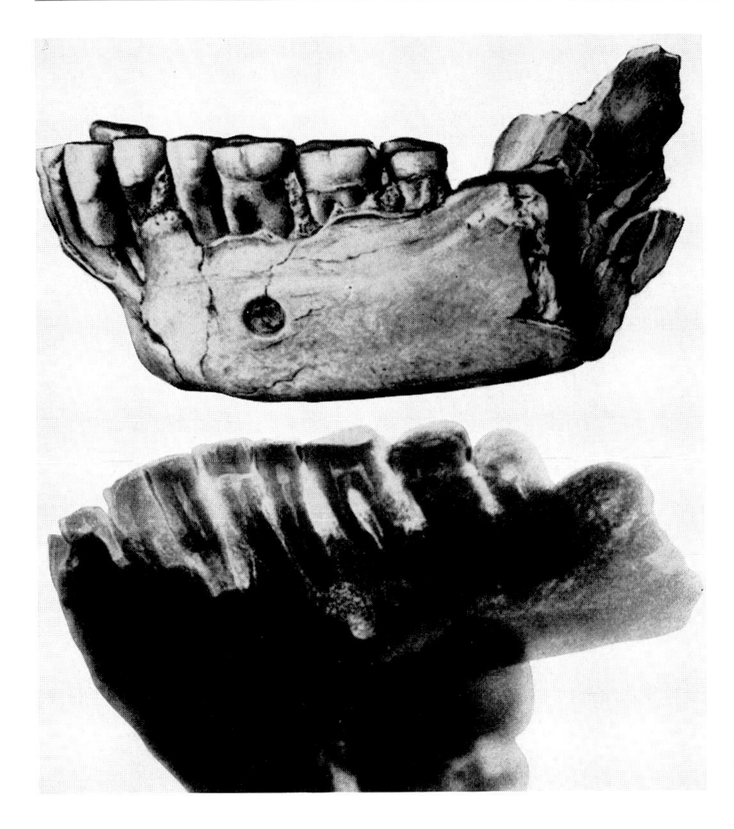

Fig. 1 *Left half of a pre-Neanderthal mandible with indications of alveolar resorption. Found at Ehringsdorf near Weimar (from Hans Virchow)*

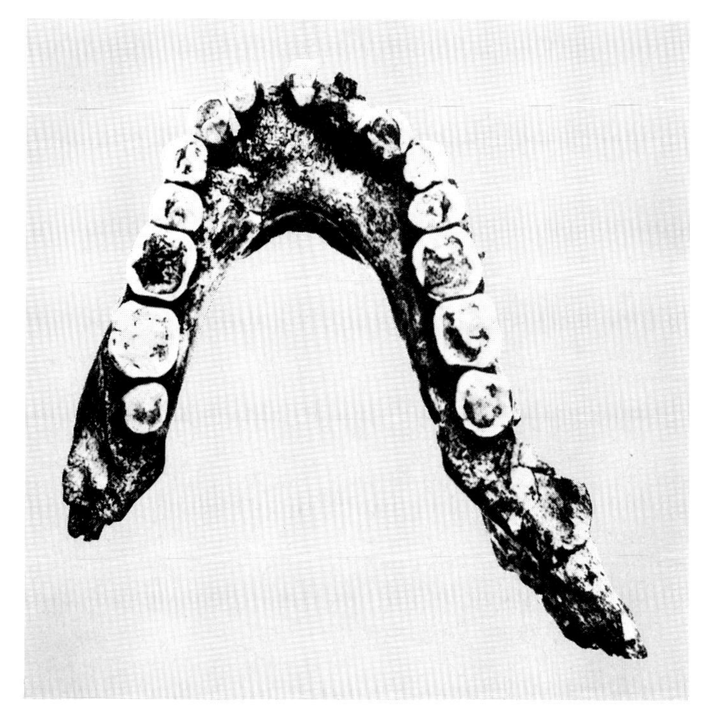

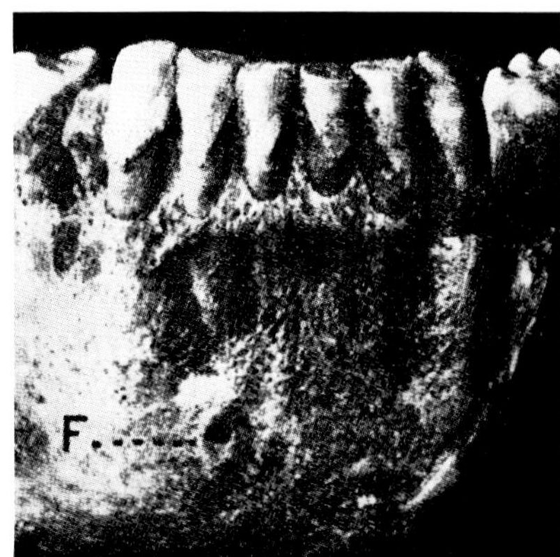

Fig. 3 *Fistula formation in the region of the chin (F), arising from a severely abraded right lateral incisor of a pre-Neanderthal. Found at Krapina, Croatia (from Gorjanowič-Kramberger)*

Fig. 2 *The molars of the Ehringsdorf jaw show severe abrasion*

References

Bouvet, Pierre
Considérations sur les lésions dentaires de l'homme aux temps préhistoriques. Rev. Stomat. 24 (1922) 567—574

Choquet, J.
Examen de l'appareil dentaire du crâne de l'homme préhistorique de la Chapelle aux Saints. Verh. V. Internat. Zahnärztl. Kongr. Berlin 1909, Vol. I, pp. 138—139

Ferrier, J.
a) Considérations sur les mâchoires et les dents d'un ossuaire de la pierre poli. Rev. Stomat. 19 (1912) 11—18
b) Étude sur les dents temporaires recueillies dans un ossuaire néolithique à Vendrest. Rev. Stomat. 20 (1913) 171—178

Gorjanowič-Kramberger
Anomalien und patholog. Erscheinungen am Skelett des Urmenschen aus Krapina. Korresp.bl. Dtsch. Ges. Anthrop. 39 (1908) 108—112

Lenhossék, M. von
Die Zahnkaries einst und jetzt. Arch. Anthrop. N.F. 17 (1919) 44—46

Morton, Friedrich, Hermann Wolf, Heribert Goll
Kiefer und Zähne in der La-Tène-Periode. Zschr. Stomat. 37 (1939) 1067—1080

Mummery, John R(idgen)
On the relation which dental caries . . . may be supposed to hold to their food and social condition. Trans. Odont. Soc. G.B. N.S. 2 (1870) 7—24, 27—80

Praeger, Wolfgang
Das Gebiß des Menschen in der Altsteinzeit und die Anfänge der Zahnkaries. Dtsch. zahnärztl. Wschr. 28 (1925) 90—99, 112—122

Virchow, Hans
a) Unterkiefer von Ehringsdorf. Zschr. Ethnol. 47 (1915) 444—449
b) Die menschl. Skelettreste aus dem Kämpfe'schen Bruch im Travertin von Ehringsdorf bei Weimar. Jena 1920

Chapter 1

The ancient Orient

Egypt

The Nile Empire appeared from the darkness of history as a centrally ruled nation around 3000 B. C., with its capital Memphis (near Cairo) to meet the need of a regulated society along the life-supporting river. The earliest recorded period of the ancient empire was initiated about 2600 by King Djoser whose vizier, Imhotep, was chief of the administration, architect—he is credited with the Step Pyramid of Saqqara—and physician. In the latter role he was attributed by later generations to have God-like qualities, comparable to the God of healing, Asclepios, in the Hellenistic aera.

In the second half of the third millennium B. C., the great pyramids appeared along the Nile as symbols of a grandiose death cult which included the custom of embalming. As the skill was practiced by primitive artisans, it was not usual to collect anatomic knowledge. Even systematic investigation was an unknown concept to Egyptian physicians. Still, they were keen observers and discovered empirically some useful drugs and sensible healing methods. These were eventually transcribed, interspersed with magic words in a difficult to decipher archaic script, and retained their validity among tradition-conscious Egyptians through the millenia.

In about 2000 B. C. the Old Kingdom disintegrated into principalities. About 200 years later the beginnings of scientific systematization and solidification evolved under strong rulers of the Middle Kingdom (2040—1785), along with a flowering literature. Because of the inroads of the Asiatic Hyksos, a dark interval commenced. This lasted until 1570, with liberation from the South introducing the illustrous New Kingdom (1552—1070). Under war-minded kings such as Thutmosis III, Egypt became the driving force of the Orient with southern Thebes as its capital. The immense temples of Karnak and Luxor dedicated to the God-King Amun Re were built. In the 1400's the attempts of Amenophis IV to break the power of the Amun priests by introducing a monotheistic sun cult failed. The weakening of the kingdom which ensued was overcome under Sethos I and Ramses II. Then a decline followed. One more final independent period was presented to the country in 600 with its center in Saïs, in the Nile delta. Here the knowledge of traditional old art and science was cultivated. In 525 Kambyses made Egypt to a Persian satrapy. By 332 it was controlled by Alexander and after his death by the Greek dynasty of the Ptolemies in Alexandria until it became a Roman province in about 30 B. C.

Already in the Old Kingdom medicine appears as a fully developed profession. In particular, in excavation of the city of the dead around the Gizeh pyramids, which reflected the Pharaoh's court city, the so-called mastabas or burial chambers of physicians were discovered. Their inscriptions reveal a good insight into sociological aspects of their status four to five thousand years ago. The Egyptian term for physician was "sjnw." It is pronounced "sinu" today. (Written Egyptian, just as Hebrew, has no vowels.) Hieroglyphically it was represented by a horizontal arrow, often with an ointment jar (Fig. 4). A hierarchy developed very early at least at court for the prominent rank which was always attached to the temple in some manner. There were chief physicians, court physicians, and highest physicians. The rank of the physicians was symbolized hieroglyphically according to title, and there was specialization. Much later, in 500 B. C., the Greek Herodotos described the specialists: *The practice of medicine is distributed among them in the following manner: Each physician limits himself to one area of disease. Physicians abound. Some specialize in eyes, others in the head; teeth; the abdomen and its parts, in internal disorders*[1].

Grapow believes that specialization as such did not exist in ancient Egypt, but that it appeared during the Egypt of Herodotos'. However, he does recognize the man who deals with teeth for the ancient era, as does Junker[2]. Often an esteemed physician had more than one title, that is, he did not specialize in just one

1 Herodotos II 84
2 Grapow III p. 91; Junker (b) pp. 69 f.

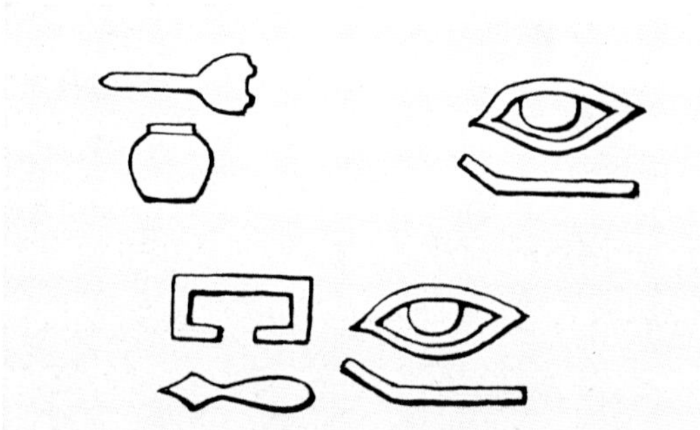

Fig. 4

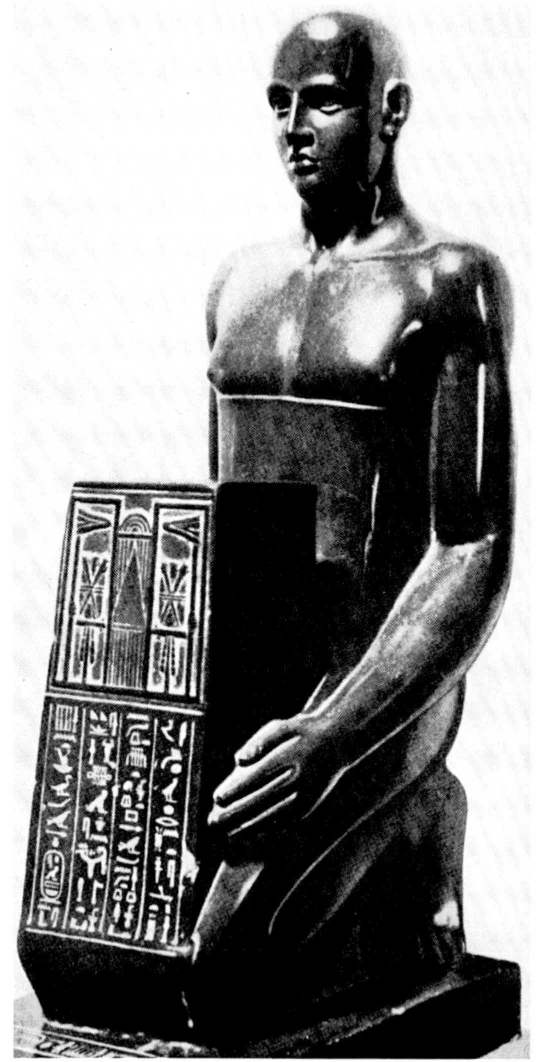

Fig. 6

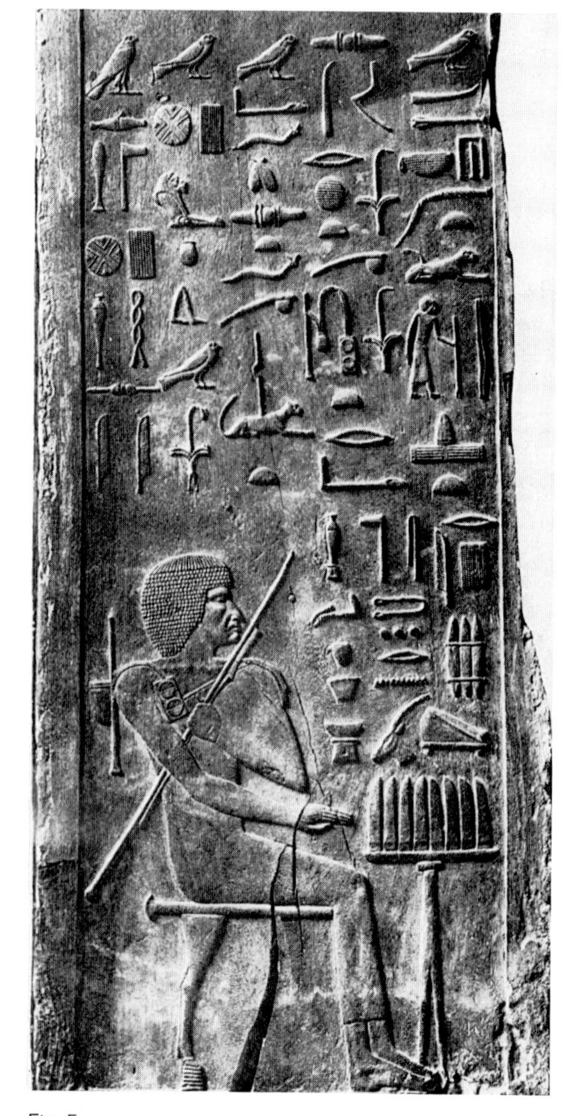

Fig. 5

Fig. 4 *Egyptian rank hieroglyphs: physician, one who deals with teeth, and one who deals with teeth at the court of the Pharaoh*

Fig. 5 *Hesy-Re, before the altar with bread. Hieroglyphs upper right: bird, tusk and arrow mean "Greatest of those who deal with teeth, and of the physicians" (from Quibell)*

Fig. 6 *Basalt statue of Psemtek-Seneb, one of the "greatest of the physicians" (first row from left, center) and one of the "greatest of those who deal with teeth at court" (third row, center), around 600 B. C. (from Jonckheere)*

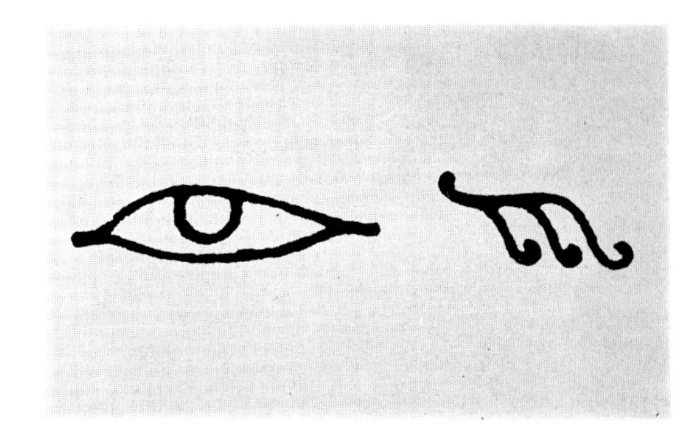

Fig. 7 *Hieroglyphs of "one who deals with hair"*

disease. A report from the Persian era leads us to assume that all physicians were trained in medical schools.

In contrast to other physicians, the Egyptian tooth practicers did not have the arrow hieroglyph and were not designated by sjnw, but characterized by an eye and a horizontal elephant's tusk, accompanied, if necessary, by the corresponding service rank symbol (Fig. 4). Early traces of "one who deals with teeth" were found in the time of the Step Pyramid of King Djoser (about 2600 B. C.) in a contemporary burial chamber. In this personal Mastaba of Hesy-Re (literally "praised by Re") five wooden panels with his titles and portraits were discovered. Junker described one of these as representing *the greatest of those who deal with teeth, and of the physicians* (Fig. 5). Hesy-Re commanded 13 official titles in addition to the medical, as, for example, director of royal records and guard of the diadem. It is difficult to imagine these high functions as those of an ordinary dental therapist[3]. Perhaps the title indicates some administrative or temple function or it could have been a meaningless honorary designation or even a sinecure.

In contrast, the tooth practicers found in the burial chambers of important persons in the group of *officials and servants* (Junker) must be recognized as active specialists even if they were available only to the upper classes. Thus one of the servants, named Nfr-irjts, of a prince at the start of the V dynasty in Gizeh is represented on the north wall of the burial chamber as one who deals with teeth[4]. For a dental specialist in the sense of a dentist, the occasionally occuring combination of the physician's hieroglyph is indicated. On the other hand the term "tooth dealer" seems proven by its similarity to the hieroglyph for "one who deals with hair" (Fig. 7) symbolized by an eye and a curl.

Apparently Egyptians cleaned their teeth in the morning[5]. Grapow indicates that the colloquial expression *for washing the mouth* became synonymous with breakfast (so common was it) and that at one point mouth cleansing and tooth cleansing became synonymous too[6]. This is not to preclude the upper classes from having special servants to care for their hair and their teeth. This arrangement held for title-happy Egyptians for over 2000 years. As recently as the Saitic Period, about 600 B. C., a basalt statue found in Heliopolis shows a greatest of the physicians specializing in dental dealing and in the latter quality even greatest at court[7] (Fig. 6).

As already noted, Egyptian physicians had little interest in anatomy. There was no description of the mouth to be found, for example only its function as the primary orifice of the body is described, other than the anus. Teeth were pictured by the well-known tusk. In addition to the monumental hieroglyphs, italics existed. These were also found on papyrus and contained the 2 words ībḥ and nḏḥ.t. However, a differentiation between anterior and lateral teeth cannot be dis-

3 Junker (b) p. 69; Kaplony p. 583. Also according to Kaplony who combines the three hieroglyphs in opposition to Junker as head (chief) dentist, "this fits poorly in the other titles of hieroglyphs of H.". Weinberger (c. p. 65) identifies Hesy-Re, perhaps under the influence of Ranke, somewhat cavalierly as "first known dentist."
4 Junker (d) pp 193 f.
5 Junker (b) p. 70
6 Grapow III pp. 7 f.
7 Jonckheere p. 40

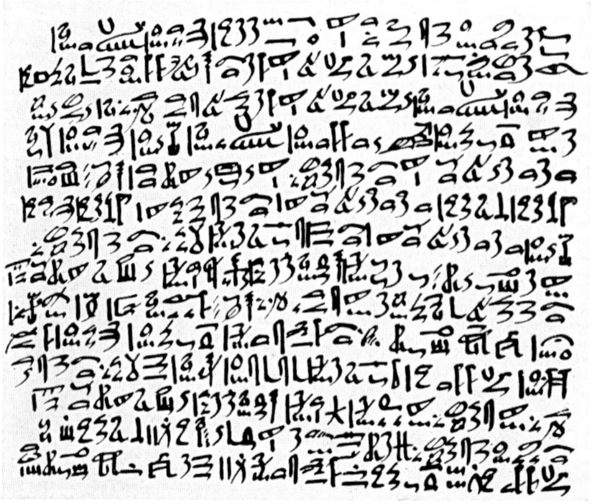

Fig. 8 *Ebers papyrus: Texts "On strengthening a tooth," about 1550 B. C.*

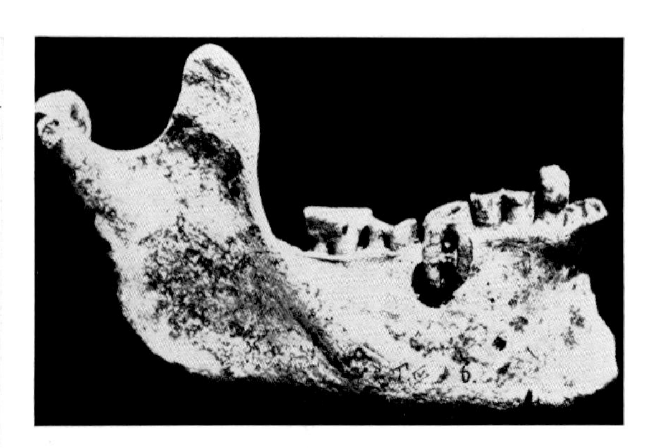

Fig. 9 *Carious first mandibular molar from the Predynastic period, with cyst formation at the distal root (from Ruffer)*

cerned therein with certainty[8]. The description of the mandible is clear. It is designated as the mastication bone: *the end of his ramus is in his temple, just as the claw of the "clawbird" grasps an object.* A clearer portrayal of how the crown and mandibular process terminates in the ascending branch under the zygomatic bone and in the articular fossa formed by the temporal bone is not possible[9].

The majority of these and the ensuing citations are taken from the seven medical papyrus rolls which were recorded during the period of about 1900—1200, but whose roots rest on a uniform concept of Egyptologists in the flowering period of medicine, in the Old Kingdom. At that time an attempt at rational-empirical therapy temporarily restrained the proliferating magic view of the ancient Near East (and not only here). We owe them the considerable information concerning Egyptian medical science. Especially interesting to us is the Ebers papyrus, dating to 1550, which is anonymous as are all the others. In the 21-meter long, by far most extensive work references to the stomatological region can be found. Even early traces of preventive dentistry can be detected in 2 prescriptions. *The basic of a remedy for strengthening a tooth: Meal of the seed grain of emmer* (a wheat-like flour)*—1; ocher—1; honey—1. The mixture is to be pressed into a tooth.*

Another (remedy)

Grinding stone powder—1; ocher—1; honey—1. This mixture is to be pressed into a tooth (Fig. 8). Also a tooth powder for strengthening a tooth was prescribed: *terebinthenic resin—1; ocher—1; malachite—1; the mixture is to be pulverized, to be applied to the tooth*[10].

Five prescriptions are for tooth abscesses. The following is an example: *Another* (remedy) *for eliminating abscesses on teeth, allowing the gingiva to grow. Cows milk—1; fresh dates—1; w'h legume—1; is to be exposed to the dew at night, the mixture is to be chewed for a time, is to spit out*[11].

Ebbell describes this disease as obviously ulcerous stomatitis, Sudhoff less convincingly as aphthous blister formation and ulceration or periosteum abscess[12].

Treatment of caries that extends to the gingival margin (?), employs another powder: *Another* (remedy) *for treating a deteriorated tooth* (or which opens into the gingiva?). *Caraway—1; terebinthenic resin—1; colocynth* (a type of pickle with a purgative effect)*—1; the mixture is to be pulverized*[13].

Caries was a very rare occurrence in the predynastic period and remained so among the common people until the time of the Ptolemies.

8 Grapow I pp. 41 f.
9 Grapow I pp. 42 f.; Breasted (b) p. 293; Westendorf p. 61
10 Grapow IV 1 p. 65; Ebbell (b) pp. 103 f.
11 Ibid. p. 66
12 Ebbell (a); Sudhoff p. 19
13 Grabow IV 1 p. 66; Ebbell (b) pp. 103 f.

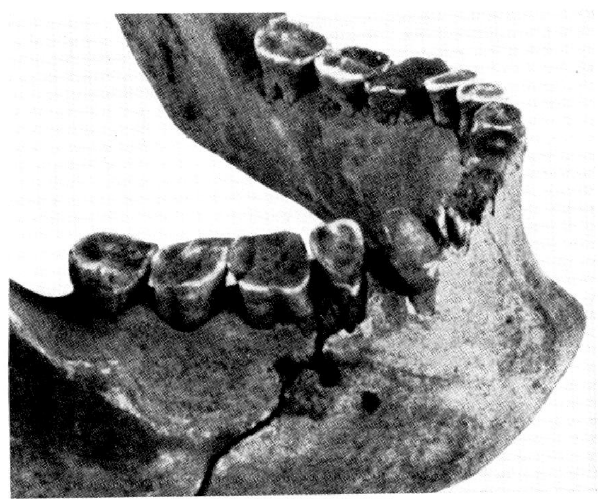

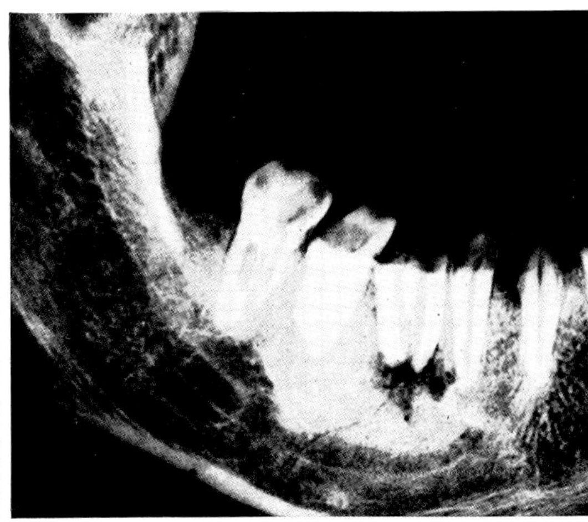

Figs. 10 and 11 *Ancient Egyptian mandible (about 2500 B. C.) with questionable bore-holes, and its radiograph (from Weinberger)*

However, apical changes and cysts were observed that were usually the consequences of pronounced abrasion (Fig. 9). Quenouille discovered 441 teeth with pulp chambers opened (3.4 %) through abrasion among 13,015. Elliot Smith found that among 500 skeletons of aristocrats in burial chambers near the pyramids, dating from about 2500, *tartar-formation, dental caries and alveolar abscesses were at least as common as they are in modern Europe today*[14]. Other methods were concerned with toothaches, and a complicated recipe with fractional components of $^1/_{32}$ and $^1/_{64}$ *for hemolysis of a tooth*. Was it the bleeding pulp polyp in an abraded tooth? In the Hearst papyrus there is a recipe for a tooth *that is ready to fall to the ground*. Was this perhaps for periodontal mobility? The harmless remedy of emmer, gum and an unknown herb would have as little effect as the fat of a black snake against grey hair.

Similarly, the Anastasi papyrus from the New Kingdom touches upon the worm cited as the source of burrowing toothache during an earlier period in Mesopotamia[15]. This is a bit of mythology that is encountered often even into the 19th century. The text reads: *One ... of the scribes is with me, who has twitching of all the veins in his face, both eyes are diseased with wst* (eye-disease) *and the fnt-worm attacks his teeth*[16].

No papyrus contains recommendations for methods of operative dentistry. Jones, a pathologist, after examining numerous skeletons from the Predynastic to the Christian and Coptic periods, reported in 1910 that *at no period do the teeth show signs of dentist's handiwork*. Likewise in 1920 Ruffer determined that his extensive examination of ancient Egyptian dentitions *have not revealed any facts that the Egyptians practiced operative dentistry*[17]. Still, Hooton claimed to have observed signs of boring in a mandible of the IV Dynasty (about 2500 B. C.) kept at the Peabody Museum in Boston. Do the 2 holes seen in Figure 10 to the left above the mental foramen actually represent borings to relieve abscesses of the root tips of abraded first molars? Can it be concluded that the borings, rarely performed nowadays, were made to provide ventilation for periapical abscesses? A radiograph of the jaw shows that there definitely was an abscess and that the left passage leads directly into it, sloping from top to bottom (Fig. 11). Obviously, those examining the bone concluded that an ancient artificial product was involved, not a natural fistula formation. At least ancient Egyptian cabinetmakers were familiar with drills according to a 100 year younger relief from a burial chamber near the Step Pyramid of Saqqara[18]. It shows a

[14] Quenouille p. 118; Smith in Smith/Jones p. 281
[15] See p. 31
[16] Grapow III p. 31
[17] Ruffer; Smith/Jones p. 283
[18] Steindorff, Pl. 133

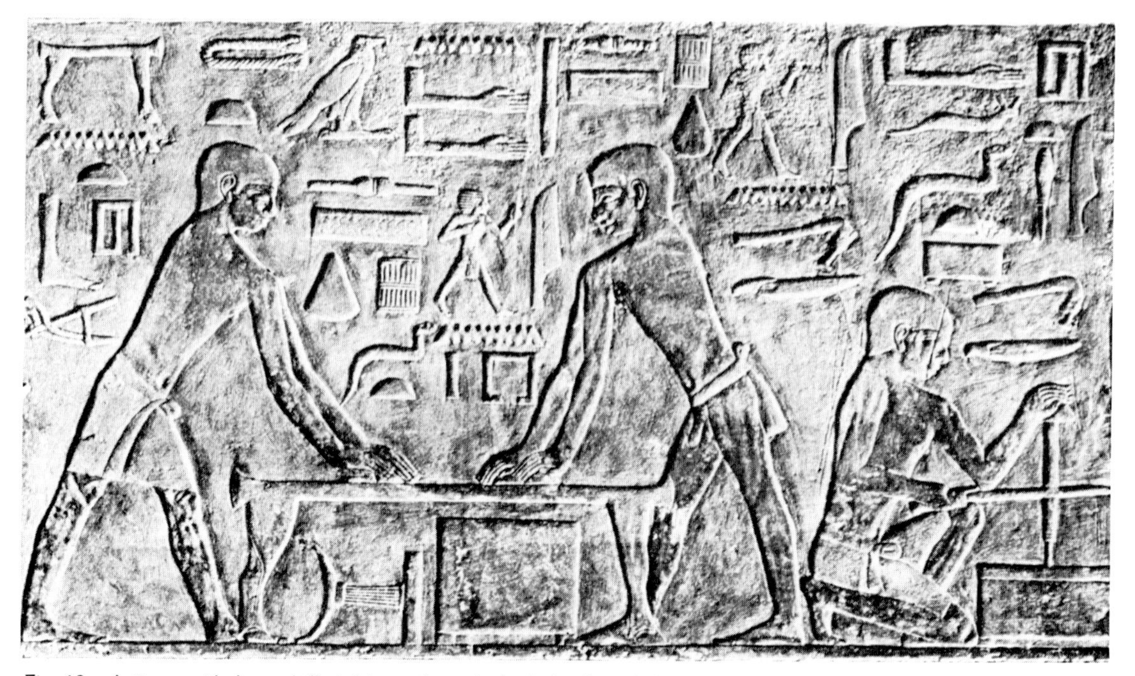

Fig. 12 *Artisan with bow drill right on the relief of the burial chamber of Ti near the step pyramid of Saqqara (Steindorff, Plate 133)*

skilled worker using a bow drill (Fig. 12), a tool that was used as dental drilling equipment into the 19th century. However, among ten thousands of excavated mummy skulls there is no mandible with traces indicating the existence of dental surgery[19].

That Egyptian doctors were continuously and successfully involved in surgery is explained in the Smith papyrus, which is of the same age as the Ebers papyrus. It deals primarily with war and accident surgery, but also with reducing a luxated mandible.

Information regarding a displaced mandible. If thou examinest a man having a dislocation in his mandible, shouldst thou find his mouth open (and) *cannot close for him, thou shouldst put thy thumb*(s) *upon the two ends of the rami of the mandible in the inside of his mouth,* (and) *thy two claws* (meaning two groups of fingers) *under his chin* (and) *thou shouldst cause them to fall back so they rest in their place. You should say to someone with a dislocated mandible: a disease which I will treat. Then you should bandage the region every day with bandages and honey until he feels better*[20].

Here an absolutely correct procedure is recognizable. Because the description of mandibular relocation resembles that of ancient Greek medicine[21], Breasted assumes that it is an example of Greek physicians as scholars of their Egyptian colleagues[22].

Quite contrary to today's standards was the advice to avoid all attempts at therapy for an infected jaw fracture: *When you examine man with a fractured mandible, find the break with your hand as it is displaced beneath your fingers. In addition, if there is an open wound over the fracture and the discharge* (?) *has stopped flowing* (?)*; he has fever as a consequence. This is a disease that cannot be treated*[23].

[19] Hooton, pp. 31 f. The bore-holes are situated on both sides of a continuously passing fracture distal to the foramen mentale. Should they perhaps have served for an early or actual attempt to join the two skeletised fragments with a clamp? These bore-holes could not have been made on a living individual without an anglepiece (at that time certainly not existent), even for reasons of topographic anatomy.

[20] Breasted (b) pp. 303 f.; Grapow IV 1 p. 187; Westendorf p. 63; Ebbell (b) p. 47. Here the more recent translation of Westendorf (1966) was used rather than the customary Breasted translation.

[21] See p. 60

[22] Breasted (b) pp. 16 f. See p. 63

[23] Breasted (b) pp. 301 f.; Grapow IV 1 p. 187; Westendorf pp. 62 f.; Ebbell (c) p. 46

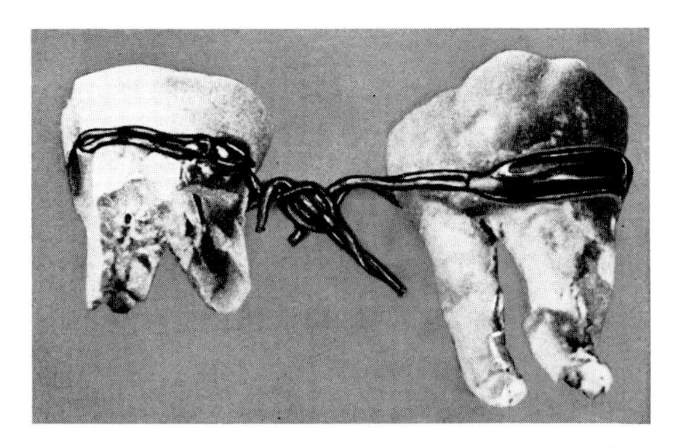

Fig. 13 *Gold wire binding with mandibular molars, approximately 2500 B. C. (from Junker, 1929)*

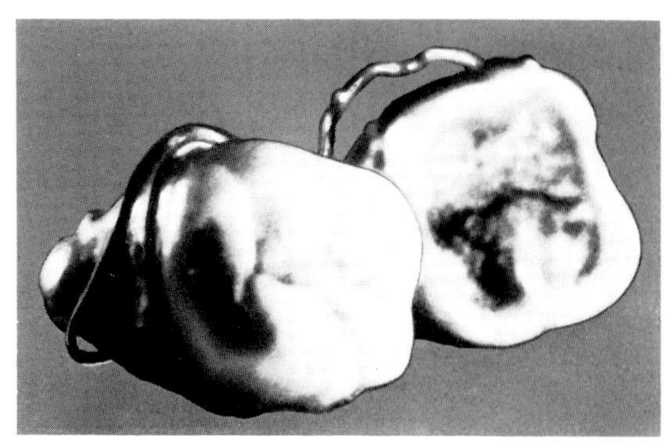

Fig. 14 *The molars, top view (Roemer-Pelizaeus Museum, Hildesheim 1972)*

Whether Egyptians concerned themselves with prosthetic dentistry is at least questionable. The first indication was a discovery by Hermann Junker in 1914. Hidden in a shaft attached to a burial chamber at Gizeh from about 2500 were 2 teeth connected by a gold wire (Fig. 13). At that time he wrote in his "Preliminary report:" *While attempting to keep the corpse intact as far as possible, another rare discovery was made: in the burial chamber of the reserve head of Nile mud 2 teeth were found artfully connected with a gold wire. An attempt had been made to secure a loose tooth by connecting it to a firm adjacent tooth. Or, the man could have worn this dental splint during his lifetime?*[24]

In the definitive report in 1928, Junker provided an expert opinion from the director of the Breslau University Dental Institute at that time, Hermann Euler. Accordingly, second and third mandibular molars of the same individual were involved, having *calculus in the cervical region*, but no concrement was described on the gold wire[25]. The crown of the second molar was severely abraded. Its roots were typically resorbed. Euler concluded that gingival margin inflammation was the cause and explained *that also today, just in such instances, one treats with wire ligatures, and connection to an adjacent tooth is used as an aid in therapy.* From this he concludes that with great probability we are dealing with splinting of two adjacent teeth intraorally. Junker consequently abandoned his 1914 position and agreed with the expert[26].

As examination (1972) revealed, the severely abraded anterior molar (Fig. 14) had a bluish discoloration, which Euler neglected to mention. The manifestation of root degeneration was probably caused by the pulp necrosis resulting from abrasion. Contrarily, the third molar has an almost undisturbed profile and a normal yellowish color. The continuity of the wire connection shown in Fig. 13 and described by Euler was broken by 1972. No calculus could be established on the wire[27].

An additional (and to date the last) dental technique was discovered by Farid in 1952 in the El-Qatta graveyard northwest of Cairo *among the crushed bones of the skull* in a Mastaba. This was from approximately the same era as the one Junker examined. As Harris and Iskander established in 1974, the discovery consists of a maxillary right canine, probably vital, encircled with a double wire forming a distal sling. Separate from this were a central and a lateral incisor connected to each other with a gold wire. In the first, the wire is drawn through

24 Junker (a) p. 169

25 Euler stated after Weinberger "that tartar was found on both the teeth and gold wire". Therefrom Weinberger infers "that the dental work was performed in the mouth of a living individual" (see Weinberger c, p. 75). Unfortunately, Leek (b) and Ghalioungui accepted this wrong interpretation of Euler's expertise by Weinberger without previously examining the German text.

26 Junker (c) p. 256

27 Leek (c). — The damage occurred probably by indirect war influence, as the museum as well as nearly the whole center of the city of Hildesheim was destroyed by fire in 1945. In 1974, the author was astonished to see that the roots of booth teeth were imbedded in a plaster cast and the teeth themselves were joined once more by an intact, clean metal wire!

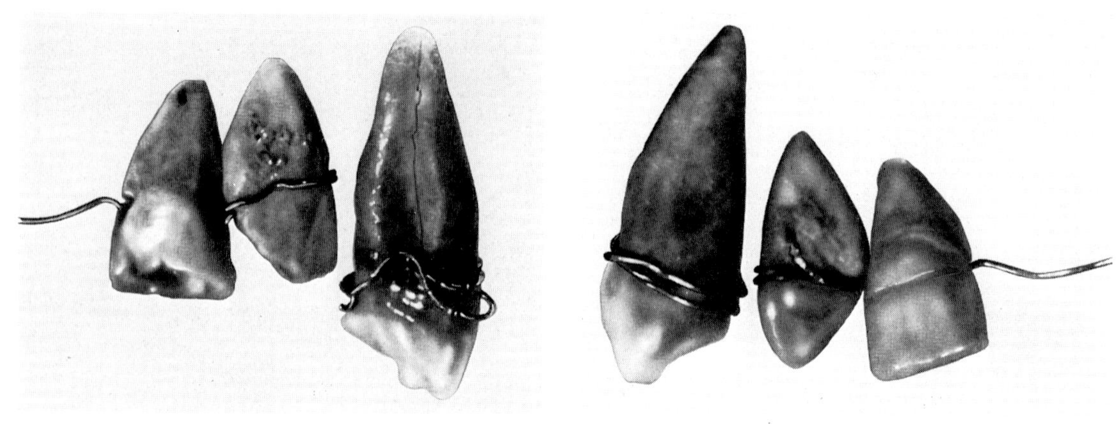

Fig. 15 Fig. 16

Figs. 15 and 16 *Gold wire ligature with maxillary anteriors, approximately 2500 B. C. (from Harris, Iskander, Farid)*

a transverse boring (Figs. 15 and 16). Parallel to the boring an artificial groove extends across the labial surface. The lateral incisor is encircled with the same wire resting in a labial groove. The roots of both incisors are artificially polished by scrapers. The lateral has calculus (Fig. 15). It can be assumed rightfully that the incisors were secured as intermediate pontics on the wire loop of the right canine and in place of the lost left central incisor[28].

Thus, among tens of thousands of skulls from ancient Egyptian excavations two examples of dental work have been found. Both belong to the period of the IV to the V Dynasty. L e e k rightfully established that chiefly Pharaohs had received dental care, but . . . *not in one royal mummy is there evidence of dental intervention to be seen, in spite of, in some cases, its very obvious need*[29]. Also newer (1973) radiographic examinations of pharaoh mummies of the New Kingdom showed no indication of tooth replacement[30]. The question remains open whether these two wire bindings should be viewed as therapeutic or cosmetic measures, that is wether they were worn by the living or served the dead as cult-related devices. Until the introduction of Christianity, Egyptians placed the highest premium on entering the dead kingdom of Osiris without bodily defects. Subsequently mummies of a later period (about 1150) received artificial eyes of variegated stones or metal[31]. In the Old Kingdom the purpose was served by binding up the prepared corpse with a resin-soaked linen wrap. At that time preparation took a predominantly simpler form: After removal of the internal organs, with the exception of the heart, by means of an incision below the rib cage, and of the brain with a hook through the nostrils (all done with special protection of the outer skin), fluids were removed by rubbing the body with sodium hydroxide. Washing with palm wine and plastering served further, but incompletely, to conserve. Therefore, the hypothesis J u n k e r presented in his 1914 "Preliminary report" and consistently defended by the Egyptological position, should not be discounted. The splinting could involve preparation of the dead, possibly to mend an injury occurring during preparation[32].

28 Harris/Iskander/Farid
29 Leek (b)
30 Harris, Kent
31 Otto
32 However, Junker's finding suggests that we certainly cannot reach a promise of even short-lived success from the wire ligature attachment of the second molar to the wisdom tooth. The ligature unearthed by Farid makes it clear that the roots of both replacement teeth were not separated from the crowns. As a prosthesis for the living, such "pontics" are completely inappropriate because of the rapidly closing alveoli. That is the reason that in ancient times and more recently, the roots of human false teeth have been shortened according to the prevailing conditions. If the luxation took place during the preparation, perhaps even shortly before death, it was a simple matter to replace the teeth in the alveoli and to fasten them to the adjacent teeth in this situation. That there was loosening of the teeth may be explained by severe root resorption in the first case and by calculus formation on two-thirds of an incisor root in the other. The wire was free of calculus in both instances. See Hoffmann-Axthelm

Accordingly, two opposing hypotheses exist which, based on the presently available material, cannot result in a definitive statement. Because in the entire ancient world the denture had no medical purpose, but was considered a mere product of skill[33], we can conclude as little from these two wire bindings regarding the existence of a dentist's position in ancient Egypt as from the traditional title hieroglyphs. These indicate a dental occupation that is unclear throughout with regard to the actual occupational methods practiced. The dental references found in the papyrus scrolls, like the ophthalmological and rhinological constituents of general therapy, are no proof of the existence of a specialty.

The doctrines of the Old Kingdom, the important period for the healing art of Nile region, remained valid until the decline, thanks to the conservative and traditional attitude of the Egyptians. The native traditions were not abolished until the third century B. C., at first by the medicine influenced by the Greeks, who earlier had been influenced by the Egyptians.

Mesopotamia

The story of Mesopotamia, the fertile plain between the Euphrates and the Tigris, progresses in a more open manner because its borders were always open in contrast to the Nile portions that were protected by the sea and desert.

The first people with a culture were the Sumerians who appeared in the beginning of the third millennium, to whom Babylonians and Assyrians were indebted for the cuneiform script. Regardless of how often the people and their rulers changed, the culture, like the medicine of Egypt, maintained a uniform character through these writings for thousands of years.

The Sumerians, who were divided into city states, were overthrown by the semitic Akkadians, the later Babylonians, under Sargon I still in the same third millennium. Their conquerors readily adopted their culture and script and cultivated the Sumerian language as their language of culture and learning. Ancient Akkadian became the language of the people and the land. Later it split into the Assyrian and Babylonian dialects. In the 18th century the great Babylonian king Hammurapi extended the kingdom from the Persian Gulf to the Mediterranean. Babylon became the capital.

The existing law was reformed by a code containing 282 paragraphs delivered to us chiseled on a stele 2.25 meter high (Fig. 17).

Meanwhile in the North the Assyrian Kingdom developed, with Assur as its capital, also composed of semitic people, and about 1200 B. C. overthrew the superior culture of Babylon for a time. Between these poles the lustrous era of Babylonian-Assyrian culture developed. The Gilgamesh epic attained its final form; astronomy and mathematics flourished, but also astrology and belief in numerology. All current information concerning astrological charts, meaning of dreams, magic numerology and amulet cults, as well as our system of measuring time in hours is based on the Babylonian sexagesimal system.

The store of Sumerian-Babylonian-Assyrian literature and science of two millennia was collected in a giant clay tablet library by the Assyrian King Ashurbanipal in 700 B. C. in Niniveh, his capital. A considerable amount of it has survived. Then for almost 100 years Babylon once again came under the rule of the Chaldeans. Nebuchadnezzar II gave the city the traditional aspect of the "Tower of Babel," the strong fortification walls and the colorful tile reliefs, the picture transmitted by Herodotos. This two-river land was incorporated by the great Kyros into the Persian Empire in 539 B. C.

Numerous medical texts were found in the library of Ashurbanipal. Among these were prescriptions for toothache, but no reports of active surgical procedures for the region of the jaws. Sudhoff concluded from this a low level of surgery in the two-river land, and attributed it partly to the stringent liability stipulations among the collection of laws on the previously described Hammurapi stele[34]. Paragraph 218 of this code stipulated that if a patient died during surgical intervention or if his eye was injured during lancing of a nearby abscess, the doctor should have his hands cut off. Still, a very good honorarium for success existed if the operation worked and the eye remained intact. The surgeon received 10 shekels of silver (1 shekel = 8.4 g). A surgical skill was undoubtedly practiced. In the law collection, which is about 3700

[33] Therefore dental prostheses are not mentioned at all in the comprehensive medical literature of antiquity, although much space is devoted to odontological problems.

[34] Sudhoff p. 31

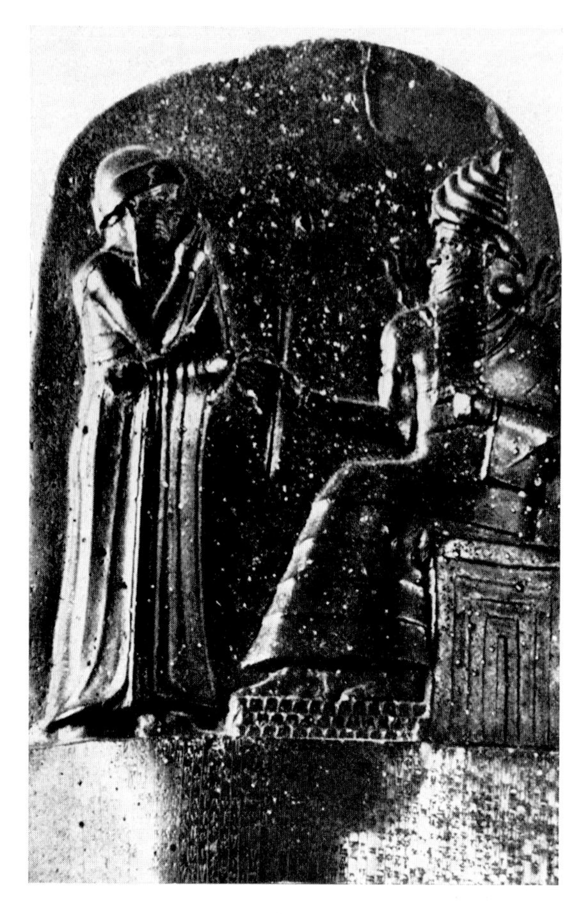

Fig. 18 *§ 200 of the Hammurapi code*[35]

Fig. 17 *Head section of the Hammurapi stele with text of law. The king stands before the Sun God who holds the staff in his hand as a symbol of power (Louvre, Paris)*

years old, we see the oldest national tariff. Additionally, the Hammurapi code shows the high value placed on a tooth in those days:
Law 196. If someone injures the eye of an equal, his own eye is destroyed.
Law 198. If someone injures the eye of a lesser, he is fined a mine of silver (= 505 g).
Law 200. If someone knocks out the tooth of an equal (šinnu in Akkadian), *his own tooth is knocked out* (Fig. 18).
Law. 201. If someone knocks out the tooth of a lesser, he is fined 1/3 *mine of silver.*
Although a tooth is worth only 1/3 as much as an eye, considering the high value of an eye this is still a substantial evaluation. Obviously, these laws remind us of the Old Testament statement, "an eye for an eye, a tooth for a tooth." This can be continued in Exodus XXI, 27: "And if he smite out his bondsman's tooth ... he shall let him free for this tooth's sake".

Practitioners of medicine were divided into 2 classes in ancient Mesopotamia. The educated of a higher social order in 1000 B. C. who were court conjurers (Akkadian—*āšipu*) probably evolved from the priesthood and assumed a difficult-to-classify position between priest and physician. The origin of these therapists corresponded to their belief in omens and demons (Fig. 19), in astrology and numerology. They sought to heal patients primarily with conjuring done at a specific hour and recited a given number of times. The other type was the practicing therapist (Akkadian—*asû*). They, whom we consider the practicing physicians of the time, conducted an essentially symptomatic therapy using herbs that had proven valuable in practice. Besides this, they practiced surgery. Their methods were better than those of the official magicians, caus-

[35] This text is inverted in the works of Sudhoff (p. 24), Weinberger (p. 32), and Proskauer/Witt (Fig. 11)

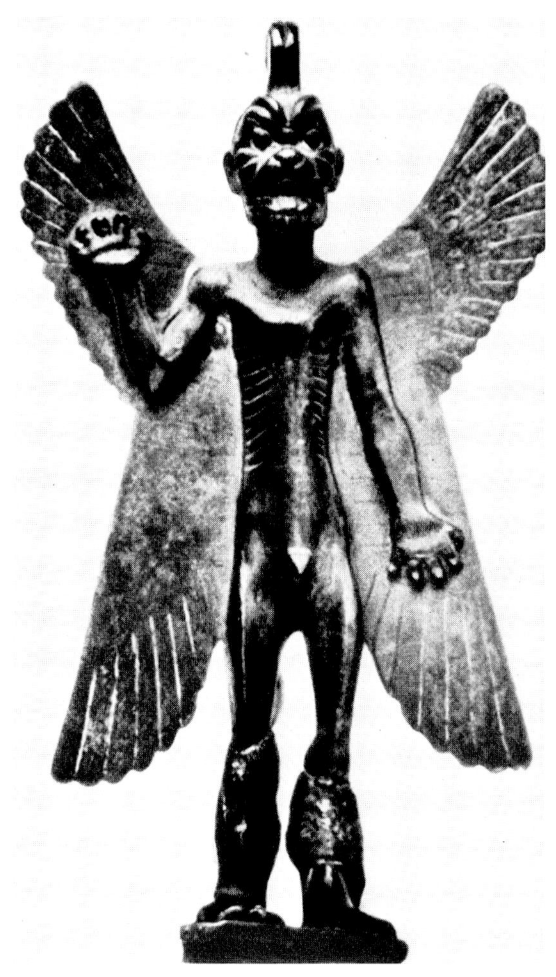

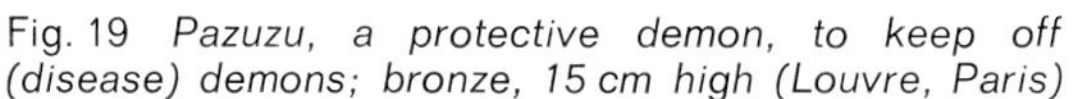

Fig. 19 *Pazuzu, a protective demon, to keep off (disease) demons; bronze, 15 cm high (Louvre, Paris)*

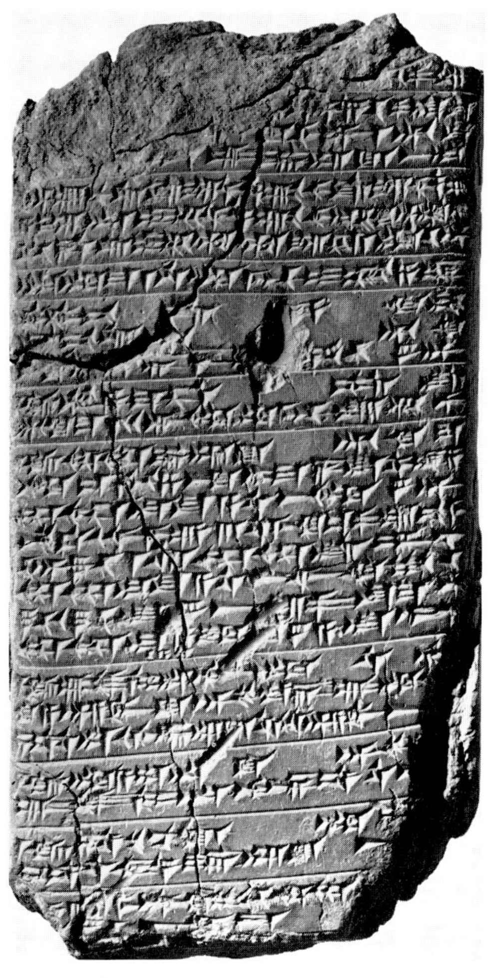

Fig. 20 *Cuneiform text with incantations and instructions (Köcher I 30)*

ing the latter to change over to them in a more recent period (some time after 1200 B. C.) and to add prescriptions from practical medicine to their conjuring. Examples thereof will be given. Educated conjurers had an extensive literature at their disposal. Many of these works still exist. Most of the literature is from the library of King Ashurbanipal in Niniveh. Other significant areas of discovery were Assur, Babylon, Nippur and Uruk.

A compilation of tablets devoted exclusively to diagnosis and prognosis had the title "When the conjurer goes to the house of the sick." It consisted of 40 tablets, 26 of which were found although several of them were quite damaged. According to the work, the diagnosis was based on the symptoms as was the prognosis given. The work was arranged systematically from skull to toe. Of the prognoses, 13, located between lip and tongue symptoms, are determined through the teeth:

If one of his teeth aches and saliva flows, (. . .)
If his teeth are white, he will become well.—
If his teeth (are) *X, his disease will be . . . long in duration.—If his teeth* (. . .)
If his teeth are dark-colored, the disease will last a long time.
If his teeth are crowded together, he will die.—

If his teeth (fall out, his h)*ouse will collapse.*
If he grinds his teeth, the disease will last a long time.—If he grinds his teeth and loses consciousness (?) *the disease will last a lo*(ng time).
If he grinds his teeth, his eyebrows are loose, his eyes, eyebrows and (. . .)*: he will die.*
If he grinds his teeth and his hands and feet have black spots, touch of the spirit of death; he will die.
If he grinds his teeth and his hands and feet shake: Hand of the moon god[36]*, he will die.*
If he grinds his teeth and his head falls back: Hand of the Goddess Ištar.
If he grinds his teeth and his head is thrown back: Hand of the Goddess Ištar.
If he grinds his teeth and his hand is reverted: Hand of the Goddess Ištar.
If he grinds his teeth and his (saliva) *flows from his mouth, he will die: Hand of the Goddess Ištar.* (Special) *diagnosis: Contact.*
If he grinds (his) *teeth continuously and his face is cold, he has contracted a disease* (?) *through the hand of the Goddess Ištar*[37].
These omens were limited to diagnosis and prognosis. Apparently another clay tablet existed which completed the missing therapeutic recommendations. The following cited methods, for which information Franz Köcher is to thank, are for treating those diseases having tooth grinding as a symptom (Fig. 20). They are based on a fragmentary conjuration:
(This is a) *text* (to recite) *when a person grinds his teeth.*
Ritual direction: Red salt and juniper are combined and pulverized; apply it to his teeth cleaning purposes.
If the same (symptom, namely tooth grinding) *exists, take a human skull*
and spread a cloth of apple colored wool across a chair.
That skull you place on it.
For 3 days, both morning and evening bring a sacrifice and
recite 7 times the conjuration (indicated above) *into the skull.*
The skull should be kissed 7 and 7 times by the patient,
before retiring; then he will become well.
Other prescriptions on the tablet describe herbal and mineral remedies which were ground and placed in leather pouches. These were worn around the neck by the patient as a prophylactic talisman:

If the same (symptom) *existed: harmunu herb, algal mud,*
black sulfur, barley flour, sumac,
Asafetida (stimulant and anthelmintic)—*male and female—amilānu herb and yellow sulfur in leather* (pouches)[38].
Thereupon followed the instruction for making an amulet chain of 4 magic stones, and an additional skull conjuration.
A collection of practical medicine prescriptions, free of magic accessories, was discovered on tablet VAT 8256. It contains 16 prescriptions for teeth. It is arranged in 3 columns. The first contains the medication, the second the indication and the third the method of application. The 16 lines are divided into divisions of various sizes according to indication (with one exception). An example follows:

Male pillû plant	*Drug for toothache*	*apply to tooth*
Root of the false carob which should not be exposed to sunlight when pulled from the ground	*Drug against* (tooth) *worm*	*apply to tooth*
Root of the camel's thorn, not exposed to the sunlight while it is pulled from the ground	*Drug for an affected tooth*	*dry, pulverize, mix with oil, apply to the tooth*
Galbanum resin	*Drug for loosened teeth*	*apply to the teeth*
Alum, mint and aromatic ṭurû	*Drug to clean teeth*	*clean his teeth before meals*[39]

Of special interest here is that the (tooth) worm is combated by other means than is toothache. In those days, it was probably not held responsible for toothache but for caries, or vice versa. As a typical creation of the Mesopotamian medicine the toothworm rose to new proofs during the first half of the second century B. C. A tablet

[36] That is, a disease brought upon mankind by the moon-god Sin.
[37] Labat I pp. 60—61
[38] Köcher I 30

excavated in Nippur[40] contained as addition to a prescription for jaundice the following instructions. They appeared to be the basis for the oldest methods of dental therapy in the two river land.

If a person's tooth has a worm,
pulverize (water) *weed in fine oil.* (You should proceed as follows:) *If the tooth is diseased on the right side, pour the mixture on the left side and it will become well.*
But if the tooth is diseased on the left side, pour it on the right side and it will be healed.

The third prescription is on the back of the tablet following instructions for dog bite:

If the tooth of a person has a worm,
take the bark of an X-tree
and apply it, and it will become well.

For some time two opinions existed regarding the first mention of the toothworm. Sudhoff accepted the toothworm mentioned in the Egyptian Anastasi[41] papyrus as a manifestation taken over from the Euphrates[42]. Weinberger agreed with Townend who saw the Anastasi position as the first mention of this worm ascribing it to the Egyptians[43]. We thank Köcher for the above text dated about 1800 B. C., upon which rests clearly the primacy of the Mesopotamian cultural era according to present day knowledge.

Easily the most significant contribution of Babylonian-Assyrian dentistry is the treatment entitled: "When a person has a toothache." It is recorded on two large, although very fragmented, clay tablets. These are from the library of the Assyrian king Ashurbanipal. The treatment, based on many therapeutic procedures, also has an entire series of conjurations and magical prescriptions. It incorporates the medical-therapeutic knowledge of practicing physicians in that of conjurers, the result of more than 1200 years accumulation.

F. Köcher has the well-founded opinion that these two tablets do not represent a single work of the ancient Mesopotamian therapeutic literature, but that they are a two clay tablet chapters of a greater therapeutic table. This seems possible because the beginning line of the first chapter reads, "When a person's head is hot from fever". Despite the many gaps it shows, in addition to tooth diseases, this chapter of the work also deals with diseases of the nose and respiratory tract[44].

The chapter's first tablet[45], which is in poor condition, contains more than 35 prescriptions with 7 conjurations. The long-recognized "toothworm conjuration" is intact. Probably established in ancient Babylonia (about 1800 B. C.), it is contained in several prescriptions of the new Assyrian (about 650 B. C.) and new Babylonian (about 550 B. C.) eras. The frequently translated conjuration describes the origin of the toothworm in the form of a legend of creation. It reads as follows:

Oath: The God Anu (existed and)
[.]
After Anu (had created heaven),
Heaven had created (the earth),
The earth had created the rivers,
The rivers had created the canals,
The canals had created the marsh,
(And) *the marsh had created the worm—*
The worm went, weeping, before Shamash,
His tears flowing before Ea:
"What wilt thou give for my food?
What wilt thou give me for my sucking?"
"I shall give thee the ripe fig
(And) *the apricot."*
"Of what use are they to me, the ripe fig
And the apricot?
Lift me up and among the teeth
And the gums cause me to dwell!
The blood of the tooth I will suck,
And of the gum I will gnaw its roots!"
Fix the pin and seize its foot.
Because thou hast said this, O worm,
May Ea smite thee with the might
Of his hand!

The immediatly following passage, with ritual direction describing local lenitive application in the tooth is interesting:

This is a text (to be recited) *against toothache. Ritual direction: Emmer mixed beer, cracked malt and sesame oil you combine, the incantation you recite thrice over that place* (the mixture) *on his tooth.*

[39] Köcher I 1
[40] Jena HS 1883 = Köcher IV 393
[41] See p. 23
[42] Sudhoff p. 21
[43] Weinberger (c) p. 25; Townend (a)
[44] A larger number of the associated text fragments from Niniveh has been published in the Assyrial Medical Texts by R. C. Thompson (London 1923) and translated in the Proceedings of the Royal Society of Medicine, vol. XIX 3 (1926) pp. 56 f. A new edition of these texts in cuneiform writing may be found in Köcher, vol. VI.
[45] Thompson 28, 1, and others

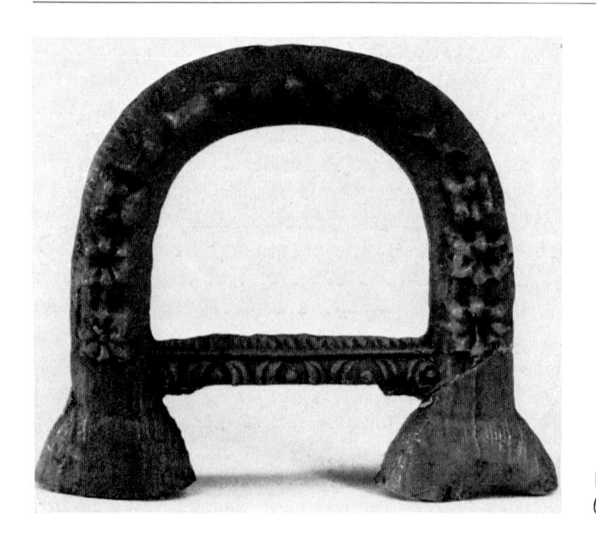

Fig. 21 *A wax votive of a jaw, end of the 19th century (Deutsches Museum für Volkskunde, Berlin)*

A discernible section among the numerous gaps in the first chapter of the text is fragment K. 2450[46]. Here at the conclusion of a not very well understood (other) incantation of the toothworm are instructions for the preparation of a jaw model. Because this is unique, a translation by F. Köcher follows:
Ritual direction: You prepare a jaw of clay, fasten emmer seeds to the seals of his teeth. Fasten a black emmer seed to the diseased tooth, fill his mouth with fine oil. He blows it onto the jaw. You recite the above incantation three times. Place (the jaw) *in a hole at sundown, stuff it with clay and straw,* (and) *seal his opening with a seal* (stone) *of jasper and a matfinished hematite.*
The Akkadian word *kunukku* can mean both (seal) stone and (seal) impression. Because it is difficult to accept that impressions were made of teeth in ancient Mesopotamia, the expression "seals of teeth" could refer to the impression of the roots in the jaw, that is, alveoli. The root of the tooth is not meant for it was designated by a special term.
The fact that this is the first indication of the preparation of a dentulous jaw model for ritual use makes this text particularly valuable. In antiquity, copies of this sort were found as consecrated gifts or donations. They can still be seen nowadays as votives in some Catholic churches (Fig. 21, see Fig. 48).
Tablet 2 of the chapter[47], which is in considerably better condition, begins with the following description of symptoms: *When all of a person's teeth are loose and inflammation (?) is present.* This disease should be treated with three (not yet identified) herbs combined with black alum and pulverized in a mortar. The mixture should be placed on a piece of linen coated with honey. The teeth are rubbed with this mixture until bleeding starts. Also lion or fox tallow was eaten. Other prescriptions were for weak or bleeding teeth or for occurrence of yellow exudate, that is, the early signs of purulent inflammation of the periodontium.
The library of Niniveh is also the source of several physician's letters from the New Assyrian period (700 B. C.) which deal with stomatological problems. Letter K. 1102 is of special interest[48]. Unfortunately, the introductory lines are broken off, causing the writer, probably a magician, and the recipient, an Assyrian king, to remain unknown. The text of the latest translation by Simo Parpola (1970) is a follows: *The "burning" wherewith his head, arms* (and) *feet were "burnt" was because of his teeth: his teeth were to come out. Because of that he felt burnt* (and) *transferred* (it) *to his innards. Now he is very well;* (the gods) *bless him*[49].
This text indicates rather clearly that a concerned royal father requested a report from the court

[46] Köcher VI 542
[47] Thompson 21, 1 and others; Köcher VI 543
[48] Harper VI 586
[49] Parpola I p. 161, 216

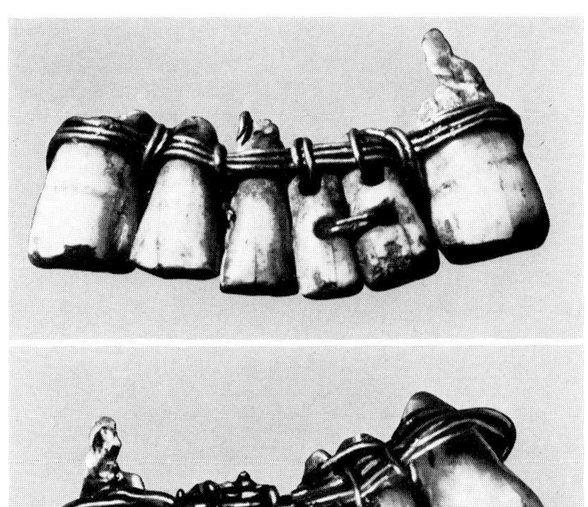
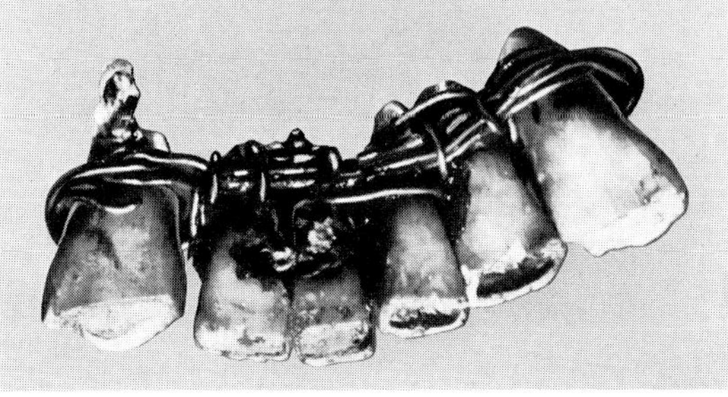

Fig. 22 *Front and back of a maxillary prosthesis found in ancient Sidon. 6th—4th century B. C. (Louvre, Paris)*

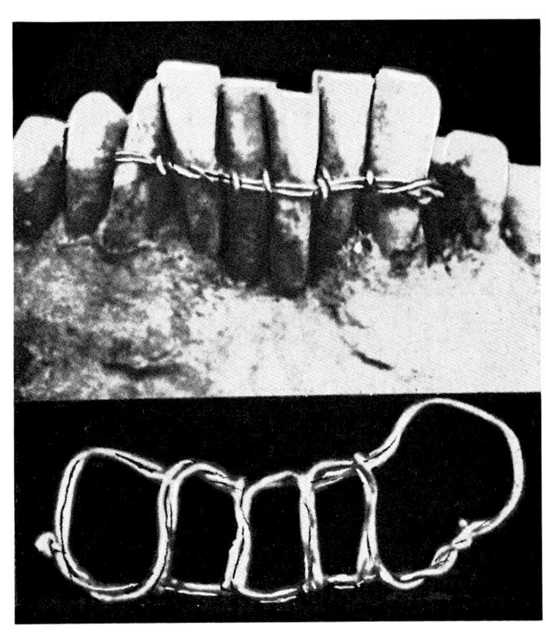

Fig. 23 *Gold wire ligature of mandibular anterior teeth, Phoenician (from Weinberger)*

physician about his son's illness. He tells the king in archaic words that the fever was caused by tooth eruption[50]. The educated magician was able to refer to a specific text for his diagnosis. This particular one can be found on tablet 40 of the aforementioned diagnostic-prognostic work entitled: "When the conjurer goes to the house of the sick." Here among numerous diagnoses and prognoses of infant illnesses is the following observation: *When the infant's head is hot from fever, his body does not have a high fever and he does not sweat, his hands and feet are immobile, saliva flows and he cries vigorously, when he vomits all food intake, then the infant is teething. The discomfort and dejection lasts 15 to 20 days*[51].

Equally significant is another letter from the royal library. The sender, a court physician of the Assyrian king *Asarhaddon* in 700 B. C., was known as Urad-Nanâ. The interesting letter had the following text: *As regards the cure of the* (aching) *teeth about which the king wrote to me, I will* (now) *begin with it; there is a great lot of remedies of* (aching) *teeth*[52]. We can only assume from the general regretful tone that the letter contains no word about methods of treatment.

As is the case with incantations and prescriptions the letters contained no indication of surgical intervention. This condition with regard to an aching tooth and the use of extensive new medical knowledge was strengthened through fear based on the paragraphs of the Mesopotamian laws. This was observed in Egypt and will be experienced with Greek, Roman and Islamic medicine, generally in every cultural circle.

50 B. W. Weinberger (c, p. 33) used the older translation of R. C. Thompson (1920) although a translation similar to the one used here by G. G. Cameron (1943) was known to him from the publication of J. B. Denton. The critical place he reads as follows: "The inflammation wherewith his head, his hands (arms), feet (legs) are inflamed, is due to his teeth. His teeth must be drawn: it is on this account that he was inflamed; he will reduce (it [?]) through internal (channels) (?). Then will be well . . ." Weinberger concluded from this, with the British dentist B. R. Townend, that the Assyrians had already dealt with the problem of oral sepsis; he emphasized this by placing the title "An Assyrian Concept of Focal Infection" on the section (Weinberger [c] p. 32; Townend [b]; Denton). Sigerist (p. 435) moved away from this position in 1951; today we can only say that this text has nothing to do with focal infection, from the Assyriological nor from the odontological points of view.

51 Labat p. 218, lines 10—12

52 K. 532, 12, Harper I 109; Parpola I p. 195, 250

Palestine and Syria

Traces of Mesopotamian culture along with medicine extended as Far East as India. Even stronger were the influences to the west coast of Asia Minor (via the Hittites?) on the Greek tribes. Also, the Israelites residing in the land spanning the distance between Egypt and the two-river land made reference to the "tooth for a tooth" of both the Hammurapi stele and the biblical Exodus and Deuteronomy. Unfortunately, the great amount of literature of these people rarely alludes to medical and never to dental therapy. Of course, some biblical passages praise the beauty of teeth. From a later period, the Talmud claims that an edentulous person is unfit to serve as a priest. Still, there is no reference to the practice of dentistry. The practice of medicine by doctors (binders) was also transitional on the "rophe." The first reference to artificial teeth of gold, silver or natural materials was in the order of the Sabbath of the Hellenic period. These were only worn by women[53]. In 300—400 A. D. several prescriptions and indications appeared in the Talmud. These did not transcend the knowledge of the period in any way. There is also reference to a "tooth of gold" to beautify a marriage (bride) candidate[54].

In the region of the northwestern neighbor of Israel, the Phoenicians, a female maxilla was found with anterior teeth held together by a gold wire. The discovery was made by Gaillardot in 1862 at a gravesite of about 400 B. C. of ancient Sidon, now known as Saida in Lebanon. Today it has been established definitely as a prosthesis for 2 maxillary incisors[55] (Fig. 22). Based on the remains of a dozen Egyptian statues of gods, a scarab and other ceramics[56] as well as a certain similarity in technique with the corresponding find on some corpses at the Gizeh gravesite, this tooth replacement is traced back to Egyptian influence[57]. Moreover, the earlier rules for the binding technique are conspicuous here. This indicates a learned hand. A similar discovery from about the same period at Sidon in 1901 revealed a gold wire splint for periodontally mobile mandibular anterior teeth. The wire was hidden in situ[58] (Fig. 23). It would be difficult to establish a relationship to Egyptian construction. More than 2,000 years lay between the Nile discovery and the Phoenician splint.

53 Nobel
54 Kotelmann; Mittwoch
55 Renan pp. 472 f. Guerini p. 30; Sudhoff pp. 34 f.
56 No mention is made in Renan's original text of a neck ribbon with illustrations of the figures, as reported by Guerini and by Weinberger after him. Only "un grain de collier en verre bleu" is mentioned!
57 Guerini p. 31; Weinberger (c) p. 103; see p. 25
58 Weinberger (c) pp. 103 f.

The author thanks the former director of the Egyptian Museum in Berlin who is now director of the Cairo division of the German Archaeological Institute in Cairo, Prof. Dr. Werner Kaiser, for his intensive scrutiny of the Egyptian manuscript, and the late Prof. Dr. Hermann Grapow for his critique of the text.
The Babylonian-Assyrian section could not have been written without the diligent aid of Dr. Franz Köcher of the Institute for Medical History of the Free University of Berlin. He is thanked for the translation of formerly unknown cuneiform texts on dentistry.

References

Breasted, James Henry
a) A history of Egypt . . . London 1906
b) The Edwin Smith surgical papyrus. Vol. I, Chicago 1930

Denton, George B(ion)
A new interpretation of a wellknown Assyrian letter. J. Near Eastern Studies 2 (1943) 314—315

Ebbell, B(endix)
a) Die ägyptischen Krankheitsnamen. Zschr. Ägypt. Sprache 63 (1928) 71—75
b) The Papyrus Ebers. Copenhagen 1937
c) Die altägyptische Chirurgie. Oslo 1939

Ghalioungui, P(aul)
Did a dental profession exist in ancient Egypt during the 3rd millennium B. C.? Med. Hist. 16 (1972) 404—406

Grapow, Hermann u. a.
Grundriß der Medizin der alten Ägypter. I. Anatomie und Physiologie. Berlin 1954. III. Kranker, Krankheiten und Arzt. Berlin 1956. IV 1. Übersetzung der medizinischen Texte. IV 2. idem, Erläuterungen. Berlin 1958

Guerini, Vincenzo
A history of dentistry. Philadelphia, New York 1909

Harper, R. C.
Assyrian and Babylonian letters belonging to the Kouyunjik Collection of the British Museum. Vols. I—XIV, London, Chicago 1892—1914

Harris, James E.; Zaki Iskander; Shafik Farid
Restorative dentistry in ancient Egypt: an archaeological fact! J. Michigan Dent. Ass. 57 (1975) 401—404

Harris, James E.; R. Weeks Kent
X-raying the pharaos. London 1973

Herodotos of Halikarnassos
The nine books of the history of Herodotus. Transl. Peter Edmund Laurent, Oxford 1837

Hoffmann-Axthelm, Walter
Is the practice of dentistry in Ancient Egypt an archaeological fact? Bull. Hist. Dentistry 27 (1979) 71—78

Hooton, E. A.
Oral surgery in Egypt during the Old Empire. Harvard African Studies 1 (1917) 29—32

Jonckheere, Frans
Les médecins de l'Egypte pharaonique. Bruxelles 1958

Junker, Hermann
a) Vorbericht über die 3. Grabung bei den Pyramiden von Gizeh, Jänner—April 1914. Anzeiger Wiener Akad. Wiss. Phil.-hist. Klasse 51 (1914) 140—183 (p. 169)
b) Die Stele des Hofarztes 'Irj. Das Spezialistentum i. d. ägypt. Medizin. Zschr. Ägypt. Sprache Altertumskd. 63 (1928) 68—70
c) Giza I. Vol. I. Die Mastabas der IV. Dynastie . . . Akad. Wiss. Wien, Phil.-histor. Klasse 69 I; Wien, Leipzig 1929
d) Giza II. Vol. II. Die Mastabas der beginnenden V. Dynastie . . . Wien, Leipzig 1934

Kaplony, Peter
Die Inschriften der ägyptischen Frühzeit, Vol. I. In: Ägyptolog. Abh., Vol. 8, Wiesbaden 1963

Kazenelson, L.
Die normale und pathologische Anatomie des Talmud. Hist. Studien Pharmak. Inst. Univ. Dorpat, V pp. 164—296. Halle 1896

Köcher, Franz
Die babylonisch-assyrische Medizin in Texten und Untersuchungen. Vols. I—VI, Berlin 1963—79

Kotelmann, L.
Ist das künstliche Auge schon im Talmud erwähnt? Mitt. Gesch. Med. Naturw. 6 (1907) 243—249

Labat, René
Traité akkadien de diagnostics et pronostics médicaux. 2 Vols., Paris, Leyden 1951

Leek, F. Filce
a) Observations on the dental pathology seen in ancient Egyptian skulls. J. Egyptian Arch. 52 (1966) 59—64
b) The practice of dentistry in ancient Egypt. J. Egyptian Arch. 53 (1967) 51—58
c) Did a dental profession exist in ancient Egypt during the 3rd millennium B. C.? Med. Hist. 16 (1972) 404—406

Mittwoch, Eugen
Ist das künstliche Auge schon im Talmud erwähnt? Mitt. Gesch. Med. Naturw. 6 (1907) 514—517

Nobel, Gabriel
Zahnheilkunde in Bibel und Talmud. Leipzig 1930

Oefele, Felix von
Zwei medizinische Keilschrifttexte. Mitt. Gesch. Med. Naturw. 3 (1904) 217—224

Otto, Eberhard
in: Gustav Korkhaus, Eberhard Otto, Mumienuntersuchungen im Zahn- und Kieferbereich. Schweiz. Mschr. Zahnhk. 85 (1975) 681—719

Parpola, Simo
Letters from Assyrian scholars to the kings Esarhaddon and Assurbanipal. Part I, Neukirchen-Vluyn 1970

Quenouille, Jean-Jacques
La bouche et les dents dans l'antiquité égyptienne. Thèse Chir. Dent. Lyon 1975

Quibell, J(ames) E(dward)
Excavations of Saqqara. Vol. V, Le Caire 1913

Ranke, Hermann
Medicine and surgery in ancient Egypt. Bull. (Inst.) Hist. Med. 1 (1933) 237—257

Renan, Ernest
Mission de Phénicie et la campagne de Sidon. Paris 1864

Ruffer, Sir Armand
Study of abnormalities and pathology of ancient Egyptian teeth. Am. J. Phys. Anthrop. 3 (1920) 335—382

Sigerist, Henry E.
A history of medicine. Vol. I, New York 1951/1955

Smith, G. Elliot; F. Wood Jones
The archaeological survey in Nubia. Report 1907—1908, Vol. 2. Report on the human remains. Cairo 1910

Steindorff, Georg
Das Grab des Ti. Leipzig 1913

Sudhoff, Karl
Geschichte der Zahnheilkunde. 2nd ed., Leipzig 1926

Thompson, R. Campbell
Assyrian medical texts from the originals in the British Museum. Oxford 1923

Townend, B(ernhard) R(obert)
a) The story of the tooth-worm. Bull. Hist. Med. 15 (1944) 37—53
b) An Assyrian dental diagnosis. Iraq 5 (1938) 82—85

Weinberger, Bernhard Wolf
a) Further evidence that dentistry was practiced in ancient Egypt, Phoenicia and Greece. Bull. Hist. Med. 20 (1946) 188—195
b) The dental art in ancient Egypt. J. Am. Dent. Ass. 34 (1947) 170—184
c) An introduction to the history of dentistry. Vol. 1, St. Louis 1948

Westendorf, Wolfhart
Papyrus Edwin Smith. Bern/Stuttgart 1966

Chapter 2

India

The enormous mass of land forming the fertile Indian peninsula even to this day has had no true development as a centralized nation; it has no common religion or language and no uniform culture. Early inhabitants can be traced back to the third and fourth millenia B. C. as members of the so-called Indus culture. They left no written documents, but from approximately 2300 B. C. we know of the admirable hygienic arrangements for densely populated cities. Current interpretations hold that the dark-skinned early population was subdued in about 1500 B. C. by a fire and sword invasion of light-skinned Aryan herdsmen. The new masters segregated themselves from the remaining population through a caste system that remains to the present. The priestly caste, the Brahmins, assumed spiritual guidance. To them we owe the earliest written Sanskrit documents, the Vedas (Veda = knowledge). These contain, among other topics, prescriptions of medicinal herbs incorporated in magic conjuring formulas, and general rules of hygiene too, concerned, among other things, with care of the oral cavity. This Vedic period, in which the healing arts were purely priestly medicine, ended around 600 B. C.

The subsequent Brahmanic period marked the zenith of ancient Indian medicine. It ended violently with the advent of Islam around 1000 A. D. Its beginnings in the second half of the sixth century B. C. were marked by the historically significant appearance of Gautama Buddha, whose teachings of redemption led, around 250 B. C., to the formation of a great religious empire. After its decline Hinduism rose again, the Brahmins ultimately removing Buddhism from its native land.

The earliest traces of medical writings are those of the so-called Bower manuscript, inscribed on birch bark approximately 400 A. D, which includ 6 prescriptions for care of the teeth and mouth. A gargling solution, for example, is concocted of Barringtonia (a tree whose sap is used in diarrhea, catarrh, etc.)[1], mustard, Bengal pepper, ginger, alkaline ash, and salt. A pill is described for use against inflammations of the oral and respiratory mucosa (Fig. 24): *Take extract of Asiatic barberry, bark of Chaba pepper, and long pepper, carefully weigh them out in equal portions, grind them with water, and hold the pill* (made of this pulp in your mouth). *It cures* (morbid) *blood*[2] (in the oral region as manifested in) *stomatitis, tonsillitis and pharyngitis.*

During the first six centuries A. D., a true professional class of physicians developed from the Brahmin caste, one which adheres to some of the ancient traditions even today. At approximately the same time the physicians' schools were compiling the collected works of the legendary authors Caraka and Sushruta. Later the

[1] Dragendorff p. 464

[2] Blood, like water, bile and mucus, has the significance of a juice that elicits diseases, in the Bower manuscript. Hoernle part II, fol. 2^r, 41—42. Transl. Claus Vogel

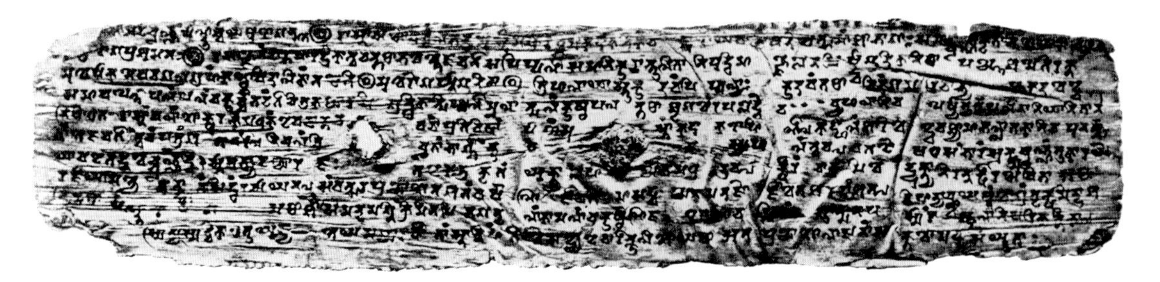

Fig. 24 *Page from the Bower manuscript. Rows 2 and 3 contain a prescription for a pill against oral diseases (Hoernle)*

Ashtângahridaya-Samhitâ of Vâgbhata (Samhitâ = collection) summarized the knowledge of the previous centuries. These textbooks are divided into portions dealing with pathology and others with therapeutics. These, in turn, are arranged topographically. No longer is the prevailing procedure that of observation and waiting, at best providing a magic potion. Rather, the beginnings of a true empirical system based on experience and observation are seen. Here, with limited knowledge of anatomy, are described remarkable surgical procedures such as the "Indian" method for reconstruction of the nose. A pedunculated skin and fatty-tissue flap from the forehead was taken as the material to wrap about the freshened nasal defect. The technique was used primarily in the restoration of defects resulting from the cutting off of the nose and ears as punishment.

Training was provided in firmly structured form. The student, depending on conditions, was required to be a member of a higher caste. He had to be young, prosperous and of high character. His teacher, who selected him, initiated him in a ritual ceremony with a pledge of obedience and readiness to provide aid to all seekers of health except hunters, criminals, unaccompanied women and those who were terminally ill[3]. He was trained systematically in surgery on animals and phantoms, learning to use a well-developed range of instruments. The position of an Indian physician was highly esteemed because of his origin and his training.

Internal diseases, the chief concern of the Caraka collection, were treated with herbs and minerals, plentiful and varied in the region. Dietetic measures were used also. India has enriched the pharmaceutical treasures of the occident with a variety of medicinal plants, most recently with Rauwolfia.

The more surgically oriented Sushruta-Samhitâ describes 67 diseases of the mouth and teeth alone: classified as 8 diseases of the lips; 15 of the tooth root, actually affections of the periodontium, such as gingivitis and periodontitis; 8 of the teeth; 5 of the tongue; 9 of the palate; 18 of the throat; and 4 of the entire oral cavity, which consist essentially of blisters and aphthous diseases of the mucosa. These diseases have been collected in special chapters by Sushruta and in about 650 A.D. by Vâgbhata, an author relating to the Sushruta tradition. He recognizes as many as 75 oral diseases, although his descriptions in the subject of interest to us are less precise, just as we notice in his work a general decline of the art of surgery[4]. Some of the diseases are ascribed etiologically to disproportions of the three fundamental humors (Dosha): wind (Vâyu), bile (Pitta), and mucus (Kapha, Shleshman), in accordance with the fundamentals of Indian-Brahmin medicine. Wind, incidentally, here represents a sort of vital breath.

The similarity to the Hippocratic humoral teachings permits consideration of a possible direct influence by the Greek tradition (Alexandrian conquests). An example is shown in the translation of a Sanskrit text from the Sushruta-Sâmhita (Fig. 25): *The seven natures* (of man) *originate in the humours* (of the body, which may act) *singly, by pairs, and jointly.* (A person's) *nature is determined by that humour which is produced in excess at the union of sperm and* (menstrual) *blood. Accept my definition of it! Amongst* (men) *the wind-natured one is sleepless, averse to cold, ugly, thievish, envious, dishonorable, fond of music, has chapped hands and feet, a thin and rough beard, nails and hair, is violent and grinds his teeth.* (He is) *unrestrained, unstable in his friendship, lean, rude, covered with* (visible) *veins, garrulous, quick in his gait and speech, emotionally unstable, and hastens through the air in his dreams. Uncertain of his resolutions, fickle-eyed, lacking in stocks of jewels and money, and* (poor) *in friends, he talks just incoherent stuff. This* (is) *the wind-natured man*[5].

All forms of gingival inflammation are described exactly by Sushruta in the pathological section. In the therapeutic part we find that they are cured with laxatives and emetics, scarification, application of herbal infusions and pastes with bases of butter or honey. Take scurvy (Shitâda) as an example: *The gums of the teeth suddenly bleed and become putrified, black, slimy, and emit a fetid smell. They become soft and gradually slough off. The disease has its origin in the deranged condition of the local blood and slimy substance* (Kapham)[6]. As to therapy, we read that the gingiva is made to bleed and then gargling with a decoction of five

[3] Esser; in the translation of Bhishagratna II p. 101.2—3, there are only 65 but "according to others 67" (footnote)
[4] Müller (a)
[5] Bhishagratna Vol. II p. 154, 59—60
[6] Bhishagratna II p. 102, 14

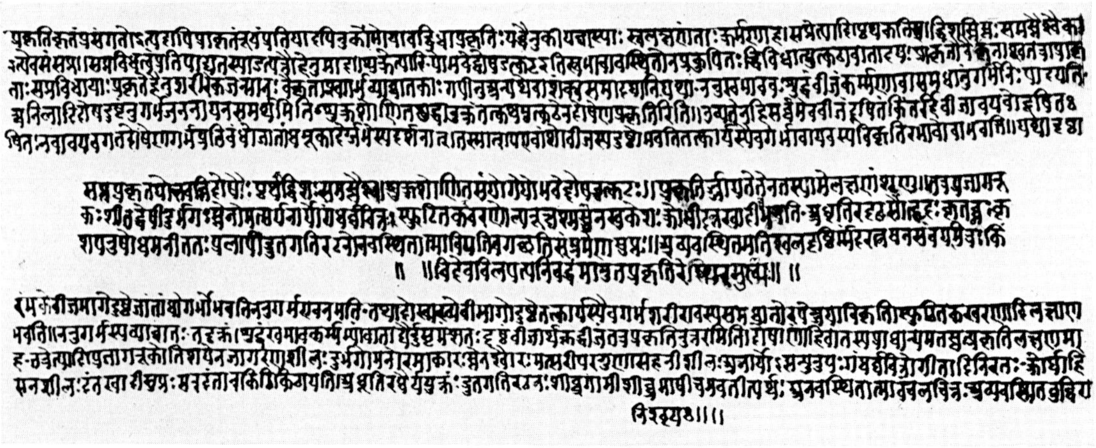

Fig. 25 *Sanskrit text from an undated paper manuscript (written between 1774 and 1799 at the latest) of the Sushruta Samhitâ (Chambers Collection No. 577, fol. 18v; State Library, West Berlin)*

astringent herbal drugs is employed, followed by application of a similarly complicated plant-butter paste [7].

In Danta-veshtaka *the teeth become loose in the gums, which exude a discharge of blood and pus. This disease is due to the vitiated blood of the locality.—The disease which is marked by the advent of an additional tooth through the action of the deranged Vayu* (wind) *with a specific excruciating pain of its own, is called Vardhana or eruption of the wisdom tooth. The pain subsides with the cutting of the tooth.* The course of this eruption with an extremely painful tumor is called Adhimânsa (excess flesh). In this case, *the additional fleshy growth about the roots should be removed* (with a knife), treated with a compound of astringent botanical drugs, sodium and potassium carbonate, *pasted together with honey.* Fistulas (Nâdi) are cauterized. The responsible tooth, according to Vâgbhata, is principally removed but, according to Sushruta, is left in the maxilla because of the danger of hemorrhage which may have blindness, facial paralysis, or other dangerous affections (convulsions) as a sequela [8].

The disease conditions, thus far described, are given by the translator as diseases of the roots of the teeth; more properly they are diseases of the periodontium. *Diseases of the teeth proper* follow. In toothache (Dâlana), the tooth appears to be cleft by the tremendous pain, *the origin of which is ascribed to the action of the aggravated state of the bodily Vâyu* [9]. In the description of caries, the toothworm reappears: *If the marrow is dried out because of Dosha through the predominance of the wind after it has entered the tooth and the root,* (and) *the tooth has become hollow and filled with food and dirt, fine worms arise through the decay, and there results severe pain or its diminution without reason. If the tooth has become black and loose with itching, it is called Pralûna* (cut off); *if it has a* (flow of) *blood and pus, it is called Krimidantaka* (worm-tooth) [10]. Treatment consists of sweating, scarification, ointments, gargling, sneeze-inducing materials, and foods that drive wind away. Vâgbhata also suggests local therapy: he fills the cavity with treacle or wax and then burns it out with a heated probe, or overcomes the worms and stabbing pains with a filling of sap of two plants. If this or many similar things do not help, the tooth must be pulled even if it is firm in its socket. Sushruta is more careful here, and extracts only the loose tooth. In general the reaction of the pulp to various stimuli is differentiated clearly: *The disease in which the teeth cannot bear the heat, cold or touch is Dankaharsha* [11].

The symptomatology of the disease identified as Kapâlikâ is not quite clear: *in which the preced-*

[7] Ibid. p. 463, 9—10
[8] Ibid. pp. 103 f., 16 and 20—24; p. 465, 17—21; Vogel-Brauer
[9] Ibid. p. 104, 23
[10] Hilgenberg and Kirfel VI 21, 18—19
[11] Bhishagratna II p. 104, 28

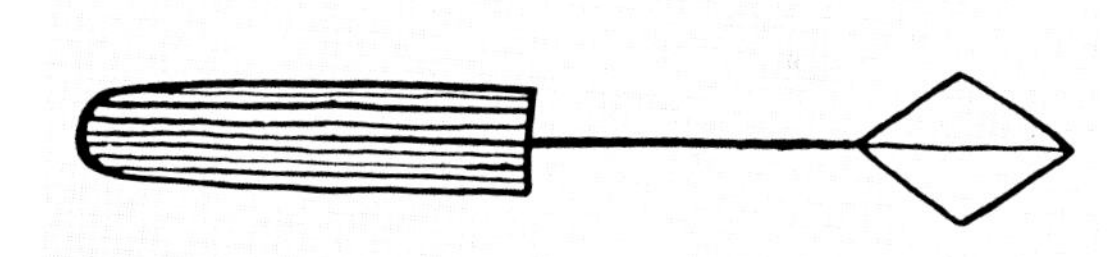

Fig. 26 *Dental hygiene instrument (Dantalekhana or Dantashanku)*

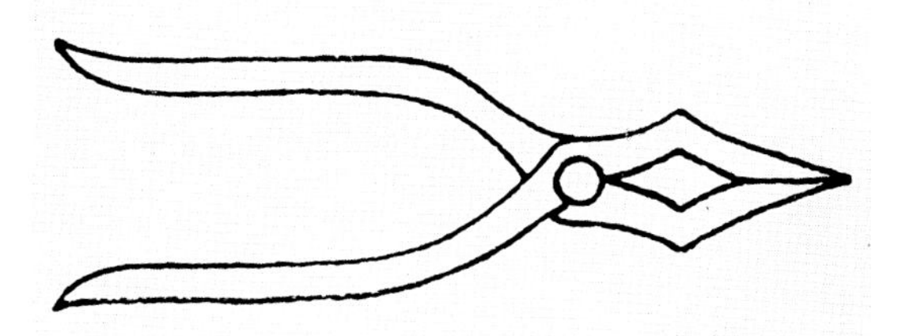

Fig. 27 *Forceps (Samdamsha)*

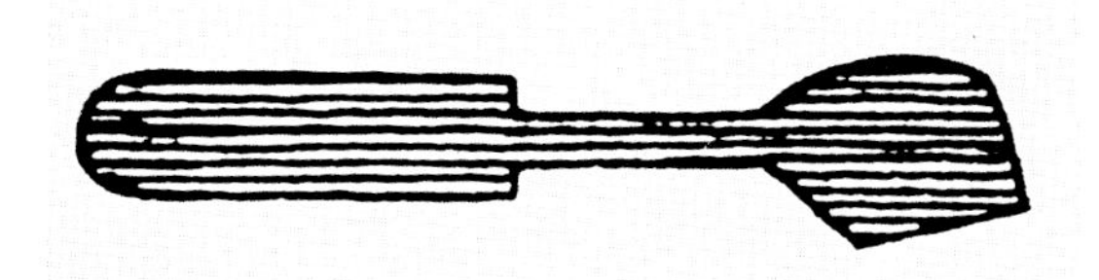

Fig. 28 *Extraction instrument similar to a lever, "Instrument with an arrow tip" (Sharapunkhayantra)*

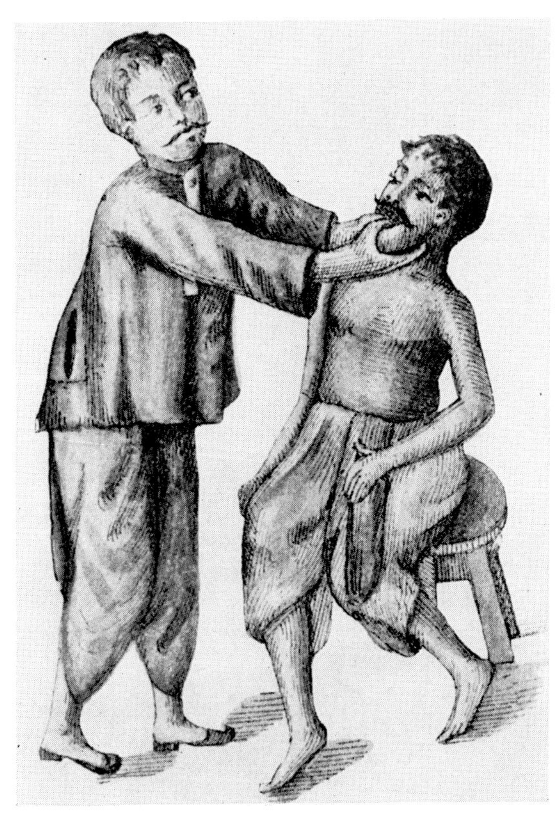

Fig. 29 *Mandibular reduction (Mukhopādhyāya)*

ing cristallized deposits get cemented together and afterwards separate from the teeth taking away a part of their coating . . . which naturally makes an erosion into the teeth and destroys them[12]. This observation of Sushruta is important because perhaps for the first time it is noted here that the tooth crown has an (enamel) coating[13]. Vâgbhata writes: *Kapâlikâ leads to the exfoliation of the teeth as minute bone splinters*[14]. Is this calculus so adherent that the enamel is damaged in its removal? Or is it cervical caries covered with calculus? Both conditions are thorougly unusual.

The removal of calculus (Sharkarâ) is undertaken with a rhombus-shaped instrument (Fig. 26), the periodontium being protected. Tooth extraction with a forceps (Samdamsha) or a kind of lever (Sharapunkhayantra), which however, like the pes caprinus or punch of our own time, is used for loose teeth only (Figs. 27 and 28).

There is no special description of fracture of the jaw, although Sushruta uses bamboo splints to immobilize fractures generally, covering them with a setting mixture of flour and glue. Luxations of the jaw are treated by heating the region of the joint and bringing the bones (the plural is used) into the correct position (Fig. 29). Then a chin sling is applied and a sternutative agent given to dispel wind. Curiously, luxations of the jaw are not described in the section devoted to fractures and luxations, but rather in that about to "Diseases of the Teeth Proper." The cause again is "wind," here elicited by loud speaking, chewing of hard substances, and immoderate yawning[16].

12 Ibid. p. 105, 31
13 Artelt
14 Hilgenberg and Kirfel VI 21, 17
15 Vogel-Brauer
16 Bhishagratna II p. 284, 37; p. 105, 33

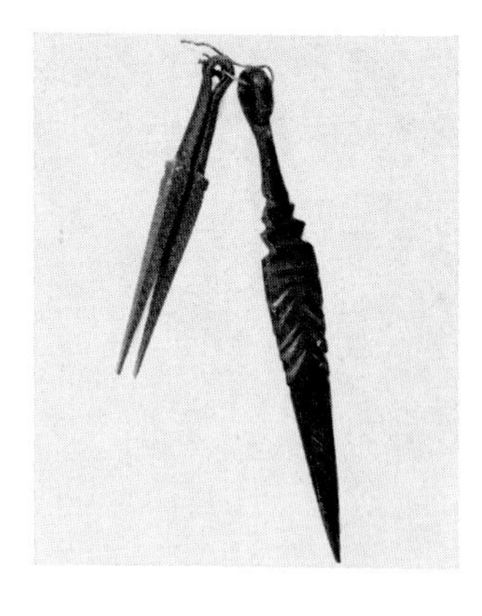

Fig. 30 *Beard tweezers and toothpick, Delhi (Museum für Völkerkunde, Berlin)*

The luxated tooth finds its discussion among the fractures. In young people, if not broken but loosened, it should be treated from outside of the mouth after the collected blood has been removed from the alveolus by pressing. Then water is used to cool the region and drugs are given. The patient should drink milk with the aid of a lotus reed [17].

Disturbances of eruption are discussed in Vâgbhata among the diseases of childhood: *The eruption of teeth may be the cause even of all diseases, especially those of fever, diarrhea, coughing, vomiting, excessive twitching* (cramps), *Pothaki* (discharging pustules on the eyelids), *and erysipelas. When cats arch their backs, peacock's tailfeathers become erect, and children's teeth erupt, these are storm signals* [18]. Treatment consists of local application of pulverized Bengal pepper in honey. Vâgbhata also advises: *Dried ground quail or partridge meat mixed with honey quickly elicits the cusps of children's teeth . . . In all diseases of the teeth, the activities of the child should not be too much restricted because diseases of eruption fade away by themselves.* The latter is a rather sensible piece of advice, especially when compared to the suggestions of some European surgeons and dentists of the 18th and 19th centuries [19].

Much is made of dental hygiene: *Early in the morning a man should leave his bed and brush his teeth.* Thus Sushruta introduces his chapter about bodily hygiene. The toothbrush consists of a fresh, worm-free twig, its end frayed into fibers, and its length, thickness, and especially the type of wood to be used is carefully specified. The wood variety was selected according to the time of year and the Dosha dominating the user, i. e., his temperament. A mixture of honey, oil, powdered Bengal pepper, cinnamon, ginger and salt was used as a dentifrice. The gingiva must not be injured during cleansing. Such dental care is specifically forbidden during the course of certain gingival diseases. Finally, the tongue should be scraped with a metal scraper. Later metal devices were used as toothpicks (Fig. 30).

Not a single word is to be found in the Sanskrit literature about the replacement of extracted or crumbled teeth, but that is not evidence that skilled craftsmen did not know how to overcome such defects discreetly.

Space permits only some examples of the comprehensive dental learning of ancient Indian medicine to be described here. In their separation of etiology and symptomatology, in their systematic pharmacology and in their significant surgical accomplishments, but in the arrangement and clarity of exposition also, they attained a level far beyond that of contemporary European medicine. Still, the stream of knowledge ran its own course; its contacts with ancient Greek, Islamic (Gondeshapur) [21] and modern medicine were too passing to affect its development decisively.

[17] Ibid. p. 284, 35
[18] Hilgenberg and Kirfel VI 2.25—28
[19] Ibid. VI 2.36
[20] Bhishagratna II p. 482, 3
[21] See p. 90

The author thanks Dr. Claus Vogel, professor of Indology at the University of Bonn, for revising and correcting the manuscript and its English edition, and for providing some of the illustrations.

References

Artelt, Walter
Geschichte der Anatomie der Kiefer und Zähne bis zum Ausgang der Antike. Janus 33 (1929) 199—212, 281—300, 310—336

Bhishagratna, Kunjalal
An English translation of the Sushruta Samhita. Vol. II, Calcutta 1911

Dragendorff, Georg
Die Heilpflanzen der verschiedenen Völker und Zeiten. Stuttgart 1898

Esser, A. Albert M.
Altindisches Arzttum. Münch. Med. Wschr. 81 (1934) 758—763

Hilgenberg, Luise; Willibald Kirfel
Vagbhatas Astangahrdayasamhita, ein altindisches Lehrbuch der Heilkunde. Leiden 1941

Hoernle, A. F. Rudolf
The Bower Manuscript. Calcutta 1893—1912

Kutumbiah, P.
Ancient Indian medicine. Madras 1962

Müller, Reinhold F. G.

a) Indische chirurgische Instrumente. Sudhoffs Arch. Gesch. Med. 30 (1937) 91—97

b) Grundlagen altindischer Medizin. Nova Acta Leopoldina, Vol. XI, Nr. 74, Halle 1942

Mukhopadhyaya, Girindranath
The surgical instruments of the Hindus. Vol. II, Calcutta 1913/1914

Sanyal, P. K.:
A story of medicine & pharmacy in India. Calcutta 1964

Vogel, Claus
Vagbhata's Astangahrdayasamhita. The first five chapters of its Tibetan version. Wiesbaden 1965

Vogel-Brauer, Anneliese
Die Zahn- und Zahnbetterkrankungen in der altindischen Medizin. Stoma 17 (1964) 126—140

Chapter 3

The Far East

China

The history of the Chinese kingdom is that of its ruler dynasties. These were usually dissolved after centuries of power into interval periods which often were characterized by dissipating into feudal states. During one of these interim reigns in the 6th century B. C., a time of philosophical brilliance evolved: The teachings of the legendary Lao-tse recommended renunciating worldly possessions and yielding to Tao, the laws of nature. Confucius (K'ung-tse) strove for an aristocratic order, a return to earlier patriarchal circumstances and established the roots of the ancestral culture and family ethics. He was responsible for the expression that all diseases enter through the mouth.

In 221 B. C. the king of Ch'in, a component state, united the kingdom as its first emperor into a centralized state of officialdom. This he secured to the northwest against restless factions of central Asia by means of an earth wall, the forerunner of the Great Wall of China. During the following Han Dynasty (206 B. C.—220 A. D.), Buddhism, originating in India, gained a foothold in China. Again there was splintering, invasion by Turks, Tibetans and Mongols in 400 A. D., and extension of Buddha's teachings. Then the kingdom attained its position as a great power under the T'ang emperors (618—906). The conquest of China by Genghis Khan began in 1211 and was followed by a hundred years of Mongolian rule with Peking as capital, whose brilliancy was described by Marco Polo. In 1368 the Ming Dynasty came into power, constructed the wall which exists today, gathered knowledge of the times together in a formidable encyclopedia and left considerable western spiritual influence into the country. After a slow decline the Ming were deposed by the Manchu in 1644. They occupied the throne until 1912. With the Manchu emperors China reached its pinnacle of power. Several encyclopedic collections of prescriptions and medical textbooks originated during their reign. These give us less of an insight into the development of medicine than of its level at that time. Generally, these are epochs more of collections and recordings than progress.

According to the history of the empire, Chinese medicine evolved in complete seclusion even from neighboring India until the 3rd century B. C. Its beginnings were entirely different from those of earlier cultures whose medicine was mixed with religious ideas and at least in its early stage lay entirely in the hands of priests and priest physicians. In the Middle Kingdom the earliest medical disclosures such as the "Nei Ching" were traced to the emperor authors in the 3rd millennium B. C. This classic work on internal medicine was attributed to the mythical "yellow emperor" Huang-ti. He is said to have reigned from 2696—2598[1], however, the names and dates are completely legendary. The traditions were developed and amplified primarily by court physicians who belonged as a group to a very low official class, or by recognized scholars and high officials who pursued them as hobbies. The social standing of a free practicing physician was still considerably lower than that of any other official.

Chinese medicine was also intermingled with magical concepts. Thus, a binding relationship was found between the 5 organs of liver, heart, spleen, lungs, kidneys, and the 5 elements of wood, fire, earth, metal, water, the 5 planets, the times of year, colors, emotions and so forth, all based on the dominant number 5. The "Nei Ching" contains information concerning the development of the body that is reminiscent of the Hebdomaden teachings of followers of Hippocrates[2]. The first chapter deals with the development of women. At the age of 7 the teeth and hair become long, at age 14 menstruation and the ability to give birth commence, at 21 development is completed, etc. The development of man is treated similarly using the guide number of 8 in the following section[3].

Anatomic and physiological knowledge, limited to cultural reasons, was replaced with speculative conclusions. Although based on incorrect

[1] Veith pp. 4 f.
[2] See p. 62
[3] Veith pp. 20 and 99

theories, often successful therapeutic recommendations resulted. Through experience, Chinese physicians learned to use the rich plant and mineral stocks of their land. Drugs were used in manifold combinations, often sufficiently mixed with the products of the so-called junk apothecary such as cicada shells, turtle urine and pulverized horns, etc. But, scattered throughout these were modern directions for gymnastics and breathing exercises which must have evolved from Buddhist influences. Highest value was placed on an excessively accurate pulse registration which was the base for decisive conclusions regarding diagnosis. Second in place the condition of the tongue was used as a base[4].

In the "Golden Mirror", a gigantic encyclopedia begun at the close of the 18th century by the emperor's decree to collect historical and the most ancient knowledge, caries was designated as toothworm traveling from one tooth to another. Pulpitis pain is lessened with a warm drink. When carious teeth bleed, presumably from an injured pulp polyp, therapy involves use of mixed pulverized rhinocerus horn, earth and the peel of the fruit of 2 types of peonies taken simultaneously with tea, and external application of the sediment from human urine. Such nonsense is diametrically opposed to absolutely rational recommendations such as the application of arsenic to the tooth cavity as a genuine causal therapy for toothache, and an early reference to this devitalization material still in use today. Hübotter reports that arsenic is rubbed into the stomach of a small perch-like fish. The fish is air-dried and the white material obtained is used to devitalize the pulp[5]. The first use of a toothbrush and of amalgam for cavity filling are attributed to Chinese medicine[6].

Amalgam is first mentioned as a silver dough in the Materia Medica of Su Kung, 659 A. D. during the T'ang Dynasty. It is mentioned again in the "Ta-Kuan Pent-ts'ao" of T'ang Shen-wei in 1107. In the Ming Period, Liu Wen-t'ai in his writings "The Essentials of Materia Medica" in 1505 discussed amalgam, as did Li Shi-chen in 1596. The former also made known its exact composition: 100 parts mercury, 45 parts silver, and 900 parts tin. These are mixed in an iron pot[7], and he added that cavities in anterior and posterior teeth could be filled[8]. We can assume that amalgam was known as a filling material for carious teeth in China probably since the 7th and certainly since the 16th century, that is, at about the same time as in Europe[9]. In both places the early amalgam prescriptions were forgotten.

That is the extent of reports on the practice of dentistry in China. Hübotter observed that even today in special stalls at markets, teeth which have become loosened through aging or inflammation, are removed using the fingers, without the aid of instruments. Elevators were used only if the tooth was firm. This is probably the result of European influence[10]. Dai reports that toothworm removers practised their trade in rural areas using slight-of-hand tricks to produce the worm. Tooth cleansers bleached the anterior teeth with hydrochloric acid[11]. Obviously, none of these were doctors, but were therapeutically comparable to the tooth-drawers of the yearly markets in Europe.

Since the Mongolian Dynasty, about 1280, medicine had been divided into 13 special areas, among which dentistry was included. Acupuncture played a significant role. It consisted of insertion or hammering in of needles of various calibers into specific points to prescribed depths for a period of time based on the number of respirations. Even in ancient times, a complete system had been developed for the procedure, reminding the occidental physician immediately of Head-zones (Fig. 32). This was based on the restoration of a disturbed circulation, a type of "pneuma" especially of "Ch'i," which builds the vital force and is situated in the large intestines of the body as a gas-like element. Definite times were forbidden for the treatment of certain organs, for example, the 10th day of each month for teeth and the 2 hours between 7 and 9 o'clock in the morning for neck and mouth. Some puncture points were close to the organs being treated while others were in remote regions. Thus, *tooth wind with swollen face and jaw separation* was treated between the middle bones of the hand, the mandibular teeth at the heel of the foot, precisely at the distal end of the 4th bone of the middle foot.

4 Hübotter (b)
5 Hübotter (a) p. 101
6 Huard/Wong (a) pp. 144 f.
7 Chu Hsi-T'ao; Huard/Wong p. 35
8 De Maar
9 See p. 156 f.
10 Hübotter (c)
11 Dai

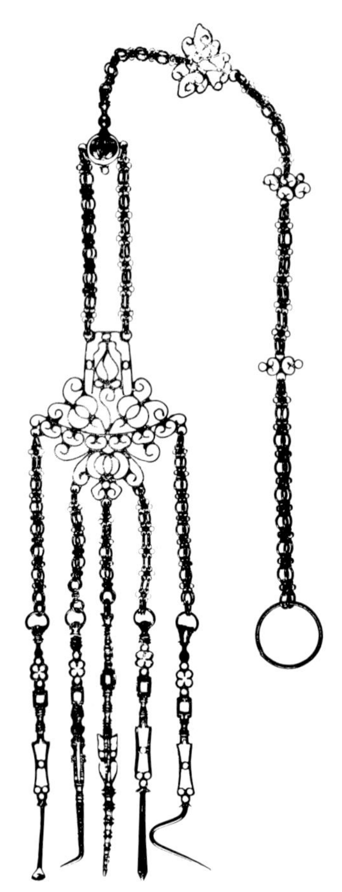

Fig. 31 *Silver filigree jewelry with ear wax remover, knot breaker, nail cleaner, and toothpick, from the boundary region between the Chinese Yunan province and Tibet (Museum für Völkerkunde, Berlin)*

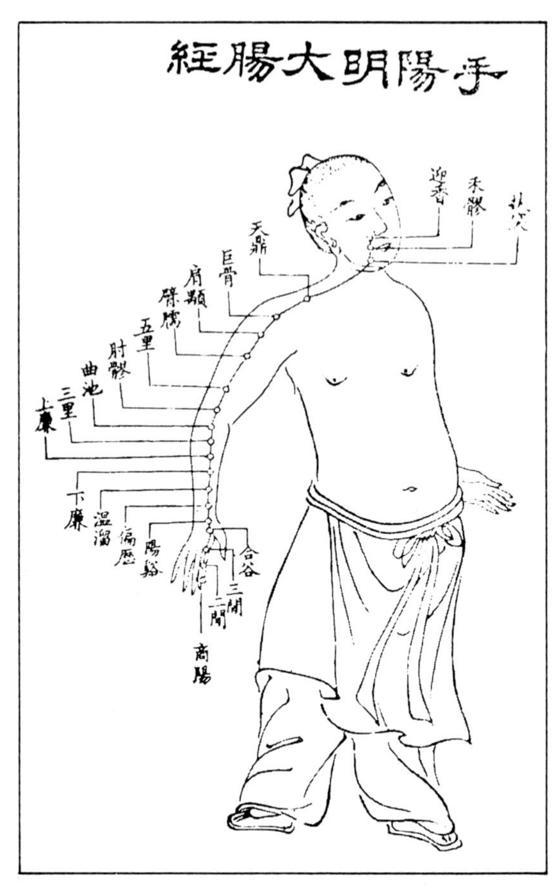

Fig. 32 *Acupuncture picture in the time of the Ming dynasty (from Huard/Wong)*

The aforementioned "Nei Ching" contained the following very ancient prescription: *If the patient can tolerate the touch of cold water in his mouth, puncture at the point of the meridian of the stomach, if he cannot tolerate it, puncture the meridian of the large intestines*[12]. The use of moxibustion is similar. This involves the burning of cones of plant fibers at points on the skin corresponding essentially to acupuncture points[13].
Accordingly, Chinese medicine was limited by a structure of rules and systems which made a vital development for millenniums difficult for the conservative attitude of a people virtually isolated from the outside world.

Japan

The spread of Chinese medicine traveled almost exclusively in an eastern direction, across Korea to Japan. As was the case with the entire Japanese culture, the medicine of the island kingdom was based on the Chinese medicine in about 700 A. D. and developed a more unique character in 900 with separation from the continent. Several folk remedies against toothache came from Japan: The dental arch is clearly drawn on a piece of paper shaped like the outline of two

[12] Chamfrault I p. 837
[13] Hübotter (a)

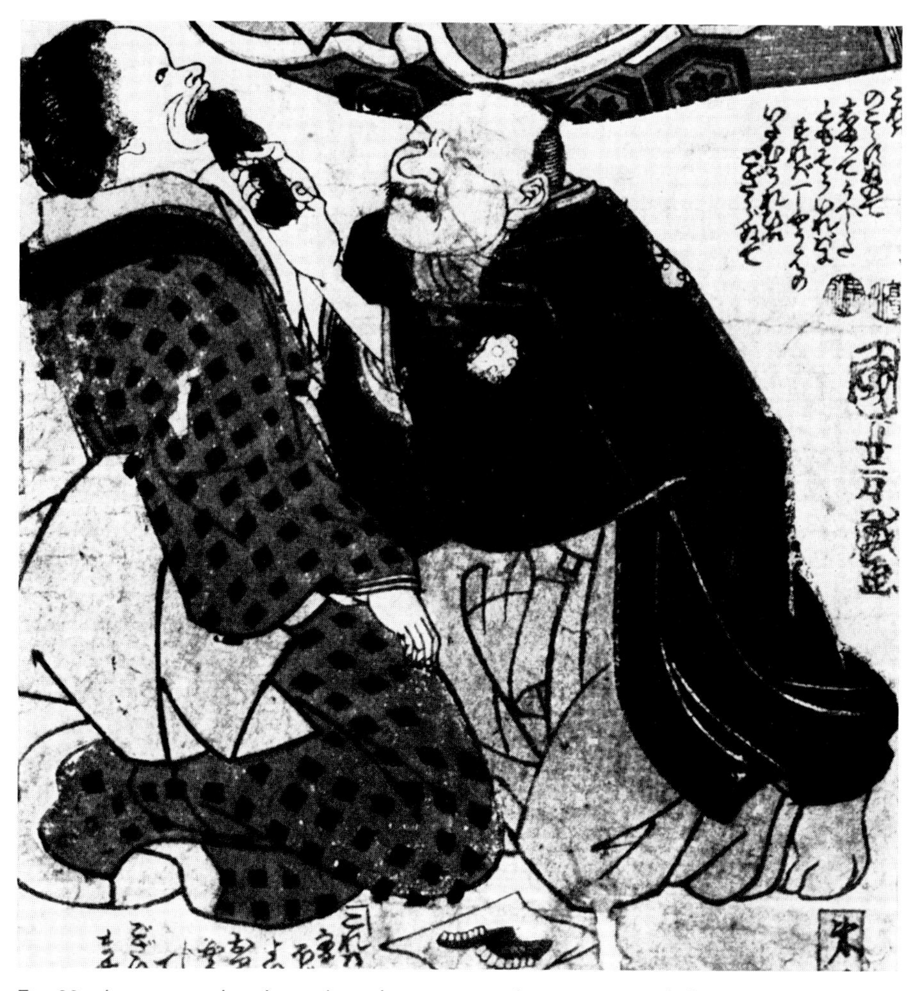

Fig. 33 *Japanese colored woodcut showing a tooth extraction with forceps; prosthesis in the foreground, around 1820*

feet. This is nailed to the doorway post, the nail piercing the aching tooth, or it is thrown in the river with the tooth colored black. The use of sorcery to transfer toothache to another object was prevalent on Europe[14]. In order for a child to have strong, sharp teeth he was, at the age of 120 days, given a type of fish to eat that had sharp spines on the oral and back fins[15]. Pulse diagnosis, acupuncture and moxibustion were practiced with slight variations from the Chinese. Teeth were also removed with the fingers. This procedure was first practiced diligently using wood flakes. Later, in the early 19th century, as is depicted in a wood carving, the European influence had brought in the use of forceps (Fig. 33). Also, skillful dentures were carved from hard wood with nailheads as grinding surfaces, and flint or mother of pearl platelets were set in as anterior teeth (Figs. 34 to 36).

[14] See p. 133
[15] Kleiweg

The author thanks the late Prof. Franz Hübotter, MD, PhD, for review of the manuscript and for generous advice.

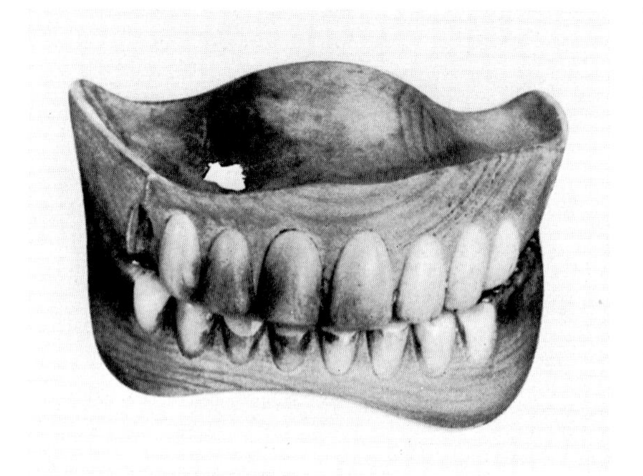

Fig. 34

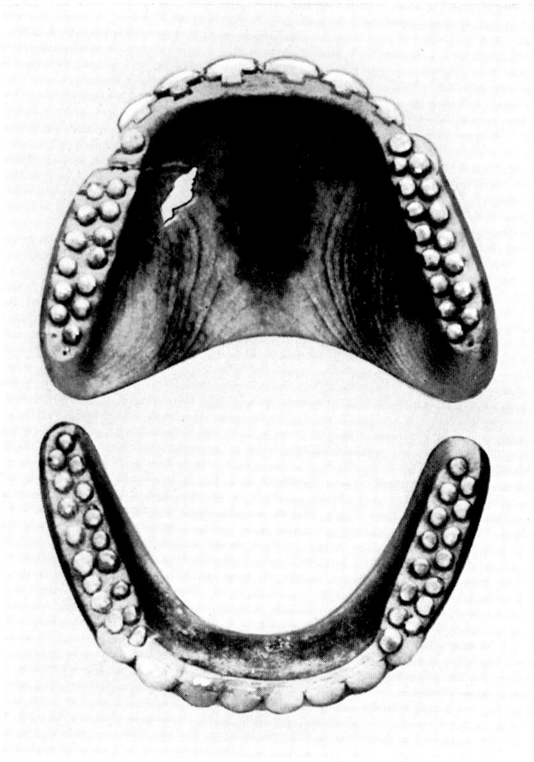

Fig. 35

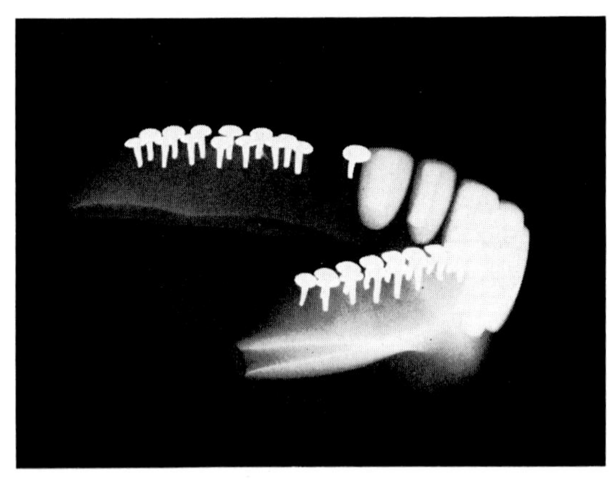

Fig. 36

Figs. 34 and 35 *Japanese carved wooden denture with flint teeth and nailheads as occlusal surfaces (from Homma)*

Fig. 36 *Radiograph of the illustration above (from Homma)*

References

Chamfrault, A.
Traité de la médecine chinoise. 5 Vols., Angoulême 1957—1961
Vol. I, 2nd ed. 1964

Chu Hsi-T'ao
The use of amalgam as filling material in dentistry in ancient China. Chin. Med. J. 76 (1958) 553—555

Dai, David S. K.
Dentistry in China—past and present. J. Amer. Dent. Ass. 30 (1943) 219—223

Huard, Pierre; Ming Wong
a) La médecine chinoise au cours des siècles. Paris 1959
b) Chinesische Medizin. Transl. Hannes W. Schoeller, München 1968

Hübotter, Franz
a) Die chinesische Medizin zu Beginn des XX. Jahrh. und ihr historischer Entwicklungsgang. Leipzig 1929
b) Chinesische Medizin. Ciba-Zschr. 8 (1959) 3110—3137 (Wehr)
c) Personal Information to the author (3. 3. 1966)

Kleiweg de Zwaan, J(ohan) P(ieter)
Völkerkundliches und Geschichtliches über die Heilkunde der Chinesen und Japaner. Natuurkundige Verhandelingen van de Hollandsche Mij der Wetenschapen, 3. Assembling, part 7, Haarlem 1917

Maar, F. E. R. de
Wie introduceerde het zilveramalgaam in de tandheelkunde? Ned. tschr. Tandheelk. 75 (1968) 395—404

Shindo, Satohisa; Kuninori Homma
The History of the customs of dental cosmetics as shown in the Ukiyoe art of painting. Tokyo 1978 (in Japanese)

Veith, Ilza
The yellow emperor's classic of internal medicine. New Ed., Berkeley, Los Angeles 1966

Chapter 4

Pre-Columbian America

After all that archeologists have discovered in the American continent, and more importantly, have not discovered, it can be concluded that the first humans of the New World arrived from Northeast Asia 30,000 to 40,000 years ago. Their entry as perfect homo sapiens took place across an ice bridge in the region of the Bering Straits. This is assumed because no fossils of human intermediate stages have been found. Also, the New World apes remained in a former evolutionary stage; they have broad noses and 3 premolars. This contrasts with the Old World apes which are narrow-nosed and have human-like dentitions. The original American Indian population is characterized by the presence of shovel-shaped upper incisors, a mongoloid race characteristic also found in Chineses, Japaneses, and Eskimos (Fig. 37). Additional immigrants followed, probably as small hordes of nomadic hunters. Their descendants spread southward across the isthmus of Panama to Tierra del Fuego and development markedly different ethnic and linguistic roots.

When the Spanish conquistadors conquered the mainland in the first half of the 16th century, they found 3 main cultures: The Aztec in the Mexican hills, south of there—centered on the Yucatan peninsula—the Maya in the process of becoming extinct and in the South American Andes, the Inca. These populations were mutually in highly organized cities with theocratic rule and significant accomplishments in the area of construction skills, working essentially with stone age equipment. The cultural maturing in both Americas, however, cannot be measured against the evolutionary stages of the Old World. This continent remained in a continuous Stone Age, with occasional splashes of bronze casting.

The Aztec

After extended wanderings, the Aztec settled in the lake region of the Mexican highlands after 1200 and came under the moderating influence of the neighboring races, whose culture they adopted. The cultural foundations rested on the accomplishments of the pre-Christian period of the Gulf residents, the Olmec and especially their descendants, the Toltec and Chichimec. Under capable rulers the Aztec race achieved hegemony and gradually expanded its area of dominance from the Pacific Ocean to the Gulf of Mexico. In 1519 the Spaniards under Hernando Cortes invaded the mainland. The ruler of the land, Moctezuma II, died in Spanish captivity in 1520, ending the empire with complete disruption of the capital, Tenochtitlan, which is now Mexico City, in 1521.

As was the case with ancient Asiatic cultures and the early Greeks, early Mexico had a rational and a magic medicine which were partially intermingled. There were trained physicians as described for us by the prominent chronologist and Franciscan monk, Bernardino de Sahagún, who had command of the Aztec language. The following excerpt is from his report on the Indian people (translated from a 1570 Aztec text). *The physician,* [ticitl] (is) *a curer of people, a restorer, a provider of health. The good physician* (is) *a diagnostician, experienced —a knower of herbs, of stones, of trees, of roots. He has* (results of) *examinations, experience, prudence.* (He is) *moderate in his acts. He provides health, restores people, provides them splints, sets bones for them, purges them, gives emetics, gives them potions; he lances, he makes incisions in them, stitches them, revives them, envelops them in ashes*[1].

Prophets played an important role. They predicted the course of a disease from a calendar There were also surgeons with good anatomic knowledge. Treatment of toothache belonged to a very primitive class of medicine which understood how to take the worm (ocuilin) from the eyes and teeth. There were also tooth specialists among them[2].

The medical books "tici-amatl" collected by Sahagún contain a vocabulary for individual organs of the mouth, with some physiological and pathological remarks. The teeth were desig-

[1] Sahagún (b) p. 77; (c) p. 30
[2] v. Gall p. 112; Dietschy (a); Busch p. 24

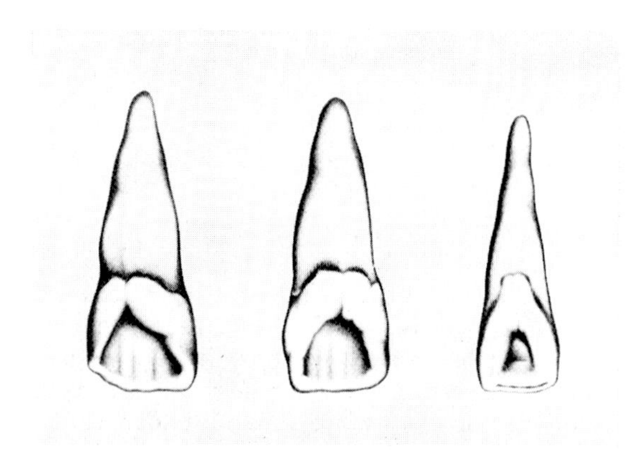

Fig. 37 *Indian shovel-shaped incisors (from Fastlicht)*

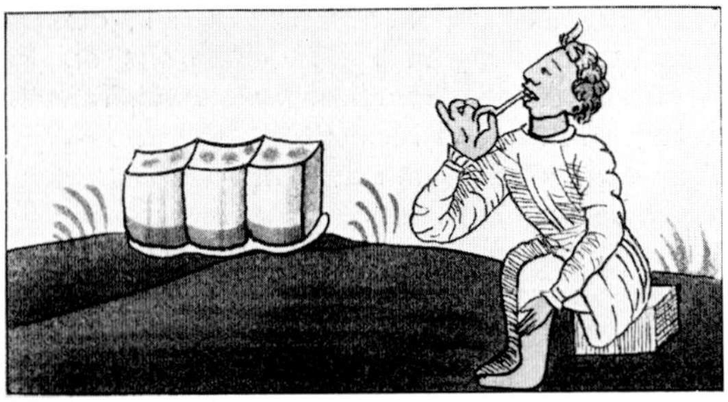

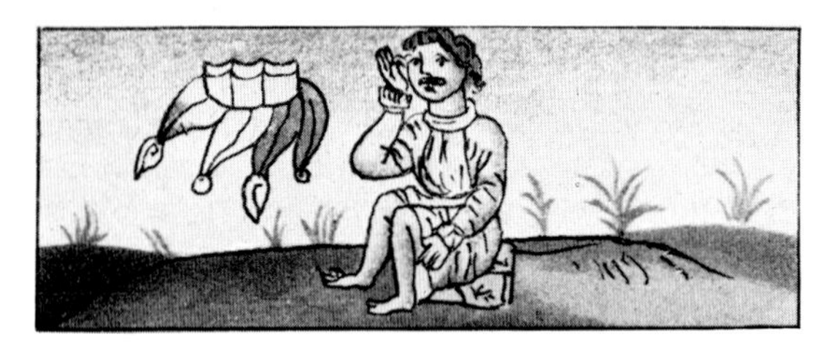

Fig. 38 *Sahagun illustration for the "tooth anatomy" section, 1570*

Fig. 39 *Sahagun illustration for the "toothache" section, 1570*

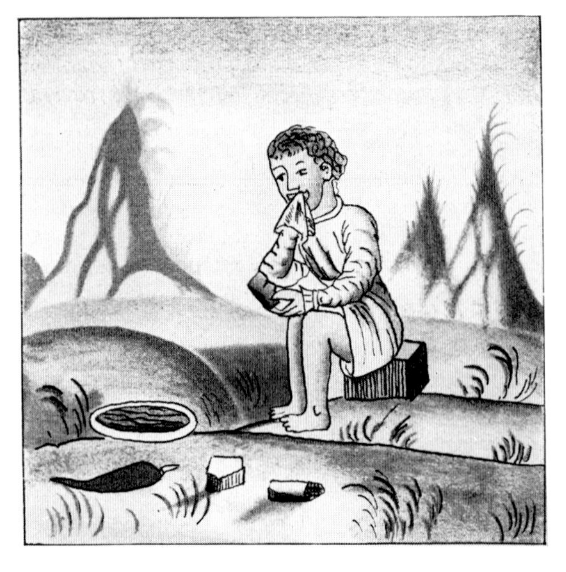

Fig. 40 *Sahagun illustration for the "tooth care" section, 1570*

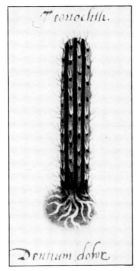

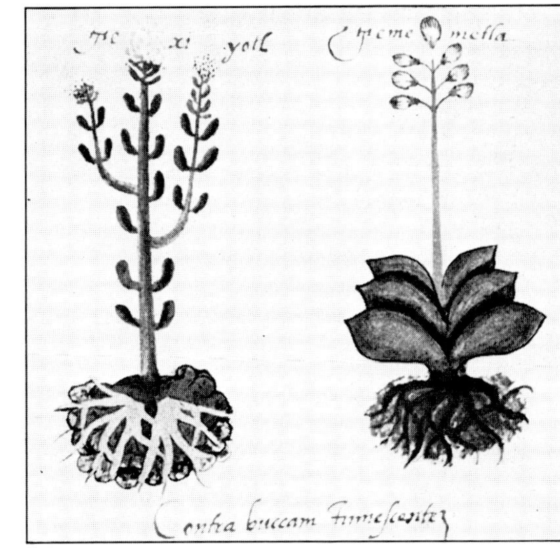

Figs. 41 and 42 *Medicinal plants from the so-called Badianus manuscript of Martinus de la Cruz, 1552*

nated as "tlantli": *tlantli, teeth: The teeth are bones; white, chalk white, white as chalk, yellow, yellowish, like ripe corn, like cornmeal, entirely white, like a snail shell, dark violet, black, cleaned, red from cochineal, colored red; (large, small, tiny), narrow, strong, round, natural, round, like a stone whorl, like a spinning whorl, pointed like a thorn, very sharp like a thorn, broad, pointed, filed to a point, mobile, very mobile, fractured, decayed, eaten by worms, abscessed* (at the root), *porous, like decayed corn, full of debris, full of tooth debris, mealy, full of coarse meal, decayed at the root, narrow at the root, they bite, teeth decompose, shred thoroughly, grind thoroughly (grind fine); it is tasty, it is eaten; they are like decayed corn, are dark violet, are colored red; they fracture, abscess, splinter, are mobile, rotate, fall out; I clean my teeth, I make my teeth beautiful, I wash my teeth, I dye my teeth, I file my teeth.*

Tlancochtli: Buccal teeth; (very) round like a ball, like a spinning whorl, whorl-shaped, whorl-like; they grind, grind very much, a strong mill-stone with which one grinds fine, with which one grinds, with which one minces, with which one pulverizes; (they mince), they pulverize; they replace themselves, they meet, change; they grow, increase, become stronger, become longer, become larger.

Coatlantli tocoatlan: Incisors; our incisors; round like a file, pointed in front; they pierce, grow, are round like files, are pointed in front.

Tlanixquatl totlanixqua: The tooth surface, our tooth surfaces are broad, extend broadly, hard as copper, sharp, sharp-edged; with which one bites; they bite, they grind; one minces with the teeth; as one whistles with the teeth, whistles with the teeth; (as one whistles with the lips, whistles with the lips), he whistles with the teeth, I whistle with the teeth; I cut with the teeth, I grind fine, I whistle with the lips; he bares his teeth[3] (Figs. 38—40).

Here teeth are showed at every age and condition, also filed and dyed. Moreover, there is a nomenclature for caries, toothache, calculus, for fractured and loose teeth as well as mucosal inflammation. Only children born during an eclipse of the moon have hare lip *because our man in the moon was a rabbit for the Mexicans*[4].

To fight caries caused by the worm, they wore the herb tlepahtli (Plumpago scandens L.)[5] and chewed hot chili (Polygonum hydropiper L.). A cavity was filled with a powder of snail shells, sea salt, the herb tlalcacaoatl (Arachis hypogaea L.) or picietl, tobacco[6]. Chewing tobacco or pop-root (Baccharis sarothroides)[7] were used to ease toothache. Among the assortment of healing plants, the root of chilmecatl (Clematis spec.) was the most effective. Prescriptions from

[3] Sahagún (c) p. 109 f.; v. Gall pp. 144 f.
[4] v. Gall p. 211
[5] The Latin designations for plants have been taken from Busch's dissertation; he took them in part from W. Eschrich of Bonn.
[6] F. A. Flores, cited by Busch p. 24
[7] v. Gall p. 100

an herb book compiled by a baptized Aztec, Martinus de la Cruz (author) and translated by Johannes Badianus into Latin, wavering between magic and rational treatment. It has many pictures of various plants. It is called the Badianus manuscript of 1552. Here is the treatment for toothache: *First the sick and decayed teeth should be tapped with the tooth of a corpse. Then the root of the long perennial teonochtli* (Pachycereus spec.) (Fig. 41) *is ground and burned thereon with hartshorn. The precious stone yztac quetzalitztli* (white feather obsidian). *chichiltic tapachtli* (red coral shell) *and a small amount of coarsely ground flour are heated with salt. The mixture is wrapped in a towel and should be pressed against the tooth for a short time, especially against any that ache or are carious. Finally, white incense and a type of salve known as xochiocotzotl* (Liquidambar styraciflua L.) *are burned upon glowing coals. A thick piece of cotton is saturated with the smoke and held close to the cheek, exactly in the center and bound tightly*[8].

A remedy against buccal swelling (*contra buccam tumescentem*) is also given: *The swollen cheek is healed if one drinks a liquid composed of water with ground tememetla leaves* (Echeveria fulgens Lem.), *from the marrow of texiyotl* (Sedum burgaei), a type of Crassula (Fig. 42) *and white earth. This liquid is lightly herbal and contains sticky resin from a resin-containing shrub known as Nocheztli* (Nopalea cochinillifera). *The ground root of the tlatlacotic plant* (Baccharis saligna) *heated in water is useful for those who cannot open the mouth widely. When this fluid is drunk, the patient vomits from the taste, expelling mucus which causes the mouth to open*[9].

Additional stomatological prescriptions in the herb book were for halitosis[10], gingivitis[12], mouth dryness[12] and other disorders.

Sahagún describes a bit of Aztec junk apothecary. It is recommended that a worm be ground, mixed with oil of turpentine and painted on the cheek[13]. At the same time heated pepper is placed on the tooth in which a grain of salt has been placed. An incision is made in the gingiva and the herb tlalcacaoatl (Arachis hypgaea L.) is placed on it. *If nothing reduces* (the infection), *the tooth is extracted; salt is inserted*[14]. Actually this is the only reference to tooth extraction in Aztec writings. Still these warlike people did practice wound surgery: *Laceration of a lip: While still fresh, it is sewed with hair. Salted maguey sap is applied. And if the scar or the cut persist, it is cut or burned along the sides of the lip laceration. Then the wound lips are joined; it is sutured with hair. Salted maguey sap is applied*[15].

The frequent reference to the detrimental influence of hot and cold food in the medieval literature of the Old World was also made here: *..., in order that the teeth should not become infected, one should eat* (and) *drink things not very hot; only tepid. And if* (something) *hot is eaten, one should not immediately eat* (something) *cold; one should not immediately drink cold water*[16].

Calculus removal was considered important. Sahagún reports that the concrement was impregnated with quautepuztli (Budleia spec.), and the crusts softened in this manner were removed with a copper instrument[17].

Also, for other mucosal manifestations, such as aphthous (*oral ulcers*), herpes labialis (*blisters of the lips* caused by sun, wind and cold), ulcers and blisters of the tongue, there were special drugs[18].

Ancient Mexicans seemed to place a great deal of importance on dental care as they were also concerned with an exemplary body hygiene. *And then the eaten food is picked from the teeth;... Especially meat should not be left in our teeth, for small particles of meat in the teeth consume them; .... The teeth are to be washed with cold water; polished with a cloth* (Fig. 40), *rubbed with* (powdered) *charcoal; cleaned, made attractive, with salt ... And the teeth are to be dyed with tliltic tlamiaualli herbs* (Espiga negra); *however, these blacken the teeth. Or one will proceed washing* (them) *with urine*[19]. — Fauchard still recommended this in Paris in the 18th century.

According to Sahagún's dental description, the teeth were colored dark violet and red (with cochineal). The dyes, which as v. Gall reported, also have a preventive effect, served an

[8] de la Cruz fol. 17v (p. 48)
[9] Ibid. fol. 22v
[10] Ibid. fol. 21v
[11] Ibid. fol. 17r
[12] Ibid. fol. 19v
[13] Sahagún (c) p. 146; v. Gall p. 235
[14] Sahagún (b) p. 647; (c) p. 146; v. Gall p. 234
[15] Sahagún (c) p. 146; v. Gall p. 232
[16] Sahagún (c) p. 146; v. Gall p. 234
[17] Sahagún (c) p. 147; v. Gall p. 236
[18] Sahagún (c) p. 146; v. Gall 232 f.
[19] Sahagún (c) p. 147; v. Gall pp. 235 f.

essentially cosmetic, perhaps even a cultural purpose, as did the simultaneously mentioned filing and veneering of the anterior teeth with semi-precious stones.
Tooth mutilation, especially filing of the tips to resemble those of rapacious animals is found also among native Africans and Asians. Still, nowhere were they finished in the unique artistic style of ancient America using round polishing stones, perhaps with the aid of quartz powder (Fig. 43). From archeological discoveries it was possible to determine that these procedures were performed already about 200 B. C.[20]
Romero (1951) reported the existence of 51 different artifacts and incrustations which could be separated into 3 groups: 1. Filing of the tooth contour (Fig. 44 A—C), 2. filing and inlays on the anterior surface (D, E) and 3. combinations (F, G). Stones set in the surface of the anterior teeth were not discussed by the chronologists. It was no longer practiced during the Spanish conquest.
The pulp was generally protected. This was an indication of the anatomic knowledge of Indian specialists and the skill with which they knew how to manipulate their polishing stones and burrs (Fig. 45). Of the mostly round inlays, which were never found in carious regions, it can be assumed that they were secured by some type of cement[21]. Hematite and jade were the stones used.
Preponderantly in the realm of magic there was a conjuration for toothache, particularly for molars, wording and combination with rational therapy are reminiscent of a corresponding text from the two-river land. In combination with numerous similar formulae, it was preserved in the Aztec language by the spiritual Hernando Ruiz de Alarcón. In 1629 it was translated into Spanish and annotated; however, here a modern translation from the Aztec is presented[22]. In the Ruiz Spanish accompaniment parallel healing measures are listed which, as in the Old World to this day, consisted of the customary cauterization of painful pulp:
Treatment of pain in teeth or molars: Usually only copal (resin of several tropical trees) *is used for pain of teeth or molars. This was the forerunner of piciete* (tobacco) *or tenexcu* (lime). *In these instances it was placed in the tooth followed by conjuration, which was originally directed at piciete:*

Come
Little tobacco
Nine-convoluted
Nine-grounded!
Come
Black tooth worm
Come
Woman similar to me
White woman
Enter to pursue
The green pain
Do not disgrace yourself
Be on your guard, prepared:
You should drive out the green pain
Which wants to disturb my protective order.
Come
Five signs possess!
We will dispell
The green pain.
What already disturbs
My bewitched grind stone (molar)
In its function,
In my occupation of grinding
Because it has broken down
The protective wall?
During this (incantation) *they burned the molar or the tooth which aches with heated drops of copal resin. This, combined with the heat, suffices to soothe the pain, then they add this to the words.*

In another text there is an interpretation of the tobacco and lime combination which seems to have been used in this instance to still pain: *There is also another plant with divine properties. It is known as tobacco or tenechiete*[23]. *To this they add lime. The tobacco is treated by rubbing it between the hands with the lime. They call it "Brown possessed person, seven times beaten" because of the frequency with which it is rubbed between the hands. It is either spread over or rubbed on the patient. It is said of* (it) *to give the mouth strength*[24].

The Maya
The Maya who resided south of the Aztec had played their political state almost 100 years

[20] Fastlicht (a)
[21] See p. 53, footnote 26; Fastlicht (d) p. 57
[22] Ruiz p. 203. Unpublished translation of the Aztec text by Walter Lehmann (Ibero-Amerikanisches Institut, Berlin, signature Y 697)
[23] From the Aztec "tenex" (chalk) and "yetl" (abbreviated form picietl, tobacco)
[24] Serna p. 388

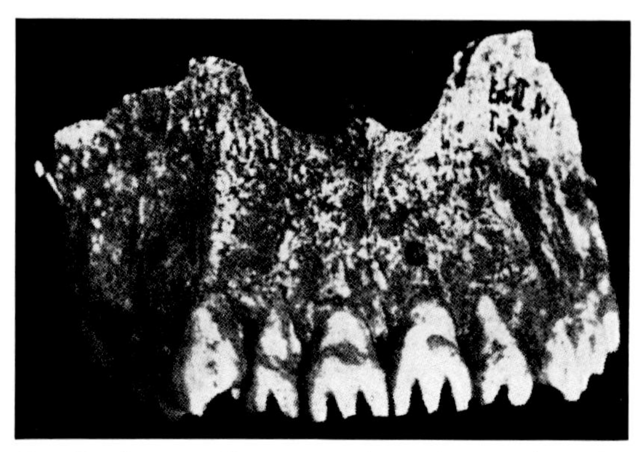

Fig. 43 *Ancient Mexican tooth mutilations (from Romero)*

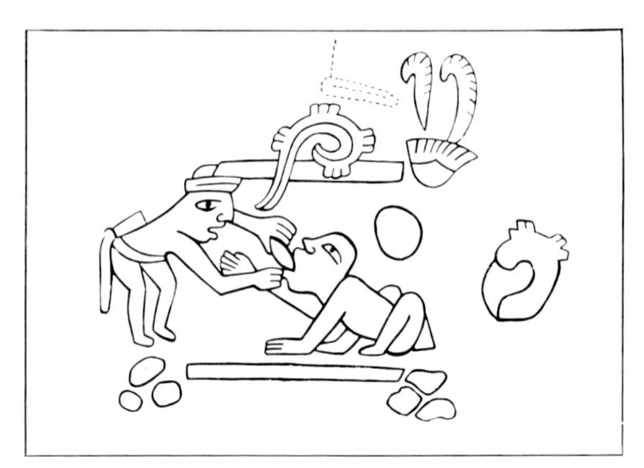

Fig. 45 *Redrawing, from colored frescoes, presumed to show the filing of teeth, in the "Earthly Paradise" of Tepantitla, Teotihuacan, Mexico*

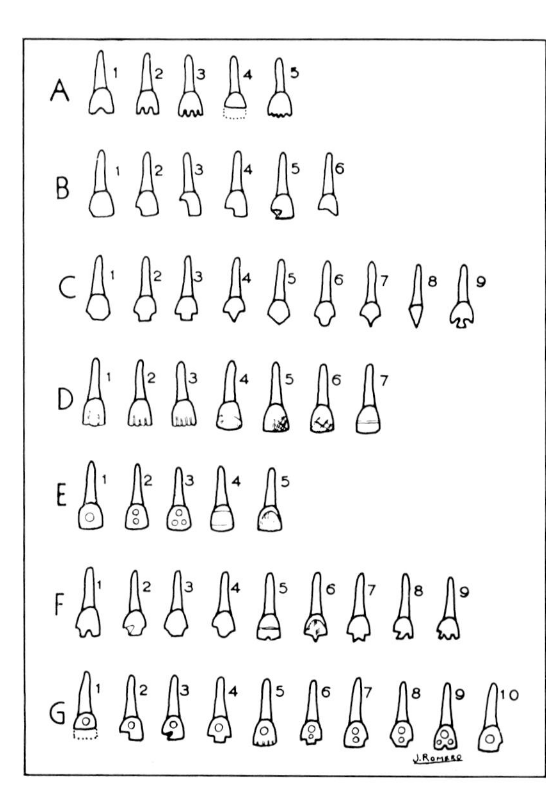

Fig. 44 *Classification of pre-Columbian dental mutilations: A 5, D 7, and F 5 were found only in North America; E 3, F 7, F 8, F 9, G 1, and G 3 in Central America; E 4, E 5, and F 6 in South America; all others in the entire continent (from Romero)*

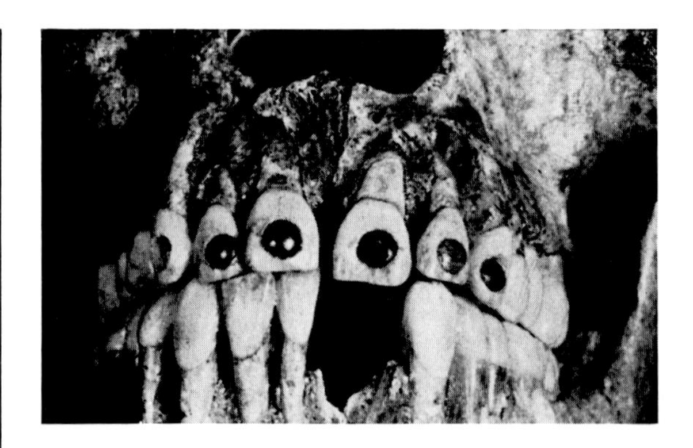

Fig. 46 and 47 *Four hematite inlays and one jade inlay (left lateral incisor) of a Maya jaw (National Museum of Anthropology, Mexiko) with a radiograph thereof on which periapical changes can be seen (from Fastlicht). A proof that drilling was done on living subjects.*

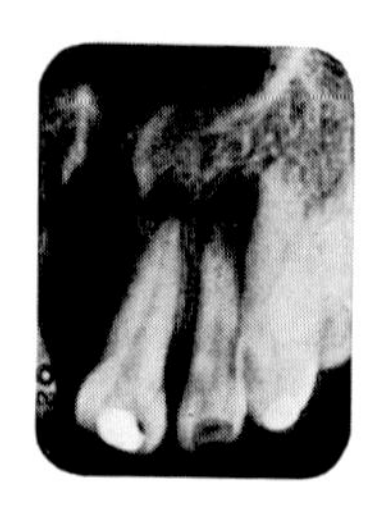

before the land was invaded by the Spaniards. The inhabitants of the city states described as the "Greeks of America" were spread over the entire southwest of today's Mexico and Guatamala during the first millennium A. D. At the close of the so-called classical period in the 10th century, they shifted their cultural weight to the northern portion of the Yucatan peninsula for reasons unknown. Splendid stone structures and singular steles are still found in ancient excavations, but the number of inscriptions available to us today is unfortunately very limited. Consequently we are essentially dependent on the Spanish chroniclers of the conquest, such as the bishop of the Yucatan, Diego de Landa. This prince of the church, who allowed most valuable illustrated scripts to be burned because of their pagan significance, we have to thank for the singular report on the technique of tooth filing of the Yucatan Maya. *They had the habit of allowing their teeth to be filed like those of a saw. It was done for reasons of vanity. The skill was practiced by elderly women using certain stones and water*[25]. The insertion of semiprecious stones such as turquoise, jade, jadeite and hematite was most highly developed among the Maya. It was even believed that the Aztec learned the art from them (Figs. 46 and 47). An analysis of Fastlicht of the substance used as cement gave approximately the following figures: calcium 23.5 %, phosphorus 30.4 %, aluminum 0.35 %, silicon 1.51 %, iron 2.8 %, magnesium 1.5 %, manganese 0.055 %, traces of copper and strontium[26].

A reddish material which was found in 1957 on teeth from "classical" period is worth while noticing. It was identified spectrographically as needle iron ore (goethite). It is assumed that this substance in the form of iron pyrite powder (markasite) mixed with an unknown substance was placed in a cavity in plastic condition to replace lost stones[27].

There were also references to teeth adorned with precious stones in "Popol Vuh", the holy book of the Quiché Indians, a southern Mayan race living in today's Guatemala. In the text of the original story a demon appears, called Vucub Caquix[28] who believes himself to be above the gods. Therefore the Celestial Heart decides to let him perish. First the demon glorifies his splendor: *For my eyes are of silver, bright, resplendent as precious stones, as emeralds; my teeth shine like perfect stones, like the face of the sky*[29]. Then 2 youths (actually gods) seal his downfall. Using a blowgun, one of them shot Vucub-Caquix in the jaw but then he pulled his arm off. Then they both withdrew and took shelter as a trick. They sent an aged couple (they were old magicians) to Vucub-Caquix. He was plagued with toothache and asked the aged for help: *I earnestly beseech you to have pity on me. What do you know how to cure? the lord asked them.*

And the old ones answered, "Oh Sir! we only take the worm from the teeth, cure the eyes and set bones."

"Very well. Cure my teeth, which are really making me suffer day and night, and because of them and of my eyes I cannot be calm and cannot sleep. All of this because two demons shot me with a pellet (from their blowgun) *and for that reason I cannot eat. Have pity on me, then, tighten my teeth with your hands."*

"Very well, Sir. It is a worm which makes you suffer. It will end when these teeth are pulled and others put in their place". "It is not good that you pull my teeth, because it is only with them that I am a lord and all my ornaments are my teeth and my eyes."

"We will put others of ground bone in their place." But the ground bone was nothing but grains of white corn.

"Very well, pull them out, come and relieve me," he replied. Then they pulled Vucub-Caquix's teeth; but in their place they put only grains of white corn, and these grains of corn shone in his mouth. Instantly his features sagged and he no longer looked like a lord. They removed the rest of his teeth which shone like pearls in his mouth. And finally they cured Vucub-Caquix's eyes,

25 de Landa XXXI pp. 216 f

26 Fastlicht (b). Prof. Rehberg, of Leverkusen, remarked in a 1969 letter about these values: "1. The cited analysis is incomplete, because it is given in percentages without the total being 100 %. 2. The cited values do not even approximate a known cement. 3. The high levels of Ca and P appear more similar to those of bone-like hard tissue, or soluble Ca-salts were mixed with phospheric acid, which usually contains traces of Al, Fe and Mg. The 1.5 % Si are surely impurities, like the other trace elements; whether intended or accidental is unknown. I am not familiar with any reaction that could make a cement from this composition. Sigvald Linné, in 1950, in his study of traces of Aztec cements, came to the conclusion that "dental cement —at least that used in Sweden—has a very different composition." (Linné b)

27 Fastlicht (b)

28 Vucub Caquix is translated by Schultze (Jena) as "Sieben-(Seven-)Arara", a type of parrot that here (according to Prowe) may symbolize the rainbow. Popol Vuh (b) p. 19; Prowe

29 Popol Vuh (a) p. 93

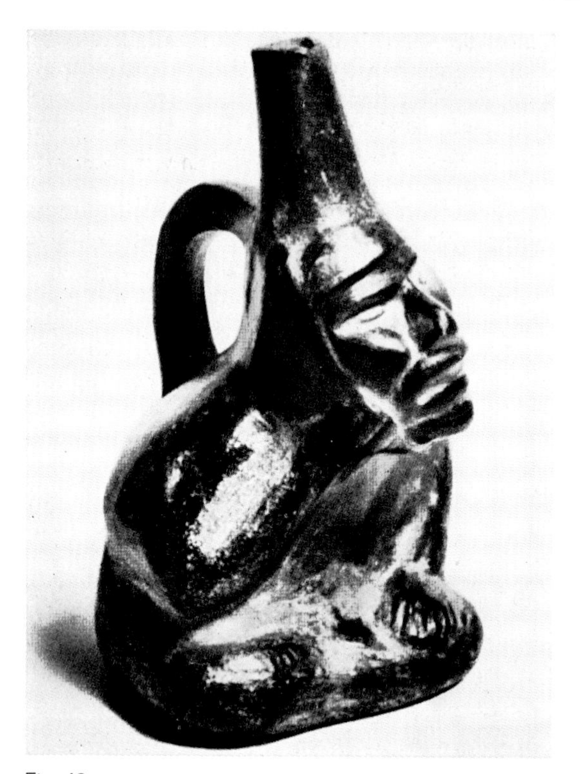

Fig. 48

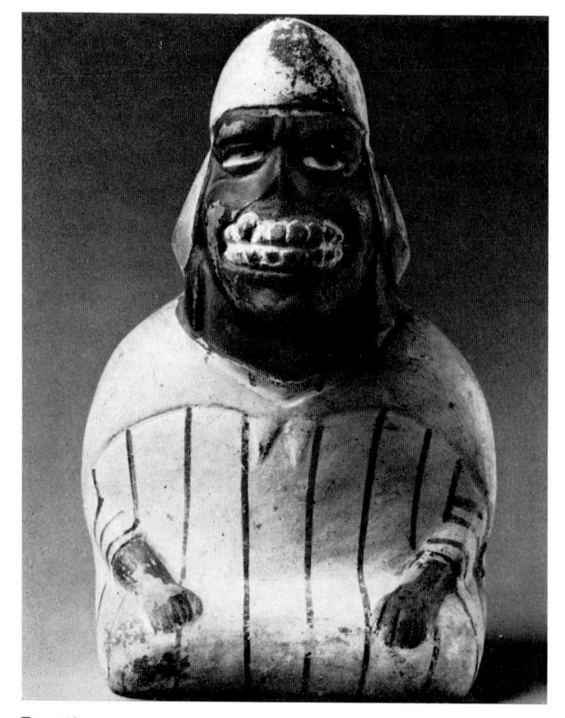

Fig. 49

Fig. 48 *Moche vessel showing a painful swelling of the cheek (from Wassermann-San Blas)*

Fig. 49 *Moche vessel showing a man with a nasolabial defect, presumably in consequence of leishmaniasis, syphilis, or lupus vulgaris; the canine is displaced to the outside (Museum für Völkerkunde, Berlin)*

piercing the pupils of his eyes, and they took his riches[30].
Vucub-Caquix died. The aged reset the youth's arm. Both had simply carried out the judgement of the celestial heart.
Several facts are obvious from this myth: The high value placed on teeth adorned with precious stones—their extraction caused death of Vucub-Caquix—and the reference to the tooth worm. Then there was the substitution of corn kernels for the teeth which reminds us of the Mesopotamian jaw phantom with emmer kernels[31]. Finally, the indication of tooth replacement by bone, which touched upon an ancient tradition, in the time of the conquistadors, fixed in a manuscript in the Quiché dialect.

The Inca

Similar to the Aztec, and also almost simultaneously (about 1430), the dynasty of the Inca began establishing their position on the South American continent in the southern Peruvian highlands. Their warriors descended on the domain of Pacific inhabitants, came under the yoke of the culturally superior Chimú population in northern Peru and pushed south to the center of Chile. Among the forebears of the Chimú, in the middle of the first millennium A. D., the Moche culture blossomed. Manifestations of this are the valuable artistic ceramic accomplishments of nowadays. Pitcher-like receptacles, which served as burial decorations often displayed the shape of a head. They also depicted entire episodes from the people's lives. Some of the representative types showed signs of illness, as for example, facial paralysis, buccal swelling (Fig. 48), cleft lip, and very often, lip and nose defects as complications of a mutilating disease (Fig. 49).
The kingdom of the Inca, which had existed since the middle of the 15th century, was conquered in 1523 by Francisco Pizarro with remarkable lack of consideration. Their culture stemmed from numerous earlier races. The state of the Inca was scientifically organized to the finest detail. The warriors carried bronze weapons. For documentation the Inca had only a knotted script for recording numbers. As all Indians, they did not use the wheel. Learned physicians existed among the Inca. They corresponded to some extent to the theorizing doctors of the European Middle Ages. There where socially lower but practically skilfull surgeons and herb collectors and also men of magic medicine[32]. Because illness was officially viewed as a consequence of sin, therapy involved confession to special priests. Here also, there was indication, as in earlier cultures, of the usual mixture of ritual, magic and rational measures in the practice of medicine. The rational involved the use of plant drugs predominantly. The Spanish conquerers made use of these.
The same held true for the stomatological field. One of the chroniclers, the Inca descendant Garcilaso de la Vega, relates that the rainbow is responsible for loose teeth and decay: *. . . and owing to the veneration they felt for it, when they saw it in the air, they shut their mouths, and put their hands over them, for they said that if they exposed their teeth it would decay and loosen them*[33], a custom that is still observed in Peru today. However, the tooth worm is not mentioned by the Inca. The burning out of carious processes was also reported. Dental treatment was done with picks of special wood as well as the pulverized bark of the quinaquina tree, the supplier of Peruvian balsam. These were also used to treat diseases of the gingiva. The resin of the guarango tree (Acacia macrantha) had a similar effect as had numerous other drugs.
Garcilaso reported on the cauterization of inflamed gingiva. A root was heated to glowing and splitted with the teeth, *and when it was very hot they pressed it on the teeth, putting one part on one side of the gums, and the other on the other, and left it there until it was cool.* At first the gingiva was like burned flesh. The patient couldn't eat, but after 3 to 4 days it was pink and healed. The chronicler attempted this himself *without necessity, but dropped it because I could not endure the burning of the heat roots*[34]. Treatment of toothache was accomplished primarily with locally applied plant drugs, possibly also with sulfur and arsenic-containing minerals[35]. The most effective pain killing substance was the leaf of the Coca bush. But this was considered holy, monopolized by the Inca and accessible only to the upper class.

[30] Ibid. (a) p. 98
[31] See p. 32
[32] Dietschy (b)
[33] Garcilasso (sic) III 21 (Vol. I p. 276). Gantzer (p. 53) translates from the Spanish original here ". . . wears them down and loosens them."
[34] Garcilasso II 25 (I p. 188)
[35] Gantzer p. 60

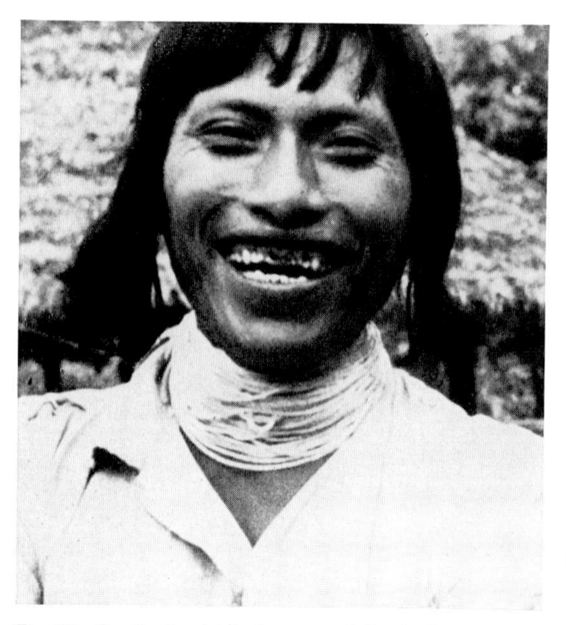

Fig. 50 *Teeth dyed black, in an Achual of the upper Amazon region (from Roggensack)*

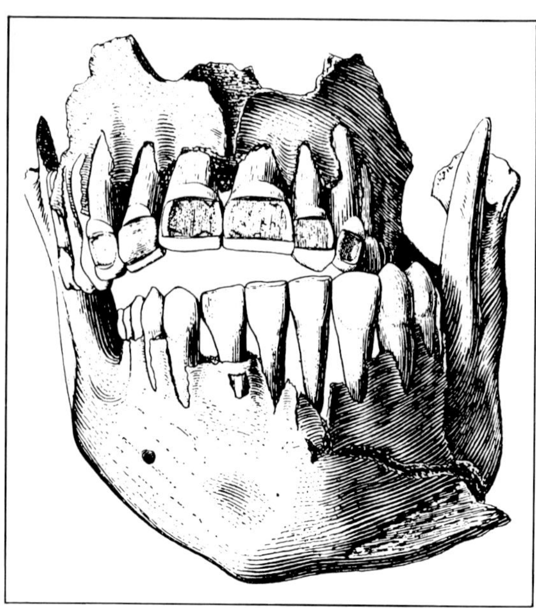

Fig. 52 *Right-angled gold inlays, of which only that of the right lateral incisor has been retained (from Saville)*

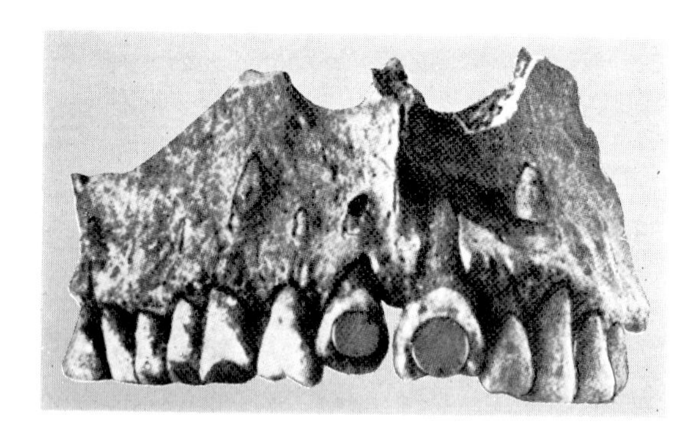

Fig. 51 *Alleged replanted and resected upper right central incisor with round gold inlay (from Saville)*

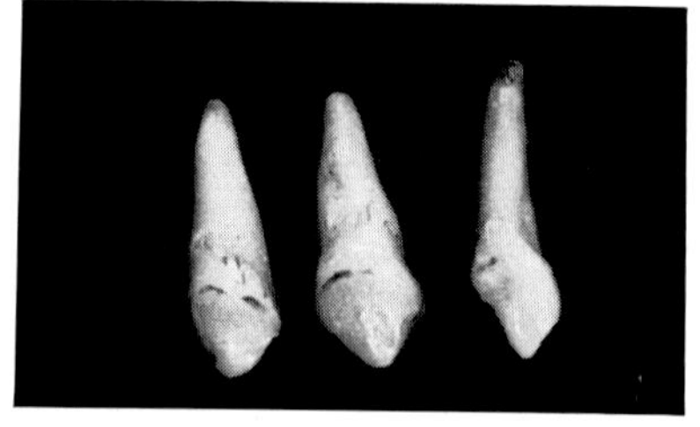

Fig. 53 *Mutilated incisors of the Ticuna of the upper Amazon region, extracted because of caries on the chiseled lateral surfaces (from Roggensack)*

Among the Chiribichi Indians settled in the northernmost Inca region of the Caribbean Sea, Venezuela today, the papal Protonotar Petrus Martyr Anglerius reported in the eighth decade, written before 1525, of his "De orbe novo" (On the New World) about a ritual using plant substances for caries prevention. This was based on the current reports of the time. During puberty, ages 10 to 12 years, the developing youths chewed tree leaves without eating or drinking until their teeth were as black as burned-out coal. The Spaniards, who loved white teeth, they called women and children. They retained their teeth for a lifetime. They never caused pain nor did they decay *(putrescunt unquam)*. The leaves are somewhat larger than those of the myrtle tree and soft as those of the terebinth

[36] Anglerius Octava decas, Caput VI.
a) pag. 109r
b) Tomus II pp. 416 f.
c) p. 686
d) p. 368

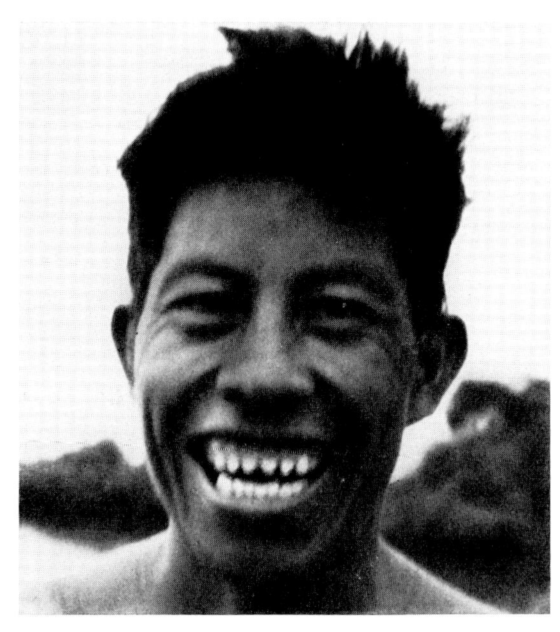

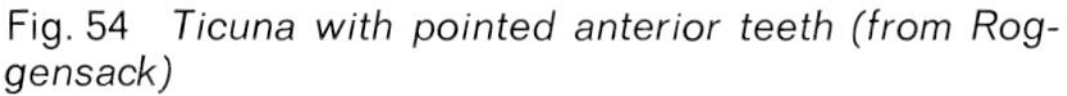

Fig. 54 *Ticuna with pointed anterior teeth (from Roggensack)*

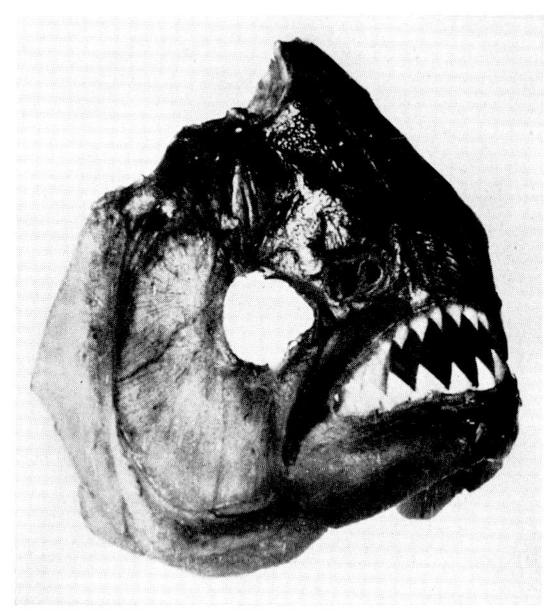

Fig. 55 *Piranha skull*

tree[36]. Moreover, the Dominican de la Casas, in Ecuador as a dentist, was of opinion that the men *chewed a specific type of herb all day long. And, although their teeth were generally very white, they became coated with a crust that was blacker than pitch*[37].

In 1960 Dobkowsky, who spent 10 years in Ecuador as a dentist, was of opinion that the Indians of the Amazon region pursued systematic caries prophylaxis using the berries of the Nashumbi bush and leaves of the Piyu tree, which is of the Rubiaceae: *The Indians chew the plants several times early in the morning while fasting and spit them out. For a short interval they do not partake of hot food or drink. The dentition looks like it is covered with a blackish veil that is darker at the cervical margin. The discoloration last 4 to 7 months and is then reapplied*[38]. Von Gall observed a similar purpose in the tooth coloring of the Aztec. But they never dyed their teeth black, only dark violet, as reported by Sahagún[39].

Similar to Dobkowsky the Berlin dentist Bruno Roggensack reported in 1969 of the Achual tribe of the upper Amazon region (Rio Pastaza): *It is a custom among the men to blacken their teeth with leaves from the Piu and Nashumbi bushes. The leaf is folded, held between the fingers, rubbed along the teeth and chewed vigorously.* The occlusal surface remains light, the crown of the tooth develops a black coating (Fig. 50). *The extent to which this custom contributed to the conservation of teeth cannot be determined without analysis. Probably it was the tabus* (eliminating sweets before and during the hunt) *and firmer foods that were responsible for the good condition of the men's teeth*[40].

According to a third contemporary report from Ecuador, the Uitoto Indians from the eastern part of the country blackened their teeth by chewing the leaves of the yanamuco bush. *The color fades in time and after a long interval during which they appear stippled, they seem whiter than before. These leaves obviously contain a substance against tooth decay (caries). Moreover, among several groups of Indians of East Ecuador between Rio Napo and Rio Cor-*

[37] Cited by Nordenskjöld p. 86
[38] Dobkowsky
[39] v. Gall p. 235 f.; Sahagún (c) p. 147
[40] Roggensack

rientes, the resin of a tree identified as a mulberry tree, Chlorophora tinctoria L. Gaud, is used to extract teeth painlessly[41].—Here also, the idea of loosening teeth through the use of caustic plant materials seemed to play an important part, as was described in the literature of the Middle Ages of the World.

Tooth extraction was mentioned by two chronologists without giving a description of the method[42]. In contrast Moodie insisted that the ancient Peruvians had no knowledge of operative dentistry. *Even the simplest curative effort, that of extraction seems never to have been thought of by them*[43]. It is difficult to make a decision in this respect. Possibly a technique that is still prevalent in the region today was used. After preparing the patient with chewing of coca leaves, a wooden spatula placed against the dental neck is struck a blow. This loosens the tooth enough so it can be removed[44].

The hypothesis of Saville (1913) of the implantation of a lateral incisor in the alveolus of a right central incisor, which was amplified by Weinberger (1948) with a apicectomy on the same tooth (Fig. 51), was disproved by Fastlicht. He assumed rightly that a foreign tooth of different shape was implanted in the jaw[45].

The Inca themselves did not ornament their teeth, but in Ecuador Marshall Henry Saville found round and rectangular inlays which are worthy of attention. They were probably the first gold inlays, although not for therapeutic use. Their first mention was by Kriegsmann and chronologist Pedro de Cieza de León who observed between 1540 and 1550 that in some Ecuadorian villages the caciques and chiefs fastened bits of gold to their teeth[46]. Possibly these corresponded to the gold ear pegs of an earlier group of Inca. It could have been a kind of privilege or distinction. Saville also referred to this relatively infrequent decoration.

Rectangular inlays adorn the anterior surfaces of the anterior teeth. A groove is recessed in the cutting edge and the gingival margin. The enamel layer is carefully removed (Fig. 52). A single inlay in situ also encloses the lateral surfaces of the teeth. Questionable remnants of cement were found in the empty cavities. As communicated by F. J. Dockstader, Director of the Museum of the American Indians in New York to Gantzer, the object obviously consisted of cold hammered gold[47]. The surface of the inlays is polished.

Tooth truncation was not prevalent in pre-Columbian South America. Von Ihering believed that this custom was imported with the first Negro slaves from Africa. In 1969, however, Roggensack observed such artifacts among a race of Ticuna in the vicinity of Leticia in the laguna region of the Amazon River. *They still file their teeth, in part, even today . . . In the 8th or 9th year of life this procedure was considered a ritual. The medial and distal edges were broken off by hitting a machete placed against the tooth with a stone. The edges were then polished with pieces of wood and wet sand. Combined with earlier nutrition this was practiced without detriment. I use teeth that I have extracted for comparison*[48] (Fig. 53). Not to be overlooked is the similarity between this type of anterior tooth truncation and the dentition of the feared, rapacious local fish, the piranha (Fig. 54 and 55).

The knocking out of entire teeth observed by the Patagonians is a type of tooth truncation, according to von Ihering. Others saw these practices, also observed in Africa and Australia, as a type of offering or a painful test of courage for youths[49].

In conclusion, it can be observed that the Indians as early as the first millennium A.D. knew how to insert inlays, that they may even have used some type of cement, that the Maya seemed to possess a plastic filling material which has lasted for hundreds of years, but that this knowledge never was used for therapeutic purposes. The successful healing measures of the herb physicians deserve special attention without a doubt. With the exception of the coca leaf, accepted by the occidental pharmacy, the entire pre-Columbian knowledge of the New World has remained without significance toward the development of dentistry. This is unfortunate with reference to several plant drugs.

[41] Written communication from Dr. Günther Hartmann, Museum für Völkerkunde, Berlin, dated June 1, 1972.
[42] Gantzer p. 62 f.
[43] Moodie (b)
[44] Iwaki, quoted by Gantzer
[45] Saville: Weinberger (b) p. 178; Fastlicht (b); (d) pp. 39 f.
[46] Cieza de Leon p. 196
[47] Gantzer p. 77
[48] Written communication, Roggensack, Jan. 8, 1970
[49] v. Ihering; Lasch

The author thanks the late Prof. Dr. Gerdt Kutscher and Dr. Anneliese Mönnich of the Ibero-American Institute in Berlin for reviewing and correcting the manuscript and for referring him to the Popol-Vuh text.

References

Agrinier, Pierre
Nuevos casos de mutilaciones dentarias procedentes de Chiapas, México. An. Inst. Nac. Antrop. Hist., México 15 (1962) 229—243

Anglerius, Petrus Martyr
De orbe novo.
a) Alcalá 1530
b) Ed. Joachim Torres Assensio, Tomi 2. Matriti 1892
c) Trad. Paul Gaffarel, Paris 1907
d) Transl. Francis Augustus Mac Nutt, New York. London 1912

Busch, Herbert
Die Zahnheilkunde innerhalb der aztekischen Medizin, Med. Diss. Düsseldorf 1966

Cieza de León, Pedro de
La Crónica de Perú. Madrid 1922

Cruz, Martinus de la
Libellus de medicinalibus Indorum herbis, . . . 1552. Trad. Johannes Badianus. Reprint Mexico 1964 (Ed. Inst. Mex. del Seguro social)

Dietschy, Hans
a) Aztekische Ärzte und Zauberer. Ciba-Zschr. 4 (1937) 1448 — 1456 (Basel)
b) Die Heilkunde im alten Peru. Ciba-Zschr. 7 (1957) 2746—2776 (Wehr)

Dobkowsky, Teodoro
Kariesprophylaxe im Urwald. Dtsch. Stomat. 11 (1961) 50—54

Emmart, Emily Walcott
Concerning the Badianus manuscript, . . . Smithsonian Misc. Coll. 94, Nr. 2, Washington 1935

Fastlicht, Samuel
a) Tooth mutilations in pre-columbian Mexico. J. Am. Dent. Ass. 36 (1948) 315—323
b) Dental inlays and fillings among ancient Mayas. J. Hist. Med. 17 (1962) 393—401
c) Incrustaciones dentarias entre los mayas. Recientes hallazgos. Rev. As. dental mexicana 20 (1963) 609—625
d) Tooth mutilations and dentistry in Pre-Columbian Mexico. Berlin 1976

Gall, August Freiherr von
Medizinische Bücher (tici-amatl) der alten Azteken aus der ersten Zeit der Conquista. Quellen und Studien Gesch. Naturw. Technik 7 (1940) 81—260

Gantzer, Joachim
Die präkolumbischen Kulturen des Inkareichs aus der Sicht der Zahn-, Mund- und Kieferheilkunde. Med. Diss. Düsseldorf 1969

Garcilasso de la Vega
First part of the Royal Commentaries of the Yncas. Transl. and ed. Clements R. Markham Vol. I, London 1871

Ihering, Hermann von
Die künstliche Deformierung der Zähne. Zschr. Ethnol. 14 (1882) 213—262

Kutscher, Gerdt
Chimu, eine altindianische Hochkultur. Berlin 1950

Landa, Diego de
Relation des choses de Yucatan. Paris 1928

Lasch, Richard
Die Verstümmelung der Zähne in Amerika. Mitt. Anthropol. Ges., Wien 31 (1901) 13—22

Linné. S(igvald)
a) Dental decoration in aboriginal America. Ethnos 5 (1950) 2—28
b) Dental decoration in ancient Mexico. II Ethnos 15 (1950) 166—173

López, Alonso Sergio
Cinco craneos procedentes de Tanquian, S.L.P. An. Inst. Nac. Antrop. Hist., Mexico 17 (1964) 181—197

Moodie, Roy L.
a) Studies in paleodontology. I. Materials for a study of prehistoric dentistry in Peru. J. amer. dent. Ass. 15 (1928) 1826 — 1850
b) Studies in paleopathology. XXIII. Surgery in pre-columbian Peru. Ann. med. Hist. New series 1 (1929) 698—728 (p. 723)

Nordenskiöld, Erland
The changes in the material culture of two indian tribes under the influence of new surroundings. Göteborg 1920. P. 85—91

Popol Vuh, the sacred book of the ancient Quiché Maya
a) English version by Delia Goetz, Sylvanus G. Morley from the transl. of Adrián Recinos. Oklahoma 1950
b) Transl. and ed. by Leonhard Schultze Jena, Quellenwerke zur alten Geschichte Amerikas, Vol. II. Stuttgart, Berlin 1944

Prowe, Hermann
Altindische Medizin der Quiché. Zschr. Ethnol. 32 (1900) 352—354

Rippen, Bene van
Pre-Columbian operative dentistry of the indians of middle and south america: . . . Dental Cosmos 59 (1917) 861—873

Roggensack, Bruno
Zivilisation und Gebißverfall am oberen Amazonas. Zahnärztl. Mitt. 60 (1970) 21—25. — Personal communications

Romero, Javier
a) El arte de las mutilaciones dentarias. Mexico 1951
b) Mutilaciones dentarias . . . Mexico 1958
c) Recientes adiciones a la colección de dientes mutilados. An. Inst. Nac. Antrop. Hist., Mexico 17 (1964) 199—256

Romero, Javier, Samuel Fastlicht
El arte de las mutilaciones dentarias. Enc. Mex. de Arte 14, Mexico 1951

Rubín de la Borbolla, Daniel F .
Types of tooth mutilations found in Mexico. Am. J. Phys. Anthrop. 26 (1940) 349—362

Ruiz de Alarcón, Hernando
Tratado de la supersticiones y costumbres gentilicas . . . Anales del Museo Nacional, vol. VI, pp. 123—223, México 1892

Sahagún. Bernardino de
a) Histoire générale des choses de la Nouvelle-Espagne. Trad. D. Jourdanet-Rémi; Siméon, Paris 1880
b) Gliederung des alt-aztekischen Volkes in Familie, Stand und Beruf. Aus d. Aztekischen übers. Leonhard Schultze Jena. Quellenwerke zur alten Geschichte Amerikas. Vol. V. Stuttgart 1952
c) Florentine Codex, Book 10, transl. Charles E. Dibble; Arthur J. O. Anderson. Utah 1961

Saville, Marshall H(oward)
a) Archaeological researches on the coast of Esmeraldas, Ecuador Verh. 16. Internat. Amerikanisten-Kongr. II. Wien 1908
b) Pre-columbian decoration of the teeth in Ecuador . . . Am. Anthropol. 15 (1913) 377—394

Serna, Jacinto de la
Manual de ministros de Indios. In: Anales del Museo Nacional vol. VI, pp. 261—275

Wassermann-San Blas, B. J.
Cerámicas del antiguo Perú . . . Buenos Aires 1938

Weinberger, Bernhard Wolf
a) Ancient dentistry in the old and the new world. Ann. med. Hist. 6 (1934) 264—279
b) An introduction to the history of dentistry. Vol. I, pp. 165—192, St. Louis 1948

Chapter 5

Greco-Roman Medicine

The Greek Region

The quite highly developed Indian and Chinese medicine had no perceptible influence on occidental medicine. In contrast, extensions of the ancient Egyptian and Assyrian cultures were incorporated significantly in the neighboring Greek cultural circles. Here, from the region settled by the Hellenic people, lie the significant foundations upon which the structure for today's medicine was built.

The Greek people became known during the great migrations of the Indo-Germanic races who invaded the southern portion of the Balkan peninsula from 2,000 to 700 B. C. in several waves. They came in contact here with Cretic culture in a disruptive and acquisitiving fashion. Propagation across the Aegean islands followed to the coast of Asia Minor and further to the shores of the Black Sea and in a western direction toward Sicily and southern Italy and the coasts of Spain and France. This resulted a contact with the ancient cultures of Egypt, Babylon and Phoenicia and acceptance of the medical experience of these peoples.

The motherland, cleft by numerous mountains, was settled in just as many city states. Of these, usually one maintained control. After the triumphant repulsion of the Persian invasions, Athens and Sparta became temporarily allied. This was followed in the fifth century by the classical period of Greek tragedies, building and sculptur skills in Athens. Simultaneously in the Ionic island region, Hippocrates developed the first scientific medicine of Europe.

This highpoint of ancient medicine was preceded in the sixth century by a separation from the old belief in gods and miracles developed with the introduction of pre-Socratic philosophy. Greek medicine was also a magic-religious priest medicine in ancient times. It included many healing gods. Gradually the original Thessalonian earth god, Asclepios, was chosen. He was venerated in special cult places, for instance in Epidauros. The sick made pilgrimages with offerings to Asclepios. He sought healing during sleep from the hand of the god represented by priests (Fig. 56), or through dream interpretation, a mixture of medicine and magic as was characteristic of the early medicine of almost all cultures. This still holds true for nature people even today. Greek temple medicine had maintained itself—*The miracle is the most beloved child of faith*—with the development of real medicine running a parallel course until late antiquity. It attained a position comparable to today's pilgrimage places of such as Lourdes. True medicine started even in the time of Homer (about 900) to remove magic trappings and to learn therapeutic procedures from experience. Its pinnacle was the appearance of the "Father of Medicine" Hippocrates (Fig. 57) who conducted a school for physicians on the coast of Asia Minor on the island of Cos. Here he taught a rational medicine based on accumulated knowledge. Thus, he completed the separation of Greek medicine from the magic-religious realm, but he recognized godliness as the guiding principle.

From this school originated essentially the "Corpus Hippocraticum", a collection of medical writings of which several were certainly authored by the master himself. Most represent the work of contemporary scholars and associates and additions of later centuries. All the texts from the fifth and following centuries B. C. have a singular physiological and pathological basis. In the "Hippocratic oath", also probably the product of a later spiritual direction, the ethical duties of the physician were fixed in an exemplary manner: Obedience and loyalty to the teacher and his followers, forbidding euthanasia and abortion, prescribing proper behavior when visiting the sick, and the professional discretion.

When a disease was examined, not only symptoms were registered. The etiology was explored and as a result, the prognosis and therapy were based on the sum of this knowledge and experience. The pathophysiological framework was based on the study of juices of the body (Latin: humores) on which life depends. Among these humors gradually prevailed the following four: blood, phlegm, yellow and black bile which possess the four qualities: hot and moist, cold and moist, hot and dry, cold and dry. They cor-

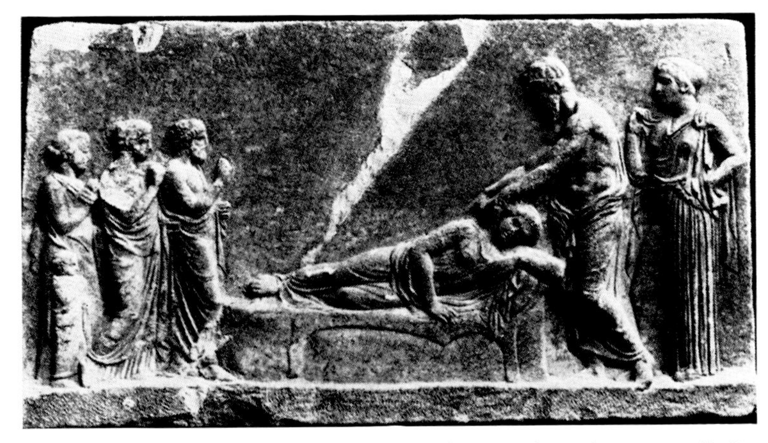

Fig. 56 *Asclepios healing a sleeper in the temple, 4th century B. C. (Relief in National Museum, Athens)*

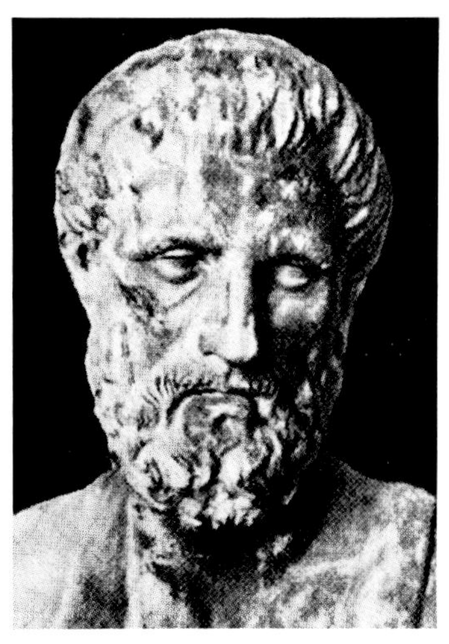

Fig. 57 *Bust of Hippocrates (?), found in Odeion of Cos in 1929, dated to 4th century B. C. (Museum of Cos)*

respond to the four cardinal elements: air, water, fire and earth, of which—according to earlier teachings of the natural philosopher and physician in the 5th century B. C., Empedocles—all material substances in the world are composed. The level of health depends in the physiologic concept of the Hippocratic physicians on the right or wrong mixture (eucrasia or dyscrasia) of these four humors. This "Humoral Pathology"—ascribed essentially to Hippocrates' son-in-law Polybos—governed theoretical medicine until the middle of the 19th century, when in 1858 the great pathologist of Berlin, Rudolf Virchow, published his revolutionizing "Cellular Pathology." This work established a complete new conception of the causes of health and disease by placing the cell into the center of all physiological and pathological circumstances. But remnants of the old ideas of humoralism still exist even today.

Stomatological problems were not collected in special chapters as in Indian literature. Instead they were discussed as ancillaries of other disease pictures. Within a disease history of the 4th book on epidemic diseases, we discover that the Greeks had a tooth numbering system which in principle corresponded to ours. The complete text follows:

In the boy with painful mouth erosion, the lower teeth loosened first, then the maxillary anteriors. They leaved left in the bone.

Among those who lose bits of bone from the palate, the nose sinks in the middle. If the anterior teeth fall out, the nose flattens.

The 5th tooth, counting from the anterior teeth, had 4 roots paired in combination. Their tips were bowed inward as are those of both adjacent teeth. Abcesses occured more frequently on the 3rd tooth than on any of the others. The thick nasal discharge and the pain experienced during sleep are primarily caused by this tooth. It was decayed, but more often the 5th. This had a cusp in the center of the crown and 2 towards the anterior. The small first cusp inward from the other two was decayed. The 7th tooth had a single, thick pointed root[1].

From this report on ulcerous stomatitis, probably even noma, considering the special and consequent manifestations in general, we assume that the Hippocratic method of tooth numbering started with the lateral incisor. The central, known as "the anterior" (ἐυπρόσθιοι euprósthioi), was not included in the numbering. The 5th tooth men-

[1] Hippocrates Epidemics IV 19. 5, 156, 4—15 Littré

tioned is thus the first upper molar, although the root description fits that of the mandibular. The 3rd tooth, that is the first upper premolar, had apparently infected the maxillary sinus (unknown at that time). This caused the thick nasal discharge. The upper third molar, usually designated here as the 7th (ἕβδομος, hébdomos) had only one root in this instance. In another part of the text, the third molars had the name of teeth which impart wisdom (ὀδόντες σωφρονιστῆρες, odóntes sophronistéres)[2]. Our designation of wisdom tooth derives from this. The development of teeth, which seemed to occur later than that of other bones, as was always mentioned in ancient literature, was reported in the book on flesh: *Growth arises from the bones of the head and both jaws. The colloids and fats found there are dried and burned by heat and the teeth that originate in this manner are harder than the other bones because they are not exposed to cold. Teeth grow in the child, the first are nourished in the mother's body, after birth by the mother's milk, and when these have been lost, by food and drink. Teeth originating with the first nourishment fall out when the child is 7 years old, in some even earlier ... I have said ... that of all bones, only those of the jaw contain veins. This causes more nourishment to be drawn to the jaw than to the other bones.* From this it can be concluded that Hippocratics were aware of the entrance of vessel-nerve bundles into the mandible at the mandibular foramen, even of the outlet at the infraorbital foramen of the maxilla. *And that they take up more nourishment and have a richer supply of blood, they are able to grow more strongly as long as the person grows generally. They have reached their full growth when signs of maturity appear. These appear between 7 and 14 and during this period the largest teeth grow. ... In the 4th hebdomad*[3] *most persons get 2 teeth, the so-called wisdom teeth*[4]. From other writings in the Corpus Hippocraticum with its preference for the number 7, we recognize remains, perhaps of Babylonian origin, number magic which also in a proper scheme of development are reminiscent of ancient China[5].

One single book has the title "Tooth Eruption". But in sparse sentences it communicates far more than the actual experiences on tooth eruption of the newborn: *Those who while teething have their bowels moved are less subject to convulsion than those who have them moved seldom.—Those who while teething are attacked by acute fever seldom suffer from convulsions.—Those who while teething are lethargic while remaining well-nourished run a risk of being seized with convulsions.—Those who are teething in winter, other things being equal, fare better.—Not all children die who are seized with convulsions while teething; many recover.—Teething is protracted when complicated by a cough, and emaciation in such cases is excessive while teeth are coming through.—Children who have troublesome time while teething, if they are suitably attended to, bear up more easily against teething*[6].

Folklore seems responsible for the following saying: *Those who live long have more teeth*[7].—Irregular teeth and pointed palates were mentioned in connection with a malformation syndrome: *Among those with pointed heads, some have a straight neck, are strong in other parts as well as in the bones. Others suffer headache and ear discharge, have a hollow palate and irregular tooth development*[8]. As shown in the last sentence of the following text, the pathology of dental and oral diseases was only partially incorporated in the humoral teachings: *When it comes to toothache, if* (the tooth) *is decayed and mobile, extract it. But, if it is not decayed and mobile and still aches, it must be dried out through cauterizing. Chewing materials are also useful. Pain results where mucus accumulates under the tooth root. The mucus disrupts and decays the teeth in part, as does food, when they are naturally weak, hollow and poorly fastened in the gingiva*[9].

Caries etiology was for the first time ascribed to two endogenous factors, disposition and mucous, and nutrition as the exogenous factor, instead of the toothworm. The various types of pulpitis are not yet differentiated. They were included in periodontal pathology as toothache. Therapy is purely local, that is, it does not include total care which is unhippocratic, probably of the school of Cnidos. For loose teeth it consisted of extraction; for fixed teeth it was cauterization to dry out the mucus. From this it can be concluded that the pulp was still unknown. Extraction of loose teeth had no high place in Hippo-

[2] Ibid. Flesh 13. 8, 602, 11 Li.
[3] Period of seven years
[4] Ibid. Flesh 12—13. 8, 593, 5—602, 11 Li.; Deichgräber pp. 45 f.
[5] See p. 42
[6] Hippocrates Dentition 6—12. 8, 544, 11—24 Li. Transl. II pp. 323 f.
[7] Ibid. Epidemics II 6, 1. 5, 132, 16 Li.
[8] Ibid. Epidemics VI 1, 2. 5, 266, 7—9 Li.
[9] Ibid. Affections 4. 6, 212, 18—24 Li.

cratic surgery. In the book of physicians there is a description of the procedure. It is considered superfluous *as the instruments for tooth extraction and the pincer pliers can be handled by an associate. Their use seems very simple*[10].

General and local therapy were usually combined for gingivitis: *Melesandros had overgrown gingiva, very painful and swollen. One gave him bleeding of the lower arm; Egyptian alum at the height of the suffering brought relief*[11]. This customary Hippocratic derivation of pathogenic humors, which according to their concept involved bleeding and purging, influenced therapy more than over two thousand years and not always positively.

In the book dealing with women's diseases, the thoroughly indicated animal charcoal was recommended as the "Indian" remedy, but in such a way that is vividly reminiscent of the later junk apothecary: *When a woman has bad breath and the gingiva is dark, having an unhealthy appearance, burn the head of a hare and 3 mice, each by itself—we remove the contents of the body cavity of the mice, except for the liver and kidneys—, pulverize marble or white stone in a stone mortar and sieve it*[12].

Teeth and gingiva were to be rubbed with this and other mixtures. Combined with this was a general fasting measure with occasional enjoyment of very nourishing food.—In 2 instances of noma, as can be predicted, neither excision of the deteriorated tissue nor the administration of purgatives could stay the advent of death[13].

The following sentence from the book of prognoses would still be appropriate for any textbook on dentistry of our days: *Persons who have chronic alteration on the tongue's margin should be examined for a sharp tooth*[14].

Serous inflammations of the mouth were brought to a head with warm applications. Then the spontaneous expulsion of pus was expected, as for example, with a palatal abscess[15]. Sometimes the area was lanced, as for an abscess at the floor of the mouth[16]. Hippocrates' followers considered pus a decayed humor, here actually the mucus which is normally found in the cranial cavity and flows down through the holes in the base of the skull in some diseases.

An odontogenic osteomyelitis resulted in necrosis of the mandible: *The boy of Metrodoros had gangrene of the mandible after toothache; in addition, the gums were hypoplastic with a little suppuration. The grinders fell out and later the mandible*[17].

Jaw luxation and fracture are described in the book on joints[18] with a clarity and minuteness of detail not elsewhere encountered. The anatomy of the jaw joints is clearly described, as is the attachment of the masticatory muscles and the relationship of the movable mandible to the fixed maxilla. Interesting is the observation that *this joint by its contraction gives the first indication of cramps and rigid cramps.* This is obviously a reference to jaw cramps (trismus) as an early symptom of tetanus. The fact that the symptoms of tetanus at that time were known results from the disease history of Skamandros of Larissa. He suffered from the typical clinical signs of a hardened jaw. He died on the 8th day during a cramp[19].

When repositioning the dislocated lower jaw, it is best to place the patient on his back with the head supported by a leather cushion, or: *someone should hold the patient's head while the operator grasping the jaw with his fingers inside and out near the chin*[20]. This is as it appears in the Nicetas codex of Apollonios of Citium[21] (about 100 B. C.) surely resting on an antique (3rd century B. C.) source written in Byzantium before 1000 A. D. (Fig. 58). The actual intervention proceeded while the patient relaxed, by correcting the lateral displacement and applying pressure from the back; the treatment was concluded with a light fixation band.

The procedure for double luxation without lateral displacement, as has been clearly established, was similar. If the adjustment fails, life becomes endangered through fever and a killing sleep. These patients then die about the 10th day[22]. This unusual prognosis, accepted by the Arabs and passed on through scholastic medicine will be met at the start of modern times through the words of Ambroise Paré[23].

In the description of fractures of the mandible to be found, for example, on boxers in the

10 Ibid. Physician 9, 216, 1—3 Li.
11 Ibid. Epidemics VII 66. 5, 430, 8—12 Li.
12 Ibid. Diseases of women II 185. 8, 366, 6—10 Li.
13 Ibid. Epidemics V 4. 5, 204, 20—206, 6 Li.
14 Ibid. Prognostic II 11. 9, 32, 12—14 Li.
15 Ibid. Diseases II 32. 7, 48, 20—49, 3 Li.
16 Ibid. Diseases II 31. 7, 48, 17 Li.
17 Ibid. Epid. VII 113. V 460, 21—462, 2 Li.
18 Ibid. Joints 30—34. 4, 140, 5—158, 3 Li.
19 Ibid. Epidemics V 15. 5, 214, 7—19 Li.
20 Ibid. Joints 30. 4, 144, 7—9 Li.; Transl. III. p. 253
21 Apollonios pp. 5 f.
22 Hippocrates Joints 31. 4, 146, 10 Li.; Transl. p. 257
23 See pp. 100 and 149

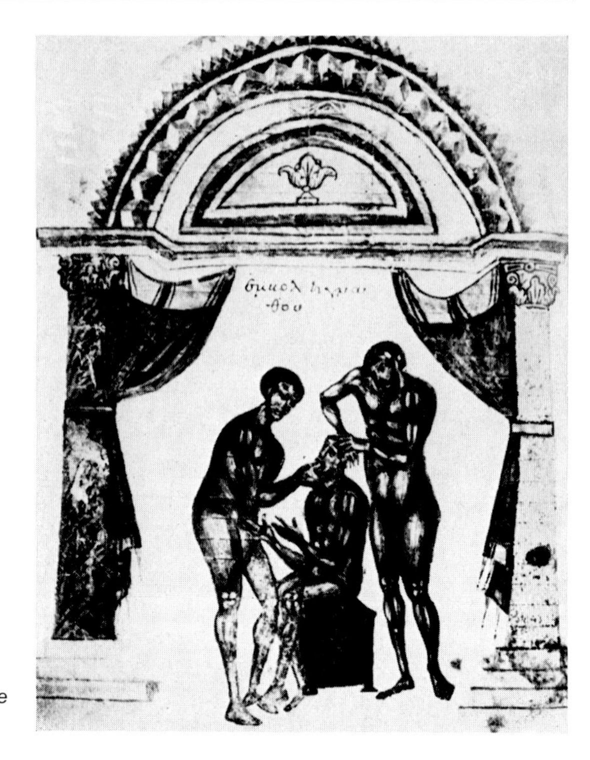

Fig. 58 *Reduction of mandibular luxation, from the Nicetas Codex of Apollonios of Citium*

palestra, frequent distinctions were made between partial and complete fractures. Therapy in both instances consisted of manual repositioning, *by making suitable lateral pressure with the fingers on the tongue side, and counter-pressure from without. If the teeth at the point of injury are displaced or loosened, fasten them to one another, when the bone is adjusted, not merely the two, but several, preferably with a gold wire, but failing that, with thread, till consolidation takes place*[24].

This is followed by loose bandaging with wax plaster or linen bindings, from which the author rightly expects little, and he returns to the discussion of repositioning: *One should make frequent palpation on the tongue side, and hold the distorted part of the bone adjusted with the fingers for a long time. It would be best if one* could do so throughout; but that is impossible[25].

From this it is obvious that the wire ligature mentioned is not a splint in the same sense of our wire splint binding. Actually it is a fixation for loosened teeth which also served to fix the fracture according to the description of the interrupted continuity: *After adjustment you should fasten the teeth together as was described above, for this will contribute greatly to immobility, especially if one joins them up properly and fastens off the ends as they should be ... Next, one should take Carthagian leather; if the patient is very young, the outer layer is sufficient, but if he is an adult, use the skin itself. Cut a 3-finger breadth, or as much as may be suitable and, anointing the jaw with gum—for it is more agreeable than glue—fasten the end of the leather to the broken-off part of the jaw at a finger's breadth or rather more from the fracture. This is for the lower part. Let the strap have a slit in the line of the chin, to include the chin tip. Another strap, similar or a little broader, the same interval from the fracture as the former, let it also be split to go around the ear*[26].

The author of this book, which is among the oldest material of the Corpus Hippocraticum,

[24] Ibid. Joints 32. 4, 146, 14—19 Li.; Transl. pp. 257 f.
[25] Ibid. Joints 32. 4, 148, 4—7 Li.; Transl. p. 259
[26] Ibid. Joints 33. 4, 148, 10—13 Li.; Transl. pp. 259 f.

had the right approach to treatment of a fractured mandible. Unfortunately, he didn't understand it completely and did not develop the method consequently. That remained for the 19th century.
Still valid today is the Hippocratic critique of conventional bandaging of jaw fractures as they are applied by some physicians who lack insight: *But any bandaging of a jaw fractured in this way tends to turn the fragments inward at the lesion rather than bringing them to their natural position*[27].
In describing a fracture at the center of the chin, the author introduces the anatomic error to the literature, that a connecting point, a symphysis, is found here, as he had observed in lower animals. He transferred this to man by analogy: *When the lower jaw is torn apart at the symphysis which is at the chin . . .*[28]. Human dissections were not performed by Hippocratic physicians. This error was copied in good faith without examining its basis, with the exception of Celsus, by one author from another. The Arabs copied from the Greeks, the physicians of the Middle Ages from these, until 1543 when the great anatomist Andreas Vesalius brought it to an end[29].
Nonetheless, the excerpts from the book on joints were superior to anything previously written on the subject of fractures and luxations of the jaw. They are also the highpoints of Hippocratic medicine's contribution to the field of stomatology. The therapy of dental diseases per se appears, as it reads in one of the texts, to be a question of practice that requires no written description.
After the battle of Chaironia in 338 B. C., the Greeks were required to submit to the hegemony of Macedonia, whose young king Alexander started his reign 2 years later. The great Aristotle had introduced him to science. Aristotle, beginning as student of Plato, had gradually turned to empirical thinking. Natural science was given a first rank in his teaching system.
His extensive writings on the animal kingdom contained references to comparative anatomy and physiology as well as numerous odontological notes. He introduced the world to the error that males among humans, sheep, goats and pigs have more teeth than females. And another one, that humans with supernumerary teeth live longer, he adopted from Hippocrates[30].
The 4 incisors are called "the anteriors" (πρόστιοι próstioi), the "canines" (κυνόδους kynódous) as still called in some areas today, premolars and molars were identified as peg teeth and for the wisdom teeth which erupted at age 20 he used the name "finisher" (κραντῆρες krantéres). *Instances have been known of women whose wisdom teeth have erupted at the age of eighty or more, at the very extremity of life, causing much pain in so doing. The same has occured in men also. This occurs in persons whose wisdom teeth have not erupted in youth*[31].
Aristotle was aware of the blood supply of the teeth: *Of the remaining blood vessels which divide off from the one just mentioned, some encircle the head, others find their terminus in the sense organs and the teeth in extremely fine blood vessels*[32].
He was also the first to describe the alveoli: *In the jaws are the teeth, which consist of bone and are partly perforated, partly not. This is the only bone which resists the carving too*[33].
In contrast, he erred in his statement that the teeth were the only bones to grow for a lifetime. He believed the reason to be that they *take an oblique direction and fail to come into contact with each other*[34]. Aristotle seems to have been led astray by the fact that vital teeth without antagonists grow out of the alveoli[35]. In the book, "On the Members of the Creatures," we find the remark that the human dentition has a median position between tame and wild animals, or as we would formulate it, between herbivores and carnivores. The significance of teeth in speech and among animals for grasping and defense were understood clearly[36].
Aristotle made no therapeutic recommendations. However, the "Mechanics," which employs his name, refers to tooth forceps of iron (ὀδόντάγρα odontágra) as an instrument of the physician: *Why can physicians pull teeth more effectively using tooth forceps than with the fingers alone? Possibly because the teeth slip out of the fingers more easily than from tooth forceps? Or, doesn't the iron slide out more readily*

[27] Ibid. Joints 33. 4, 154, 9—11 Li.
[28] Ibid. Joints 34. 4, 154, 12—158, 3 Li.; Transl. III p. 263
[29] See p. 137
[30] Aristotle Hist. an. II 3 p. 501 b 19—21; 501 a, 22 f. See p. 62
[31] Ibid. Hist. an. II 4 p. 501 b, 3—29
[32] Ibid. III 3 p. 514 a, 21—23
[33] Ibid. III 7 p. 516 a, 25—27
[34] Ibid. Gen. an. II 6 p. 745 a, 25 f.
[35] Ibid. p. 745 b, 5 f.
[36] Ibid. Part. an. III 1 p. 661 b, 6—15

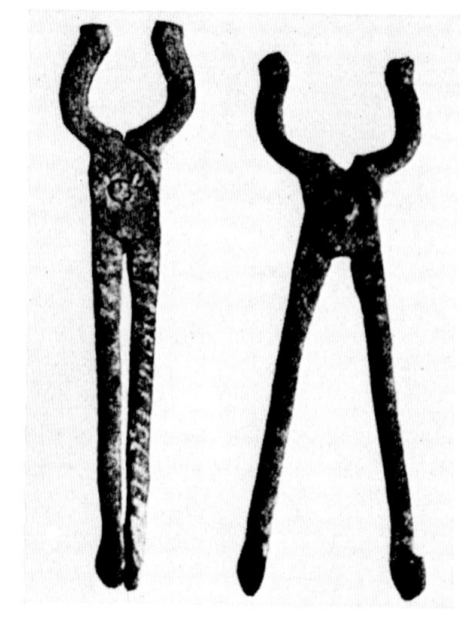

Fig. 59 *Tooth forceps, full size (National Museum, Athens; from Sudhoff)*

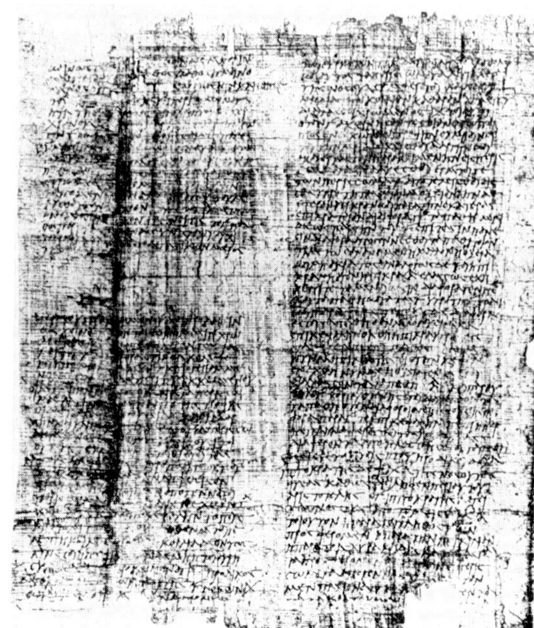

Fig. 60 *"Anonymus Londinensis" papyrus*

than the fingers and encircle the tooth? The flesh of the finger is soft. The forceps hold more strongly and cling better. Moreover, the 2 levers of the tooth forceps oppose each other and find their meaningful point of support in the lock of the forceps. Thus, the instrument is used for extraction because it mobilizes (the tooth) *more easily . . . Once he* (the physician) *has loosened it, he can remove it more easily with his hand than with the instrument*[37].

A representative history of tooth extraction was related later by Erasistratos, one of the great men in the school of Alexandria in the 3rd century B. C. The Roman physician Caelius Aurelianus[38] in 500 A. D. reported the fact that tooth forceps of lead were displayed in the Apollo temple at Delphi. Erasistratos indicated that as a rule only such teeth should be extracted as can be removed with an instrument made of this pliable material. This is a sign that Greek doctors did not take tooth extraction as lightly as we were led to believe by the Hippocratic writings. The forceps, 64 mm long, shown in the photograph, are from the Athens Archeological Museum and could hardly be used to remove a normal molar (Fig. 59). In addition to the actual tooth forceps, the "odontagra," the Greeks had special root forceps, "rizagra", as reported by the Roman Celsus in 100 A. D.[39] Further anatomic-physiologic references to the dental system are found in "Anonymus Londinensis," a fragment which in part is founded on a textbook by Menon (Fig. 60), a student of Aristotle. Although this idea probably did not originate with Menon, we find the first reference to today's tooth designation based on function: *This* (the nutriment), *when taken, undergoes a first stage of digestion in the mouth, being cut up by the front teeth* (τομείς tomeis), *called incisors and ground by the molars* (μύλαι mylai = millstones, molars)[40].

Diocles of Carystos had the honor of being considered another Hippocrates in Attica about 300. He touched upon the problems of actual tooth treatment. In his hygienic specifications is found the recommendation that after early rising the teeth should be cleaned with the fingers and the juice of pulverized mint. In 200 A. D., that is 500 years later, Galen quoted a prescription by Diocles for toothache: *gum*

[37] Ibid. 21 p. 854 a, 16—31; see Grundmann p. 18
[38] Caelius Aurelianus Chron. II 4, 84
[39] Celsus VII 12 1 F
[40] Anonymus Londinensis XXIV 20—24; Transl. p. 93

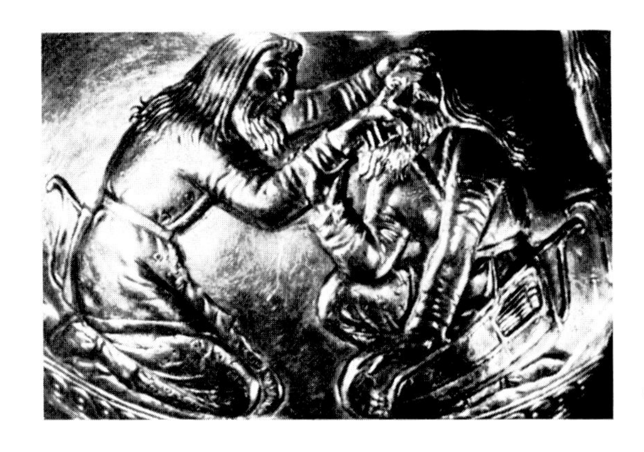

Fig. 61 *Oral treatment by a Scythian warrior, depicted on a metal vase relief found in the Crimea. 4th century B. C. (from Artamonov)*

resin, opium, pepper, wax, lousewort, Cnidic grains of Daphne mezereum, always one drachma (4.367 g) *by weight, mix with wax and paint on the tooth*[41].

Similarly attributable to the Greek cultural influences of the fourth century B. C. is the stomatological scene seen on a vase found as part of the grave contents of a Scythian mound grave on the Crimean peninsula; the work is without doubt that of an Ionic settler. The small vessel, made of a natural gold-silver alloy (electrum), bears four reliefs of Scythian warriors, one of which shows the painful—as indicated by the subject's defensive position—manipulation in the oral cavity of the bow and quiver-equipped person by one of his comrades (Fig. 61). This may well be one of the oldest renderings of oral surgical efforts, but we should be satisfied with the facts alone. Any further interpretations about the type and circumstances of the procedure are pure speculation and without any consequence to medical history[42].

After the death of Alexander the Great in 323 B. C. a new intellectual center developed for the Mediterranean world on the Egyptian shore in Alexandria. Here the Diadochian dynasty of the Ptolemies exerted a generous patronage of arts and letters; here the entire writings of the Greek culture were assembled in gigantic libraries, making refuge and research possibilities available to the world of learning. Here the physicians Herophilos and Erasistratos were able to dissect corpses, very probably also living humans (adjudged to death), making this period of the earlier Hellenism to a period of the greatest advances in anatomy, and consequently in surgery. Unfortunately, with the exception of the writings of Apollonios of Citium, very few direct sources of Alexandrian medicine were given us.

In 30 B. C. Egypt and Alexandria were incorporated in the Roman Empire by Octavianus, later Emperor Augustus. One hundred years previously Greek skills and science had made their entrance into Rome. However, the medicine of this culture had not penetrated the capital city of the world extensively at that time.

The Roman Empire

The historical epoch of the Appennine peninsula began about 1000 B. C. with the invasion of Indo-Germanic Italics in central and southern Italy. Approximately simultaneously during the 8th century B. C., Etruscans, whose origin was probably Asian, penetrated Tuscany, and the Greeks settled in Southern Italy and Sicily. Eventually the Etruscans, who, similarly to the Greeks, never established a unified state, moved further north to the plains of the Po and southward across Rome, the home of the Italian princes, which they subjugated and whose last kings were Etruscans. Shortly before 500 B. C. the Romans freed themselves of these foreign dynasts, established the republic and deposed the Etruscans in the course of the 4th century.

Very little is known regarding the medicine of that time. In a healing temple in the Etruscan city of Veji, innumerable offerings of burned clay representing all possible organs, were found. There was also a complete arch of teeth, a sign that such was on the wish list of the Etruscans

[41] Diocles 12. 141 p. 178, 8—11; Galen (a) De comp. medicam. sec. loc. 5, 5. XII p. 880, 3—5 Kühn
[42] Schuchardt; Kurtz; Artamonov

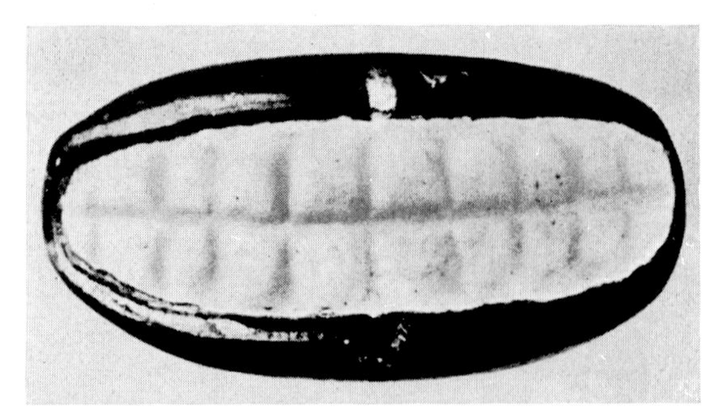

Fig. 62 *Etruscan Donar with complete dentition, found in a temple in Veji*

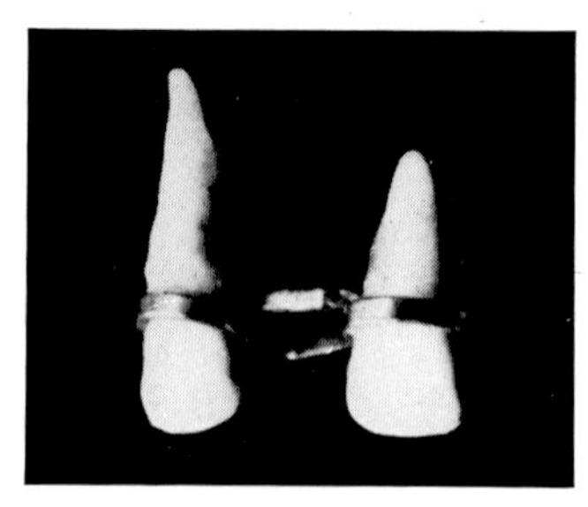

Fig. 65 *Etruscan gold wire ligature to support a lateral incisor*

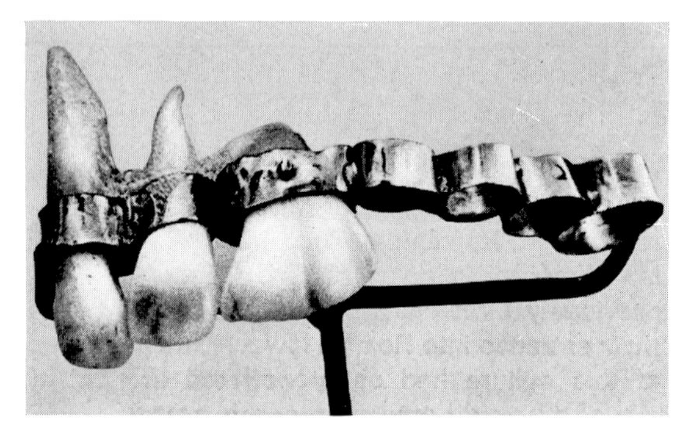

Fig. 63

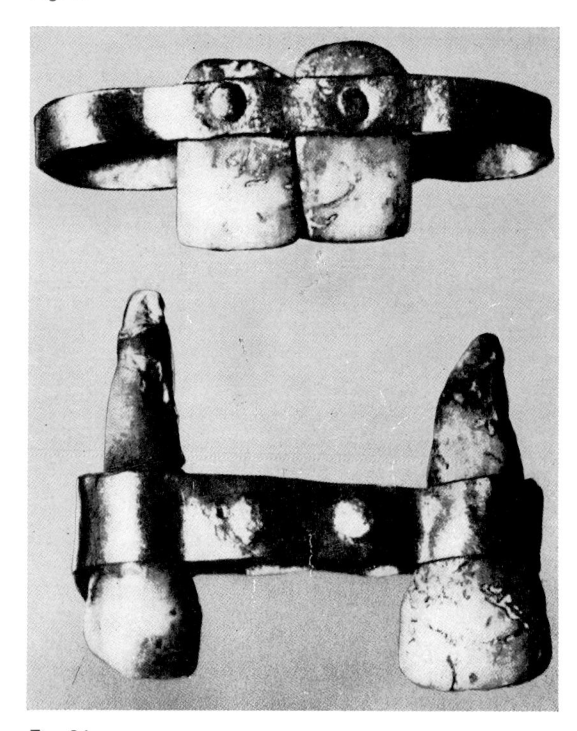

Fig. 64

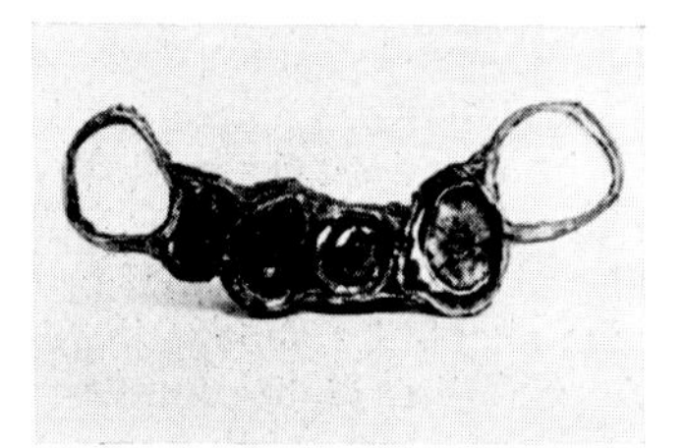

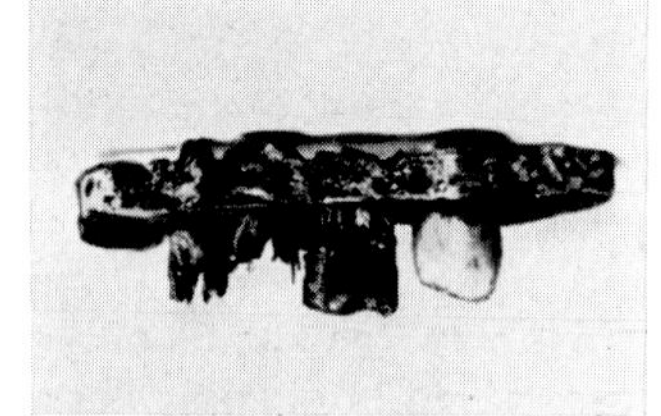

Fig. 66 *Roman gold band denture, from Teano in the Campania, southern Italy (Berlin)*

Figs. 63 and 64 *Etruscan gold band dentures (from Tabanelli)*

(Fig. 62). These people communicate with us primarily through their death cult, as did the Egyptians. From the representations in their tombs we can assume that there was considerable Greek influence in their culture, that they had well-developed gold smithing skills and that this accomplishment was made available to dental cosmetics. Here we encounter a high level of the technique of prosthetics. This surpassed the Syrian standard and also the efforts made about 2,000 years later. The abutment teeth were encircled with flexible gold bands, 3 to 5 mm wide. The artificial teeth, removed from humans or calves, were riveted with pins to now mostly empty intermediate rings. Several excavated examples are depicted here. Most of them fell prey already to ancient grave robbers (Fig. 63 and 64).
Such prosthetics served cosmetic purposes and speech, but hardly the function of chewing. Gold wire bindings of the early Syrian and Greek types were used only to splint periodontally loosened teeth (Fig. 65). This is shown in a discovery of the early Etruscan Cerveti.
The mechanical skill was adopted by the Romans. The gold denture shown in Fig. 66, worked in the Etruscan technique, was found in a grave from 300 B. C. in Teano, at that time already conquered by the Romans. Dieck adds: *Jewelry was found next to the denture including a diadem of tooled gold leaf. Thus, it can be assumed that the wearer was very fashionable or at least wealthy*[43]. Apparently at the time of this burial with the golden diadem the Roman Law of the Twelve Tables was no longer rigidly enforced. The 10th table specifically forbade burial with gold jewelry. Only gold on the teeth was left to the corpse: *But when the teeth were bound with gold, this was permitted for burial or cremation*[44]. Gold dentures were so important even in the early republic that they are found on the law tables placed in the Forum around 450 B. C.
In Roman medical literature they were considered simple products of mechanical skill for essentially cosmetic purposes, with no reference to serving a useful purpose. This caused the satirists to vent their ire all the more. Thus, a poem by the satirical Martial (V 43) goes as follows:
Thais habet nigros, niveos Laecania dentes.
Quae ratio est? Emptos haec habet, illa suos.
(Thais has black, Laecania snowy teeth.
What is the reason? One has those she purchased, the other her own.)
And of an elderly whore named Galla, he says that in addition to removing her silk dress at night she also removed her teeth and curls (IX 37).—From a verse about a certain Aegle we even learn something about the material (I 72):
Sic dentata sibi videtur Aegle
Emptis ossibus Indicoque cornu;
(So Aegle imagines she has teeth
when she has purchased bone and ivory;)
Ivory, a material new in the realm of the Roman Emperors, was used for this purpose until the 19th century.
The earlier author, Horace, also refers to tooth replacement. He tells of two old women running from a ghost. One loses her teeth, the other her wig (I 8). All these references indicate a pronounced spread of tooth replacement at least among the upper class. Ancient Italic medicine, as all primitive medicines known to us, was a mixture of folk and priest medicine, empirical, magic and debris apothecary as Pliny reports, and as the poet Catullus sings regarding Spanish custom (39):
Nunc Celtiber (es): *Celtiberia in terra,*
Quod quisque minxit, hoc sibi sole mane
Dentem atque russam defricare gingivam
Ut que iste vester expolitior dens est,
Hoc te amplius bibisse praedicet loti[45].
(You come from Spain. Spaniards use their morning urine for tooth-wash. To us that blinding mouthful means one thing and one only—the quantity of urine you have swallowed.)
Contact with Greek medicine first occurred when the special slaves came to Rome after the conquest of Corinth in 146 B. C. They served as servi medici (slave physicians), later as freed physicians, and established the basis for the position of doctor, little recognized because of its origin. Later perigrini (wanderers) were found among them such as Asclepiades from Prusa, the first Greek who was able to practice the scientific medicine of his homeland in Rome. He immigrated in about 91 B. C. The prerequisites were favorable, for in the person of Asclepiades a highly cultured, clever personality entered Rome and quickly made friends with the leading men. He was a leader against the

[43] Dieck
[44] Cicero (a) II 60
[45] Horatius Sermones I 8, 48—50

excessive use of bloodletting, purgatives, etc. and introduced simple natural methods of healing. He is also responsible for the first description of a tracheotomy.

The sum of the medical knowledge originating from Greek roots, from Cos and Cnidos and especially from Alexandria of the third century was represented in the first half of the 1st century A. D. by the Roman encyclopedist Aulus Cornelius Celsus. Only the 8 volumes on medicine of the work "Artes" (Arts), which encompassed the total knowledge of his time, are left intact. It is said that Celsus was not a physician. His disease aspects are described with such clarity that he must have had at least medical training and probably some practical experience. The sentence most familiar to us is that of the 4 classic signs of inflammation: *Now the signs of an inflammation are 4: redness* (rubor) *and swelling* (tumor) *with heat* (calor) *and pain* (dolor)[46].

The 9th chapter of Book VI concerns toothache *which by itself also can be counted among the greatest torments*[47]. Wine must be cut off entirely. Food should be eaten sparingly. A complete set of prescriptions with symptomatic remedies is given: Application of heat to the jaw, mustard plasters for the shoulder, pastes containing poppy juice tears for inside or outside the tooth. One should not be agitated during tooth extraction, but should attempt to alleviate the pain with medication. *But, if pain compels its removal, a peppercorn, without the tegument, or an ivy berry without the tegument is inserted into the cavity of the tooth, which splits it and the tooth falls out in bits. Also the tail spine of the flat fish which we call pastinaca and the Greeks, trygon, is roasted, pounded and taken up in resin, and this, when applied around the tooth loosens it. Also shredded alum and . . . put into the cavity loosens the tooth. However, it is better to insert this wrapped up in a flake of wool, for it thus relieves the pain whilst preserving the tooth.* This quotation includes the sensible and the absurd: an early notation of medicated tooth removal which will follow us to the 18th century, and a pain-relieving temporary filling. *These are the remedies recognized by the medical practitioners.* In contrast, Celsus recommends the farmer's remedy of inhaling peppermint steam, *and this ensures good health always for a year and often longer*[48].—The Hippocratic suggestion that a tooth must be polished if a lateral tongue lesion exists, is adopted[49].

Parulis should be treated first by rubbing it with salt, cypress and catnip, as well as rinsing. If intraoral treatment is impossible because of swelling, steam should be applied externally same as with purulent swelling. *If suppuration shows itself, the steaming is continued longer, and hot honey wine in which a fig has been boiled down is held in the mouth; and before the abscess is quite mature it should be cut into, for fear that the bone may suffer if the pus should be retained longer*[50], a very sensible recommendation. A diseased tooth or jaw bone (osteomyelitis) is considered responsible for fistula formation: *When this is the case, the place must be laid open, the tooth extracted; any projecting scale of bone is to be removed; and any carious bone scraped away*[51].

In Book VII, devoted to surgery, chapter 12 discusses mouth diseases requiring surgery. The first section recommends cauterization of the gingiva with a glowing iron for periodontally loosened teeth. The chapter on tooth extraction is almost like a chapter in a modern textbook: *But if a tooth gives pain and it is decided to extract it because medicaments afford no relief, the tooth should be scraped round in order that the gum may become separated from it; then the tooth is to be shaken. And this is to be done until it is quite moveable: for it is very dangerous to extract a tooth that is tight, and sometimes the jaw is dislocated. With the upper teeth there is even greater danger, for the temples or eyes may be concussed. Then the tooth is to be extracted by hand, if possible, failing that with forceps. But if the tooth is decayed, the cavity should first be filled, whether with lint or with neatly fitted lead (bene adcomodato plumbo) so that the tooth does not break in pieces under the forceps. The forceps (forfex) are to be pulled straight upwards, lest if the roots are bent, the thin bone to which the tooth is attached should break at some part. And this procedure is not altogether free from danger, especially in the case of the short teeth, which generally have longer roots, for often the forceps cannot grip the tooth, or*

[46] Celsus III, 10, 3; Transl. I p. 273
[47] Ibid. VI 9, 1; Transl. II p. 247
[48] Ibid. VI 9, 6—7; Transl. II p. 251
[49] Ibid. VI 12. See p. 63
[50] Ibid. VI 13, 2; Transl. II p. 261
[51] Ibid. VI 13, 4; Transl. II p. 261

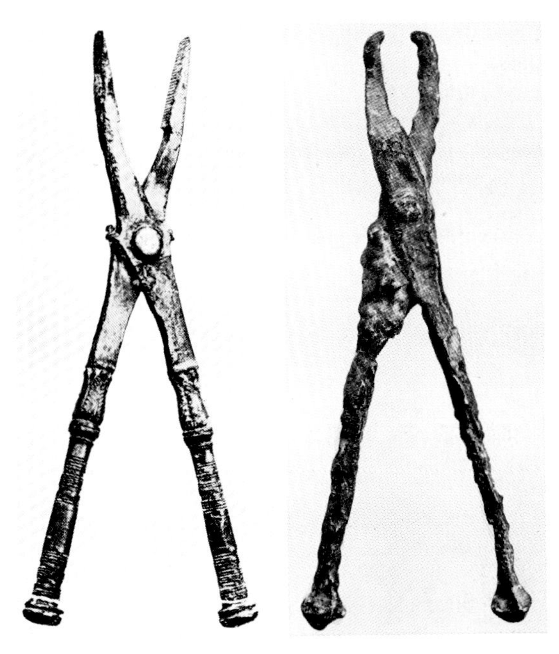

Fig. 67 Fig. 68

Fig. 67 *Iron forceps, approximately 100 A. D. (Saalburg-Kastell, Germany)*

Fig. 68 *Bronze forceps from a Roman camp in Comitat Aranayos, Hungary (National Museum, Budapest)*

does not do so properly, they grip and break the bone under the gum. But as soon as there is a large flow of blood it is clear that something has been broken off the bone. It is necessary therefore to search with a probe for the scale of bone which has been separated, and to extract it with small a forceps. If this does not succeed the gum must be cut into until the loose scale is found. And if this has been done at once, the jaw outside the tooth hardens, so that the patient cannot open his mouth. But a hot poultice made of flour and fig is then to be put until pus is formed there: then the gum should be cut into. A free flow of pus also indicates a fragment of bone; so then too it is proper to extract the fragment; sometimes also when the bone is injured a fistula is formed which must be scraped out[52].

This is a classical description of tooth extraction, which can be traced to good Alexandrian sources and even describes an actual "toothfilling." It did not have the anticipated direct significance before the Renaissance as a consequence of the minor effects of Celsus in the Middle Ages. However, Paré adopted the works in the 16th century almost word for word[53] (Figs. 67 and 68).

Celsus also took a position on caries therapy: *But a rough tooth is to be scraped in the part which has become black, and smeared with crushed rose petals to which a 4th part of ox gall and the same amount of myrrh has been added*[54]. These treatment principles were maintained into the 18th century.

Hippocrates[55] had established the splinting of loosened teeth with gold wire. Questions of tooth replacement are not mentioned. A completely accurate description of an orthodontic procedure for an ectopically erupted tooth was an innovation. The only primitive method was use of a finger: *In children too if a second tooth is growing up before the first one has fallen out, the tooth which ought to come out must be freed all round and extracted; the tooth which has grown up in the place of the former one is to be pressed upwards with a finger every day until it has reached its proper height. And whenever, after extraction, a root has been left behind, this too must be at once removed by the forceps made for the purpose which the Greeks call rhi-*

52 Ibid. VII 12, 1 A—D; Transl. III pp. 369 f.
53 See p. 147
54 Ibid. VII 12, 1 E; Transl. III p. 391.
55 See p. 64

zagra (stump forceps)[56]. Celsus ended the chapter on teeth with this description.

The VIIIth Book on fractures and luxations is introduced by bone description. *The lower jaw* (here still maxilla) *is a soft (molle) bone and a single one, of which the chin formes the middle and lower portion.*

Here the mandible is described as a single bone. This exception is probably the result of efforts on the part of the Alexandrian school. *It alone is moveable, for the cheek bones (malae) with all that bone which produces the upper teeth are immobile.*[57] In discussing incisors Celsus Latinizes the Greek tomeis to tomi. The canine (dens caninus) follows and the 5 maxillares, whose root count is generously given as 2 to 4. Celsus also includes the following disputable information regarding the roots: *Generally the longer root produces the shorter teeth; the straight tooth has a straight root; a crooked tooth a crooked root*[58]. Moreover, the pulp is unknown to him.

While the authors of the Corpus Hippocraticum gave much thought to tooth development, Celsus only came to the foolish conclusion that new teeth develop in children from the same root, usually pushing out the earlier only, occasionally appearing above or below them[59].

For the treatment of fractures the Hippocratic teachings essentially are followed[60]. The fragments are repositioned using 2 fingers, then *tie together with horsehair the two adjacent teeth, or if these are loose, tie them to teeth further away*[61]. Going further than the Greeks, who only tied the loosened teeth, Celsus recommended a ligature for fracture fixation. After treatment consisted of applications of wine, oil, white flour and incense soot, and abstinence from drinking wine. Nutrition was liquid for a prolonged time, converting to easily chewed vegetables, *until the formation of callus has rendered the lower jaw quite firm*[62].

The method prescribed by Celsus for adjustment of a luxated mandible is still used today. Thumbs were wrapped with linen bands (to protect against biting), the jaw was grasped from inside. The remaining fingers were used externally to simultaneously press the chin upward holding the head steady. The bones were repositioned and the mouth closed. Post-treatment included liquid meals and restricted speech. In case of complications bleeding[63].

In brief, this is essentially our legacy from Celsus regarding the stomatological region. If the question of sources is still generally unclear, they are probably primarily Greek science and experience, among which the advances beyond the Corpus Hippocraticum were essentially the merit of the Alexandrian physicians.

Although we have no information concerning the life of Celsus, we know that Cajus Plinius Secundus, who lived a little later, served simultaneously as a soldier, official and writer; he died at the age of 79 in Stabiae as he steered his ship through the rain of ashes from Vesuvius while pursuing his scientific interests and fulfilling his duties as a navy commander. This was the same eruption that buried Herculaneum and Pompeii. Of his manifold works only the last and largest, the 37th volume, is left. "Naturalis historia" is an encyclopedia of applied science combining alternately the read and the experienced, the overheard and the self-observed.

His anatomic observations closely resembled those of Aristotle. But for the molars, Pliny used the conventional designations dentes genuini (gena = cheek)[64], which prevailed since Cicero[65]. He also criticized the Greek assertion that longevity meant excess teeth[66]. Instead, he maintained that men, rams and boars had more teeth than their female partners[67]. He established rightly that some people are born with teeth, as Curius, for example, who was called Dentatus for that reason. Others were said to have a bone in the maxilla at birth, such as the son of King Prusias of Bithynia[68]. The Greek writer Plutarch reported a similar occurrence almost simultaneously, about King Pyrrhos of Epiros[69].

The surprising assertion by Pliny, that human teeth contain poison, appears only once in the literature: ... *for they dim the brightness of a*

[56] Ibid. VII 12, 1 F; Transl. III p. 371
[57] Ibid. VIII 1, 7; Transl. III p. 479. There is reason for the conjecture that "molle" resulted through the erroneous copying of "mobile" (movable).
[58] Ibid. VIII 1, 10; Transl. III p. 481
[59] Ibid. VIII 1, 10; Transl. III p. 481
[60] See. pp. 63 f.
[61] Ibid. VIII 7, 2; Transl. III p. 525
[62] Ibid. VIII 8, 6; Transl. III p. 527
[63] Ibid. VIII 12, 2—4; Transl. III pp. 565 f.
[64] Plinius (Pliny) XI 166
[65] Cicero (b) II 134
[66] Plinius XI 274
[67] Ibid. XI 167. See p. 65
[68] Ibid. VII 68—70
[69] "He had not many teeth, but his upper jaw was one continuous bone, on which the usual intervals between the teeth were indicated by slight depressions" (Plutarch, Pyrrhos 3). Perhaps this relates to an example of especially hard calculus formation

mirror when bared in front of it and also kill the fledglings of pigeons[70].

Many remedies for toothache and loose teeth are given. Part of these are thoroughly rational, consisting of the herbal ingredients of the ancient drug box but in part also of the often obnoxious materials of folk medicine such as earthworms, frog hearts and rabbit brains mixed together. This decoction was applied to the tooth or trickled into the ear on the aching side. Raven dung wrapped in wool and placed in a hollow tooth is described[71]. Ivy sap was supposed to burst a hollow tooth while those adjacent were protected by wax. The alleged splitting capacity of the ivy berry we had already learned from Celsus[72].

The after-effects of "Naturalis historia" in the Middle Ages were slight to the extent that such nonsense prescriptions were not entered in the "Medicina Plinii," a collection taken from the "Natural History" of late antiquity itself but also from other compilations. Pliny, in particular, shows the level of Roman medicine, to the extent that it was not a continuation of Greek material.

Roman medicine suffered from the fact that its source was the institution of slave physicians, even though Julius Caesar sought to regulate the pressing need for qualified physicians by granting citizenship to all of them. The efforts of Augustus had the same purpose: He gave freedom from taxation, as did Trajan on a larger scale in 117. Not only did this increase the immigration from Greece, but during this period Romans turned to this profitable branch for which no instruction or even state recognition were required but only in essentially lower auxiliary positions. Prominent physicians, particularly the court physicians, were and remained Greeks for the most part. The personal physician of Emperor Claudius, Scribonius Largus, was a Roman and an exception. In 43 to 48 A. D. his "Compositiones medicamentorum" evolved. He dedicated it to the emperor's favorite, Callistus. This book of prescriptions created from the empirical Greek school, contains a singularly accurate defined section on dentistry. As a warm supporter of pharmacological therapy, the author took a stand against the indiscriminate use of tooth pliers: *therefore I recommend that a tooth, even if it is partly decayed, should not be extracted immediately. The hollow portion should be cut out with a medical knife (scalprum medicinale). This procedure is painless. The remaining firm portion of the tooth has the appearance and function of a normal tooth. But, if the pain becomes constant, it is preferable to place medication in the decayed tooth because the rest of the tooth will still give good service*[73].

Among the numerous material for pain control Scribonius recommends inhaling henbane seeds (semen alterci), which has a narcotic effect, to kill the toothworm: *It is useful as well, the mouth being open, to fumigate with henbane seeds which are scattered on* (glowing) *coals and to rinse the mouth thereafter with warm water: sometimes something akin to small worms in appearance is thus rinsed out*[74]. While the Roman formulates his thoughts about the toothworm very circumspect, in the Middle Ages his much cited suggestion was expanded greatly and the worm was always described as a fact. The white threads emanating from henbane (Hyoscyaminus) seeds by steam heat were identified as toothworms by wandering charlatans in Europe until modern times, and in the Orient this practice were continued into the 20th century[75].

Scribonius recommended his tooth powder (dentifricium) especially because Octavia, the sister of Augustus, used it[76]. A powder used by Claudius' wife Messalina (murdered in 48) consisted of burned hartshorn, mastic from Chios and ammonia salt, that is, once more the use of animal charcoal with mastic as a gingival dressing for treating gingivitis[77].

For the most part the prominent physicians of Rome for the first 200 years of the Empire and beyond were Greeks, so in the second half of 100 A. D. Pedanios Dioscorides of Anazarba in Kilikia. As the military physician of Claudius he learned about the herbal, animal and mineral healing materials on trips throughout the known world of the time. He incorporated the information in a 5-volume work, which represented the dominant pharmacological textbook of his time and up to the early Middle Ages when it was translated into Latin in 600 A. D.

[70] Plinius XI 170
[71] Ibid. XXX 26
[72] Ibid. XXIV 80
[73] Scribonius 53
[74] Ibid. 54
[75] Sudhoff (b) p. 95. See pp. 145 and especially 241 f.
[76] Scribonius 59
[77] Ibid. 60

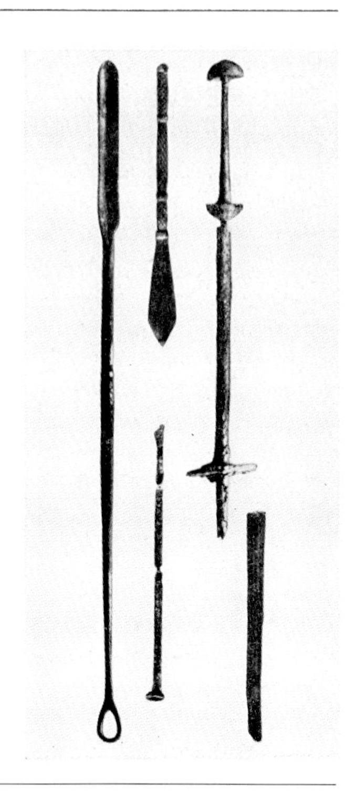

Fig. 69 *Roman instruments, including a drill bur at the upper right*

Dioscorides also conveys in his so very influential writings an excess of prescriptions against toothache: decoctions with vinegar of the roots of henbane, cinquefoil, marshmallow, plantain and pellitory, of pine splinters, hartshorn raw and burnt, sulfur with marjoram, asafetida or oak gall with salt and juniper oil, garlic fruits and incense, to give but a few examples. One is reminded of Celsus by the suggestion that the painful tooth be rubbed with the sting of a ray. *Some people place the sting into a tube and rub* (it) *therewith in the assumption that this too will lead to freedom from pain.* Stabilization of loosened teeth was served through rinses with a special decoction: 10 frogs are cooked in approximately three-quarters of a liter of vinegar with 100 g copper vitriol and 150 g mandragora root, until two-thirds of the volume are evaporated[78].

The recognized surgeon, Archigenes of Apameia in Syria, practiced in Rome around 100 A. D. As reported by Galen, he also recommended in addition to a decoction, the inhalation of henbane seeds. Galen gives us information on the use of a bur to relieve tooth pain: *When the pain cannot be alleviated by any of the mentioned materials and the pain is severe, I use the drugs after boring the tooth with a soft bur* (λεπτῷ τρεπάνῳ leptó trepáno)[79].

Archigenes perforated the painful tooth and relieved the inflamed pulp or periodontal membrane. His treatment using a bur unfortunately served only to still the acute pain, not as today to remove the carious tissue. The burs he used were probably drilling burs as had already been used by Egyptian artisans (Fig. 69; see Fig. 12).

In the second century at the time of the emperor Trajan lived Rufus of Ephesos. It is not accurately known if he worked in Rome. Like Archigenes, he was an eclectic, that is, he did not belong to one of the often dogmatic rigid Greek schools of medicine. Instead he sought the good and useful in all the writings of the period. He concentrated on anatomic nomenclature without much innovation except for the reasonable plastic designation ὁλμίσκος (holmískos, actually the position of the door hinge) and φάτνη (phátne, actually crib) for the tooth alveoli[80]. The name used for wisdom teeth since Hippocrates[81],

78 Dioscorides III pp. 177 f.
79 Galen (a) De comp. medicam. sec. loc. 5, 5. XII p. 863, 15—17 Kühn
80 Rufus Onom 55
81 See pp. €2 f.

(σωφρονιστῆρες sophronistéres), he based on their simultaneous occurrence with intelligence[82].

The therapeutic recommendations of Rufus are found in al-Hāwī by the Arabic physician ar-Rāzī (Rhazes)[83]. For toothache he recommends the application of hot cataplasm with millet or heated towels. The tooth itself should be treated with hot oil[84]. Only a loosened tooth should be pulled, and then with great care. Rightfully, he warns against surgical interventions in case of inflammation[85]. *And concerning carious lesions, insert fig milk or opium and galbanum or arsenic with wax or sharp larkspur or pepper and resin and wax. Preparation involves the use of wolf's milk and cedar resin. When there is danger of tooth fracture use cedar resin and be careful of fracture because the damage and pain are great*[86]. If this position was really taken by Rufus without Arabic contributions, then it was the first recommendation for the use of arsenic in occidental literature. Noteworthy is the justified care the author gives to the durability of the resin seal of the corrosive inlay. Generally, there are rather sensible instructions which are documented for the first time in the scientific medicine of the empire based on Greek tradition.

With Rufus we have approached the best known physician of antiquity after Hippocrates, with whom again we have a survey of a large literary work: Galenos of Pergamon, an eclectic trained in his home state, in Smyrna, Corinth and Alexandria. From 174 A. D. he was the personal physician of the emperor Marcus Aurelius, of equal excellence as army commander, administrator of the Empire and stoic philosopher. In an entirely eclectic manner Galen collected the complete medical knowledge of the ancients in a gigantic work. He embellished it with many personal research findings and experiences. He enclosed it in a system derived considerably from the ideas of Hippocrates. Still, it contains the learned opinions of various schools of medicine of the Hellenic and post-Hellenic periods. His work brought Greek medicine, insofar as it was viewed as scientific, to its conclusion, at least in occidental countries. His effect was amazing, even if not for occidental late antiquity and for the early Middle Ages. Only through Arabic intervention it became known again in the high Middle Ages and remained canonic in this form for centuries.

Galen expanded the Hippocratic humorism, and his conception of blood circulation through the body was only disposed by Harvey in 1628. Moreover, the wealth of drugs obtained from him had such an impact that we still speak today of galenic materials. The 4 inflammation signs of Celsus were expanded by him to include the "injured function" (functio laesa). His dental sections were still quoted by Fauchard in the 18th century, just as the Hippocratic works.

Galen did anatomic research primarily on monkeys and pigs. Through analogic conclusions based on those of Aristotle, several errors were included, which were first corrected by Vesalius[87]. Thoughtlessly, he adopted the representation from Hippocrates that the mandible is separated by a suture in the center of the chin and intentionally testified to it[88]. This idea was obtained from findings in lower mammals[89]. However, Galen had to admit that even if he observed this in dogs, he did not encounter it in his main subjects for dissection, the monkeys. In the portion that was translated only into Arabic he makes the observation in the preparation of a monkey that its *mandible, when carefully manipulated, has no indication of a joint. The mandible must be cooked until loosened and broken apart using force*[90]. Thus, it was only possible for him to maintain his opinion of a two-part mandibular bone by forceful manipulation, despite experimental findings.

Still, Galen is independent of Hippocratic teachings in a similar work describing brain nerve pathways. He accurately describes the insertion of the mandibular nerve in the mandibular canal *through the foramen located near the molars*[91], its course in the mandibular body and its exit on both sides of the symphysis[92] (assumed by him to exist in humans). Similarly he described the correct outlet of the maxillary nerve through the infraorbital foramen and its further course to the tooth roots[94]. However, he believes that only

82 Ibid. 51
83 See p. 95
84 ar-Rāzī III p. 97, 7—9
85 Ibid. III p. 135, 17—19
86 Ibid. III p. 136, 7—9
87 See pp. 65 and 137 f.
88 Galen (b) XI 19 p. 177. 12—14 Helmreich; XI 20 p. 170. 16—20
89 see Galen (c) II p. 546 Rep. 61; Galen (a) In Hipp. Art. comment. 2, 31. XXVIII 1 p. 460, 4 f. Kühn
90 Galen (e) X p. 49. 41—50, 2
91 Ibid. XIV p. 170. 37
92 Galen (a) 3, 3. II p. 432, 4 f. K.
93 Galen (b) IX 8 p. 26, 20—27, 8 H.; see Galen (c) I p. 443 Rep. 1
94 Galen (c) De anat. administ. XIV p. 177. 20—24

some tooth roots had nerves, others did not. And that molar roots have small nerves because they are large, while other teeth have large nerves because they are small[95].

In Galen's introductory writings, "On bones", the teeth, which he considered bones, were depicted with the known nomenclature. They were categorized according to shape, appearance and function: 10 γόμφιοι (gómphioi = peg teeth) or μύλαι (mylai = millstones) *because we use them to pulverize and grind food as millstones do the fruits of Demeter.* Molars and premolars were not differentiated. There are 2 κυνοδόντες (kynodóntes = canines) *because they resemble the teeth of a dog closely* and 4 single-root τομεῖς (tomeís = incisors) *because they cut food like a knife*[96]. The teeth are wedged into the alveoli γόμφωσις (gómphosis) to secure them[97].

Galen gave little consideration to the development of teeth, but put more importance on the throbbing, that is, pulpitic toothache, which he had experienced himself[98]. He seemed astonished that *a manifestation we call phlegmon or inflammation could occur in a single tooth consisting of a stone-like and hard substance.* It must be correctly assumed from this opinion that the author remained ignorant of the existence of the pulp.

Galen discussed dentistry primarily in his pharmacological works[99]. This in itself indicated his limited knowledge of operative measures. Furthermore we are inundated with numerous recipes for toothache and decay, tooth mobility, and gingivitis. Everything that his predecessors learned or wrote on the subject was also accurately described. This included complicated drugs placed in or on the tooth or trickled into the nose, inhalation, and individual amulets. In this respect Galen adhered to ancient tradition. The use of arsenic (ἀρσενικόν), not in today's manner of pulp devitalization, but with root of sorrel cooked in wine and used as a mouthwash for tooth decay and pain[100], was found in an excerpt from the pharmacological works of Andromachos the Younger from about 80 A. D. He was the personal physician of Nero. Incorrect data such as the conviction that milk softens the gingiva and causes caries[101], but sour milk does not[102], are rare and contradictory to his empirical attitude.

Only occasionally Galen goes beyond drug and dietetic prescriptions. His recommendations concerning the drill bur of Archigenes for dental therapy has already been discussed. Teeth protruding from the normal row he shortened carefully, using a small iron file, a procedure which if it was painful was spread over several sittings[103]. He did not use forceps much[104]. He recommended against it, joining the physician Criton from the Trajan era, in the application of various materials to the gingiva for loosening the tooth so it could be removed with the fingers[105].

It was no wonder that Galen generally found no actual solution for surgical problems. The subject of jaw surgery he touches upon only in his commentary on the Hippocratic writings "On the joints". Although he was six hundred years removed from the flourishing season of the Cos school from which these writings stemmed, he was barely able to bring a new viewpoint with reference to luxation and fracture treatment. The application of a leather chin strap was explained in detail. He dwelt upon such insignificant aspects as the very special value placed on the Carthegian leather recommended by Hippocrates[106]. This was the condition of the essential advances in the field of anatomy and physiology by Galen, but he was one of the first to categorize the individual groups of teeth according to their function.

In a work delivered only in Latin and in an Arabic translation (De partibus artis medicativae), Galen even mentions the dentist (dentalis medicus)[107]. He jokes about the fact that in Rome during his time there was a freely growing multitude of specialization: Soon there will be more doctors than parts of the body and each disease will have its own doctor. His one consolation was that these conditions existed only in Rome and Alexandria because in other areas the profession did not support its men. In the time of the Emperors in Rome, a dentist did not have the status of a significant specialist. This was

95 Galen (b) XI 7 p. 130, 5—8 H.
96 Galen (a) De ossibus 5. II p. 754, 1—5 K.
97 Ibid. 5. II p. 754, 9—12 K.
98 Ibid. De comp. medicam. sec. loc. 5, 4. XII 849, 2 K.
99 Galen (a) Vols. XI—XIV
100 Ibid. De comp. medicam. sec. loc. 5, 5. XII p. 879, 9—16 K.
101 Ibid. De aliment. facult. 3, 15. VI p. 688, 11—15 K.
102 Ibid. De aliment. facult. 3, 16. VI p. 689, 8—10
103 Ibid. De comp. medicam. sec. loc. 5, 5. XII p. 872, 2—15 K.
104 Galen (d) In Hipp. Epidemics VI comment. 2, 9 p. 68, 7—14 Wenkebach
105 Galen (a) De comp. medicam. sec. loc. 5, 5. XII p. 883, 11—884, 3 K.
106 Ibid. In Hipp. Art. comment. 2, 25. XVIII 1 p. 454, 1—10 K.
107 Galen (f) 2, 2 p. 26, 23 Lyons = 2, 2 p. 120, 19 Schoene-Kollesch

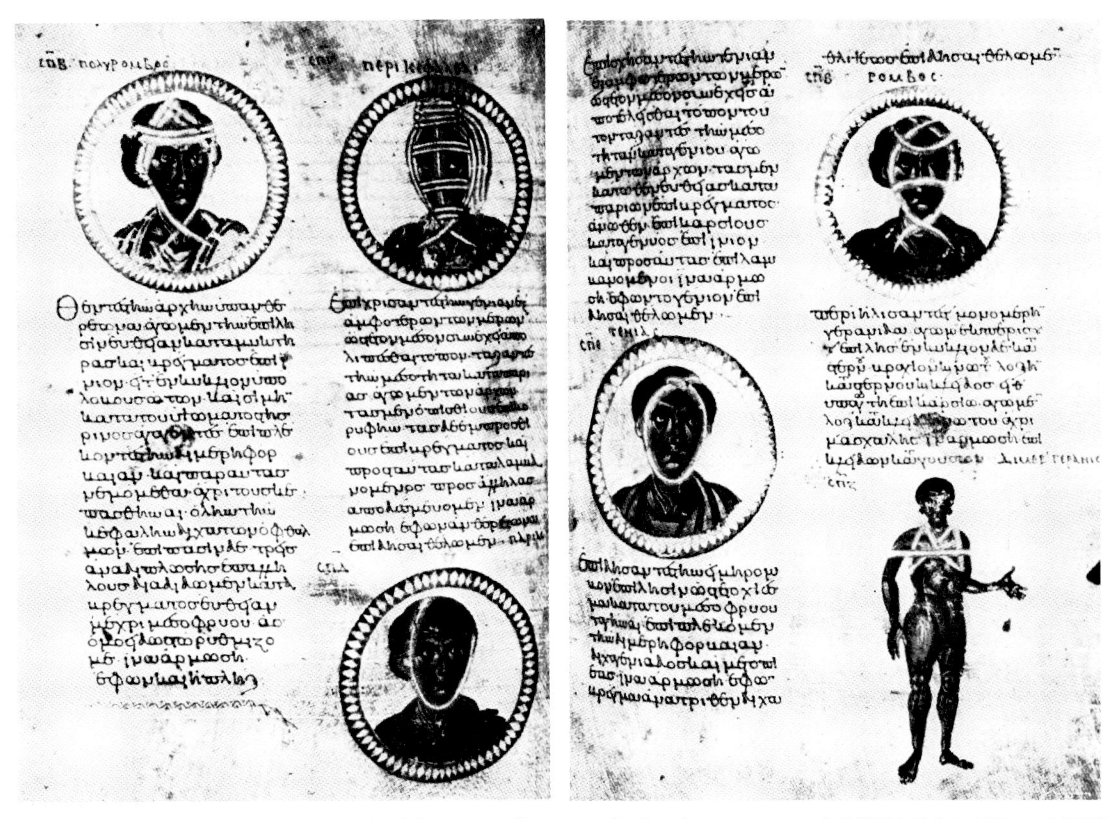

Fig. 70 *Head bandages from a work of Soranos (Florence, Codex Laurentianus pl. LXXIV, 7 fol. 232ᵛ and 233ʳ)*

only the result of striving towards a small profit. Organ specialization stemmed from positions having little recognition and not from the physicians belonging to the scientific Greek medicine. A specifically named dentist was the subject of bitter jokes by Martial:
Eximit aut reficit dentem Cascellius aegrum[108].
(Cascellius removes the diseased tooth and puts it back.)
Also these specialists had no followers[109], beginning with the decline of society in late antiquity. With Galen the scientific medicine of Rome finally found its completion and its connection to Greek knowledge practised mostly by Greeks. What followed had a two-fold significance and presented a true picture of the decline of antiquity. Medical works were written essentially in Latin because of the decline of culture. As it affected at least the physicians of North Africa in 400 to 500, it did not remain under the level of the times. Among these, the first was Vindicianus Afer, the personal physician of Emperor Valentinian I, to name a compatriot and friend of the priest Augustine who converted him to Christianity. His short anatomic-physiologic manual entitled "Gynaecia," created from Greek sources and not Galen's work, was the chief basis of anatomy for the early Middle Ages.
Completely different from Galen, Vindician believed that teeth were not bones because they have no marrow. The pulp was unknown to him, though. *When teeth are extracted or fractured* (in contrast to bones), *they cannot be returned to their place*[110]. The alveoli were discussed in a form obviously based on the Greek "gomphosis" (per confossos dentes)[111]. The teeth were called organs of speech: *A child*

[108] Martialis X 56, 3
[109] Baader
[110] Vindicianus (a) 23 (P) p. 459 a, 24—26
[111] Vindicianus (b) 2 p. 13. 37

who has no teeth squeaks, as soon as it has (2) *or 3 it stammers and with a mouthful of teeth it speaks*[112]. He also believed that men had 32, women 30, but castrated men 28 teeth[113].

Also among African physicians, compendia limited to collections of prescriptions prevailed in the fifth century. Vindician's student Theodorus Priscianus, delivered a work "Euporiston" (easy to obtain), in which a chapter is devoted to the teeth. Among others inhalation of alcyonium root, a poisonous plant[114], or the burned tooth of a dog are described[115].

A contemporary practitioner, Cassius Felix worked in North Africa around 400. He described the molars as being particularly susceptible to caries and having 4 roots which were called tetrazius by the Greeks[116].

From the same period and region came the physician Caelius Aurelianus. He once again sought a connection to the scientific Greek medicine. His main work "On Acute and Chronic Diseases" was based predominantly on the writings of the Greek, Soranos of Ephesos (Fig. 70) who worked in Rome in the second century. In the chapter, "Toothache"[117], he recommended complete bedrest with the head elevated, massages, bleeding and purgatives[118], that is general means of treatment in accordance with the methodic school of Soranos but besides a multitude of locally applied remedies.

The gingiva should be scarified or loosened from the tooth with an iron instrument that he called a pericharacter. Wool with olive oil, as hot as the patient can tolerate, should be applied to both sides of the gingiva[119]. Inhalation, which only stills the pain but does not heal, is considered as useless as trickling into the ear and nose[120]. In agreement with Galen, he rejects extraction which is not without danger especially when the tooth aches[121]. He tells the already quoted story of Erasistratos and the lead pliers of Delphi[122]. All this is well suited to maintain the basic methods. Caelius Aurelianus must have practiced tooth extraction himself for he included instructions on tooth extraction (detrahendus est) in the section on "Medical questions"[123].

Scientific medicine ended with the African doctors, mutually and finally with the Western portion of the Empire. In summary it can be established that authors of the first to the fifth centuries were able to contribute no new viewpoint. Their timidity concerning tooth extraction was important, as was the complete lack of prosthodontic procedures, of which we find a literary reference even in 100 A. D. During the middle ages therefore, this ancient Italic contribution to dentistry was entirely forgotten.

Concerning actual innovations, the dying Roman epoch gave us the first reference to the bur, used by Archigenes during the Trajan period, as well as several anatomic facts. Most of the information is contained in the comprehensive works of Celsus and Galen. However, not these, but the surfeit of useless prescriptions from folk medicine and the late antiquity compendians were first to be applied in the aftermath of antiquity in the early Middle Ages.

112 Vindicianus (a) 22 (C) p. 459 b, 3—7
113 Ibid. 7 (D) p. 435 a, 2—16
114 André p. 23
115 Theodorus Priscianus I 46
116 Cassius Felix 32 p. 63, 18 f.
117 Caelius Aurelianus Chron. II 4
118 Ibid. II 4, 71—74
119 Ibid. II 4, 74
120 Ibid. II 4, 79—82
121 Ibid. II 4, 83
122 See p. 66
123 Ibid. II 4, 84

Thanks are owed by the author to the late Prof. Dr. phil. Konrad Schubring and Dr. phil. Gerhard Baader of the Institute for the History of Medicine of the Free University of Berlin for critical review of the section on Greek medicine. Furthermore, Dr. Baader revised the section entitled "The Roman Empire" and checked translations and references.

References

André, Jacques
Lexique des termes de botanique en latin. Paris 1956

Anonymus Londinensis
Ex Aristotelis iatricis Menoniis . . . eclogae (Suppl. Aristotelicum III) Berolini 1893. Transl. W. H. S. Jones, Cambridge/London 1947

Apollonios von Kition
Kommentar zu Hippokrates über das Einrenken der Gelenke (Corpus medicorum graecorum XI 1, 1). Ed. Jutta Kollesch and Fridolf Kudlien, Berlin 1965

Aristotle
Opera. Ex recensione Immanuelis Bekkero, ed. Academia regia borussica. Berolini 1831. Part. editions:

a) De generatione animalium. Recognovit H. J. Drossaart Lulofs, Oxonii 1965.
b) Historia animalium. Ed. and transl. by A. L. Peck, Vol. I. London/Cambridge (Mass.) 1965.
c) Generation of animals. Ed. and transl. by A. L. Peck, London/ Cambridge (Mass.) 1963

Artamonov, Michael I.
The splendor of Scythian art. New York 1969

Baader, Gerhard
Spezialärzte in der Spätantike. Med. hist. J. 2 (1967) 231—233

Caelius Aurelianus
On acute disease and on chronic diseases. Edited and transl. I(srael) E. Drabkin. Chicago 1950

Cassius Felix
De medica ex graecis logicae sectae auctoribus liber translatus . . . (anno 447). Ed. Valentin Rose, Leipzig 1879

Catullus, Gaius Valerius C.
The poems of Catullus. Transl. Peter Whigham, Berkeley/Los Angeles 1969

Celsus, A(ulus) Cornelius
Corpus medicorum lat. Vol. I, A. Cornelii Celsi quae supersunt rec. Fridericus Marx. Lipsiae et Berolini 1915. Transl. W. G. Spencer, Vols. 1—3. London/Cambridge (Mass.) 1960—1961

Cicero
a) Traité des lois. Ed. and transl. Georges de Plinval, Paris 1959
b) De natura deorum libri. Ed. Arthur Stanley Pease, Cambridge (Mass.) 1955/58

Deichgräber, Karl
Hippokrates, Über Entstehung und Aufbau des menschlichen Körpers. Leipzig, Berlin 1935

Dieck, Wilhelm
Das Zahnärztliche Institut der Universität Berlin im Rahmen der Entwicklung der Zahnheilkunde als Universitäts-Lehrfach. Dtsch. Zahn-Mund-Kieferhk. 1 (1934) VII—XXIV

Diocles of Carystos
Die Fragmente der sekilischen Ärzte Akron, Philistion und des Diokles von Karystos. Ed. Max Wellmann (Fragmentsammlung d. griech. Ärzte I), Berlin 1901

Dioscorides
The Greek herbal of D. Ed. Robert T. Gunther, New York 1934

Galen
a) Claudii Galeni opera omnia. Ed. C. G. Kühn, 20 Vols., Leipzig 1821—1833
b) De usu partium. Ed. Georgius Heimreich, 2 Vols., Leipzig 1907—1909
c) Galen on the usefulness of the parts of the body. Transl. Margaret Tallmadge May, 2 Vols., Ithaca/New York 1968
d) In Hippocratis Epidemiarum librum VI commentaria I—VIII. Ed. Ernst Wenkebach and Franz Pfaff (Corpus medicorum graecorum V 1 I, 2, 2), Berlin 1956
e) Sieben Bücher Anatomie. Hrsg. n. d. Handschriften einer arab. Übersetzung des 9. Jahrh. n. Chr. Transl. and com. Max Simon, Vol. II, Leipzig 1906
f) Galen on the parts of medicine on cohesive causes on regimen on acute diseases on accordance with theories of Hipp. Ed. of the Arab. versions by Malcolm Lyons . . . (= Corp. Med. Graec. Suppl. orientale II) Berlin 1969

Grundmann, Gerhard
Zahnärztliches aus den Werken des Aristoteles und seiner Schüler Theophrast und Menon. Med. Diss. Leipzig 1922

Heyne, Rudolf
Zähne und Zahnärztliches in der schönen Literatur der Römer. Med. Diss. Leipzig 1924

Hippocrates
Œuvres complètes. Transl. and ed. E(mile) Littré, Vols. I—X. Paris 1839—1861.
Transl. W. H. S. Jones and E. T. Withington: Hippocrates. Vols. 1—4, Cambridge (Mass.)/London 1923—1931

Horatius
Opera. Tertium recognovit Fridericus Klingner. Bibl. scriptorum Graecorum et Romanorum Teubneriana. Lipsiae 1959

Kurtz, Michal; Cindy R. Kurtz
The mystery of the Kul Oba Vase: a Scythian treasure. Bull. Hist. Dent. 23 (1975) 19—24

Martial
Epigrams. Transl. Walter C. A. Ker, 2 vols., London/Cambridge (Mass.) 1961

C. Plinius Secundus
a) Natural history. Transl. H. Rackham, London/Cambridge (Mass.) 1966
b) Histoire naturelle. Vol. XX, Texte établi Jacques André, Paris 1965

Plutarch
Lives. Transl. Bernadotte Perrin, London/Cambridge (Mass.) 1968

ar Rāzī (Rhazes)
Kitāb al-Hāwī fi t-tibb. (Continens) Vol. III, Haiderabad 1955

Rinne, Felix
Das Rezeptbuch des Scribonius Largus. Historische Studien aus dem Pharmakologischen Institut der Kaiserl. Univ. Dorpat, V pp. 1—99, Halle 1896

Rufus d'Ephèse
Œuvres. Transl. Ch(arles) Daremberg and Emile Ruelle, Paris 1879

Schuchardt, B.
Über Darstellungen von chir. Operationen und Verbänden aus dem Althertume. Langenbeck's Arch. klin. Chir. 30 (1884) 681—683

Scribonius Largus
Compositiones. Ed. Georgius Helmreich, Leipzig 1887

Soranos of Ephesos
De fasciis. Ed. Johannes Ilberg, Corp. med. graec. IV, Leipzig and Berlin 1924

Sudhoff, Karl
a) Zahnzangen aus der Antike. Arch. Gesch. Med. 2 (1908) 55—69
b) Geschichte der Zahnheilkunde. 2nd ed., Leipzig 1926

Tabanelli, Mario
La medicina nel mondo degli Etruschi. Firenze 1958

Theodorus Priscianus
Euporiston, Libri III . . . Ed. Valentin Rose, Leipzig 1894

Vindicianus Afer
a) Expositiones membrorum quae reliquae sunt: I. Gynaecia. In: Theodorus Priscianus, Euporiston. Ed. Valentin Rose. Lipsiae 1894, pp. 424—466
b) Schipper, Josef, Ein neuer Text der Gynaecia des Vindician . . . Med. Diss. Leipzig 1921

Chapter 6

Aftermath of Antiquity in East and West

Byzantium

The Roman Empire of the West came to its final conclusion in 476 A. D., shaken by internal crises and destroyed by the unexhausted strength of Germanic tribes. Developments in the Eastern portion of the Empire took a different course. Displacement of power towards the East was anticipated by the strong ruler Diocletian. In 285 he divided the empire into western and eastern portions and maintained the latter for himself. However, it remained for Constantine the Great, under whom Christianity became the state religion, to give the Eastern Empire a permanent center. In 330 he made old Byzantium the capital, naming it Constantinople. In this way, the groundwork was completed for the development of the Byzantine kingdom. Here the continuity of antiquity progressed entirely differently than in the Occident. It ended only in 1453 with the conquest of Constantinople by the Turks.

As hardly possible otherwise Byzantine medicine was based almost exclusively on Greek tradition, as even the Alexandrian medical school had belonged to the Empire until 642. Only this period will be discussed here. There was not much innovation in dentistry. Still, numerous prescriptions from the ancient doctors were given us only through the works of Byzantine compilers of the period 400 to 700.

The first of these was Oribasios, the personal physician of the Emperor Julian, who was trained in Alexandria. Julian earned the sobriquet the Apostate (the Unfaithful) for his vain efforts to return his empire from Christianity to a Neoplatonism with a predominance of cults of mystery including the Asclepian cult among others.

Of the 70 books comprising the works of Oribasios, written in 360 to 363, which have the descriptive title "Physician's collection" (synagogai), he himself wrote a synopsis in nine volumes 20 years later. In addition, he compiled the "Euporista" (complete: Pharmacopeia) of easily obtainable materials between 392 and 395.

Oribasios followed Galen's anatomy faithfully, including the story of the divided mandible almost verbatim[1]. With the exception of extraction, which was mentioned only once as a procedure of Antyllos for fistula therapy, dental disease therapy received much attention. But there were no original ideas, only quotations from Antyllos and Galen[2].

About 200 years after Oribasios, Aetios worked in Byzantium. He was from Amida in Mesopotamia, trained in Alexandria and became the personal physician of Emperor Justinian. His 16-volume encyclopedia does not yield much in dentistry. As an example, the section regarding the filing of teeth was taken word for word from Galen[3], enriched by only one sentence: that the tip of the file should be rounded *in the shape of a kernel and as smooth as possible*[4]. Tooth extraction using forceps was not mentioned at all. Just as with Galen, the fingers were recommended as implements after loosening with drugs. Innovations consisted in part of repulsive materials[5] such as the application of a cabbage worm or the ashes of an earthworm[6]. These are indications that superstition and junk apothecary played more important roles with Aetios than at the same time in occidental countries. In contrast, the drill of Archigenes, described by Galen[7], was never mentioned, although Aetios quoted both authors frequently.

A later, decidedly more significant contemporary of Aetios was Alexander of Tralles (in Caria, Asia Minor), brother of the builder of the Hagia Sophia consecrated in 537. He wrote his "Therapeutica" as an old man in Rome. In his chapter on diseases of the teeth[8], he also adhered to Galen, as he admitted himself. But he had stronger opinions regarding inflammation of the jaw, recommending tooth extraction. This was again to be done with the fingers after loosening the tooth with an application of a mixture of rose oil, crabapple, cracked alum, sulfur, pepper,

[1] Oribasios Collectiones XXV 7, 1 p. 54, 35—37; Artelt p. 197. See pp. 75 f.
[2] Ibid. Euporista IV 56—58; Collectiones X 36; see Heinecke p. 13. Antyllos was an important surgeon of the Roman imperial era.
[3] See p. 76
[4] Aëtios VIII 32, p. 445, 122 f. See Lehmann p. 39
[5] Ibid. VIII 36
[6] Ibid. VIII 36 p. 451, 2—4; 12 f.
[7] See pp. 74 and 76
[8] Alexander I 134

cedar resin and wax. Compiled in a similarly complex fashion are numerous prescriptions for toothache and loosened teeth[9].

The Byzantine Theophilos presumably lived in the 7th century. His anatomic work "De hominis fabrica" contained the Aristotelian opinion that females had fewer teeth than men, as Vindician[10] had expanded this idea to include eunuchs. From an unknown source comes the opinion that the wisdom teeth were involved. *These develop, according to physicians after the age of 14. Those individuals who became eunuchs before their 14th year had no wisdom teeth, but only as many as the female sex, namely 28*[11]. The compilation of ancient information may be based entirely on observations of considerable proband material available at the time[12], but not today. Theoretically, it is within the realm of possibility that third molars are retained if castration occurs before puberty.

Paulos of Aigina, a prominent surgeon and primarily a gynecologist of the middle 700's, learned and taught in Alexandria, then still a part of the Byzantine Empire. His 7 volumes, "Medical Abstract" are an anthology of older physicians. In his own words, he depended essentially on Galen and the compiler Oribasios. The conventional, mostly botanical mixtures and decoctions were prescribed against inflammation of the teeth and gingiva. It is interesting that the chapter "On Affections of the Mouth"[13] contains a sharp distinction between inflammatory parulis and tumorous epulis. This was already found in Aetios[14], even if not so precisely formulated. Paulos' description corresponds completely to contemporary clinical practice: *Parulis is an inflammation in a part of the gums, which not being resolved, suppurates. Having suppurated, and being divided with a scalpel, it is to be kept separate with a tent. Epulis is a fleshy excrescence from inflammation on the innermost dens molaris*[15].

This is supplemented by the therapy prescribed in the surgical book: *Epulis is a fleshy excrescence which forms upon the gums beside one of the teeth; but parulis is an abscess which forms near the gums. The epulis, then, we raise with the flesh forceps or a hook, and cut out, but the parulis we divide circularly and fill the incision with tents*[16]. The comprehensive comparison of parulis and epulis by Paulos became classical terms of surgical literature until well into the 18th century.

The subsequent chapter on "Tooth Extraction" represented a mere variation of the indications of Celsus:[17] *And since sometimes supernumerary teeth are formed, those that are fixed in the socket we must scrape down with a graving-tool, but those that are not so fixed we must extract with a tooth-extractor*[18]. Paulos adheres closely to the Hippocratic writings "On the joints"[19] for splinting of mandibular fractures. Added to this in the intervening thousand years was the misleading indication that a complicated fracture should be probed, bone splinters removed with an instrument, and the edges of the wound brought together with sutures[20]. It has been clearly established that the chapter on reduction of the luxated mandible[21] was quoted almost verbatim.

The destiny of Paulos of Aigina led to a new epoch of medicine. This was brought about by a fundamental shift of power to the Near East. For several hundred years a balance of power had existed between Byzantium and the Persian Empire, antagonists under the command of the Sassanians. This was interrupted when the Bedouins, who had been insignificant, were united through the Islamic religion into a primary political power. In 642, Alexandria, the city in which Paulos worked, fell into the hands of the Arabs without a struggle. He remained, even as the officials of Byzantium fled, and was highly honored by the new holders of power. However, in the next several centuries, the Islamic states determined the spiritual and political destiny of the Eastern Mediterranian. Greek medicine experienced a revival in its cultural sphere 200 years later through translations of the Arabic scholars.

Western Europe

While a continuous, although somewhat sterile, survival of antiquity could be established even in the area of medicine for the early Middle Ages in Byzantium, the western portion of the Empire

[9] Ibid. I 135 f. 16 b^r—16 a^v; see Monzlinger p. 10
[10] See p. 78
[11] Theophilos IV 29, 4 pp. 178, 10—179, 3
[12] See Schubring (b)
[13] Paulos III 26
[14] Aëtios VIII 26, p. 435, 18 f.
[15] Paulos III 26, 6
[16] Ibid. VI 27
[17] See pp. 70 f.
[18] Ibid. VI 28
[19] See pp. 63 f.
[20] Ibid. VI 92, 3
[21] Ibid. VI 112, 2—3

experienced a fundamental upheaval. As a result, the medicine of this epoch was completely under the influence of the grave events outwardly manifested by the fall of the Western Roman Empire and the confusion of the age of the migration of people. The political changes, more specifically the social and economic conditions caused in this manner, are difficult to imagine. For medicine it signified the end of attempts by Roman-North African authors in the 5th century to develop a new Latin medical literature from the period of the decline in Greek culture[22].

In the 6th century as Germanic Empires formed around the western Mediterranean, the Longobardic medical literature originated in the East Gothic realm in the region of Ravenna: Poorly trained physicians translated ancient Greek writings and also Byzantine compendiums for their ignorant colleagues into very vulgar Latin. These remained the hallmark of medical writings for the next centuries. It made no difference that the translations dealt with anonymous tracts or pseudoepigraphs[23]. The material formed the exclusive curriculum of Cassiodor, the chancellor of the East Gothic King Theodoric. This was after his withdrawal from open life to found the "Vivarium" monastery in Calabria. At first glance only the writings kept there had the possibility to survive the dark ages, particularly the 8th century. Medicine had never, as it is known, been among to the "Artes liberales," the 7 free arts[24] which had formed the foundations of instruction during the entire period of the Roman Empire and beyond.

Therefore only a limited amount of medical knowledge was incorporated in the educational material of the cloister and presbyterian schools. This is found primarily in the large encyclopedic work of Bishop Isidore of Seville, a scholar who worked in the Spanish West Gothic kingdom in the 6th century. For a long period he was the last to compile the available knowledge of antiquity. Odontologically there was only a passing reference to tooth anatomy. The incisors he designated, contrary to the usual designation, as "praecisores" (precutters), a theological usage originated by the Father of the Church, Augustine; the canines conventionally as "canini." The additional term used for these was "colomelli" (small columns), a colloquialism. This lives on in Spanish as "colmillo" and is a distortion of the correct term "dens columellaris", repressed in the vulgar Latin professional writings of the period of Emperors. Isidore also mentioned the molars which, as usual, had not been differentiated from the premolars. His assertion that men had more teeth than women was founded by Aristotle[25]. Moreover, the incorrect etymology of the gingiva as *gingivae a gignendis dentibus nominatae (the gingiva bears the name indicating breeding of teeth)* was used at the start of the fourth century by Lactantius, a priest employed in the training of princes at Constantine's court[26]. Isidore's entire writings[27] were a reiteration of known terminology not even typical for medical professional literature. This material lived on into the ninth century with the important Abbot of Fulda and later the archbishop of Mainz, Hrabanus Maurus. It was merely expanded with allegoric interpretations from biblical glossaries using such designations as "church teacher" or "tongues of slander" for the teeth[28] and in old high German glossaries[29] such as the "Glossae latino-barbaricae de partibus humani corporis" (Latin-German glossaries of human anatomy) by the scholar, poet and the later abbot on the Isle of Reichenau in the Lake of Constance, Walahfrid Strabo. His later writings seem to have stemmed from an earlier work[30] of Hraban from 826 to 829. Similarly, an anonymous tract of the 11th century[31] is based almost exclusively on Isidore, in terms of the etymology as well as on his grammatical writing, "Differentiae" (Differences)[32].

These encyclopedias were not the only ones for actual medicine. Vindician[33] was preferred but he was a source of little value. A compendium of the early middle ages called, "Ars medicinae" (Art of Medicine) uses his designations for teeth. The incisors were "divisores" or "incisores," the molars, "molae."[34] Another compendium, "Sapientia artis medicinae" (Wisdom of Medicine) indicated in connection with expanded

[22] See pp. 77 f.
[23] Works said to be those of well-known ancient authors, which, however, is surely not the case.
[24] Grammar, dialectics, rhetoric, arithmetic, geometry, music and astronomy, studies open to free men, as they do not serve in earning a living.
[25] See p. 65
[26] Lactantius 10, 18
[27] Isidor (a) IV 11, 52—54
[28] Hrabanus VI 1 col. 15A/B
[29] Glosses or glossaries are annotations or commentaries placed between the lines or in the margin as supplement to the text.
[30] Langosch col. 742
[31] Beccaria p. 224
[32] Isidor (b) II 59
[33] See pp. 77 f.
[34] Laux 5 p. 422, 9—12; Vindician (b) pp. 13 f.

Aristotelian representation of Vindician that men had 32 teeth and women only 30[35]. A tract from St. Gallen entitled, "De ipso homine" (About Humans) contains a note that women and eunuches have only 30 teeth[36]. All this indicates that the limited knowledge of tooth anatomy was propagated far from reality and in a purely literary way. "Ars medicinae"[37] contained the same definition for parulis as proffered by Celsus[38]. Its treatment cannot be substantiated in the early Middle Ages. Knowledge regarding instruments was no better. Although tooth and root pliers are found in a list of instruments in "Ars medicinae"[39] it is in such a distorted manner by Graeca that practical application cannot be imagined.

In the 8th century the Anglo-Saxon church scholar, Beda Venerabilis, of whom we have also scientific writings, recommends bloodletting beneath the tongue for toothache[40]. As earlier, the therapy of this period consisted of collections of prescriptions, primarily of antidotes in the ancient tradition. The more popular remedies were also from earlier Practica. A few examples of these follow. For toothache, well established ancient poly-drugs were recommended: Galen's Hiera (holy material), a salvation material, a holy plaster, an Antidotum Hadrianum, that is, a poison antidote purported to have been used by Roman Emperor Hadrian and so-called Amazon pills to be placed in hollow teeth.

Actually, simple remedies were used in practice: For toothache, wine cooked with incense and bay leaf, with fig bark, roots of wild asparagus and ivy, dried violets, pepper, ash or vervain root were used as well as nettles cooked in vinegar. Asafetida dissolved in water should be inserted in the ear. Vinegar, savory and salt in hot water should be held beneath the shoulder. Applications of mallow root, thyme and pellitory or pulverized cyprus grass are aids, as well as rinsing with a drink of pellitory and honey. Green fennel, pellitory or cabbage should be chewed. Cleaning the teeth with a vervain root decoction alleviates toothache. For molars especially, camomille should be trickled into the ear or common sorrel root should be chewed. Spurge sap, goat's milk with galbanum, ashes, ground black caraway and sometimes the juice of all-heal herb is applied. Hemostatic agents or quince decoctions should help in gingival bleeding. Spurge sap was recommended only once for drug-induced extraction while sanguinolent extraction was not mentioned. Prophylactic measures for loose teeth were chewing of pimpernel root and rinsing with box tree leaves cooked in vinegar or horehound cooked in water. The latter should be followed by introducing the smoke of henbane seeds into the mouth by means of a funnel according to the established position of Scribonius Largus[41]. Pumice stone, as still today, served to clean the teeth, or the scales of the cuttlefish with burned hartshorn and a mixture of alum, vervain and glasswort were used[42].

Much of this is traditional ancient material or of late antiquity as in a "Botanicus" of St. Gallen of the ninth century. It used a well-known late Latin "Herbarius" which was falsely identified as the work of the Roman writer Apuleius in the second century (pseudo-Apuleius). Beyond this the author recognizes a remedy for toothache consisting of a plaster of rue, salt and vinegar, cooked parsnip, cooked cress, horsetail cooked in vinegar, pulverized burr and "pelorden"[43] cooked in wine, this is a neo-Latin plant name. A hollow tooth can be loosened by inserting parsnip and raven dung. The latter by itself was an old remedy from Pliny as in Medicina Plinii[44], but also from a pharmacopeia of St. Gallen[45]. The use of henbane root cooked in wine for toothache is not only found in "Botanicus" by St. Gallen, but also in a formulary of the same origin and in an antidote book from Cambridge[46]. This prescription stems from the herbal of pseudo-Apuleius[47] as does that in St. Gallen's formulary[48] that yarrow root should be chewed. From the writings falsely attributed to Antonius Musa (pseudo-Antonius Musa) the personal physician of Augustus, "De herba vettonica liber" (Book of the Betony) derive emerging prescriptions for rinsing with betony[49] cooked in old wine or vinegar in the prescriptions from St. Gallen[50] and England[51].

[35] Wlaschky I 12 p. 106, 17
[36] Rathje p. 13, 11 f.; see Schubring (b)
[37] Laux 7 p. 427, 5
[38] See p. 69
[39] Laux 6 p. 424, 10
[40] Beda col. 160C
[41] See pp. 73 f.
[42] See Jörimann, Sigerist, Rathje, Ferckel
[43] Landgraf 33, 2
[44] Medicina Plinii I 13, 10 and Index p. 163. See p. 73
[45] Jörimann
[46] Sigerist
[47] Pseudo-Apuleius 4, 3
[48] Jörimann
[49] Pseudo-Antonius Musa App. 48
[50] Jörimann
[51] Rathje

In addition to these herbals, it is also possible to detect actual translation from Longobardic literature of the 6th century, especially the translations of Dioscorides.[52] If this is the source of such prescriptions as that for ivy sap which served Pliny to burst a hollow tooth[53], or mixed with vinegar and salt, it is placed in the nostril opposite the aching tooth while cinquefoil cooked in vinegar or wine is held in the mouth, or applying mashed asparagus root[54], in some instances the writings are almost identical. In a prescription from St. Gallen[55] garlic cooked in vinegar is recommended for toothache in strict adherence to Dioscorides[56], as is chewing of plantain root. An antidote book from St. Gallen[57] recommends the use of rose oil.

This indicates the obvious, that the literature of remedies of the early Middle Ages was largely based on the tradition of late antiquity or was further developed on this base. The practica of the early Middle Ages followed a similar pattern. Two of these will be examined in detail: the so-called "Esculapius," the knowledge of which the early Middle Ages owed thanks to Soranos[58], and the "Practica Petrocelli."

In "Esculapius," an anonymous tract in vulgar Latin from the 7th century[59] (Fig. 71), according to Vindician[60], toothache travels from the head to the tooth root and causes all tooth ailments. This hypothesis is partly based on the Corpus Hippocraticum[61]. For toothache the heating of a cold wet poultice with burned salt, and oral rinsing with cooked rose wine are recommended. For the same purpose roots of henbane, nightshade or asparagus are cooked in vinegar water. Insertion of henbane seeds, pellitory and spurge roots should also help, as would trickling the sap of ivy into the ear on the side of the aching tooth.

Extraction was recommended by the unknown author of "Esculapius" only as a last resort. Blood letting was recommended first for swelling and loose teeth to remove fluid and blood. Then the tooth should be extracted, but only if it is loose. As a chilling example, the story is told of a philosopher who died after the extraction of a securely held molar because the physician had torn out the marrow of the tooth, this stemming from the brain and extending to the lung. Here marrow does not mean pulp. For pulpitis, whose etiology was unknown, the tooth root was treated with a branding iron heated in oreganum mixed with coal[62]. The author recommended a portion of mastic or anthera antidote cooked in vinegar to be retained in the mouth for gingivitis. Also recommended was rinsing with water mead or applying a mixture of mulberries. He recommended mastic root for cleaning the gingiva and rubbing with desiccated salt powder. For bleeding gums bloodletting under the axilla.

A tract of the early Middle Ages, "Practica Petrocelli"[63] attributes toothache to watery or cold mucous, in the Hippocratic manner. This fluid on the gingiva causes the teeth, especially the molars, to become hollow, decayed and black, causing them finally to fall out with the roots left in place. Treatment of toothache proceeds as in "Esculapius": with a poultice of burned salt, with pills of lousewort as well as chewing of mastic, hedge mustard and pellitory to stimulate the flow of saliva. Henbane root cooked in wine, familiar from the herbal book of pseudo-Apuleius, combined with vervain help, as do rubbing with pepper, alum, leek seeds, salt and honey. Also, incense and laurel berries in heated honey should be retained in the mouth. A cloth dipped in egg white, mixed with a powder of mastic, incense, aloe, sulfur, caraway and asbestos should be placed on the jaw. When the gingiva covers the teeth, as in hypertrophic gingivitis, pulverized date pits, pepper and honey or dessicated salt and pepper are rubbed on the gingiva until it shrinks. An abscess of the gingiva is opened with a bloodletting instrument. Recommendations against periodontal diseases included rinsing with leek juice cooked in wine, and for loose teeth vinegar cooked with wild leek juice and honey.

The "Practica," which appeared under the name of Petrocellus first in 1400, is also a handwritten manuscript from the 9th century of northern French origin and preserved in Paris. This was important evidence for the blossoming of early Middle Ages' medicine in this area[64]. The cathedral school at Chartres was of eminent

[52] Dioscorides II 179, 2
[53] See p. 73
[54] Rathje
[55] Jörimann
[56] Dioscorides II 152, 3; Transl. p. 164
[57] Sigerist
[58] See p. 78
[59] Esculapius 10
[60] Vindician (a) 24
[61] See p. 63
[62] Esculapius 10
[63] Practica Petrocelli I. See Schubring (a)
[64] Beccaria p. 166 f.

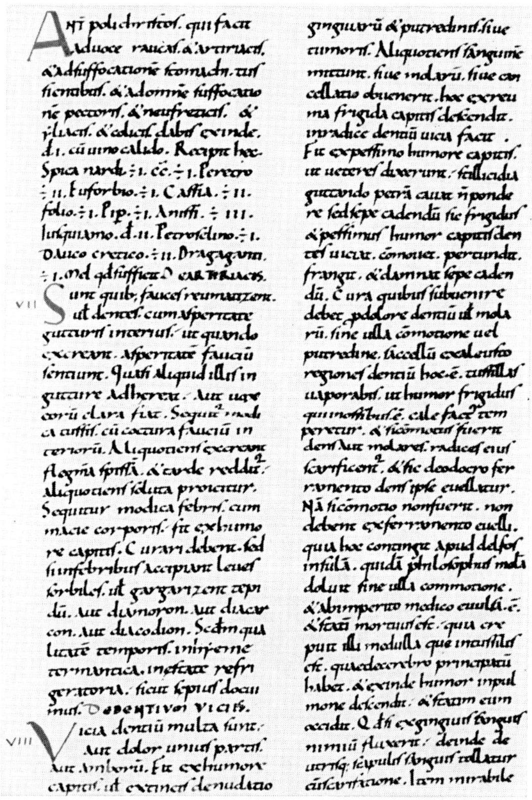

Fig. 71 *The chapter about toothache in the "Esculapius" (Bibl. Municipale Vendôme, Ms. 175 fol. 10r) Carolinian minuscule of the 11th century. The initials are written in red in the original*

significance in the circle of medical studies for the tenth century[65]. Of course, it hardly touched upon the training for medical practice, only book learning was given to supplement the "liberal arts."

The historian Richer of Reims reported from Chartres that he went there to learn from Heribrand not only the translations of the aphorisms of Hippocrates, but also the "Concordia Yppocratis Galieni et Surani" which induced *dinamidia, farmaceutica, butanica atque cirugica*[66]. A manuscript of Fleury from the 9th century, partly preserved today in Paris and partly in Bern also belongs to Chartres. This contains parts of the Longobardic translation from the 6th century of the works of Oribasios, "Ad Eustathium" (To Eustathius), the "Therapeutica" of Alexander of Tralles and of Dioscorides[67].

The manuscript is attributed to Odo of Meung, a cleric of the eleventh century from the Loire region. In a poem entitled, "De viribus herbarum" (Of the Vigors of Plants), later known as "Macer Floridus," he brought a large portion of the Longobardic Dioscorides translations into hexameter. However, he also employed Oribasios. Thus most of the herbs for toothache, such as plantain, pennyroyal, balm, celandine, black sneezewort, henbane and pellitory came from Dioscorides. From Pliny comes the recommendation for buckthorn root[68] or trickling cress juice[69] into the ear, from early medieval collections of prescriptions the application of mallow root. The rubbing in of onion juice and the use of parsnip for toothache does not seem to stem from earlier

[65] MacKinney p. 108 f.
[66] Richer IV 50
[67] Beccaria p. 157; MacKinney pp. 111 f.
[68] Plinius (a) XXV 167
[69] Plinius (b) 20, 129

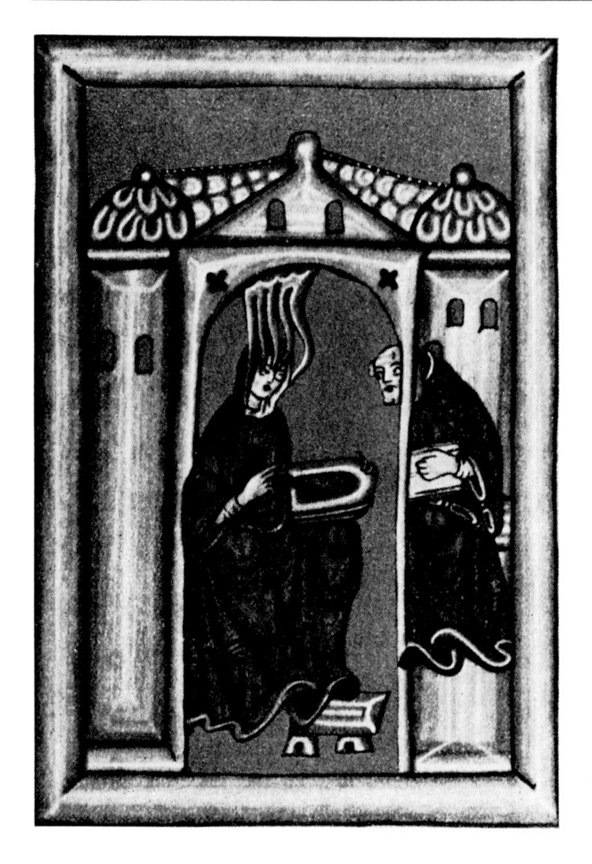

Fig. 72 *Hildegard of Bingen, writing her visions on a tablet, and the monk Volmar, correcting her Latin: "In the year of our Lord Jesus Christ, son of God, 1141, when I was 42 years and 7 months old, a fiery light came down from the open sky with lightning flashes" (from a copy of the Scivias Codex of Rupertsberg, Table 1, missing since 1945). Hildegard (d) p. 89*

documents. The application of pulverized marjoram as well as rinsing with a common sorrel decoction were repeated here under the popular name "paratella" (French — "parelle")[70].

Another landmark of medical life formed in southern Italy. The first physicians can be traced to Salerno in 848. In the 10th century their fame had spread far. Richer of Reims reported an anecdote from a physician of Salerno at a French court from the second half of the tenth century. We also know that around 985 Bishop Adalbero II of Verdun consulted the physicians of Salerno. The first Magistri Salernitani are known from the 11th century. It is a time for collection of the known ancient medical information in Salerno, as much as the early Middle Ages provided. Gariopont[71], a magister of the middle eleventh century compiled the "Passionarius Galieni" in a smooth and orderly fashion from such sources. It consisted primarily of a rewritten version of the main portion of the vulgar Latin translation of Galen's "Therapeutica ad Glauconem", and also contained the "Esculapius"[72]. Gariopont took the dental chapter from the latter. New are only the recommendations that pulverized leek be applied to the aching side of the pulse, and that pulpitis, whose etiology was still unknown, be cauterized with a heated copper rod[73].

In contrast to the beginnings of this school of medicine, which sought to combine the medical knowledge of the times with actual practice, stood the monastic medicine North of the Alps. Folk medicine also started to proliferate, especially those texts that were written in the national languages. Among these were incantations of toothworms from the old Nordic, where meaning-

[70] Odo of Meung 2002—2005
[71] Kristeller pp. 143 f.
[72] Baader
[73] Gariopontus I 17 p. 15^r, 7—9; 24

less words were interchanged with legendary reports of Christian coloring or the soothing use of henbane[74] from ancient sources. Still, there was a medical literature in middle English that was entirely based on late antiquity and early middle ages. For example, the chapter on teeth in the anonymous script, "Peri didaxeon" (About Science) is largely a translation of "Practica Petrocelli" and otherwise dependent on Vindician[75].

In the period of early Middle Age medicine basing between late antique sources and folk medicine, the appearance of Hildegard of Bingen is important. This learned woman and devout seeress descended from noble lineage of Bermersheim near Alzey, and from 1147 the Abess of the convent on Rupertsberg near Bingen in the West of Germany had extensive interests in nature. An example is in the primarily theological writings in the "Liber divinorum operum simplicis hominis" (Book of the Divine Workings of Simple Humans), in which brain physiology is based on humoral pathology[76], as is the wellknown belief of Vindician that teeth have no marrow[77]. However, Hildegard seems to have had knowledge of the alveoli.

The actual works in which dental problems were discussed are the "Physica" (Nature Studies), indicating a good understanding of the flora and fauna of the region and the "Causae et curae" (Causes and Treatment). The question of sources is unclear, as with most of Hildegard's writings[78]. Her anatomic-physiologic representations go back to Aristotle in part. Both of them describe thin arteries leading to the teeth[79] which cause toothaches if they are filled with decaying blood or foam. This occurs when the brain is cleansed[80]. An addition to this humoral pathological interpretation, the toothworm is also mentioned[81] although for Hildegard it was more a part of folk medicine than borrowed from Constantinus Africanus. For toothache, nightshade warmed in water overnight is applied to the jaw[82]. Filtered and sugared wormwood and vervain extract is cooked in wine for drinking. The warm leaves are applied as a poultice to the outside of the jaw[83]. For suppuration of teething and mobility or fractures of teeth, pulverized salmon bone and burned salt should be placed around the tooth at night[84]. If the gingiva becomes infected, Hildegard recommends washing the gingiva and teeth with wine containing the warm ashes of the grapevine[85].

Hildegard cured the toothworm with the smoke of aloe and myrrh. From these prescriptions it is obvious that she used animal and vegetable materials, but avoided intoxicating drugs and those of junk apothecary. She also knew prophylactic measures. In mentioning the toothworm she attributes it lo lack of rinsing with cold water. She recommended cleansing the mouth in the morning with clean clear water to soften the bluish tooth coating *(livor circa dentes).* Then the teeth should be rinsed frequently with the same water to retain their health[86].

Hildegard's only reference to oral surgery is abscess lancing: She recommended that a bloodletting knife or the thorn of a bramble should be used to lance the gingiva allowing the pus to escape[87].

The question of source for Hildegard's natural science writings must remain open, even on the base of the dental sections. Naturally, she must have been very familiar with the medicine of early Middle Ages. The mention of the toothworm indicates familiarity with folk medicine. In any case, an independent mind practiced rational symptomatic therapy within the limitations existing North of the Alps at a time when medicine in South Europe was influenced by the Latin translations of Islamic authors. These governed the medical knowledge of the entire continent at the height and decline of the Middle Ages in a hardly imaginable manner.

74 Fonahn
75 Cockayne; Schubring (b)
76 Hildegard (a) 23 col. 820C—821A
77 Ibid. 41 col. 836B
78 Schulz p. 9; Schipperges pp. 43 f.
79 See p. 65
80 Hildegard (c) 2 p. 94
81 Ibid. 3 p. 173
82 Hildegard (b) I 121 col. 179B
83 Hildegard (c) 3 p. 173
84 Hildegard (b) V 5 col. 1274D
85 Ibid. III 54 col. 1244B/C
86 Hildegard (c) 3 p. 173 f.
87 Hildegard (c) 3 p. 173; (b) I 169 col. 1193C. (Add. ed. pr.)

As for the Greco-Roman chapter, Dr. phil. Gerhard Baader checked the present "Byzantium" chapter. His cooperation in the section dealing with the early European Middle Ages cannot be valued greatly enough. Here the author provided the framework that Dr. Baader fleshed out with his comprehensive knowledge of the healing arts of the early Middle Ages.

References

Aëtios
Libri medicinales V—VIII. Ed. Alexander Olivieri (= Corpus medicorum graecorum VIII 2) Berlin 1950

Alexander of Tralles
Practica cum expositione glose interliniaris magistri Iacobi de Partibus necnon Ianuensis in margine additis. Venetiis 1522

Artelt, Walter
Geschichte der Anatomie der Kiefer und Zähne bis zum Ausgang der Antike. Janus 33 (1929) 199—212, 281—300, 310—336

Baader, Gerhard
Zur Überlieferung der lateinischen medizinischen Literatur des frühen Mittelalters. Forsch. Praxis Fortb. 17 (1966) 139—141

Beccaria, Augusto
I codici di medicina del periodo presalernitano. (= Storia e letteratura 53) Roma 1956

Beda
De minutione sanguinis. In: Patrologiae cursus completus, series Latina. Ed. Jean-Paul Migne, tomus 90, Parisiis, col. 959—962

Cockayne, Thomas Oswald
Peridìdaxeon. In: Lechdoms, wortcunning and starcraft of early England, vol. II, 2nd. ed., London 1961

Constantinus Africanus
a) Practica. In: Ysaac Opera omnia, Lugduni 1515, pp. 58r—144r
b) Chirurgia. In: Opera, Basileae 1536, pp. 324—341

Dioscorides Longobardus
(Cod. Lat. Monacensis 337). From: T. M. Aurachers Nachlaß. Hrsg. Hermann Stadler. Romanische Forschungen, 1 (1882) 54—105; 10 (1899) 117—127, 184—247, 372—446; 11 (1901) 5—121; 12 (1902) 162—242. Transl. Robert T. Gunther, New York 1934

Esculapius
In: Experementarius medicinae. Argentorati 1544

Ferckel, Christoph
Medizinische Marginalien aus dem Cod. Trevirens Nr. 40. Arch. Gesch. Med. 7 (1913) 129—143

Fonahn, Adolf
Orm og ormmidler. I. Nordiske medicinske skrifter fra middelalderen. Cristiania 1905

Gariopontus
Ad totius corporis aegritudinis remediorum praxeon libri V. Basileae 1531

Heinecke, Willy
Zahnärztliches aus den Werken des Oreibasios. Med. Diss. Leipzig 1922

Hildegard von Bingen
a) Liber divinorum operum simplicis hominis. In: Patrologiae cursus completus, series Latina. Ed. Jean-Paul Migne, tomus 197, Parisiis 1882, col. 739—1038
b) Physica. In: Patrologiae cursus completus, series Latina. Ed. Jean-Paul Migne, tomus 197, col. 1117—1352
c) Causae et curae. Ed. Paul Kaiser, Lipsiae 1903
d) Wisse die Wege. Scivias. Transl. Maura Böckler, 5th ed., Salzburg 1963

Hrabanus Maurus
De universo libri viginti duo. In: Patrologiae cursus completus, series Latina. Ed. Jean-Paul Migne, tomus 111, Parisiis 1852, col. 9—614

Isidorus of Seville
a) Etymologiarum sive originum libri XX. Tomi II, Oxonii 1911
b) Differentiarum sive de proprietate sermonum duo. In: Patrologia cursus completus, series Latina. Ed. Jean-Paul Migne, tomus 83, Parisiis 1862, col. 9—89

Jörimann, Julius
Frühmittelalterliche Rezeptarien (= Beitr. Gesch. Med., H. 1) Zürich, Leipzig 1925

Kristeller, Paul Oskar
The school of Salerno. Bull. Inst. Hist. Med. 17 (1946) 138—194

Lactantius
De opificio dei: In: Opera omnia, pars II (= Corpus scriptorum ecclesiasticorum Latinorum, Vol. XXVII). Ed. Samuel Brandt et Georgius Laubmann, Pragae, Vindobonae, Lipsiae 1883/1897, pp. 1—64

Landgraf, Erhart
Ein frühmittelalterlicher Botanicus. Kyklos 1 (1928) 114—146

Langosch, Karl
Walahfrid Strabo. In: Die deutsche Literatur des Mittelalters. Verfasserlexikon, Vol. IV. Ed. Karl Langosch, Berlin 1953. col. 734—769

Laux, Rudolf
Ars medicinae. Kyklos 3 (1930) 417—434

Lehmann, Alfred
Die zahnärztlichen Lehren des Aëtios aus Amida. Med. Diss. Leipzig 1921

Mac Kinney, Loren C.
Early medieval medicine with special reference to France and Chartres (= Publications of the Inst. Hist. Med. John Hopkins University III 3) Baltimore 1937

Medicina Plinii. (= Corpus medicorum Latinorum III) Berlin 1964

Monzlinger Eduard
Zahnheilkundliches bei Alexandros von Tralleis und späteren Ärzten der Byzantinerzeit, Med. Diss. Leipzig 1922

Odo of Meung
Macer Floridus, de viribus herbarum. Ed. Ludovicus Choulant, Lipsiae 1832

Oreibasios
Ed. Ioannis Raeder. 5 Vols. (= Corpus medicorum graecorum VI 1, I—VI 3). Leipzig, Berlin 1926—1933

Paulos of Aigina
a) Ed. J. L. Heiberg (= Corpus medicorum Graecorum IX 1—2) Leipzig, Berlin 1921—1924
b) The seven books of Paulus Aegineta. Transl. Francis Adams, London 1844

C. Plinius Secundus
a) Naturalis historiae libri XXXVII. Post Ludovici Iani obitum ed. Carolus Mayhoff, Lipsiae 1892/1909
b) Histoire naturelle. Livre XX. Texte établi par Jacques André, Paris 1965

Practica Petrocelli. In: Collectio Salernitana. Ed. Salvatore de Renzi. Tomo IV, pp. 185—286, Napoli 1856

Pseudo-Antonius Musa
De herba vettonica liber. In: Pseudo-Apuleius, Herbarius (= Corpus medicorum Latinorum Vol. IV). Ed. Ernst Howald et Henry E. Sigerist, Lipsiae, Berolini 1927, pp. 3—11

Pseudo-Apuleius
Herbarius (= Corpus medicorum Latinorum, Vol. IV). Ed. Ernst Howald et Henry E. Sigerist, Lipsiae, Berolini 1927, pp. 22—225

Rathje, Heinrich
Zahnheilkundliches aus der Übergangszeit zum Mittelalter. Med. Diss. Leipzig 1922

Riethe, Peter
Der Weg Hildegards von Bingen zur Medizin unter Berücksichtigung der Zahn- und Mundleiden. Med. Diss. Mainz 1951. Also abrev. in: Zahnärztl. Mitt. 42 (1954) 779—782, 804—806

Schipperges, Heinrich
Hildegard von Bingen, Heilkunde. Salzburg 1957

Schubring, Konrad
a) Johann Petrizonelli und die Urheberschaft der „Practica". Sudhoffs Arch. Gesch. Med. Naturw. 46 (1962) 364—366
b) Zur Zahnanatomie und -physiologie der Spätantike und des Mittelalters. Med. Hist. J. 1 (1966) 144—148

Schulz, Hugo
Ursachen und Behandlung der Krankheiten (causae et curae). Panopticum Med. Vol. IV, Ulm 1955

Sigerist, Henry E.
Studien und Texte zur frühmittelalterlichen Rezeptliteratur (= Stud. Gesch. Med. XIII) Leipzig 1923

Theophilos Protospatharios
De corporis humani fabrica. Ed. Guilelmus Alexander Greenhill, Oxford 1842

Vindicianius Afer

a) Expositiones membrorum quae reliqua sunt. I. Gynaecia. In: Theodorus Priscianus, Euporiston. Ed. Valentin Rose, Lipsiae 1894, pp. 425—466

b) Schipper, Josef: Ein neuer Text der Gynaecia des Vindician . . . Med. Diss. Leipzig 1921

Walahfrid Strabo
Glossae latino-barbaricae de partibus humani corporis. In: Patrologia cursus completus, series Latina. Ed. Jean-Paul Migne, tomus 112, Parisiis 1864, col. 1575—1578

Wlaschky, M.
Sapientia artis medicinae. Kyklos 1 (1928) 103—113

Chapter 7

The World of Islam

The Islamic world is rooted in the Semitic tribes of the Arabian Peninsula, which were fused into an active unit in the 7th century by a member of their nation, the prophet Muḥammad (Mohammed). Muḥammad gave to these previously scattered and feuding tribes a strictly monotheistic religion, Islam, which included Jewish, Christian, and Bedouin ideas. These concepts were spread quickly by the Prophet's successors, so that soon Palestine, Syria, Persia, and parts of the North-African coast with Egypt, followed later by Sicily and southern Italy, all came under Arabian control. In its prime the Islamic world extended from Spain, which was almost completely conquered in the middle of the 8th century, all the way to India.

Although the Arabs were energetic in conquest, they were at the same time tolerant toward the conquered and converted peoples, readily absorbed the intellectual treasures available to them from all sides, and amagalmated them in a magnificent synthesis.

This brilliant cultural growth included the healing arts. Initially, Islamic medicine was based almost entirely on the works of Greek physicians. We already know Alexandria as one of the transfer points of classical learning[1]; about in 700 there, however, medical life ceased and was transferred to Syrian Antioch and, above all, to the Persian school of Gondēšāpūr, a center of Christian-Hellenic spiritual life formed by the sect of the Nestorians exiled from Byzantium in 489. Here, the works of Hippocrates, Aristotle, and Galen, but those of Indian physicians as well, were translated, first into Persian and then, after conquest by Islam in the 7th century, into Arabic. The Hippocratic spirit joined with Christian brotherly love in the medical centers used for clinical education. Only when Baghdad, established in 762 in the ancient civilization center of the Tigris-Euphrates, grew under the great Caliph-dynasty of the Abbasids (750—1258) (which included Charlemagne's contemporary Hārūn ar-Rašid as a member) to be the shining metropolis of the nation, the spiritual life of Islam was concentrated there. Soon, however, great schools sprang up in Damascus, Samarkand, and Cairo as well, where astronomy, mathematics, chemistry, and medicine were taught.

Muḥammad himself always showed interest in medical problems, and this knowledge was helpful to his believers later in hygienic-ritual regulations such as washings, fasting laws, exercise, etc. His statements, collected in the so-called Ḥadīṯ works, concern themselves, insofar as they touch on medicine, more with particular problems. Thus, as a remedy for toothaches, the Prophet recommended cupping at the middle of the head, or simply pressing with the fingers on the painful spot[2]. In particular, he stressed care of the teeth: *Clean your teeth after eating and gargle with water, this is proper care for the incisors and molars . . . gargle after milk, it is fatty*[3].

For cleansing his teeth, Muḥammad used a small brush-like frayed stick, the siwāk (or miswāk), made from Salvadora persica, the arāk tree, also called the toothbrush tree[4] (Fig. 73). Even in pre-Islamic times, Arabs used this dental cleanser, and it is in use up to the present day in the Orient, where numerous other aromatic types of wood are available, such as mountain olive, balsam and caper shrubs, and others[5]. We have also found similar customs among the Indians. *A prayer before which a toothpick is used is worth more than 75 ordinary prayers;* such is the instruction from the sayings

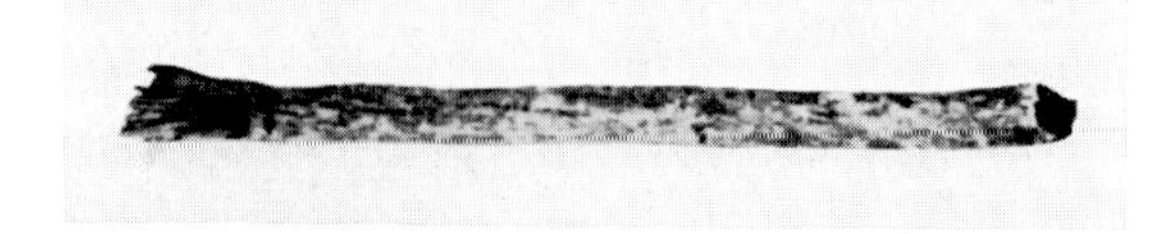

Fig. 73 *The "siwāk"*

[1] See p. 81
[2] Rasslan
[3] Ibid.
[4] Rasslan; Khalifah and Haddad
[5] Wiedemann (b and c)

of the Prophet, who was said to have cleaned his teeth even on his deathbed. Abū Bakr, his father-in-law and first successor (i. e. Caliph) supposedly said: *The siwāk is a cleanser for the mouth and a pleasure to God*[6]. Because of these great examples, care of the teeth among Muslims became an almost ritual activity; it is not surprising that with the spread of the religion, also the use of the siwāk was made so much a part of foreign cultures that it is still used today.

Tooth mutilation through filing, as it was cultivated in Africa, Asia, and above all in pre-Columbian Mexico[7], and presumably customary in pre-Islamic Arabia, was rejected by Islam as an alteration of God's creation.—The compensation for a knocked out tooth came to five camels, a twentieth of what was paid for the life of a man[8].

In the voluminous body of Islamic literature which was so important for the development of western hygiene, there are, in contrast for example, to treatment of the eyes, practically no works only on stomatology. Most texts do, however, deal with problems of dental medicine, often in individual chapters[9].

From the Gondēšāpūr school came in the first half of the 9th century the man who was personal physician to a caliph in Baghdad, and was known in the western Middle Ages as the elder Mesuë: Abu Zakarīyā' Yuḥannā ibn Māsawaih. Only a few odontological quotations of him survive, passed on by ar-Rāzī. We find more in western literature of the middle and modern ages about a younger Mesuë. Toward the end of the previous century, Arabic scholars and medical historians both came to the conclusion that this second Mesuë did not exist at all; they believe instead that concealed behind this name were 13th century physicians writing in Latin and relying on Arabic sources[10].

One of the oldest of medical writings which has survived to date comes from the Persian 'Alī ibn Sahl Rabban aṭ-Ṭabarī, whose book "Firdaus al-hikma" (Paradise of Wisdom), written around 850, was based mainly on Greek sources. It also mentions the Indian text books of Caraka and Sušruta. The odontological texts are collected in a chapter of five pages. The formation of teeth was explained by aṭ-Ṭabarī as follows: the excess nutriment, from which hair grows also, forms the teeth and nails on the way to the gums and fingers. *The teeth are hard and isolated because their substance is dry and because the place where they grow is hard.* As peculiar as this sort of formation might seem to us, hair and nails do have one thing in common with tooth enamel, even according to our presentday understanding, in that all are ectodermal products. The functions of the different teeth are briefly described, followed by the story known since Aristotle about the ancient woman who was still growing teeth. It dealt with a 120-year-old slave woman from Samarra, whose already whitened hair, furthermore, turned black again.

The therapy for unpleasant mouth odor is excellent and completely valid even now. There is a sharp distinction made, in modern terms, between odor arising within the mouth (fetor ex ore) and odor arising from processes outside the mouth (halitosis): *Unpleasant mouth odor comes from the putrescent and odoriferous fluid which forms in the stomach, or from festering of the gums or of rotting bits of food between the teeth. Therefore, when the cause lies in the stomach, it must be cleaned with a purgative and an electuary, or the patient must gargle with a gargle containing pellitory* (or bertram, popular still today against rheumatism and toothache) *and yellow Myrobalan* (astringent). *If, however, the mouth odor is caused by loose and diseased gums, then medications that strengthen and toughen the gums can be useful, as well as gargling with pellitory and marjoram and vinegar and mustard seeds ...*

If the unpleasant odor stems from bad teeth—this is indicated by yellow coloration and by corroded and hollow teeth—then the rotten tooth is extracted. The corroded teeth are filed with a file, so that the surface of the teeth become even, and the roots in the gums are cauterized by branding[11]. The customary dentifrices and toothache medications with complicated formulas are to follow, and a little superstition is furnished as well with the recommendation that the patient hang the right molar of a hyena around his neck with some lizard skin. Purging and bleeding below the beard is also helpful.

The Persian Abū Bakr Muḥammad ibn Zakarīyā' ar-Rāzī, who was temporarily active in Baghdad in the beginning of the 10th century, was

[6] Wiedemann (c)
[7] See p. 51
[8] Spies. See pp. 28 f.
[9] Ullmann pp. 215 f.
[10] See pp. 125 f.
[11] Spies

said to have been a student of aṭ-Ṭabarī. He is better known to us as Rhazes, the name under which his books appeared in the West. He is regarded as a great clinician of the golden age of Islamic civilization, although a definitive judgement on his actual importance cannot yet be reached. His most comprehensive work is "al-Ḥāwī" (Lat.: Continens), first issued after his death by his students. The name means a "collection" of all the medical knowledge of his time, collated by numerous quotations from Greek and Arab authors, and interspersed with records of his own observations. With these, the work provides for the first time an survey of Islamic medical scholarship from both traditional Greek and contemporary Arabic sources which includes the area of dental medicine.

Of the Greek physicians, Rufus, Oribasios and Paulos are quoted most frequently; also quoted are the presbyter Ahrun (Aaron), an Alexandrian physician of the 7th century, and Šem'ōn de Ṭaibūtā, a Nestorian physician and monk near the end of the 8th century. A great deal of this had become available to ar-Rāzī only through the work of the great translator Ḥunain ibn Isḥāq (Johannitius).

More important than these, however, are the quoted Arab authors, a group which also includes Ḥunain, with an independent work on dentistry. Some others of importance besides him were Hārūn ar-Rašīd's personal physician Ǧibrīl ibn Baḫtīšū', named Gabriel in the west, Masīḥ ad-Dimišqī, likewise a contemporary of the great Caliph, and Māsawaih (Mesuë), of whom we have already heard; furthermore, there was the Syrian Yuhannā ibn Sarābiyūn, author of a large medical compendium (879), Yūsuf al-Qass as-Sāhir, who lived in the beginning of the 10th century, and a man designated as Yahūdī, who was presumably one and the same as the important physician and philosopher Isḥāq al-Isrā'īlī (Isaac Judaeus). Ar-Rāzī made an effort to include, over and above the quotations, his own remarks, which are often designated as such.

The Hippocratic concept, that the teeth grow through nutritional supply, is evident with ar-Rāzī. He extends this with the assumption that discoloration of the teeth comes about through excess nutrition, and adheres to the Aristotelian observation that teeth lacking antagonists take over that nutriment and thus, and because of insufficient abrasion, grow abnormally large[12]. Like Galen, he too recommends the filing-down of such teeth; this procedure was served also to ease the pain[13].

Ar-Rāzī does not discuss the substance of the teeth any more closely in the "al-Ḥāwī", he reaffirms, however, frequently their *characteristic dryness* which must be maintained for their preservation[14]. Therefore, for care of the teeth and as a prophylactic measure, he uses, in addition to the siwāk mentioned, a cleansing tooth powder which must contain desiccating elements such as ashes of hartshorn[15], mastic[16], salt[17], alum, and myrrh[18], all usually in connection with honey, whose advantages as a cleansing agent were particularly praised[19]. Blackened or unclean teeth were treated by ar-Rāzī with brightening dentifrices, for which the following composition may serve as an example: birthwort, ocean crab and mussel ashes, salt burned with honey, soda, borax, juniper incense, pumice, glass, emery, mugwort, and burned wild thyme[20]. These are in part strongly abrasive ingredients. Oiling the teeth before going to sleep was supposed to protect them from caries[21], but so was the selection of foods, to which he refers in following Ḥunain. Ḥunain warned against both sweet and particularly sour things, against chewing hard nuts and against quickly perishable foods such as milk products and salt fish. He similary confirmed that an immediate change from hot to cold foods is damaging to the teeth, and recommended careful but gentle cleaning of the teeth after every meal[22].

When deciduous teeth begin to erupt, they require conscientious treatment to facilitate the process. Ar-Rāzī describes minutely how the nursemaid must massage the child's gingiva *so that the harmful moisture, the cause of the pain, flows away*[23]; he describes smearing with rabbit brain, chickenfat, and grape juice with rose oil, as well as wool packings around the

12 ar-Rāzī (a) III p. 94, 1—3; p. 112, 3—7. See p. 65
13 Ibid. III p. 98, 7 f. See p. 76
14 Ibid. III p. 101, 9—12
15 Ibid. III p. 109, 8
16 Ibid. III p. 115, 20
17 Ibid. III p. 101, 11
18 Ibid. III p. 99, 11 f.
19 Ibid. III p. 117, 1—9
20 Ibid. III p. 113, 8—12
21 Ibid. III p. 114, 1—3
22 Ibid. III pp. 107, 14—108, 5
23 Ibid. III p. 105, 10

neck and head, trickling of oil into the ear and elimination of diarrhea or constipation[24]. Elsewhere, in accordance with Yahūdī, he recommends the all-healing barley in conjunction with butter[25]. A magic method, however, is also revealed: if the "Fahlnās" mussel is bound in a piece of leather to the upper arm of the child. Then the pain will subside immediately[26].

With regard to the etiology of toothache, the author shares the Hippocratic assumption[27] that mucus penetrates into the roots of the teeth, citing Šem'ōn de Ṭaibūtā. Other causes can be tumors of the gingiva, caries, strong cold, or, as with the teachings of Hippocratic physicians, an excess of humors which comes in this case likewise from the head[29]. Sometimes, however, it comes from the lungs or the stomach[30]. With reference to Ahrun, he also regards air sealed into the roots as responsible for it, air which cannot escape[31].

As a remedy against toothache, in accordance with Šem'ōn, ar-Rāzī prescribed flushing with a brew made from the fruit of the colocynthis in vinegar[32]. When the cause is air sealed in the teeth, he recommends colocynthis pulp, opopanax, resin, myrrh, and borax[33]. He recognized, in addition, toothache as a result of extreme heat or cold, and prescribed against these purging of the entire body with laxatives and purging of the head through vomiting[34]. For further means to ease pain, he cites a preserve of pellitory and wolf's milk mixed with styrax resin, or of opium and henbane seed boiled in wine or honey[35]. He was familiar with the use of opium from Ğibrīl ibn Baḫtīšū'[36], but warned against narcotic agents, because they delay the intake of nutriments through prolonged sleep, and are damaging to the stomach[37]. He preferred gargle with caper boiled in vinegar[38].

If neither the purgative nor the coagulative treatments have an effect, then cauterization must take place, as already noted in the Corpus Hippocraticum. From Yūsuf Sāhir, ar-Rāzī derived the method of heating two needles in oil treated with marjoram and rue[39]. He himself was using an actual cauterizing iron[40], but also satisfied himself with the use of boiling oil alone, the region around the tooth being protected with cloths[41].

Another method is fumigation of the diseased mouth, without, however, any mention of the henbane seeds recommended by the Romans for fighting toothworms, although ar-Rāzī almost always used them for toothache[42]. He also recommends the method transmitted by Galen from Archigenes[43] of opening the tooth with a drill, which, if it does not ease the pain alone, should be supplemented by repeated trickling of boiling oil into the drilled hole[44]. Referring to Galen, ar-Rāzī also speaks of throbbing pain which arises through swelling of the gingiva[45]. This pain also might be in the nerve, *which goes to the root.* Astringent agents must be used against this, such as strong vinegar, or pellitory boiled in vinegar, or colocynthis oil[46].

In the "al-Ḥāwī" are even more indications of superstition, in addition to the application of the magic mussel, such as the instructions of Māsawaih to drop the juice of the root of Turk's cap into the ear opposite the painful side[47], or on inhibiting salivation in children with fried mice[48]. Also belonging in this category are the pain-causing toothworms which are to be removed with leek seeds and pitch[49].

Ar-Rāzī cures carious defects with a wool compress dipped in boiling oil or also with a special cauterizing iron[50]. In accordance with Ğibrīl ibn Baḫtīšū', he inserts asafetida[51] or opiate[52] into the carious tooth, while in accordance with Masīḥ, he fills it with myrrh[53]. He also uses a camphor filling or red arsenic boiled in oil, which is dropped onto the root of the tooth[55].

24 Ibid. III p. 105, 8—16
25 Ibid. III p. 125, 17 f.
26 Ibid. III p. 98, 11 f.
27 See p. 63
28 Ibid. III p. 104, 17
29 Ibid. III p. 100, 3—5
30 Ibid. III p. 103, 10—12
31 Ibid. III p. 102, 2 f.
32 Ibid. III p. 104, 17—19
33 Ibid. III pp. 102, 20—103, 1
34 Ibid. III p. 94, 9 f.; p. 100, 5 f.
35 Ibid. III p. 99, 14—17
36 Ibid. III p. 130, 1—3
37 Ibid. III p. 99, 18 f.; p. 111, 11—13
38 Ibid. III p. 100, 1 f.
39 Ibid. III p. 121, 16—20
40 Ibid. III p. 139, 12—16
41 Ibid. III p. 106, 8—14
42 Ibid. III p. 96, 10 f.
43 See pp. 74 and 76
44 Ibid. III p. 138, 9 f.; p. 96, 10 f.
45 Ibid. III p. 93, 13—16
46 Ibid. III pp. 137, 15—138, 3
47 Ibid. III p. 134, 7 f.
48 Ibid. III p. 154, 10 f.
49 Ibid. III p. 131, 16 f.
50 Ibid. III p. 101, 13 f.; p. 140, 1—3
51 Ibid. III p. 136, 16 f.
52 Ibid. III p. 130, 1 f.
53 Ibid. III p. 126, 1
54 Ibid. III p. 101, 4
55 Ibid. III p. 107, 4 f.

In the case of gingival abscesses, the patient, according to the Hippocratic method, should be bled and given purgatives in order to eliminate the excess humor, but cupping is also said to be helpful[56]. Strong astringents such as gallnut and alum are useful above all for loose teeth of old age[57]. If this does not help, one turns to application of boiling oil or scarification[58]. Cauterization with calcium and red arsenic boiled in vinegar strengthens the gums[59].

Like Galen, ar-Rāzī is hesitant about tooth extraction. With teeth already loose, he tries at first to make them firm with astringent agents, and if that does not help, to cauterize them and provide them with gold wire ligatures[60]. If extraction is unavoidable, however, he applies agents which loosen the tooth so that it may be removed without pain by hand. As a cauterization agent, he specifies mulberry bark, pellitory, and capers boiled in vinegar[61], root of squirting cucumber with vinegar[62], or wolf's milk together with galbanum. More powerful means are a mixture of vitriol, squirting cucumber, sulfur and larkspur, or yellow arsenic together with aloe and mulberry bark, the adjacent teeth being protected by wax[63].

Referring to Ḥunain, ar-Rāzī also recommends extraction as a remedy for periodontitis. *Ḥunain: If a patient feels pain in the roots of the tooth, then removal will ease the pain for him; this occurs, if the nerve which belongs to it rests from expansion, and the humors, as well as the remedy, easily dissolve, and if the remedy comes in contact* (with it)[64]. Thus, for the first time, the nerve is made responsible here for toothache, while it can remain uncertain whether it is assumed to be within or underneath the tooth[65].

Ar-Rāzī is also responsible for the first mention of a measure as perpetual as it was senseless. It appears in the west, e. g., almost literally in John of Gaddesden, and keeps reappearing like a cliché: *It is said that frog fat has the characteristic, if it is applied to a tooth, of making it fall out, particularly if the tooth is carious. Because large animals, when they chewed frogs which were in the grass, have lost their teeth*[66].—As late as in 1790 this nonsense was mentioned for the last time by the Viennese surgeon Plenk[67].

There is no tooth anatomy in the "al-Ḥawi", but it is to be found in another of ar-Rāzī's 213 books, in the "Kitāb al-Manṣūrī" (Liber ad Almansorem). It is so named because it is dedicated to the Persian sovereign of Kirman, al-Manṣur. Its ninth volume is known in Europe as "Nonus ad Almansorem", and was reprinted and discussed into the 17th century. In contrast to the unarranged "Continens" this therapy volume is systematically organized from scalp to toe, but contains very little that goes beyond the first-named opus. The first volume, however, contains what is probably the Arabs' first dental anatomy. Ar-Rāzī correctly states that there are 32 teeth, 16 in each jaw, and differentiates 2 central incisors (Arab.: ṯānīyatān), 2 lateral incisors (rubā' itān), 2 canine teeth (nābān) and 5 molars each on the right and left (ḍars); he is also aware, however, that there are sometimes only 8 molars. The number of roots is 3 or 4 in the upper molars, 2 in the lower molars, and only one in all remaining teeth[68]. It is correctly determined that the mandible is shifted forward in a biting movement[69]. Thus, the beginnings of a true dental anatomy can be seen here already. On the other hand, ar-Rāzī repeats the mistaken Hippocratic and Galenic bisection of the mandible[70]. The wrong Aristotelian concept, however, that women possess fewer teeth than men, is to be found neither in ar-Rāzī nor in any other Arabian author.

In 1937 Khalifah translated some interesting remarks on cavity formation and therapy from the "al-Faḫir" (The Glorious) text, which are ascribed to ar-Rāzī, although his authorship is not certain. From this, the quotation from Ṯābit ibn Qurra, a scientist active in Baghdad in the 9th century, is reproduced word-for-word: *Ṯābit says that the cause of dental decay and crumbling of teeth is an acid moisture that comes to the teeth ... If the tooth has been eaten away in part, fill it. This will prevent the moisture from getting to the tooth, destroys it,*

56 Ibid. III pp. 121, 4—8; p. 126, 16
57 Ibid. III p. 110, 15 f.; p. 94, 5 and p. 112, 16 f.
58 Ibid. III pp. 98, 19—p. 99, 1 f. and p. 150, 19
59 Ibid. III p. 128, 19 f.
60 Ibid. III p. 118, 10 f.
61 Ibid. III p. 105, 5 f.
62 Ibid. III p. 98, 4
63 Ibid. III p. 115, 2—4
64 Ibid. III pp. 138, 20—139, 3
65 See Artelt p. 44
66 ar-Rāzī (a) III pp. 152, 19—p. 153, 2
67 See pp. 127 and 238
68 ar-Rāzī (b) I 2 p. 16, 4—10
69 Ibid. I 22 p. 72, 17 f.
70 Ibid. I 2 p. 16, 1 f.

and relieves the pain. . . . If the decay is insignificant, file away the decayed part until the tooth is even, then cauterize several times with heat and with oil and marjoram water. The cause of the black stain on the tooth is the same as that of decay. According to Khalifah, "tancar" is recommended here as a filling material. He explains this as *an Arabic word meaning the material that the tinman or plumber works with, or a metallic salt that exists with gold and copper on the surface*[71] (?). This mention of tooth filling with a metal stands alone in Islamic literature, because the occasionally mentioned sealing with gold foil[72] has not yet been proven in the original literature.

In the second half of the 10th century, shortly after the death of ar-Rāzī, the Persian 'Alī ibn al-'Abbās al-Mağūsī, known in the Occident as Haly Abbas, wrote his "Kitāb al-Malakī" (Royal Book, Liber regalis), an ideally organized work on the entire healing art; the first Latin translation by Constantinus Africanus made Galenic material again available to the West, unfortunately including among this the false concept of a divided mandible[73]. Aside from this, the dental anatomy is correctly reproduced, as with ar-Rāzī[74].

The measures which 'Alī ibn al-'Abbās recommended for fighting toothache are numerous. For example, he uses for painful grinders a filling of pellitory, ammonia, and opium, agents that ease the pain, which he puts into the cavity and seals it with wax[75]. He loosens decayed molars with an application of date juice and asafetida[76]. He cites to a great extent Greek sources such as Galen, whom he expressly quotes in reference to application of a filling of henbane, myrrh, opium, styrax resin, pepper and asafetida for control of pain[77]. Ar-Rāzī or his source Yūsuf Sāhir probably used 'Ali ibn al-'Abbās as a source for the method of cauterizing painful dental pulp with two heated needles. The use of a protective cannula is one of his innovations: *Take an ounce of olive oil and marjoram and mountain rue, two dirhams of each, pound it soft, and put it in a pot. Let* (the mixture) *boil thoroughly in olive oil. Open the patient's mouth, find the diseased tooth, and place a tube of iron or brass on it, after completely cleaning the tooth of all the rotten substances which are in it. Then take two large iron needles and put them in fire, until they have become very hot. Take one of the two needles, dip it in the olive oil which has been boiled with the medication, and insert it into the tube until it reaches the molar. Put it on the hole in it and leave it there until it cools. When it is cooled off, put it back in the fire, so that it becomes hot* (again), *take the other needle, dip it in the olive oil, and do the same thing. Repeat this three or four times, and that will ease the pain. If the pain does not subside, then the tooth must be pulled*[78]. This tube protecting the soft portions of the oral cavity from the cautery iron became a component of western therapy through Trottus. We encounter it even in the 16th century in Ambroise Paré[79]. More important, however, even though it evoked less of a response, is his suggestion to use arsenic as a pain relieving filling: *Take arsenic, pulverize it, and knead it with styrax and galbanum, and place it in the molar*[80].

The "Kitāb Zād al-musāfir wa qūt al-ḥāḍir" (Provisions for the Traveller and Nutrition for the Sedentary) is a work that circulated both in the Orient and Occident, but which survived only as a manuscript. It was written by Abū Ğa'far Aḥmad ibn Ibrāhīm ibn abī Ḫālid al-Ğazzār, an Arab active in North Africa in the 10th century, and was translated into Latin in the 11th century by Constantine in Salerno under the title "Viaticum"[81]. It is conceived as a kind of therapeutic manual in seven volumes and is provided with quotations from Hippocrates, Galen, Rufus, and many others. The second book contains six dental chapters (Chapts. 18 to 23). Here, too, the assumptions about the origin of toothache are based on the Hippocratic teachings of excess humors from the head or stomach[82], which results furthermore in caries and gingival damage. From the same era is the statement that the teeth aid articulation of speech, among other functions, and for this reason must be protected. On the base of the humoral pathology, symptoms appearing in the teeth, such as pain, inflammation, and loosen-

[71] Khalifah (a)
[72] Spies
[73] 'Alī ibn al-'Abbās I, 2, 3 p. 54, 28 f.
[74] ar-Rāzī (a) I, 2, 3 p. 55, 1—15
[75] Ibid. II 5, 78 p. 302, 23—25
[76] Ibid. II 5, 78 p. 302, 33—303, 1
[77] Ibid. II 5, 78 p. 303, 2—5; see Galen Comp. sec. loc. 5, 5 XII 869, 12—15
[78] Ibid. II 5, 78 p. 302, 26—33
[79] See pp. 113 and 147
[80] Ibid. II 5, 78 p. 302, 18 f.
[81] See p. 111
[82] al-Gazzār p. 84

ing of the gingiva were treated first with bleeding from the cephalic vein, or, if the patient's constitution precluded that, from the vein under the tongue, with cupping on the neck and thorough purging in addition. Only then local therapy began.

Remedies for toothache are furnished corresponding to the causes, i. e., according to their heating, cooling or desiccating effects at the time: flushing with purslane, chickory, or plaintain root to remedy heat; massages with ginger and honey or with bitter larkspur, pellitory, hissop and black hellebore for cold; flushing with vinegar or salt, root of caper or rue dissolved in oil for moisture, and bitter larkspur together with fennel, myrrh and other things for the throbbing pain already mentioned by Galen. Such drugs reappear in the most varied combinations possible. In addition to the hot and cold humors of the body, hot and cold foods in rapid sequence can also cause tooth damage and pain, as we know from ar-Rāzī referring to Ḥunain[83].

With caries, too, purging must take place first, and then the teeth can be filled with gallnuts, dyer's buckthorn, terebinth resin, cedar resin, myrrh, pellitory and honey, or fumigated with colocynthis root. Opiates, too, can help against pain. The toothworm which causes caries usual is fumigated with mustard, henbane or a dog's tooth[84].

Arsenic compounds are recommended by al-Ǧazzār in the prescription for holes in the teeth, caries, loosening, and against relaxing of the nerve as a result of too much fluid: *Take red and yellow arsenic, a weight unit of 1 miṯqāl of each[85]; 1 dirham each of alum from Yemen, burned copper, and gall-nut[86]; ½ miṯqāl each of pumice, pellitory, and red myrrh; to this, ½ dirham each of dyer's buckthorn and gum arabic. Pound the material, strain it, and knead it with pure boiled wine. Small tablets are formed from this; pound one and affix it to the place where the disease abides. After this, flush with vinegar and sprinkle a ground red rose on the site; if it leaves with the dead tissue, then good living tissue will grow in its place, God willing*[87]. The remedial removal of a tooth which we know of from ar-Rāzī and 'Alī ibn al-'Abbās is thus put into effect here with rather drastic agents. The description is informative, of how the granulation tissue sprouts forth from the gangrenous area. Other means of loosening the teeth are wheat flour kneaded with wolf's milk or a mixture of mulberry root, pellitory, and strong vinegar. Before this, the gingiva should be scarified. *Yet care must be taken, not to spread any of this material on the healthy teeth*[88].

Decoctions of astringent agents such as gallnuts and sumac, and further alum, should, in different applications, make loosened teeth firm: *If the teeth have loosened as a result of mucilaginous moisture—not of corrosive moisture—then take 4 dirhams of alum, 2 dirhams of salt, grind it and pulverize it and put it on the teeth; or take alum from Yemen, boil it in wine vinegar, and have the patient inhale its vapor; . . . and drip hot oils into the ear which is on the side of the loose tooth.* Afterwards one should use a *tooth powder which has coagulative and desiccant effect in the same degree, God willing*[89].

A list of dentifrice prescriptions follows, one of which may serve as an example: *Take barley flour and salt, 10 miṯqāls of each, pulverize it and pound it with honey and burn it. Then take 6 miṯqāls each of mussel ashes and pumice, 2 miṯqāls each of white chalk, burned grapevine wood, Armenian paper, and white marble, 1 miṯqāl each of red sandalwood, arsenic, musk, seeds of the red rose, and spikenards, grind and strain it, and clean the teeth with it*[90].

The treatment of the different problems of the gingiva, such as bleeding, shrinkage, and loosening is divided again etiologically according to heat, cold, moisture and dryness, and treated accordingly after the obligatory bleeding and purging: plantain juice, myrtle, and sour milk as a remedy for heat[91], pellitory, honey, or sea onion vinegar for cold, vinegar in any form for moisture, and rose, fleabane, and quince seeds for dryness. In the case of gum shrinkage, take dragon's blood, incense, vetch flour, honey, birth-wort, sea onion vinegar, etc., *and that is his recovery, God willing*[92].

83 Ibid. p. 86 f.
84 Ibid. p. 88
85 Egyptian unit of weight = 4.68 g
86 Egyptian unit of weight approximately = 3.12 g
87 Ibid. p. 88
88 Ibid. p. 88 f.
89 Ibid. p. 89 f.
90 Ibid. p. 91
91 That sour milk in contrast to fresh milk was good for the teeth was already certified by Galen, see p. 76
92 Ibid. p. 92

The last chapter deals with mouth odor, which arises, as in aṭ-Ṭabari, either from rotten humor in the stomach, to be eliminated by purging, or from rotten gingiva. Al-Ǧazzār fights mouth odor with a strongly perfumed pill containing clove, cinnamon bark, nutmeg, mastic, and Indian aloe wood, among other things[94].

Of great importance for the development of practical dentistry was a man born and active in Spain, Abū l-Qāsim Ḫalaf ibn al-'Abbās az-Zahrāwī, named Abulcasim, or bowdlerized as Albucasis in the West. He received his education and also taught at the University of Cordoba, which was flourishing under the caliphate of the Omayadens. Here, he wrote his great textbook of all medicine, with the title "Kitāb at taṣrīf liman 'ağiza 'an at-tā'lif" (Literally translated: The book of enabling him to manage who cannot cope with the compilations. The implication being that it is: A self-contained manual of the medical art in all its branches; the user need refer to no other work).

The most famous is the 30th book of this work which is devoted to surgery. It is divided into three large sections: "On Cauterization", "On Operating", and "On Fractures and Dislocations". The therapy for dental and oral diseases is also distributed among these areas, whereby much was borrowed from Paulos of Aigina. Although religion imposed limitations on Abū l-Qāsim's surgery, the work still offers tested material, and the individual operations are presented with great attention to detail and knowledge of the subject; numerous illustrations of instruments are of particular value to us.

Cauterization with a protective cannula was borrowed from 'Alī ibn al-'Abbās[95] (Fig. 74). Abū l-Qāsim applied it to toothache as well as to loosening gingiva. He describes three cauterization methods: with hot oil, with a hot iron, or with cold oil and a hot iron laid thereon. These methods were recommended in Europe up to modern times[96].

In chapter 28 of the second book, Abū l-Qāsim discusses the excision of epulis, with reference to Paulos. Surely, he does not differentiate between abscess and tumor as precisely as the Greek[97], but his recommended therapy in the case of recurring epulis represents a considerable step forward: *There often grows on the gum superfluous flesh which the Ancients call 'epulis'. You should take it up with a hook or grasp it with forceps and cut it at its root and let the pus or blood flow out. Then put on the place either pounded vitriol or one of the absorbent styptic powders. And if the growth returns after treatment—for they often return—excise a second time and cauterize, it will not come back after cauterization*[98].

Chapter 29 deals with calculus, which discolors the teeth and causes formation of pus about them: *The patient should sit before you, putting his head in your lap; and you should scrape the teeth or molars on which you can discern crusts or gritty substance, till nothing remains... If they disappear at the first scraping, good; but if not repeat the scraping on the following day and the second and third until you attain your purpose. You should know that molars need scraping-tools of many diverse forms and shapes according to the character of your undertaking; for the tool with which the inner surface of the teeth is scraped differs from the tool with which the outer surface is scraped; and that for scraping between the teeth is different again. Here is a number of scrapers, all of which you will have ready with you*[99] (Figs. 75 and 76; see Fig. 144).

The 30th chapter is devoted to tooth extraction. As did the Roman Scribonius Largus[100], Abū l-Qāsim warns against premature extraction, but then he describes the exact technique: *You should treat toothache with every device and be reluctant to extract; nothing can replace the tooth when it is extracted, for it is a noble substance—until there is no means of avoiding extraction. When the patient is determined to have it out, act with deliberation till you are sure which is the painful tooth; for often the pain deceives the patient and he thinks the pain is in a tooth that is sound, so he has that one extracted; but the pain does not abate until the diseased tooth is removed. We have frequently seen this happen in the practice of the barber-surgeons. When you are quite sure which is actually the painful tooth you should cut away all round the tooth with a scalpel having a certain measure of strength, until the gum is separated all round. Then, with your fingers or with a pair of fine forceps, first move the tooth slowly*

[94] Ibid. p. 94
[95] See p. 95
[96] Abū l-Qāsim XXX 1, pp. 20 f.; English translation pp. 64 f.
[97] See p. 81
[98] Ibid. XXX 2, 28 p. 180, 1—8; English translation p. 270
[99] Ibid. XXX 2, 29 p. 180, 13—21; p. 182, 1 f.; English translation pp. 272 f.
[100] See p. 73

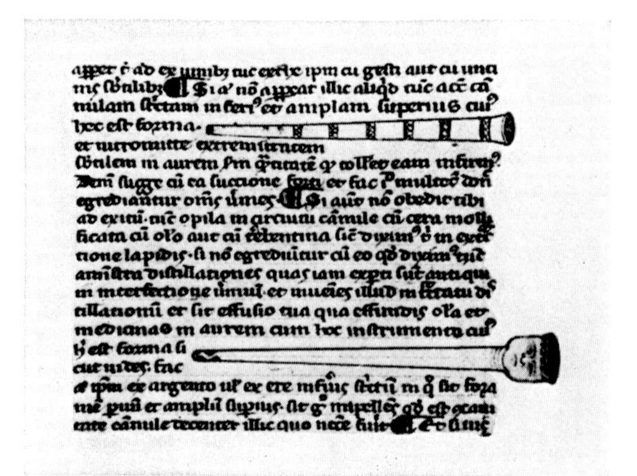

Fig. 74

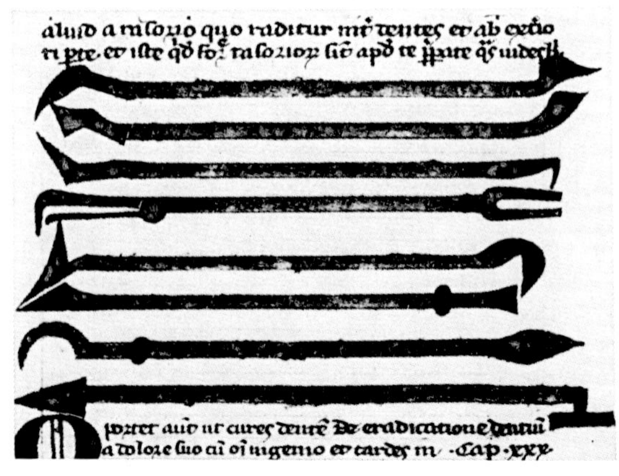

Fig. 76

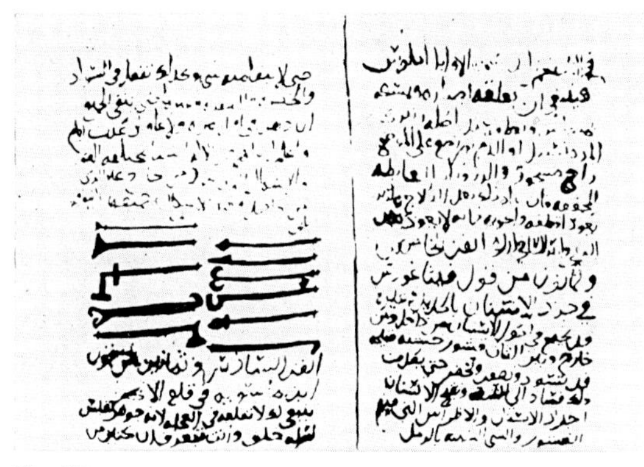

Fig. 75

Fig. 74 *Abū l-Qāsim: Cautery and protective cannula in the Latin translation of Gerard of Cremona (Stadtbibliothek Bamberg, Ms. L III 15)*

Fig. 75 *Text from the Taṣrīf of Abū l-Qāsim with scalers (National Museum of Damascus No. A/253; from Khalifah and Haddad)*

Fig. 76 *Abū l-Qāsim: Scalers in the Latin translation of Gerard of Cremona (Stadtbibliothek Bamberg, Ms. L III 15)*

and gently till you stir it; then get a good grip on it with a pair of large forceps, holding the patient's head between your knees so that it does not move. Then draw the tooth straight out so as not to splinter it. And if it will not come out, then take one of these following instruments and gradually introduce it beneath the tooth all round; then try to move it as you did before. If the tooth has a hole in it or is decayed, you should plug the hole with a rag, forcing it in with the tip of a fine probe so that it will not break when you grip it with a forceps. You must completely scarifiy all round the gum. Take the utmost care not to splinter the tooth lest a piece should remain behind and arouse the patient's ills afresh, causing greater pain than before. Take care not to do those things that the ignorant barber-surgeons do in their rashness and haste in dental extraction, neglecting to employ the methods we describe. For they often bring great troubles upon people, the least of which is to break the tooth off short, leaving the whole or part of the root behind; or to remove the tooth together with a piece of the jaw bone, as I have often seen. Then after the extraction let the patient rinse with wine or vinegar and salt. If there occur hemorrhage from the place—a common occurrence—then pound up a little vitriol and stuff the place with it. If the vitriol does not avail, cauterize[101].

Following this superb description are illustrations with explanations appended: *The shape of the fine forceps with which you first move the tooth should be with long jaws and a short han-*

[101] Ibid. XXX 2, 30, pp. 184—186, 2; English translation pp. 276 f.

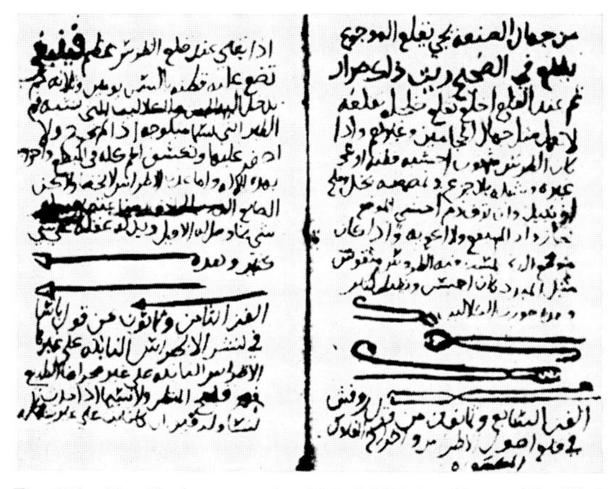

Fig. 77 *Tooth forceps in Abū l-Qāsim (from Khalifah and Haddad)*

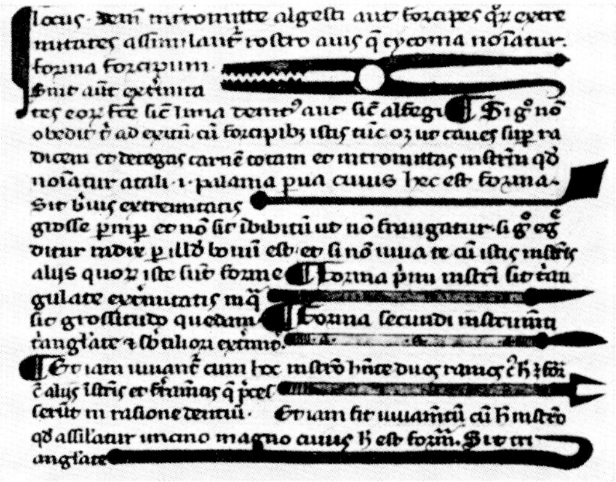

Fig. 78 *Forceps and elevator for tooth extraction in the Latin translation (Bamberg)*

dle, thick, lest they bend when you take hold of the tooth. And this is the shape of the large forceps. As you see, they have thick handles so that when you apply pressure with them they do not give or bend; and short jaws. They should be of Indian iron or of steel, strongly made, the jaws tempered and having teeth fitting into each other so that a sure and firm grip may be obtained. Sometimes the jaws are made like a file, also to give a strong grip[102] (Figs. 77 and 78).

We can see that for this epoch, Abū l-Qāsim is uncommonly active in tooth extraction, for which he seems to have used sources similar to those of Celsus[103]. But also esthetic questions occupy him: Misplaced erupted teeth appear ugly in woman and man; therefore they should be removed, cut down, or filed, the latter in the careful, protracted procedure known from Galen[104].

Teeth loosened in consequence of trauma are reinforced with silver or—better still—gold wire in the following manner: *The method is to take the wire and run it doubled between two sound teeth; then with the two ends of the wire you weave between the loose teeth, either one or several, until you bring your weaving to a sound tooth on the other side; then you repeat your weaving back to the side whence you began; tighten it gently and judiciously till they do not move at all. You should tie the wire at the root of the teeth lest it slip. Then with the scissors cut off the two ends of the wire remaining over, and bring them together and twist them with forceps and hide them between a sound tooth and a loose tooth so as to not injure the tongue, then for the future leave them thus bound*[105] (Figs. 79 and 80).

Fixation of loose teeth had, by the way, already been described in the third Caliph 'Uṯmān, of whom a later historian remarked: *His teeth were fastened with gold, which colored his beard yellow*[106]. The scholarly biography of al-Ḫaṭīb al-Bagdādī contains the observation that a cadi (religious judge) under Hārūn ar-Rašīd permitted his front teeth to be tied with gold, and in the 12th century we find the notation in al-Mutarrizī: *... he clamped his teeth with silver*[107].

In the same 33rd chapter of Abū l-Qāsim, we again find a long-lost mention of tooth prosthesis: *This can be done only by an expert and gentle practitioner. Sometimes a piece of ox-bone may be carved and made into the shape of a tooth, and placed in the site where a tooth was lost, and fastened as we have said, and it will last and he will get long service from it*[108] (Fig. 81). It was from this source that Guy de

[102] Ibid. XX 2, 30, p. 186, 4—13; English translation pp. 278 f.
[103] See pp. 70 f.
[104] Ibid. XXX 2, 32, p. 192, 4—11; English translation pp. 288 f.
[105] Ibid. XXX 2, 33, p. 194, 9—28; English translation p. 292
[106] Wiedemann (c); Spies
[107] al-Ḫaṭīb al-Bagdādī VIII, 199; Lane p. 1761
[108] Abū l-Qāsim XXX 2, 33, p. 194, 2—4; English translation p. 294

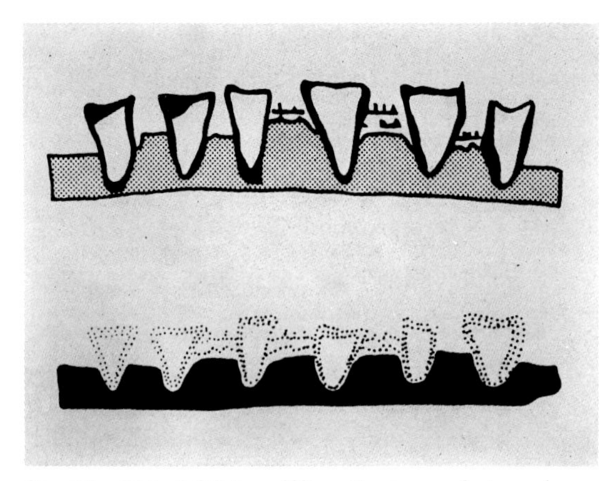

Fig. 79 *Abū l-Qāsim: Wire ligature of two loose teeth at two solid ones (Ms. Huntington, from Spink and Lewis)*

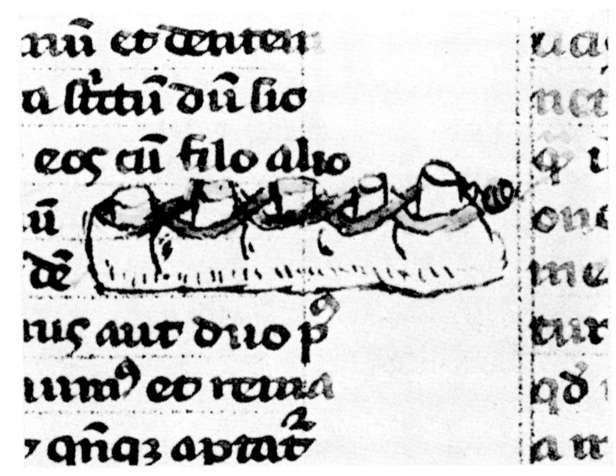

Fig. 80 *Wire splinting in Abū l-Qāsim in the Latin translation (Bamberg)*

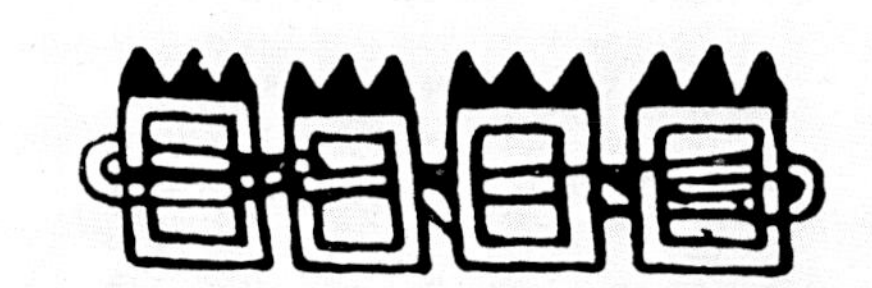

Fig. 81 *Dental prosthesis in Abū l-Qāsim in the Latin translation (Bibl. Laurentiana)*

Chauliac learned of tooth replacement by oxbone[109].

Among oral surgical procedures, the ranula operation is mentioned, being designated as frog under the tongue. If the swelling is darkly discolored and hard, it should not be touched because it is cancer. *But if it is inclined to be pale and has fluid in it, put a hook in it and incise it with a fine scalpel and free it all round; and if haemorrhage hinders you while operating apply pounded vitriol to it till the bleeding stops. Then proceed with your work till all is extracted; then let him rinse his mouth out with vinegar and salt. Then give all suitable treatment till healed*[110]. Obviously only an opening of the retention cyst, so that recurrence was certain.

Two further chapters of the third book are devoted to fractures and luxations of the mandible, referring to Paulos. At the same time, Abū l-Qāsim adopts the unique Hippocratic prognosis of mortal danger if repositioning is delayed: *If the reduction of both sides is hard when it is simultaneous bilateral dislocation, and there is no return to proper position, then thereby in many cases fevers and perpetual headaches occur; sometimes the patient's belly is loosened and he vomits actual bile. When you see this you will know that he is doomed; in most cases in which this happens death follows in ten days*[111].

So much for quotations from the work of this great representative of Arabic medicine. Even if Abū l-Qāsim recedes in general evaluation behind his somewhat later contemporary Ibn Sīnā, he is by far the more important figure in dental medicine. Although he refers to another author at the beginning of almost every article, his whole manner of expression makes it probable that he was a man versed in surgical practice, who was able thereby to raise himself far above mere compilation of his contemporaries. The "Taṣrīf" was translated into Latin by Gerard of Cremona[112] and then exerted a strong influence on western surgery, particularly on Guy de Chauliac, and thus through Paré into the 18th century.

These texts were all overshadowed in effect, however, on the European Middle Ages by the

109 See p. 131
110 Ibid. XXX 2, 35, p. 196, 22—198, 7; English translation p. 298
111 Ibid. XXX 3, 24, p. 600, 11 f.; English translation pp. 760 f.
112 See pp. 117 f.

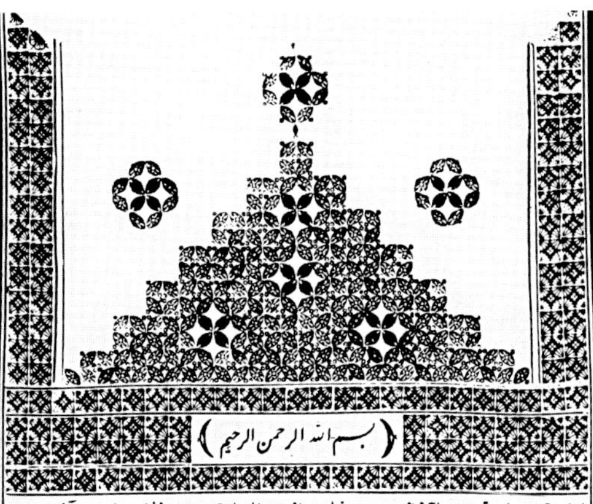

بسم الله الرحمن الرحيم

الحمد لله حمداً يستحقه بعلو شأنه وسبوغ احسانه والصلاة على سيدنا محمد النبي وآله وسلامه
وبعد فقد التمس مني بعض خلص اخواني ومن يلزمني اسعافه بما يسمح به وسعي أن
أصنف في الطب كتاباً مشتملاً على قوانينه الكلية والجزئية اشتمالاً يجمع الى الشرح الاختصار
والى ايفاء الاكثر حقه من البيان الايجاز فأسعفته بذلك ورأيت أن أتكلم أولاً في الامور
العامة الكلية في كلا قسمي الطب أعني القسم النظري والقسم العملي ثم بعد ذلك أتكلم في
كليات أحكام قوى الادوية المفردة ثم في جزئياتها ثم بعد ذلك في الامراض الواقعة بعضو
عضو فأبتدي أولاً بتشريح ذلك العضو ومنفعته وأما تشريح الاعضاء المفردة البسيطة
فيكون قد سبق مني ذكره في الكتاب الاول الكلي وكذلك منافعها ثم اذا فرغت من تشريح
ذلك العضو ابتدأت في أكثر المواضع بالدلالة على كيفية حفظ صحته ثم دللت بالقول المطلق
على كليات أمراضه وأسبابها وطرق الاستدلالات عليها وطرق معالجاتها بالقول الكلي أيضاً
فاذا فرغت من هذه الامور الكلية اقبلت على الامراض الجزئية ودللت أولاً في أكثرها أيضاً
على الحكم الكلي في حده وأسبابه ودلائله ثم تخلصت الى الاحكام الجزئية ثم أعطيت القانون
الكلي في المعالجة ثم نزلت الى المعالجات الجزئية بدواء دواء بسيط أو مركب وما كان سلف
ذكره من الادوية المفردة ومنفعته في الامراض في كتاب الادوية المفردة في الجداول
والاصباغ التي أرى استعمالها فيه كما تقف أيها المتعلم عليه اذا وصلت اليه لم أكرر الاقليلا منه
وما كان من الادوية المركبة أن ما الاحرى به ان يكون في الاقراباذين الذي أرى ان اعمله أخرت
ذكر منافعه وكيفية خلطه اليه ورأيت ان أفرغ عن هذا الكتاب الى كتاب أيضاً في الامور
الجزئية مختص بذكر الامراض التي اذا وقعت لم تختص بعضو بعينه ونورد هنالك أيضاً الكلام
في الزينة وان أسلك في هذا الكتاب أيضاً مسلكي في الكتاب الجزئي الذي قبله فاذا تم أبتوفيق

Liber ca
nonis Auicenne reuisus ⁊
ab omni errore mēdaqꝫ
purgatus summaqꝫ
cum diligentia
Impressus.
Cum priuilegio

Fig. 82 *Arabic printing of the al-Qānūn fiṭ-ṭibb of Ibn Sīnā, Būlāq near Cairo, 1294 (Hidschra) = 1877, at left; Latin translation of the Canon Medicinae of Avicenna, Venice, 1507, at right*

work by the Persian scholar and physician Abū 'Alī al-Ḥusain ibn 'Abdallāh ibn Sīnā. Ibn Sīnā, whose name we recognize in its latinized form as Avicenna, was born near Buchara in 980, and died in 1037. He was an outstanding figure, of equal importance as physician, poet, philosopher and statesman. As a philosopher, he became an interpreter of Aristotle for the Occident, and the five-volume "Qānūn fī ṭ-ṭibb" (Canon medicinae) by this "prince of physicians", as he was called, determined the medical thinking of the world for centuries, thanks to its brilliant systematization (Fig. 82). In contrast to previous medical compendia however, Ibn Sīnā's work is so stamped with scholarly methodology that its truly great merit is to be found in the collection and systematization of the knowledge of his time, while very little original material is offered.

Thus the stomatological and anatomical elaborations also offer little that is new[113]. Just as ar-Rāzī and 'Ali ibn al-'Abbās did, he correctly gave the number of teeth as 32, and likewise states the possible absence of the third molar. At the same time, however, he

[113] Ibn Sīnā I 1, 5, 1, 4/5 p. 26, 27—28, 18

accepted without question the mistaken belief in a divided mandible[114].
Ibn Sīnā explained the methods for prophylaxis and treatment of pain in great detail. Referring to this, the Qānūn reads: *He who wishes that his teeth be healthy, must observe eight things: (1) that he avoid an abundance of decay of food and drink in the stomach,* (first) *because of* (perishable) *substances in the food matter, as there are quickly spoiling things such as milk, salted fish, and small salted fish,* (and second) *because of incorrect diet, which is discussed in its place; (2) that he not vomit, above all when it is something that would be sour in vomiting; (3) that he avoid chewing all hard things, particularly if they are sweet, such as nāṭif, figs, and mastic; (4) that he avoid cracking hard things, (5) narcotic things, (6) very cold things, particularly immediately after hot, and all hot things, particularly immediately after cold ones; (7) that he undertake continuous cleaning, however,* (without too much) *thoroughness or repetition, so that it does not damage the jaw tissue or the tissue between the teeth, or pull it out, or loosen the teeth; (8) that he avoid things which can damage the teeth by their very nature, such as, for example, leeks; this is all because damage to teeth and gingiva is great, as we have said in detail*[115].
This passage brings together in collected form all that had already appeared in individual Arabic predecessors and which is generally regarded as valid. We remember aṭ-Ṭabarī's therapy for mouth odor: cleaning of the teeth and stomach of rotting substances[116]; and Ḥunain, quoted by ar-Rāzī, who set down detailed measures for quickly perishable things in the stomach, for eating sweets for the debilitating effect of hot and cold foods in sequence, and for cleaning of the teeth[118], and Ibn al-Ǧazzār, who had already agreed on the result of a sequence of hot and cold, and who warned in his chapter on mouth odor against eating *bad things such as dates and milk products and others*[119], and who prescribed cleaning the stomach of rotten liquids. All this, however, became known in the West for the first time through the Qānūn of Ibn Sīnā.
As in ar-Rāzī and al-Ǧazzār[120], toothache is caused by a diseased constellation of humors, for which—and this is apparently one of Ibn Sīnā's own conclusions—the different discolorations of the teeth are an indicator: yellow points to bile, white to phlegm, red to blood, and black to black bile as the pain-causing substance. Pain also occurs, however, with fever, through the evil worm, as it is found in ar-Rāzī's al-Hāwī, through caries and gingival swelling[121]. The cause at the time being must be researched as exactly as possible before treatment.
The treatment for toothache is correspondingly multi-faceted, beginning Hippocratically with bleeding and purging. The prescriptions are to contain "desiccating remedies", because the teeth—this is also already verified by ar-Rāzī—have a *dry nature*[122]. *And it is often necessary to drill through the tooth with a thin drill, in order to remove the damaging materia from it and to help the medication penetrate to its base*[123]. This is a practice which had been recommended first by Archigenes, later on by Galen, and ar-Rāzī[124]. Grains of mustard seed are helpful against the throbbing pain, and exterior bandages should, according to ar-Rāzī, draw the "materia" (the pus) from the jaws[125].
Cauterization also should take place, with hot oil containing solvents, whereby again trepanation before cauterization allows better deep penetration[126]. Here, too, reference must be made to ar-Rāzī[127]. If these agents do not help, then recourse may be taken to narcotic medications also. These should not, however, reach the stomach, a possibility that ar-Rāzī had already warned against[128]. These are familiar agents, such as henbane, opium, styrax fumigating resin, galbanum, asafetida, mandrake, and philonium (?), applied as a poultice on the tooth, for flushing or fumigation of the mouth: according to al-Ǧazzār's advice, rose oil is dripped into the ear at the same time[129].
A further therapy was suggested again by ar-Rāzī: *Among all the things that anesthetize*

[114] Ibid. I 1, 5, 1, 4 p. 28, 2; see pp. 94 and 95
[115] Ibid. II 7 p. 184, 20—28
[116] See p. 91
[117] See p. 92
[118] See p. 96
[119] al-Gazzār, Chapter 23, p. 93
[120] See pp. 93 and 96
[121] See p. 93
[122] See p. 92
[123] Ibn Sīnā II 7 p. 186, 13 f.
[124] See pp. 74, 76 and 93
[125] Ibn Sīnā II 7 p. 188, 19—26
[126] Ibid. II 7 p. 188, 29—189, 1
[127] ar-Rāzī (a) III p. 96, 11 f.
[128] See p. 93: Ibn Sīnā II 7 p. 186, 13
[129] See pp. 96 f.

without harm, there is cold water with ice, which cools deeply when it is taken in the mouth slowly until the tooth is deadened and the pain stilled, even if it increases at the outset[130]; ar-Rāzī had recommended the same therapy with snow[131]. Ibn Sīnā filled carious teeth with cypress grass, mastix, myrrh, or styrax, among others, with gall-nuts, dyer's buckthorn, opium, galbanum, yellow sulfur, pepper, camphor, as well as with the drugs for fighting pain which we mostly already know, just as we know of the application of wolf's milk and arsenic from al-Ǧazzār[132]. Arsenic boiled in oil should be dripped into the carious defect itself[133].

Like his predecessors, Ibn Sīnā approved tooth extraction only conditionally. At first it must be determined exactly, whether the tooth itself is causing the pain and not the gingiva, because the extraction would not help otherwise—see the regulations of Abū l-Qāsim[134]. Also, extraction should only be done for one reason: because, in the opinion of the author, the diseased tooth might infect its surroundings. Firmly rooted teeth may not be extracted at once, because fractures of the jaw, eye pain, and fever may appear. First, the surrounding area is scarified, and then loosening takes place with corrosives derived primarily from ar-Rāzī[135], such as bark of mulberry root, ground with pellitory and thickened with strong vinegar in the sun to the consistency of honey. This extract is spread daily on the root region. Or, pellitory with vinegar, steeped for four days in the sun, is dropped into the fissures; this must act for 1 to 2 hours, and afterwards be plated with wax, *then it* (the tooth) *is drawn out and removed*[136]. Further agents, made known in part by ar-Rāzī, are pellitory with squirting cucumber or arsenic boiled in vinegar[137], the mixture of fig roots—'Alī ibn al-'Abbās loosened teeth with fig juice as well[138]—colocynthis, caper, yellow arsenic, wolf's milk and similar compositions in which yellow arsenic often recurs. For the so-called painless extraction, ar-Rāzī's frogfat turns up again[139]: *With reference to how a rotten tooth is crumbled away, which is like the painless extraction: knead flour with the milk of wolf's milk. Put this mash on it* (the tooth) *for several hours, and it will thus crumble. Also, the leaves of the great bitter lablab plant must be laid upon it, and fat from the tree frog, which has a strong crumbling effect. This frog is the green one, which lives on plants and trees and leaps from tree to tree*[140]. Later, John of Gaddesden is to refer to this passage[141].

The great Ibn Sīnā also firmly maintains the stereotype of henbane fumigations as a remedy for the toothworm, just as we have already found in al-Ǧazzār[142]: *Take four grains each of henbane and leek seeds and two and a half onions, knead it with goat-fat until it is smooth, and make pills from it with a weight of one dirham; burn one pill in a funnel under a covering of the patient's head*[143].

Teeth that have grown too long are filed down, an old tradition which extends from Galen through ar-Rāzī to Abū l-Qāsim[144], but only after application of astringents[145]. Gingival abscesses are caused by the *bad materials which come to it* (the gingiva) *from the head or stomach*[146], which is explained in particular detail by Ibn al-Ǧazzār. They are treated initially by blood-letting and cooling, astringent rinses such as rose and myrtle water, olive and mastix oil, and others. *This has a restricting effect* (on the inflammation), *is mild, and is above all useful for pain*[147]. Bleeding gingiva either can be left to stop by itself, or be treated with olive leaf water, wine yeast, rue juice, or other materials applied directly. Hot, deeply situated abscesses, which cannot be treated with purgative medications, but continue to fester, are to be poulticed daily with copper acetate and gall-nut, together with a layer of burned copper or with finely chopped gall-nut and vitriol. This is all to be found predominantly in ar-Rāzī[148]. If nothing of this sort helps and the gingiva begins to atrophy, then he advises cauterization: *Take boiling oil on a small bit of rolled wool, and apply it repeatedly, until it* (the sore) *diminishes and becomes white*[149].

130 Ibn Sīnā II 7 p. 189. 22 f.
131 ar-Rāzī (a) III p. 127, 1—3
132 See p. 96
133 Ibn-Sīnā II 7 p. 190, 28—191, 2
134 See p. 97
135 See p. 94
136 Ibid. II 7 p. 192, 3—17
137 See pp. 93 f.
138 See p. 92
139 See p. 94
140 Ibid. II 7 p. 192, 30 f.
141 See p. 127
142 See p. 96
143 Ibid. II 7 p. 192, 30—32
144 See pp. 73 and 89
145 Ibid. II 7 p. 193, 5 f.
146 Ibid. II 7 p. 194, 2 f.
147 Ibid. II 8 p. 194, 10 f.
148 ar-Rāzī (a) III p. 110. 114; p. 141, 4; p. 150, 19; etc.
149 Ibn-Sīnā II 8 p. 194, 16 f.

The treatment of jaw fractures and luxations is also exhaustively described, and proceeds, in the framework of the ancient tradition, according to Paulos, as it was taken from Abū l-Qāsim[150]. For reducting of the fracture, Ibn Sīnā writes: *If it* (the jaw) *is broken inwards, but not in two pieces, then insert the index finger and middle finger of the left hand into the patients mouth if the right jaw is broken* (the corresponding fingers) *of the right hand if the left jaw is broken, and lift the arch of the fracture with them towards the outside, and receive it on the outside with the other hand and make it even; you will recognize the correct position by the straight position of the teeth which are in it*[151]. A complete fracture (*in two pieces),* on the other hand, must first be stretched and then brought into its proper position. Wounds caused by bone splinters are to be sutured after removal of the splinters. Finally a supporting dressing is put arround the jaw, head, and neck, and a light splint is applied upon it. Correct positioning of the teeth must not be forgotten here; if necessary, they should be fixed with gold wires. If sores appear, the dressing must be removed and the jaw treated with hot compresses. According to Ibn Sīnā, as well as according to Abū l-Qāsim and current experience, the healing process as a rule takes about three weeks[152].

Setting of dislocations of the jaw should take place as emphasized also by Abū l-Qāsim,[153] as soon as possible, before the jaw hardens and induces fever and sharp headaches. *And sometimes the matter is so serious, that death ensues on the tenth day*[154]. Hardening that has already appeared should first be softened with hot compresses. Resetting follows after a sudden stretching with one pull. This reduction, too, is supported with a bandage spread over with wax and rose oil[155].

These few examples from dentistry already show to what extent the Qānūn relies on the Arabic medicine of its predecessors and largely only arranges and compiles the knowledge of its time in encyclopedic fashion. Still, Ibn Sīnā was regarded both by his contemporaries and by the European Middle Ages, whose scholastic method of thought largely accomodated itself to his, as an authority in medicine as unassailable as Galen was for the ancients. The later revisions, commentaries, and numerous translations of the Qānūn by themselves form a whole library. The most famous transcription into Latin is that by Gerard of Cremona, in the second half of the 12th century, about 150 years after the author's death[156].

With Abū l-Qāsim and Ibn Sīnā, the climax of Arabic-Persian medicine had been reached. In conjunction with the gradual regression of the Islamic nation's world power, initiated by Mongol attacks and furthered by internal dissent, Arabic science thereafter declined as well. In dental medicine, there are only a few other names to be mentioned, such as that of the Jewish philosopher and physician Ibn Maimūn (Maimonides), born in Cordoba, who transferred the knowledge of Spanish-Moorish medicine to Egypt. In his works, there are herb prescriptions for toothache, for tooth extraction without forceps, and for oral and dental care[157].

It can be inferred from the "Report about Egypt", written in about 1200 in Baghdad by 'Abd al-Laṭīf, a theologian, philosopher and later opponent of Ibn Sīnā, that the wisdom of the ancients was not, after all, always unquestionably. A finding of approximately 20,000 skeletons, probably stemming from a period of famine or plague, moved the author to the following observation concerning the bones of the mandible: *All anatomists agree in saying that this jaw is composed of two bones, which are firmly united at the chin. When I say "all anatomists" here, it is actually as though I say "Galen completely alone", because he, by himself, personally carried out the anatomical investigations . . . Observation of this part of the cadaver has convinced us that the mandibular bone is a single bone, and that it has neither a joint nor a seam. We have repeated this observation many times, with over 200 heads. We have used all possible means to assure ourselves of the truth of it, and we have never found more than one single bone*[158]. Here we have therefore at last a correction of the false Hippocratic and Galenic hypothesis of the divided mandible which has not, however, been accepted.

Nor was the belief in the toothworm generally accepted, as can be seen from the report of a

150 See p. 81
151 Ibid. III 5. 3. 2 p. 211, 9—12
152 Ibid. III 5. 3. 2 p. 211, 12—25
153 See p. 102
154 Ibid. III 5. 1. 7 p. 188, 33—189, 1
155 Ibid. III 5. 1. 7 p. 189, 1—10
156 See pp. 117 f. and, e.g., 119
157 Khalifah (b)
158 Artelt

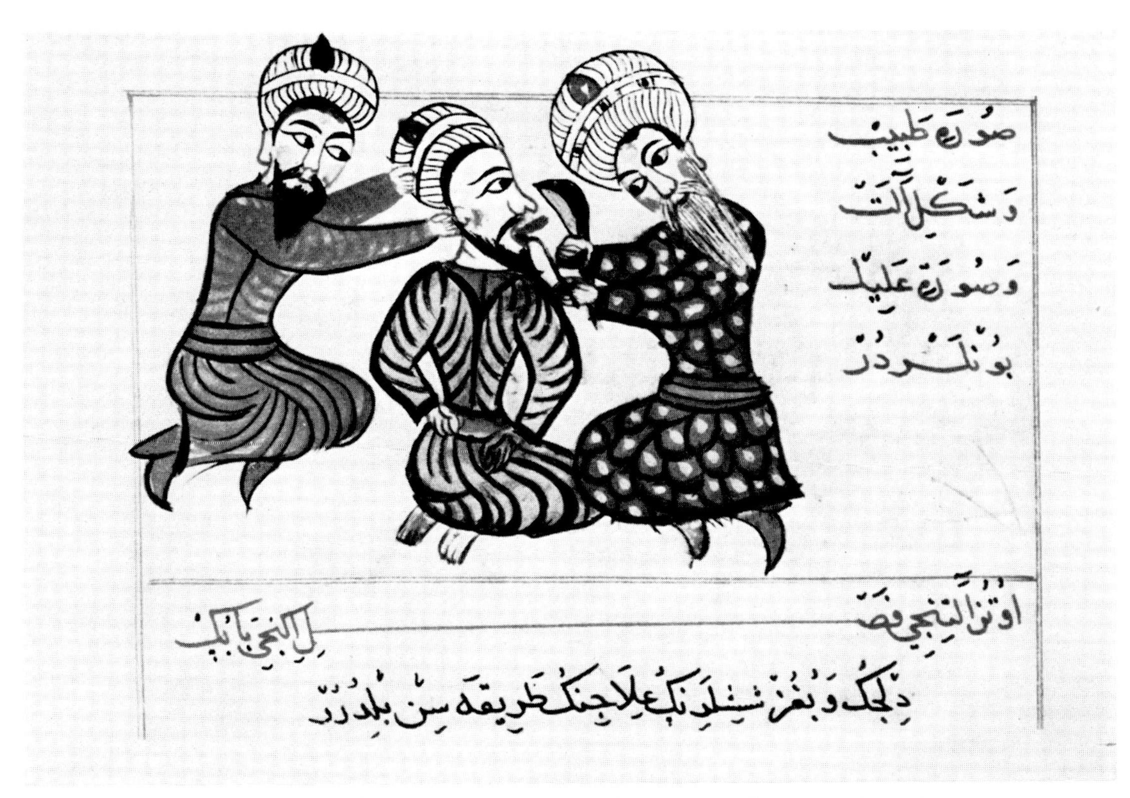

Fig. 83 *Scheref ed-Din Sabuncuoğlu: Operation for a ranula, 1465 (from Huard and Gremek)*

certain Ğ a u b a r ī, who lived around 1200. His "Book of the Elite concerning the Unmasking of Mysteries and Tearing of Veils" contains a chapter about dentistry. In it there were revealed a quantity of tricks with which pretended toothworms (fruit maggots, dissected camel sinews) were placed into the patient's mouth and then shown as the toothworms which were causing the pain. These were things, therefore, which in the opinion of the author *did not even exist*[159].

Also of some importance are the odontological chapters from the surgical textbook by I b n a l - Q u f f, who was active in Damascus in the 13th century. The section on anatomy and physiology is based almost completely on A b ū l - Q ā - s i m; here, too, the mandible is divided. In tooth extraction, I b n a l - Q u f f however, is even more cautious than his great predecessor; he prescribes first the known corrosives containing arsenic. Only if these do not help should the tooth be extracted, and then only after a preparatory blood-letting and exposure of the root *in a vertical direction* with the forceps. *Be advised, too, that sometimes another tooth can grow around the molar*, probably a paramolar; then a means must be sought to pull the tooth out[160]. Loose teeth should be bound with gold wire. *A tooth may also be taken of bone or ivory, set in the site of a tooth which has fallen out, and affixed with the tie mentioned in the fashion suggested*[161]. The cauterizing iron so preferred in Islamic medicine because it was not bleeding, should, according to 'A l ī i b n a l - 'A b b ā s, be brought to the painful tooth through a copper

[159] Wiedemann (a and b)
[160] Spies and Müller-Bütow pp. 142 f.; the authors were poorly advised when they termed the extra tooth a "dens in dente." This externally hardly perceptible invagination malformation which occurs practically exclusively on maxillary lateral incisors, was not known at a time when the existence of tooth pulp was not even known. The initial description of the malformation occured in the 19th century
[161] Spies; Spies and Müller-Bütow, pp. 144 f.

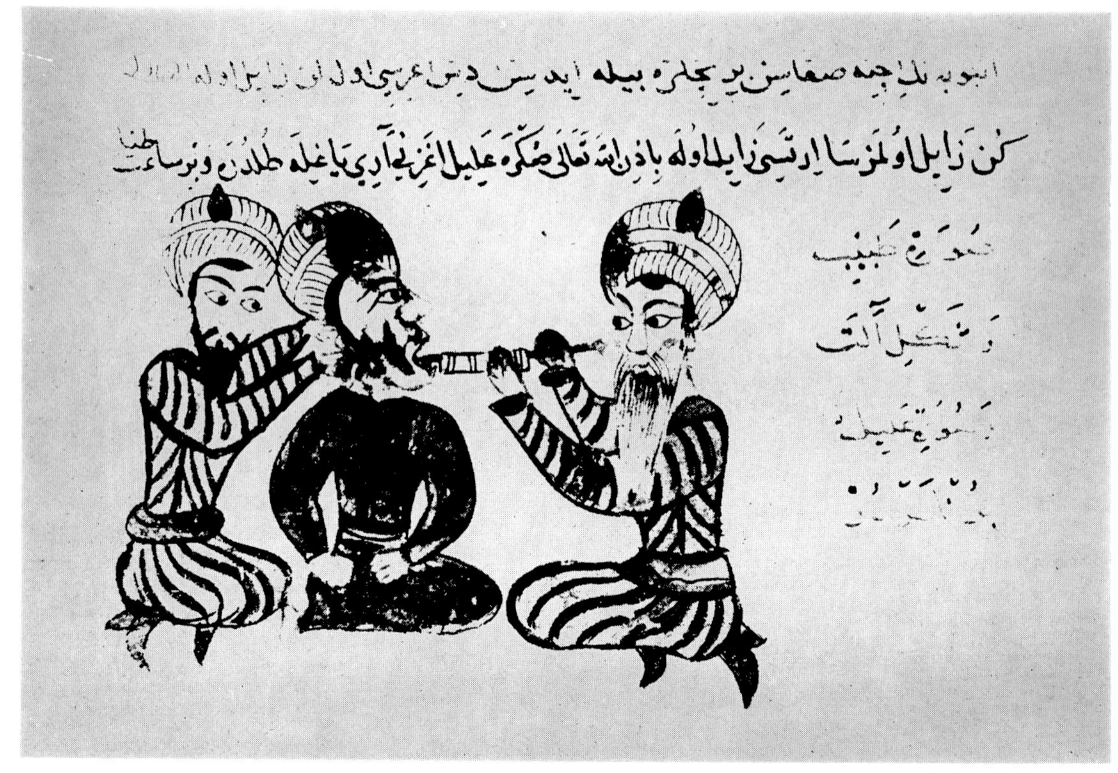

Fig. 84 *Scheref ed-Din Sabuncuoğlu: Cauterization of the dental pulp through a cannula, 1465 (from Huard and Gremek)*

tube. A collection of prescriptions included contains the customary mixtures known from ancient times, increased by some Arabic specialties.

Ibn al-Quff thus did not bring any new insights to the subject, compared with the comprehensive works of his predecessors. The reluctance to proceed with a tooth extraction, observed with few exceptions in all the ancients, remained in effect. All conceivable corrosive agents for loosening of the tooth through medication were utilized in order to avoid using the forceps.

Since the 9th century, the central Asian nomad and equestrian peoples of Turks had filtered into the Arabian world. After adopting Islam, these concentrated under the ruling clan of the Ottomans on an Asia Minor divided by power politics, and conquered parts of the decaying Byzantine Empire as well. In 1354, the Straits of the Dardanelles were crossed and extensive areas of the Balkans made to pay tribute, so that a century later (1453), a surrounded Constantinople fell to Sultan Mehmed II, the Conqueror, like a ripe fruit. Like old Byzantium, Istanbul became a political and cultural hub again, this time of the Ottoman Empire, whose armies forged their way to the gates of Vienna in the 16th century.

Under the culturally tolerant government of Mehmed II, it was even possible that in 1465 a medical work could appear, complete with human diagrams written by the Turkish physician Scheref ed-Din Sabuncuoğlu. In organization and content this adhered very closely to Abū l-Qāsim[162]. Many of the colored pictures, presumably drawn by the author himself[163], have to do with stomatological procedures, such as the excision of a ranula (Fig. 83).

[162] Huard and Grzemek
[163] Terzioglu (b)

Also represented is the cauterization of painful pulp through 'Ali ibn al-'Abbās' protective cannula (Fig. 84).

In the 16th century, in which the first books completely dealing with dental medicine appeared in Germany (1530), in Spain (1557), and in Italy (1563)[164], there is also a manuscript in the Turkish contemporary literature especially devoted to this subject. Its author was the Jewish physician Moses Hamon, a court physician of Suleiman II, the Magnificent. Hamon's father, also a physician, had emigrated to Turkey from Granada, in anti-Semitic Spain. In the 101 pages of his manuscript, Hamon preferred drug therapy for oral diseases, supporting his conclusions in part by his own experience[165].

Seen as a whole, Arabian-Persian medicine up to the end of the 12th century must be regarded as the definitive pinnacle of the medical sciences of the Middle Ages. To be sure, certain restraints were imposed on its development by the teachings of Islam, because dissection of corpses and even pictorial representations of the human body were forbidden, and thus the possibilities for anatomical research were greatly limited. Also, the aversion to blood, and the preference given to the cautery iron that stemmed from it, placed limits on surgical activity. Howewer, Islamic medical works acquire a special value because they are based on well-founded sources, i. e., on direct translations of Hippocrates, Galen, and others. Beyond this, they were able to correct anatomical mistakes and to develop therapy and extend it on their own, through which, above all, pharmacology flourished.

The particular importance of Islamic medicine for the further development of the healing arts lies in the fact that their Persian and Arabian authors repaid with compound interest the ancient treasures of the West, which they had preserved and increased. Herewith they formed the fundamental base for the European medicine of the high Middle Ages.

[164] See pp. 159 f.; 151 f.; 141 f.
[165] Hamon; Terzioglu (a)

The author wishes to thank Frau Jutta Schoenfeld, PhD, from 1970 to 1976 in the Institute for the History of Medicine of the Free University of Berlin, for her tireless aid, so that we could quote throughout from the original Arabic sources instead of from Latin translations, as previously. She also reworked the manuscript and revised the literature statements from the perspective of an Arabist.

References

Abū l-Qāsim (Albucasis)
a) De Chirurgia, arabice et latine. Cura Johannis Channing, Oxonii 1778
b) On surgery and instruments. A definitive ed. of the Arabic text with English transl. and commentary by M. S. Spink and G. L. Lewis. London 1973

'Ali ibn al-'Abbās (Haly Abbas)
Kamil aṣ-Sinā 'a at-tibbīya (= Kitāb al-Malaki) Būlaq 1294 h. =

Kamil aṣ-Sinā 'a at-tibbīya (= Kitāb al-Malaki. The complete book of medical art) Vol. II, Būlaq 1294 h. = 1877 A. D.

Artelt, Walter
"Ossa mandibulae inferioris duo". Sudhoff's Arch. Gesch. Med. Naturw. 39 (1955) 193—215

Galen
Claudii Galeni opera omnia. Ed. C. G. Kühn, 20 vols., Leipzig 1821—1833

ibn al-Ǧazzār
Kitāb Zād al-musāfir wa-qūt al-ḥāḍir (Provisions for the traveller and nutritions for the sedentary). Ms. Kopenhagen Arab. 109

Gurlt, E(rnst)
Geschichte der Chirurgie. Vol. I, Berlin 1898

Hamarneh, Sami
Thirteenth century interprets connection between arteries and veins. Sudhoffs Arch. 46 (1962) 17—26

Hamon, Moses
Kompendium der Zahnheilkunde. Ed. Arslan Terzioglu, München 1977

al-Ḫaṭīb al-Baġdādī
Kitāb Tarīḫ. Baġdād. Vol. 8. Kairo 1349 h. = 1931 A. D.

Huard, Pierre, Mirko Drazen Grmek
Le premier manuscrit chirurgical turc. Paris 1960

Ibn Sīnā (Avicenna)
a) al-Qānūn fī ṭ-ṭibb. Druck Būlāq 1294 h. = 1877 A. D.
b) Canon medicinae. Venetiis 1507

Khalifah, Elias S.
a) Arabian description of dental caries in the 10th century. J. Am. Dent. Ass. 24 (1937) 1847—1852
b) Dentistry in the 12th century as revealed in the medical writings of Maimonides. Brit. Dent. J. 67 II (1939) 133—139

Khalifah, Elias, Sami I. Haddad
Dental gleanings from arabian medicine. J. Am. Dent. Ass. 24 (1937) 944—955

Lane. Edward William
Arabic-English Lexicon, Part V. London 1874

Mayerhof, Max
Arabic tooth-worm stories. Bull. Hist. Med. 17 (1945) 203—204

Rasslan, Wassel
Mohammed und die Medizin nach der Überlieferung. Abh. Gesch. Med. Naturw. 1, Berlin 1934

ar-Rāzī (Rhazes)
a) Kitāb al-Ḥāwī fī ṭ-ṭibb (Continens). Vol. III, Haiderabad 1955
b) Trois traitês d'anatomie arabes, pp. 3—88. Ed. and transl. P(ieter) de Koning, Leiden 1903

Spies, Otto
Beiträge zur Geschichte der arabischen Zahnheilkunde. Sudhoffs Arch. Gesch. Med. Naturw. 46 (1962) 153—177

Spies, Otto; Horst Müller-Bütow
Anatomie und Chirurgie des Schädels, insbes. der Hals-, Nasen- u. Ohrenkrankheiten. Berlin, New York 1971

Sudhoff, Karl
Chirurgie im Mittelalter. Vol. II, Leipzig 1918

Terzioglu, Arslan
a) Eine bisher unbekannte türk. Abhandlung über die Zahnhk. des Moses Hamon aus dem Anfang des 16. Jahrhunderts. Sudhoffs Arch. 58 (1974) 276—282
b) Die alt-türkische Zahnheilkunde unter bes. Berücksichtigung der türk. Handschrift des Moses Hamon über die Zahnheilkunde. Zahnärztl. Mitt. 65 (1975) 179—188

Ullmann, Manfred
Die Medizin im Islam. Leiden, Köln 1970

Wiedemann, Eilhard
a) Schwindeleien des 13. Jahrhunderts mit angeblichen Zahnwürmern. Beiträge zur Gesch. d. Naturw. Erlangen 26 (1911) 223—225
b) Über Scharlatane unter den arabischen Zahnärzten und über die Wertschätzung des Zahnstochers bei den muslimischen Völkern. Korresp. bl. Zahnärzte 43 (1914) 231—236
c) Über Zahnpflege bei den muslimischen Völkern. Dtsch. Mschr. Zahnheilk. 36 (1918) 362—366

Chapter 8

High and Late Middle Ages in Europe

Around the turn of the 8th to the 9th century, the caliphate of the Abbasids reached the high point of its power. At the same time, the Occident was united into a political unit, even if only temporarily, by Charlemagne. Diplomatic contacts were established between the Emperor and Harūn ar-Rašīd, but they still did not result in an influence by the flourishing Islamic medicine on Europe.

In the 11th century, when the universal empire of the Germans under the Hohenstaufen fell into conflict with the Holy See, the Normans who had occupied southern Italy since Carolingian times expanded their national state with papal permission. In this area, the relations to Byzantium had never been disrupted, so that the early phase of the medical school in Salerno[1] was stamped with Greek influence. The connections to the Islamic world, however, also were maintained. Through this situation, an event took place which was decisive for the medicine of the high and late Middle Ages: the first acceptance of the Islamic healing arts and thus the overcoming of the monastic medicine of the early Middle Ages. Through Arabic mediation parts of the ancient authors were made newly available to the West, in particular an Arabized Galen. Here was a language capable of abstraction, which oriented itself to the written Latin of their time, and for which Gariopont[2] in Salerno and especially Alphanus, the Archbishop of Salerno, were prepared. This latter, an author of theological essays and poems, had also composed and translated medical tracts. The Latin he used then was a tool, with which medicine became scientific to the degree that was already a tradition among the "Liberal Arts" since the late ancient times. The man who made this flourishing possible in Salerno was Constantinus Africanus. Born between 1010 and 1015 in Carthage, he probably received his education in Baghdad, although we do not know of any medical training. As a widely-travelled merchant and drug trader, he came to Salerno after 1065. His contact with Alphan began there, as shown by the dedication of Constantine's essay "De stomacho" to him. Alphan must also have stimulated him to translate the works of Arabian authors into Latin, and he was also the one who recommended Constantine to Desiderius, the Abbot of the Benedictine monastery of Montecassino[3]. We know with certainty that Constantinus Africanus prepared further translations there from the Arabic into Latin as a monk, particularly of the great compendium of Arabism, the "Royal Book" (liber regalis), by 'Alī ibn al-'Abbās (Haly Abbas), which he likewise dedicated to Desiderius, and of the "Handbook for Travellers" (Viaticum), by Ibn al-Ǧazzār.

Both these works contain odontological sections too. In dental anatomy, Constantine took the correct Galenic conviction that humans had 32 teeth[4] from 'Alī ibn al-'Abbās, whereby he breaks with the assumption of the early Middle Ages, that women had only 30. The Arabian differentiation of the incisors is also found in Constantine. According to this, the middle ones are called "dentes pares" (paired), and the lateral ones "dentes quadrupli" (four-corned)[5]. The conception of the divided lower jaw taken from 'Alī ibn al-'Abbās was of Galenic derivation[6], just as the origin of toothache from hot and rotten humors which descend from the head was taken from ancient sources[7]. Thus, he continues from an Arabian source the humoral-pathological theory that was prevalent in the early middle ages. Only a small degree of originality can be ascertained, although originality was claimed in the preface to the "Theorica."[8]

In the 5th book of the "Practica", Constantine used his own translation of Ibn al-Ǧazzār's "Viaticum."[9] In contrast to this Arabic source, however, the same arsenic composition for removal of a tooth were not applied to the alveolar process, but rather put *into these*

[1] See p. 86
[2] See p. 86
[3] Creutz
[4] Const. Afr. (a) II 3 p. 6ar 18 f. Lugduni = p. 29, 8 f. Basileae
[5] Const. Afr. (a) II 3 p. 5bv 64 L. = p. 28, 29 B; see Fonahn p. 51; see pp. 95 f.
[6] Const. Afr. (a) II 3 p. 6ar, 10 f. L = p. 29, 1 f. B.
[7] Const. Afr. (b) II 18 p. 150ar, 49—51 L. = 37, 20 f. B.
[8] Const. Afr. (a) II 1 p. 1ar, 22—27 L.
[9] Nord pp. 8 f.

holes[10], as recommended by 'Alī ibn al-'Abbās[11]. Thus, we find here for the first time in the West a recommendation for an arsenic filling as pain reliever, regardless of the uncertain passage by Rufus[12]. This method was unfortunately lost and only made known in 1836 to the world again[13].

Otherwise, Constantine incorporated this and the following prescriptions of the translation of the "Viaticum" in his text from the "Practica" with the additional suggestion that the corrosive agents be put in a wax coating for protection of the neighboring teeth, in a fashion similar to what we have read in Pliny. He also mentions here the raven manure, which we know of from the same source[15], and the toothworm, this again borrowed from al-Ǧazzār[16].

The only surgical procedure found here is tooth extraction, of course, to be applied only after remedial applications have failed. He also insists that before the performance, just as with the ancients[17], the gingiva be loosened from the bone[18]. Thus, through the agency of important Arabian authors, Constantinus Africanus provided the basis for the development of European odontology and dental medicine.

In the 12th century, instruction in medicine began in Salerno on an academic level[19], which we encounter in completed form in the medical laws issued from 1231 to 1243 by the Hohenstaufen Emperor, Frederick II. These decrees are among the legislative work of this outstanding monarch, with which this man ahead of his time was able, at an intersection point of Greek, Islamic, Latin, and Norman culture, to form a modern state from the Sicilian kingdom of his grandfather, the Norman King Roger. King Roger's regulations for a physician's examination of 1140 show that these medical laws might reflect older requirements. Frederick II's statues, with their requirement of a three-year philosophy curriculum, demonstrate features of early scholasticism, but practical experience also was held to be important. This is shown especially in the inclusion of surgery in both the medical curriculum and in a comparable state examination for the Master's degree in medicine and surgery. Only those who had studied this program and also practiced medicine and anatomy naturally on animals for at least one year were allowed to practice surgery[20].

Dental anatomy, however, was not dealt with in the first Salernitan manuals on animal dissection. Only in an illustrated anatomy text rooted originally in the Greek-Oriental tradition is the number of teeth correctly stated as 32, as in Constantine[21] (Fig. 85). In the earliest Salernitan surgical text, the so-called Bamberger Surgery dating from the beginning of the 12th century, there is to be found for the last time for centuries the concept current in ancient times and in the Middle Ages (not, however, among the Arabs) that men have 32 teeth and women have 30[22]. This is planily traceable to the Vindician passage, and is, besides, so corrupted that men are called "duribarbi;" through this, we can ascertain as an exact prototype that particular edition of Vindicianus in which eunuchs were designated as "duribarbi"[23] and had, according to him, 30 teeth just as women did.

Yet all this remains the exception in Salerno. At the beginning of the 12th century, Magister Platearius designated the molars as "dentes maxillares"[24]. Remarks concerning the odontogenesis are rare. Only in one early-scholastic anatomical manual, the "Anatomy" of Magister Urso from the second half of the 12th century, the formation of the teeth is assumed to be from phlegm (mucus)[25].

In the area of therapy only Constantinian material was passed on at first. This holds true for the "Practicae" of the Salernitan Magistri Joannes Afflacius, Joannes Platearius, Archimatthaeus, Copho, Trottus, and Bartholomaeus. The reason is that the subject of dental medicine was an exception in Salerno and because it contained no actual innovations. In these authors, there are only to be found some components of Arabian pharmacopoeia, and their therapy differed at times from that of Constantinus Africanus. Johannes Platearius even claimed to have seen toothworms when the tooth was washed whith lukewarm water[26]. There

10 Const. Afr. (b) II 19 p. 150b^r, 53 L. = p. 39, 5 B.
11 See p. 95
12 See p. 75
13 See p. 312
14 Const. Afr. (c) V 48 p. 102a^v, 14—28 L.
15 See p. 73
16 Const. Afr. (b) II 19 p. 150b^r, 43 f. L. =p. 38, 36 f. B.
17 See p. 70
18 Const. Afr. (c) V 48 p. 102a^v, 18 f. L.
19 See p. 86
20 Hein Tit. 44 p. 48; tit. 46 p. 50
21 Sudhoff (a)
22 Sudhoff (b) p. 109; see Langebartels p. 19
23 See p. 78
24 Tract. de aegr. cur. p. 146, 4
25 Urso p. 42

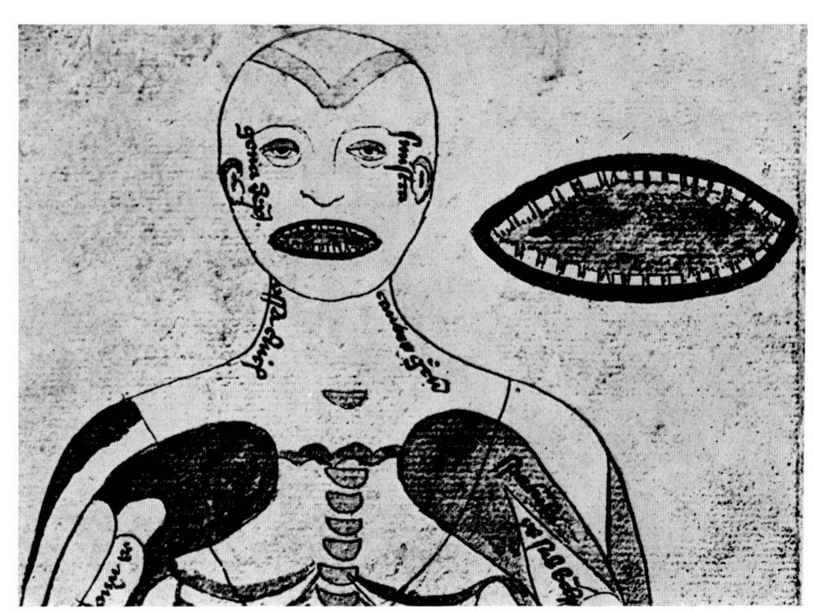

Fig. 85 *Section of the bone drawing of a Bohemian manuscript (from Sudhoff a)*

were also regulations which provide evidence for the continence of folk medicine, as with B a r t h o l o m a e u s[27]: he recommended, for example, the external use of burnt onion into which pepper powder had been put previously. Some of these practices have only been preserved for us in compilations of the so-called "Tractatus de aegritudinum curatione" (Tract on the Healing of Diseases), the famous manuscript from the Magdalen-Gymnasium at Breslau, which is unfortunately lost today[28]. This contains, surely, excerpts from C o n s t a n t i n e, such as the chapters on toothache, loosening of the teeth, and calculus, in the diction found in the "Viaticum"[29], but for the most part it concerns texts from Salerno. The excerpt from J o a n n e s A f f l a c i u s is still dependent to a great extent on C o n s t a n t i n u s A f r i c a n u s[30]. T r o t t u s recommends cauterization with 'A l i i b n a l - 'A b b ā s' protective cannula[31] for toothache, and he uses a funnel for deadening the pain as in the early Middle Ages[32] to provide vapor from henbane seeds and, additionally, from leek[33]. It is uncertain whether the midwife's instruction book from Salerno, the so-called "Trotula," may be connected with Master T r o t t u s; in this, too, the customary liniments are recommended for toothache and for strengthening loose teeth[34].

The Salernitan Master C o p h o described damage to the gingiva as a result of using white lead as a face-paint. Through accumulation of lead sulfide, a bluish-black discoloration forms on the edge of the gingiva, a symptom observed still in recent times in workers of the lead processing industry which is clinically named leadline, or halo saturninus. The medication of liniment recommended by C o p h o, with agents for depilation containing arsenic, might have effected a corrosion of the gingiva with subsequent scar tissue formation, which he expressly mentioned[35].

Otherwise cauterization and medicated tooth removal remain the rule, and extraction is recommended only when these fail. Thus, J o a n n e s P l a t e a r i u s reported on the use of glowing ash-wood or small iron rods, which were inserted in a tooth cavity previously filled with theriac. With these two, the tooth can be levered out. As drug therapy before the extraction, he

[26] Platearius IV 4, p. 176br, 7—9
[27] Bartholomaeus pp. 380 f.
[28] Sudhoff (c)
[29] Tract. de aegr. cur. p. 181, 14—183, 3
[30] Ibid. p. 178, 36—40
[31] Ibid. p. 180, 27—29
[32] See p. 84
[33] Ibid. p. 181, 3—6
[34] Trotula 54
[35] Copho p. 478, 13—16; Sudhoff (d)

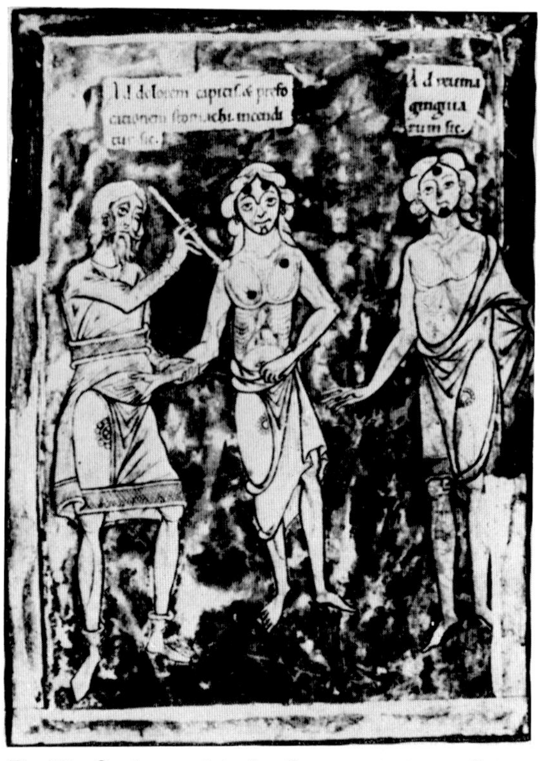

Fig. 86 *Cautery points for "reuma gingivarum" in a manuscript of the 12th century (British Museum Ms. Harley 1585, fol. 8^r)*

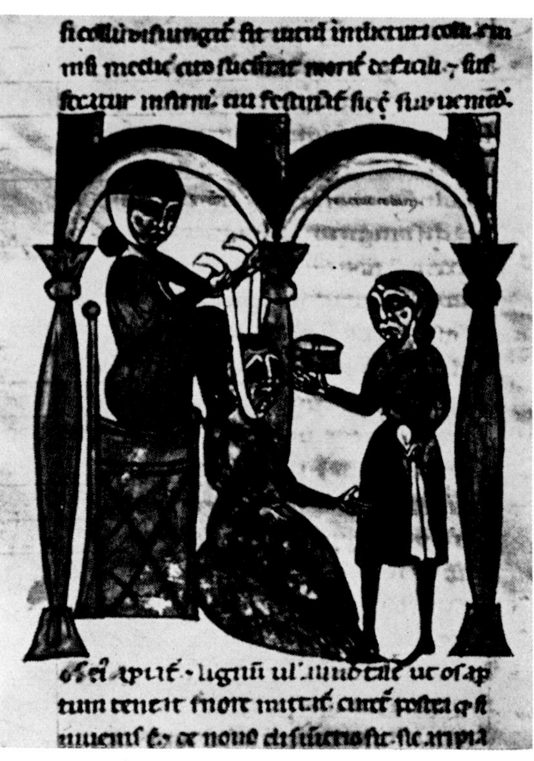

Fig. 88 *Placement of a bandage, from Roland's "Chirurgia" in a manuscript of the 13th century (Rome, Bibl. Casanatense, Ms. 1382, fol. 19^r)*

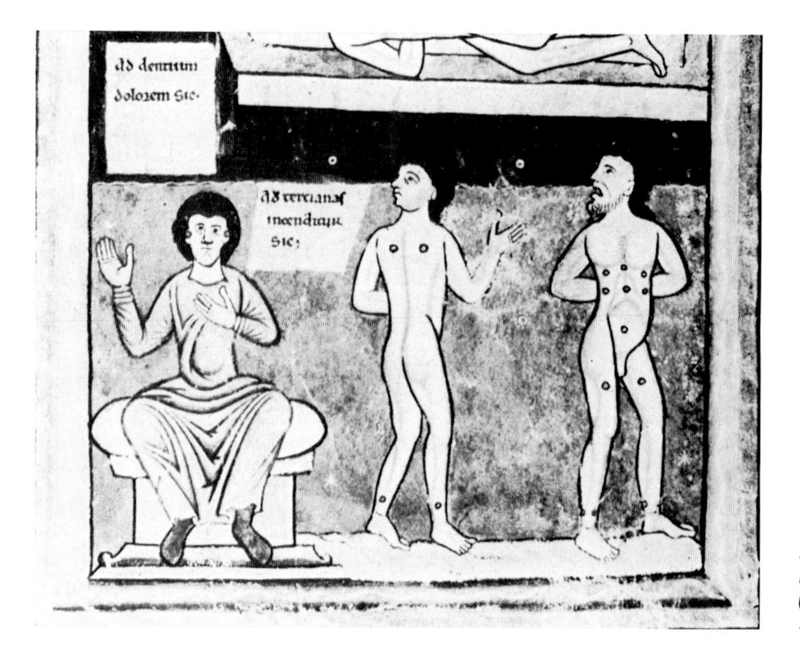

Fig. 87 *Cautery points for toothache, "ad dentium dolorem," in a manuscript of the 13th century (Oxford, Bodleian Library, Ms. Ashmole 1462, fol. 9^v)*

uses liniments with yeast, wolf's milk, and ivy or mulberry juice. He emphasizes the effectiveness of these expressly[36]. The frog-fat therapy taken from ar-Rāzī is also mentioned here for the first time in the occident. This is corroborated for Platearius in the "Thesaurus pauperum", the scanty manual by Petrus Hispanus intended for laymen: *Application of the body of the frog or its fat facilitates the extraction (evulsio) of teeth*[38]. Only when the preparatory medication has no effect Platearius extracts with forceps *correctly, with the patient's mouth open (aperto ore artificiose),* after thorough purging and bloodletting when the weather is fair[39]. In the excerpts from the "Tractatus de aegritudinum curatione," just these passages, however, have been changed. It is said of the liniments, that they never help[40], and of extraction, that it should be carried out *by a skilled workman (a perito artifice,* instead of *aperto ore artificiose).* Care also must be taken, and this is rightly added, that neither root nor stump of the tooth remain behind[41].

The mention of workmen seems to be a reference to assistance at tooth extraction by barber-surgeons. What makes it clear that the assistance is not meant here to be by surgeons is not only the designation "artifex," but also the evidence of 12th century Salernitan surgical literature, which makes no report of extracted teeth. The procedures are executed within the known limits such as, for example, cautery application to the temporomandibular joint or to the earlobe (Figs. 86 and 87).

Beyond this, the familiar henbane fumigation with the funnel is applied in the first "Chirurgie" based upon personal experience of the Salernitan Magister Roger. This procedure had become general knowledge to such a degree that it had been included even in the oldest edition of the "Regimen sanitatis Salernitanum," a late-Salernitan book of health rules which was as popular as it was primitive[44].

Thus, despite the advanced state of surgery in Salerno, no progress can be determined in operative dental medicine. Not even Roger's suggestion, deviating from customary practice, that in reducing a dislocated mandible the condyle of the joint be grasped in front of the ears and reduced, is a real advance[44a].

The surgical texts of the following century are influenced by marginal notes on the Roger text, which appeared soon after its writing. In them, cautery in the area of the tooth root is recommended, or application of a casing with ivy resin around the diseased tooth, in order to accelerate its falling out. In an extreme case, extraction should be performed, but only of a loose tooth —an already ancient requirement. Also old is the idea that tooth loosening caused by dissolving of humors and of the brain tissue[45]. These are surely no innovations, but these notes indicate that tooth extraction in Salerno was also in the hands of surgeons.

Dental materials is also found in the glosses properly of Roger, both in the "Glossulae of the four Masters" belonging to the Salerno school, and in the work of Roland of Parma, who was working in Bologna (Fig. 88). Both actually belong to the 13th century. Toothache[46], dislocation of the jaw[47] and fractures of the jaw are treated with reference to Roger. These texts do not include any new ideas, at least not in the stomatological chapters, except the recommendation of the "Glossulae of the four Masters" for repositioning of the luxated mandible by inserting a round peg on either side of the region of the molars to create fulcra[48].

Gilbertus Anglicus is occasionally quoted in Roland's work; he is not the chancellor of Montpellier, as claimed in some manuscripts, but rather a Magister Salernitanus from one of the two respected English Aquila families, who wrote his "Compendium medicinae" around 1240[49]. The stomatological chapter, to be sure, contains the old familiar henbane fumigation as a remedy for toothworm, but Gilbert also turns to extraction when the condition is advanced. He correctly regards it as possibly dangerous when pain is persistent and advises against scarification of the gingiva. If therapeutic treatment and narcotics fail to alleviate toothache, he offers the choice of either medi-

[36] Platearius IV 3 p. 176a^r, 52—176b^r, 2. The resin of the mulberry tree still is used to loosen teeth today by Ecuadorean Indians. See p. 85
[37] See p. 123
[38] Petrus Hisp. 15 p. 35^v, 6 f.
[39] Platearius IV 3 p. 176a^r, 58—61
[40] Tract. de aegr. cur. p. 172, 2
[41] Ibid. p. 176, 42—44
[42] Sudhoff (b) p. 143
[43] Ibid. p. 181
[44] Regimen san. Sa. (a) p. 242 f.; Löchel pp. 80 f. and 114 f.
[44a] Löchel pp. 74 f.
[45] Addendum to Roger's "Chirurgie" in: Collectio Salernitana, ed. de Renzi, Tomo II, Napoli 1853, p. 449, 20—22
[46] Gloss. Roger III 14 p. 677, 10—679, 23; Löchel pp. 184 f. and 150 f.
[47] Ibid. IV 9 p. 714, 28—715, 25; Löchel pp. 192 f. and 144 f.
[48] Ibid. III 1 p. 707, 19—709, 6; Löchel pp. 190 f., 146 f. and 194 f. See p. 82, footnote 29
[49] Talbot, Hammond pp. 58 f.

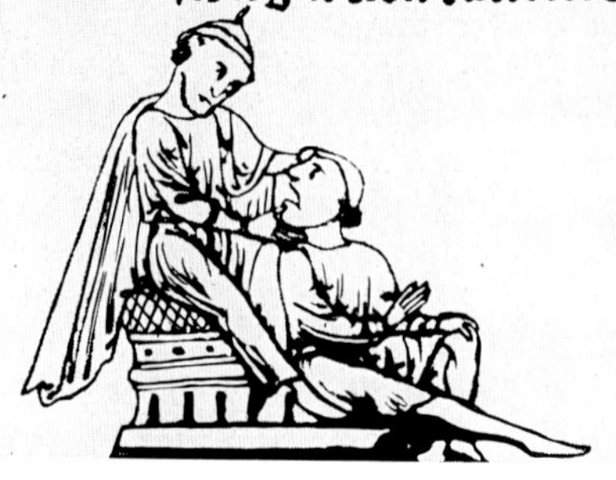

Fig. 89

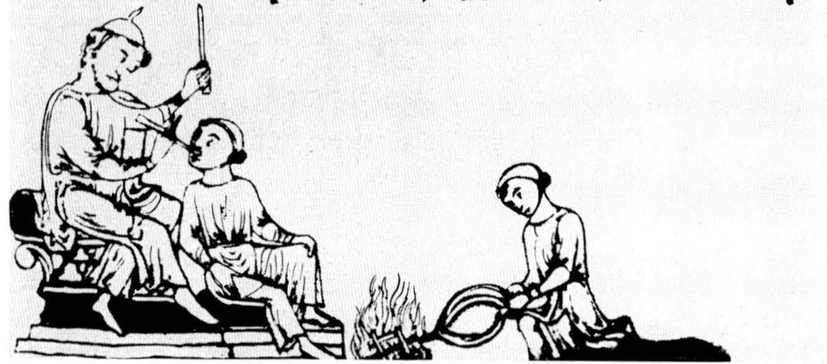

Fig. 90

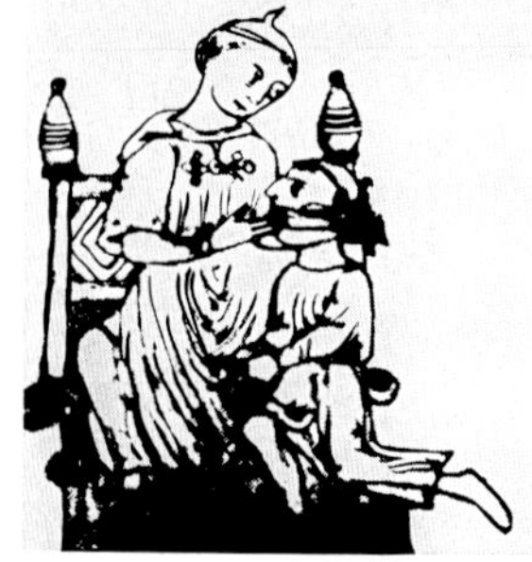

Fig. 91

Figs. 89 to 91 *Examination of the mouth, cauterization, and bandaging of the mouth in a French gloss on Roger, from the 13th century (Cambridge, Trinity College Ms. 0, I 20)*

camentous or operative tooth removal. He describes caries minutely, and his etiological differentiation makes sense: primary causes (causae primitivae), such as weaknesses in the teeth themselves, and secondary (causae derivativae), such as factors based in the organism or bits of food remaining between the teeth. He separates the secondary causes into internal and external ones. The internal ones, strictly humoral-pathologically speaking, point to a flow of evil humors from the brain or also from the stomach. This is because for Gilbert toothache is usually an accompanying symptom of other diseases.

Thus, with stomach diseases, the teeth of the mandible should ache more. This is completely in the Constantinian tradition which already attributed toothache to humors descending from the brain or ascending from the stomach[50]. Gilbert's recommendation that the juice of ground ivy be dripped into the ear opposite the painful tooth, or primrose juice be dripped into the nose, even if it was already known in ancient times, was part of folk medicine[51]. Thus, here in late Salernitan times, there is a combination of correct personal observations and arabized Galenic material, as well as folk medicine with and without ancient roots, inseparably connected.

Just as Roland's work did, other manuscripts of glosses on Roger lead away from Salerno, such as a Munich manuscript of the 13th century from Montpellier[52], the old rival of Salerno. The oldest testimony of medical studies here reaches back to 1137, and the first statutes stem from the year 1220. There is just as little fundamental innovation to be found in the gloss on Roger originating in Montpellier, with regard to dentistry, as in the "Surgery" written there by Master William of Congenis. Fumigation for toothache, as with Roger, blood-letting, treatment with the cautery iron, and extraction only as a last resort, as well as old home remedies such as the chewing of incense, the application of a linen pouch containing fleabane, pellitory and greenspan, or insertion of raven manure into the hollow tooth are quite familiar to us from the ancients[53] (Figs. 89 to 91). These are recommended just as much as antidotes: mithridatum, theriaca, or hygieia[54].

This apparent standstill is not, at least not in Montpellier, caused ultimately by the fact that surgery was never a subject of teaching, particularly at the French universities, although it had otherwise undergone a great development in the 13th century. The Hospital of the Holy Spirit, founded at the end of the 12th century, was only the site for Montpellier where it was practiced. The reason was the strict observation of the IVth Lateran Council's decree of 1215 forbidding the practice of surgery by sub-deacons, deacons, or priests in the predominantly clerical scholastic universities[55]. Particularly for France, this regulation was still only a confirmation of a condition existing for other reasons, in contrast to Salerno and North Italy. There was, as we know, a particular guild for surgeons in Paris, for which a test before the prefect from 1258 for its candidates is documented. In 1360, this "communité" was united by Charles V of France with another surgeons' guild that was founded in the meantime, the "Confrerie en l'eglise Sains Cosme et Damien"[56]. This "Fraternity at the Church of St. Cosmas and Damian", the patron saints of physicians and apothecaries, later came to be of great importance.

In Montpellier, a papal regulation of 1239 eliminated surgeons from the university statute, just as they were eliminated from university examinations. Only in 1399 a royal dispensation determined here that the surgeons had to take an examination by the Masters (Magistri) of medicine. A Magister chirurgiae, however, is not documented, and it is also uncertain whether the physician-Magistri taught surgery at all[57].

Thus, university medicine in Montpellier, just as in Paris, distanced itself definitively from the practical part of the healing arts represented by the surgeons. For the academicians, it meant an adherence to blind belief in authorities: the Qānūn (Canon) of Ibn Sīnā (Avicenna), as also Aristotelian texts, useless for medical practice, became a dogmatically binding matter of instruction.

These texts stemmed from the second great European center for the assimilation of Arabism, from Toledo, where an Arabized Aristotle

50 Const. Afr. (b) II 18 p. 150ar, 49 f. L. = p. 37, 30 f. B.
51 Gilbertus III p. 159ar, 21—160bv, 29
52 Sudhoff (b) pp. 268—294
53 See p. 73
54 Sudhoff (b) pp. 259, 278, 339
The name of "Mithridat(ic)um" is derived from Mithridates VI, King of Pontus (132—63 B. C.) who carried out experiments with antidotes on his own person. In a similar way "Theriac" can also be retraced to antique authors. Both products which, among other things, contain opium, were used as antidotes and all-healing remedies (panaceas) up to the 18th century.
55 Mansi 18 col. 1007, 8—13
56 Seidler pp. 22 f.
57 Bullough

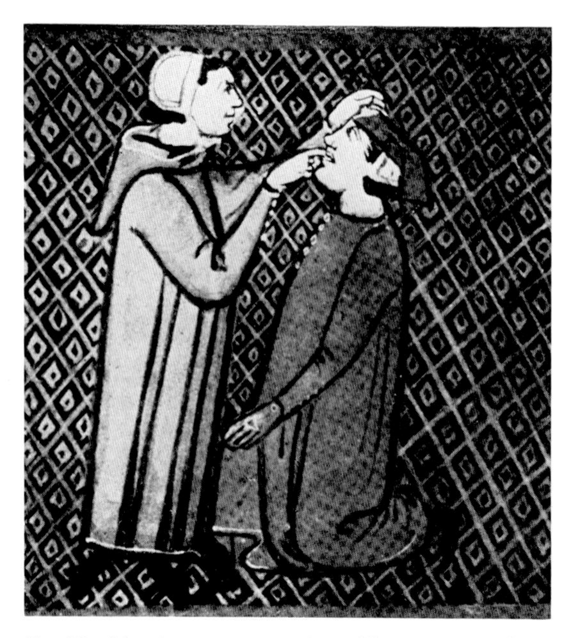

Fig. 92 *Mouth examination from Theodericus' "Chirurgia" in a 13th century manuscript (Univ. Leiden Library, Ms. Vassianus 3, fol. 117r)*

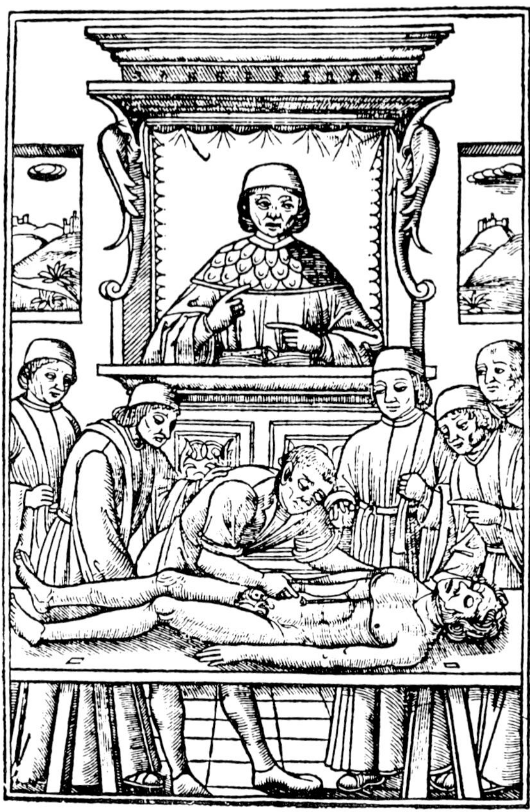

Fig. 93 *Autopsy of a human body by Mondino, the physician and anatomist (Anathomia Mundini 1316, Lyon impression 1528, fol. 1v)*

had already begun to be accepted in the middle of the 12th century. The head of this Toletan school of translation was Gerard of Cremona[58]. He came to Toledo in 1170, learned Arabic there, and then produced at least his first translations with the help of the Mozarab Galippus. Gerard died in Toledo in 1187. The comprehensive translation, which he and his "socii," as they are called in the Vita[59], produced, includes all areas of knowledge. In the area of medicine not only was ar-Rāzī's (Rhazes) "Liber Almansoris" translated by him into Latin for the first time, but also Ibn Sīnā's "Qanun" (see Fig. 82) which was very helpful in its scholastic direction to the tendencies of the following era. He also translated the section on surgery from the writings of Abū l-Qāsim[60].

Both of these last two translations were of particular importance to dental medicine: Abū l-Qāsim's for the practical part, while Ibn Sīnā's presented a dental anatomy for the first time since Constantinus Africanus. Both were mirrored in the advanced surgeons of north Italy. Among these was Bruno da Longoburgo from Calabria, who was active as a surgeon in Padua and Verona. In the chapter on toothache in his "Chirurgia magna" of 1252, he was still under the influence of the corresponding chapters of the Roger glosses[61], oriented towards Salerno, but for treatment of dislocations of the jaw he referred already to Abū l-Qāsim[62]. This chapter was taken over by Theoderico Borgognoni

[58] Schipperges (a) pp. 62 f.
[59] Sudhoff (e) p. 75
[60] See pp. 92 f., 100 f. and 97 f.
[61] Brunus Long. II 2, 3
[62] Ibid. I 20, 2

(Theoderic of Cervia) for his "Chirurgia" from him. This outstanding Bolognese surgeon, son of Hugo of Lucca, was called to Bologna in 1214 as a surgeon, soon became a Dominican, then preacher of penitence of Pope Innocent IV, Bishop of Bitonti before 1262, and then in 1266 or 1274 Bishop of Cervia near Ravenna. Such spiritual honors did not hinder him from practicing medicine and especially surgery, which had its results in a "Chirurgia" composed between 1265 and 1275 (Fig. 92). According to Theoderic, the aid of an assistant is required to hold the fragments in place by pulling while the wire ligature is placed in the case of a double fracture of the mandible[63].

Not only in Bologna was the clerical interdiction against priests practicing surgery transgressed, but surgery had its place at the university, where the study of medicine is demonstrable with Taddeo Alderotti since 1260. This is shown by a curriculum of the surgical program, first available from the year 1378, in which, in addition to translations of Arabian authors, the "Chirurgia" of Bruno da Longoburgo is to be found[64]. Yet, a personage such as the Magister William of Saliceto (Guglielmo da Saliceto) allows conjecture that there was already surgical instruction in Bologna during the 13th century, because we have not only a "Summa conservationis" (Summary of Therapy) by him, but also a "Chirurgia" dedicated to Alderotti's son-in-law. William completed this work, which he had begun in Bologna, as municipal physician of Verona in 1279. In it an innovation in surgical work is a descriptive anatomy appropriate to a time when dissection of the human body in the North Italian universities was beginning again for the first time in centuries[65] (Fig. 93).

William's dental anatomy is based on the translation of the "Qānūn" by Gerard of Cremona, from which he takes the conviction that there are men with only 28 teeth[66], namely, when the third molars are absent. The incorrect concept of the divided mandible is also found[67]. Otherwise, he reports on the surgical removal of the ranula by means of an iron hook. He fights calculus with mastix powder. In the case of a woman from the region of Piacenza, he himself performed the removal of an epulis combined with a maxillary resection, with a red-hot knife and a cotton swab for compression in March of 1279, assisted by the Magister Bernard de Grondola[68].

William describes the dislocation of the mandible in minute detail. In addition to the normal displacement of the condyle in front of the articular fossa (dislocatio ad interiora, inwards, i. e. in the direction of the oral cavity), he also mentions the rare case of displacement to the rear (exterius, to the outside in relation to the oral cavity); in the latter case, the mouth is closed, the mandibular teeth touch the palate, and an abnormal bulge appears at the site of the dislocation, that is, the condyle. He has nothing new to add to the Hippocratic material with regard to the method of repositioning. His description of the splinting of jaw fractures, however, is particularly creative. For this, he takes waxed threads of linen and silk, twisted together, and proceeds to ... *bind the teeth with it as if you were weaving a hurdle, and continue this interlacing between the teeth of the injured* (part of the) *jaw and those of the uninjured* (part of the) *jaw, going from one tooth to another in such a way that the whole jaw be immobilized.*

In the Lyon printing of 1492, there is to be found the following addition: *This done, tie the teeth of the uninjured jaw to the teeth of the injured jaw in this way.* Thus, binding of the fractured mandible to the intact maxilla is recommended here for the first time, although, since this passage is not contained in either the previously known preserved manuscripts of William of Saliceto or in the early printings based on them, except for the Lyon print, it might be an addition from 15th century[69]. In any case, such a proposal is also significant for that era because the idea was not adopted again until the middle of the 19th century.

The chapters dedicated to actual dental medicine are to be found in William's "Summa." His differential diagnosis of toothache is based on rather shaky ground. He makes a Hippocratic differentiation between pain resulting from hot and cold materia[70]. The symptoms of the first, which can be connected with a gingival abscess, are reddening, swelling of the gingiva, and in-

63 Theodoricus Cerv. II 28 p. 110bv, 35—50
64 Rashdall I pp. 236 and 246
65 Artelt pp. 19 f.; Baader (a)
66 William of Saliceto (b) 1 p. 20, 8 f.
67 Ibid. 1 p. 21, 1 f.
68 William of Saliceto (a) I 20; see Schwind pp. 22 f.
69 Ibid. III 18; III 2; see Rowe
70 William of Saliceto (c) p. 67

tense pain, which becomes even sharper with cold water. Thus, here are intermingled the pains of pulpitis with those of periodontitis. The therapy is initiated with blood letting and purging, followed by decoctions of opium, henbane, and mandrake root, i. e., a relatively reasonable symptomatic therapy. If it reaches the point of abscess formation, or if swelling of the gingiva is evident, then the abscess should be opened with a lancet. In the case of cold materia, there is found *annoying, pressing, and intermittent pain (dolor cum gravedine et ponderositate et fractione)* at the diseased site, but neither intense pain nor reddening of the gingiva. Here, purging is carried out, but no cupping, the tooth is washed in many kinds of extracts in vinegar, and the cauterization is performed with a cautery isolated by a tube[71]; this last direction stems from Trottus[72], who probably derived it from 'Alī ibn al-'Abbās.

In the following chapter, William discusses the extraction of teeth. He lists both the medicated as well as the surgical removal, but he thinks little of the former, reasonably enough, as it seems to him, *that it cannot be performed without detriment to the opinions on the subject supported by the ancients.* However, the familiar prescriptions follow, sensible ones, even if not harmless, such as liniments with realgar (red arsenic trisulfide) and wolf's milk juice, and absurd ones, such as ar-Rāzī's frog-fat therapy[73]: *Water frogs are boiled in oil, until they are dissolved. The teeth are treated with this oil for several days, the gingiva is slit, and then the tooth is pulled out.* This occurs in every case *with the iron.* Thus, for William, the medicated treatment is only secondary. In his opinion, bleeding of the gingiva stems from a materia, *which flows down from the head to the gingiva, and then to the teeth.* Finally it disturbs the substance of the gingiva, so that when it is touched and rubbed with a rough and hard object, thin, poor blood begins to flow. The treatment consists in strong corrosive agents, which contain among other things orpiment (yellow arsenic trisulfide), realgar (red arsenic trisulfide), gall-nut ash, and alum. This prescription was already known to Constantinus Africanus, known to him moreover as a devitalizing filling for fighting toothache[75].

Lanfranchi, a student of William of Saliceto, came from Milan and was also active there as physician and surgeon. Around 1290, exiled by Matteo Visconti, he had to leave his home and worked thereafter in various parts of France. He worked in Paris from 1295 on, where he probably belonged to the Confrérie St. Côme. It was there that he wrote his "Chirurgia magna" in 1296, which he dedicated to the French king, Philip the Fair[76].

This was the time in which the French nation, with its strengthened political organization, began to play a leading role in Europe, particularly after the death of the Hohenstaufen Emperor Frederick II (1250). The succeeding German kings lost their continental importance to a great extent. In Philip the Fair of France the Holy See now found a clear opponent to its claims to hegemony, to the extent that the pope's last serious attempt to establish a theocratic system failed. In 1303, the popes had to proceed to Avignon, in dependency of France.

In the center of this action, Lanfranchi found ground prepared in Paris by the surgeons, particularly by Jean Pitard. He earns credit unequivocally, however, for having transferred the contemporary leading surgical knowledge of northern Italy to the Collège de St. Côme of the Parisian surgeons' guild.

In describing jaw dislocations, Lanfranchi followed his teacher William of Saliceto in mentioning the displacement behind the articular fossa, but also provides a new method for resetting the usual dislocation: the assistant sitting behind the patient straps a strong bandage around the patient's chin, while the surgeon pushes one or two wedges, which serve as fulcra, as far as possible backwards between the dental arches. The latter was also indicated in the "Glossulae of the four Masters."[77]

William's "Summa" does not seem to have been used by Lanfranchi because, in opposition, he preferred again the medicated tooth removal[78] and also showed a more conservative stand in the treatment of ranula, following Ibn Sīnā: it should be rubbed with salt or *cum vitreolo;* only when this does not help should it be cut *cum rasorio* and then rubbed with salt[79].

[71] Ibid. p. 67
[72] See p. 113
[73] See p. 73
[74] Ibid. p. 68
[75] See pp. 111 f.
[76] Seidler p. 67
[77] Lanfranchi IV 2, 2 p. 211a^{v}, 41—60. See p. 115
[78] Ibid. III 3, 4 p. 201b^{r}, 64 f.
[79] Ibid. III 3, 4 p. 201a^{r}, 56—63

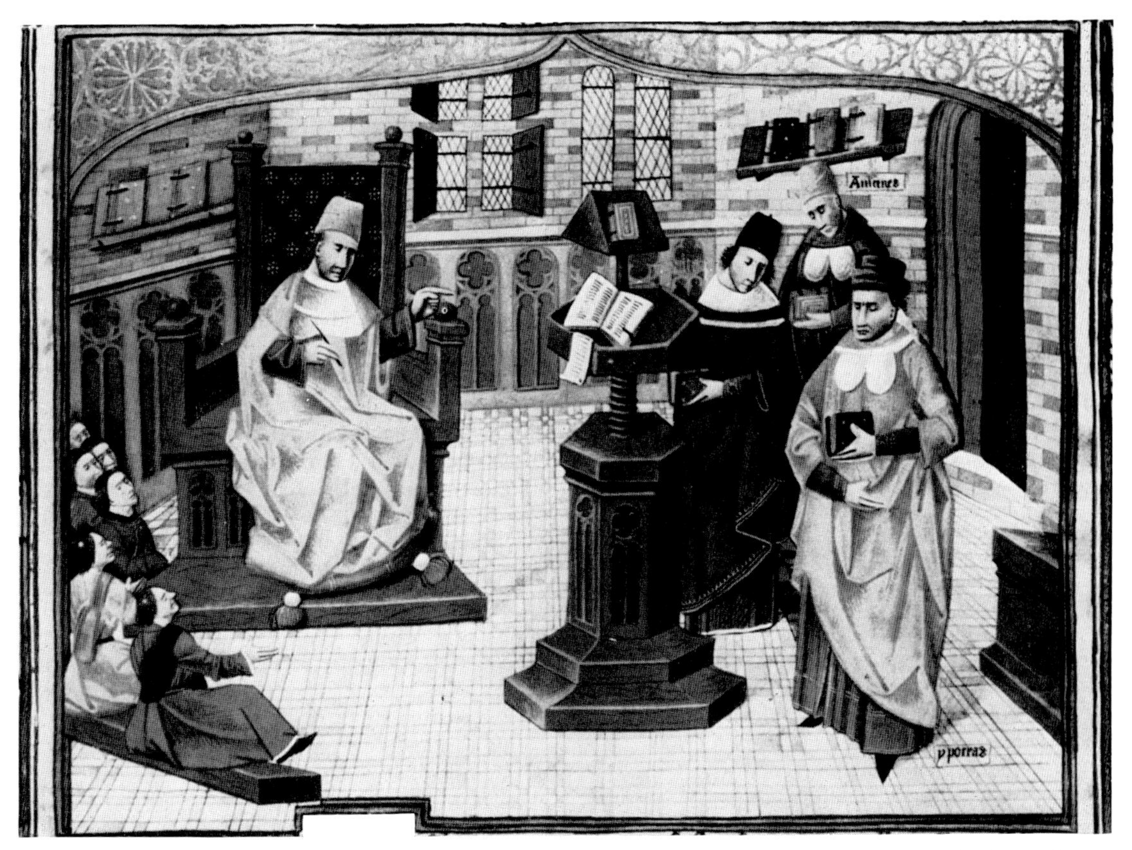

Fig. 94 *University instruction in the Middle Ages in a manuscript from 1461: Bernard Gordon, lecturing from a book from the high professorial chair, with the students showed as small at left and Galen, Avicenna and Hippocrates striding into the auditorium at right. (Bibl. nat. Paris, Ms. lat. 6966, fol. 42)*

The first important French author, Henri de Mondeville, a student of Henri Pitard, was also under Lanfranc's influence. In 1312, Henri was teaching at the Collège de St. Côme; in 1306 he began his "Chirurgia magna", in the introductory anatomical remarks of which, the most unoriginal part of the work, he followed Ibn Sīnā to a great extent. He, too, claimed, referring to Ibn Sīnā[80], that the teeth do not form from the first mixture of the humors, but rather from the excesses of nutriment, as we already found indicated in the Corpus Hippocraticum[81]. The odontological chapter he did not write, as the work remained uncompleted. Henri de Mondeville seems to have received an academic medical education in addition to his surgical one, because it is known that he studied in Montpellier. Surgery, however, as we know, was as little practiced in this university as in the one in Paris. Yet, odontological sections from masters in Montpellier are to be found in summaries by masters from the first half of the 14th century.

One of the most important masters, Bernard Gordon, is probably of British ancestry, because Chaucer, the famous author of the "Canterbury Tales", mentions him, just as Gilbertus Anglicus and John of Gaddesden did. From 1283 on Gordon was a master in Montpellier, and as such began his "Lilium medicinae", the popularity of which is attested by the large number of preserved manuscripts (Fig. 94). In dental anatomy he relies

[80] Henri de Mondeville I 3 p. 36, 9—23
[81] See p. 62

on the knowledge of his time. He, too, names the incisors (incidentes) the "anteriores."[82] It is interesting that he categorizes the teeth correctly, as did Aristotle[83], among the organs, but classed them incorrectly with the similar body parts (homoiomers)[84]. Like Gilbertus Anglicus[85], Bernard held both internal and external causes responsible for tooth disease[86], but in describing them largely relied on the translation of the Canon[87], which he further elaborated. As in this work he recognizes among the external causes of tooth decay the consumption of very hot foods after very cold ones, and vice versa, and cracking of very hard foods, or too extensive neglect of tooth care and too harsh rubbing of the gingiva, pushing it back, both of which damage the teeth. One of his original observations is that when chewed only on one side, damaging substances (plaque and calculus) will form on the other side. Among the causes of toothache enumerated by Gordon as originating from the inside[88], there is to be found, as in Ibn Sīnā, not only vomiting (of stomach acids), but also materia which stems from the head and stomach and causes pain, which had already been common knowledge since Constantine[89]. Listing fever as a side effect of toothache also came from the same source.

Bernard's individual observations, however, extend far beyond those of his predecessors. Thus, he usually advised using moderating additives with the narcotics approved by Ibn Sīnā[90], while his model only warned against excessive dosage. In cauterization with arsenic, vitriol, or tincture of cantharides he not only insists that none of it reaches the inside (of the oral cavity) but also that it be completely avoided in anterior teeth[91]. The cauterization itself may only be performed with 'Alī Ibn al-'Abbās' protective cannula[92], referring here, however, to the advice of Ibn Sīnā. As a last resort, extraction should be performed, but Gordon is hesitant about it, too, because the pain, probably the pain of the wound, returns after removal of the tooth. Therefore, he regards extraction as only an unsatisfactory treatment. Care must also be taken with the preparatory loosening, because otherwise the jaw may suffer damage, or fistula formation may occur. For that reason he recommends again the medicated tooth removal with the help of corrosive agents in a protective wax casing. The customary fumigation with henbane is advised as a remedy for toothworm[93]. Filing down of teeth which have grown too long, and the remedial after-treatment thereof[94] are made in accordance with Ibn Sīnā, as some other things[95].

The instructional material of the Montpellier school at the beginning of the 14th century represented by Bernard Gordon ist completely included within the scope of the Qanun translation and is free of Ibn Sīnā's influence only in details. And yet, its level is high, if the odontological chapters of the "Lilium medicinae" are compared with those of Arnald of Villanova's "Brevarium practicae" (Compendium of Practical Knowledge) which came out at about the same time. Teacher of this famous Catalan was John Casamicciola, personal physician to Charles of Anjou and professor in Naples[96]. Arnald, who was documented a magister in Spain in 1281 and physician to several popes in Rome and Avignon since 1300, practiced and taught partly in Montpellier. His "Brevarium" in particular proves him to be a keen observer and an experienced therapist, but this does not hold true for the odontological sections[97]; these are barely organized quotations from older authors, and contain only a few additions from personal experience. For toothache as a result of warm humoral compositions Arnald recommends, as Bernard Gordon[98], bleeding from the cephalic vein, which had already been taken from al-Ǧazzār[99] by Constantine. He uses leeches on the neck or gingiva, and follows the Canon translation[100] in its instruction to apply them under the chin as well. While Gordon recommended cauterization of the gingiva with arsenic, vitriol, and tincture of cantharides only the use of a cantharides plaster under the chin

[82] Gordon III 25 p. 410, 3 f.
[83] See p. 65
[84] Ibid. III 26, 9 p. 415, 28—33
[85] See pp. 115 f.
[86] Ibid. III 25 p. 404, 31 f.
[87] Gerard of Cremona III 7, 2
[88] Gordon III 25 p. 405, 18—24
[89] See p. 117
[90] Ibid. III 25 p. 406, 26—28
[91] Ibid. III 25 p. 406, 28—33
[92] Ibid. III 25 p. 408, 5—7
[93] Ibid. III 26, 2 p. 411, 17—25
[94] Ibid. III 26, 4 p. 413, 5—7
[95] Gerard of Cremona III 7, 22
[96] Diepgen (a)
[97] Arnald I 34
[98] Gordon III 25 p. 406, 12 f.
[99] See p. 96
[100] Gerard of Cremona III 7, 6 p. 236a^{v}, 15

is to be found in Arnald. This also had been included in more recent copies of the manuscript of the "Regimen sanitatis Salernitanum"[101].

All this obviously means a loss of substance precisely with regard to the effective methods. Arnald repeatedly quotes the prescriptions of his teacher, but only with scanty details. Of himself, he reports that he had healed toothache accompanied by swelling of the cheek, which seemed to be deadly, through flushing with nettle root boiled in wine, ginger, and pellitory, as well as a plaster of nettle roots. For medicated tooth removal, he uses the cauterizing agents introduced by Constantinus Africanus. He claims to have learned another prescription from the Romans: orpiment, ammonium chloride, and rhubarb should be ground together in equal parts, moistened with the strongest vinegar, and placed as a sort of plaster on the carious tooth. In addition to this surely effective medication, Arnald used the wax casing customary since Constantine, filled with a mixture of the bark of mulberry roots, bertram and salt, ground in vinegar, and applied to the tooth. To the realm of superstition belongs the oil of earthworms, which was dropped into the ear on the painless side while the patient lies on the ear of the painful side.

Components such as these from folk medicine are nothing new. In the previously noted "Thesaurus pauperum"[102] by Petrus Hispanus, a Portuguese scholar working in Italy, who died in 1277 as Pope John XXI, they are to be found in large number. For example in its prescriptions for toothache in addition to excerpts from Odo of Meung, Constantine of Africa, the Platearii, as well as his own personal prescriptions and apocryphal material, such as a presumed prescription from Pliny, there is the absurd instruction to touch an aching tooth with a dead man's tooth, after which the pains are certain to disappear[103].

Only in those printings of the "Thesaurus pauperum" based on manuscripts traced back no further than the 14th century St. Apollonia is confirmed as the patron saint of toothache. This is not, however, the oldest indication of this particular patronage; a corresponding annotation on a Milanese lead coin, probably dating from the 13th century, does this as well (Fig. 95). Apollonia is presented here with a forceps. She is similarly presented on the predella of a winged altar at the Church of Catherine in Pisa around 1320 by Simone Martini (Fig. 96) and at the main door of the church of the convent at Thann in Alsace around 1350[104].

We also know of prayers directed to this saint as a remedy for toothache from late breviaries from Antwerp, Mainz, Ratzeburg, and Cologne, as well as from German manuscripts from the 14th century[105], for example in the "Dudesche Arstedie" (German Pharmacopeia) and by a German Bartholomaeus[106]. A late Vita from an Utrecht manuscript reflects the same relationship: according to this, Apollonia, as she was martyred, held out the prospect of freedom from toothache and headache to all who respectfully observed the anniversary of her Passion[107].

The historical seed of this legend, however, appears to be different. The Greek ecclesiastical writer Eusebius, Bishop of Caesarea, reports the witness provided by the Alexandrian Bishop Dionysius in his "Church History", that in 249 in Alexandria, a deaconess Apollonia fell victim to the Emperor Decius' persecution of Christians: *But they also seized the worthy aged virgin Apollonia, broke out her teeth through blows to the jaw, erected a pyre of wood before the city, and threatened to burn her alive if she did not repeat with them the incantations of unbelief. Inspired by brief prayer, however, she sprang into the fire and was consumed by the flames*[108].

The ripping out of her teeth with a forceps was added only later, because both the patron sainthood of toothache and the association of Apollonia with the forceps, which seems to have been a dental forceps from the start, are undocumented before the 13th century. The connection with toothache lived on in popular belief up to the present day as shown by the customary name for henbane in Karinthia: Apollonia herb[109]. This is probably a reflection of the traditional henbane fumigation as a remedy for

101 Regimen san. Sal. (b) 3197—3199
102 See p. 113
103 Petrus Hispanus 15 pp. 34r, 26—34v, 2
104 Bulk pp. 24 f.
105 Apollonia col. 282; Wrede
106 Brodmann p. 32, 15—24; p. 39
107 Apollonia (Vita 32) col. 281c
108 Eusebius VI 41, 7. To spare Apollonia the reproach of suicide, reference is made to Augustine I 26. There, however, the discussion is quite general to the effect that saintly virgins may inflict death upon themselves by drowning to avoid dishonor; that act serves as martyrdom. Augustine I 17 speaks to the same point, as does Ambrose III 7, 32, who adds leaping into an abyss to permitted suicide.
109 Marzell II col. 932

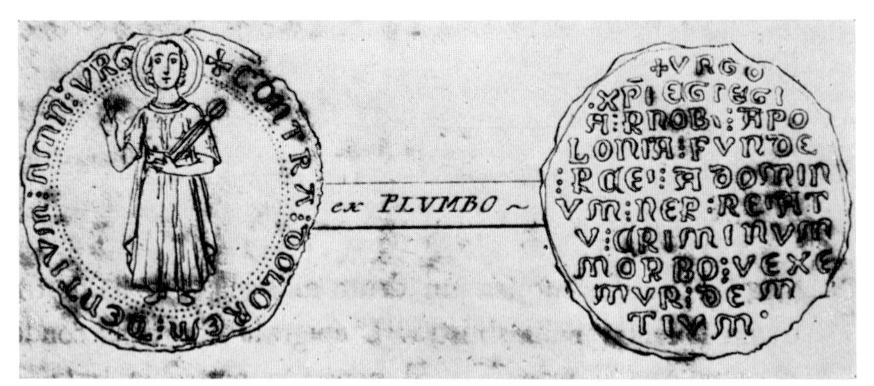

Fig. 95 *Apollonia on a lead coin, probably dating to the 13th century, preserved only as an illustration from 1812 (from Bulk)*

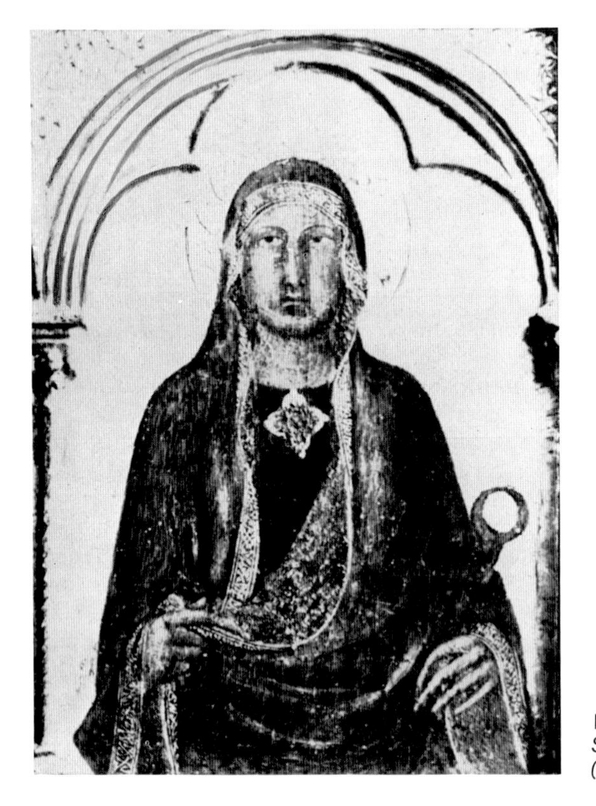

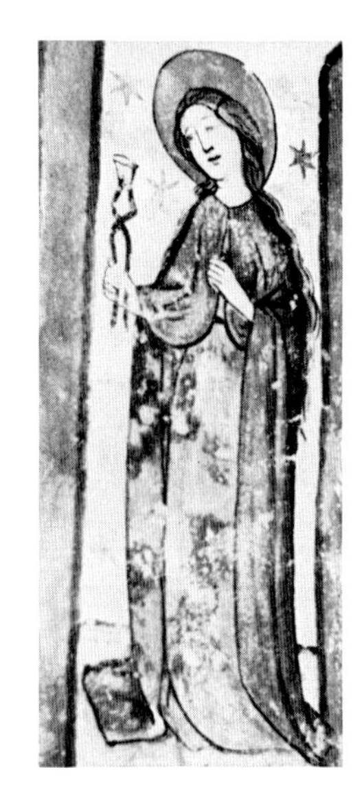

Fig. 97 *Apollonia with forceps; fresco from the Church of St. Vitus in Handschuchsheim near Heidelberg, 15th century (bricked up around 1650, exposed 1962)*

Fig. 96 *Apollonia with forceps, from a painting by Simone Martini, Catherine Church of Pisa about 1320 (from Bulk)*

toothache. In Bavaria, aconite[110], which was used in the same way, also bears the name of Apollonia.

A p o l l o n i a is connected with the idea of a patron against toothache to such an extent that in French toothache prayers of far more ancient origin, her name was substituted for that of P e t e r. The prayer in question, "Peter on the Rock," is verifiably existent in Latin since the 10th century. According to this, P e t e r sits on a rock and holds his cheek in his hands. Christ, who comes to him and asks him the reason for his sorrow, is told that it is the toothworm and is asked for the relevant blessing. Where in particular this motif came from cannot be said with

[110] Marzell I col. 107; Wrede

certainty; however, there is a stone in Jerusalem, where Peter is said to have sat after the denial of Christ, which was still being shown in the 15th century so that the conjecture of an allusion to Bible passages suggests itself[111]. German translations of this prayer to Peter are rare, and at first appear in the 15th century, a time therefore, when Apollonia had long been established as the patron of toothache (Figs. 97 and 130).

The German dental texts which have been handed down as copies of the manuscripts in the 13th and 14th century do not appear to be anything more than the sections in Petrus Hispanus' "Thesaurus pauperum." This is true even for the "Diemersche Arzneybuch" stemming from the 12th century. In it is found at least a differential diagnosis of toothache based on humoral pathology, from which the customary remedies for toothache are derived[112]. In this text, even if not in the dental sections, Salernitan concepts are contained for the first time. It differs in this respect from the low level of Bartholomaeus' "Practica", with its elements predominantly from the early Middle Ages. In it and in the "Dudesche Arstedie", there are prayers to Apollonia. The "Practica" contain additionally the advice given elsewhere in many German texts, that ground pepper dissolved in wine be given, or that an exorcising incantation be written on the cheek[113]. These two regulations are also the only remedies for toothache to be found in the Middle Low German medical book from Bremen in 1382 by Arnoldus Doneldy[114]. The "Dudesche Arstedie", however, contains Arabian influences as well[115], such as, for example, the frog-fat therapy. Parts of the Toledian translations are verifiable in the medical book by the physician in Würzburg Ortolff the Bavarian[116] from the first half of the 14th century, although almost all his odontological sections are derived from Bartholomaeus' "Practica" and similar texts. The Utrecht book of pharmacology from the same era contains nothing in the realm of dental medicine beyond the recommendation of washing the teeth with rose water as a remedy against the toothworm[117].

Thus, there is no significant trans-regional medical literature in this sphere, either in the German or the Latin language. For a long time, the tradition of the monastic medicine of the early Middle Ages was perpetuated, increased, surely, by material from the most varied sources, but without a trace of the new spirit of the universities. This new spirit only manifested itself in the works of those men who had studied at such institutions in the 13th and particularly the 14th centuries, or taught there, as in the case of the Dutch surgeon Yperman, who came from central Europe.

Jan Yperman, born in the second half of the 13th century, studied, according to his own statement, under Lanfranchi in Paris. He is known to have been in 1304 the master at the hospital "delle Belle" in Ypres and to have left Ypres only as field surgeon in 1311/12 and 1325. He probably died between 1329 and 1332[118]. His "Cyrurgie", the first in Flemish, was written after 1305, as he quotes from Bernard Gordon. In addition to Odo of Meung, the authors he mentions include the Arabic ones from Constantine to the writings of the so-called pseudo-Mesuë[119], as well as surgeons from Roger up to his own teacher, Lanfranchi, whose influence on the work is extensive.

Yperman took the dental sections to a large degree from Lanfranchi, although his presentation is sometimes more detailed, such as, for example, in the differential diagnosis of toothache[120]. From the same source were directions, such as that toothache after foods that are too hot is helped by cold foods[121], or the prescription against unbearable pain, to bean-sized pills of henbane seeds and opium moistened with vinegar upon the tooth[122]. Toothworms, which are missing in Lanfranchi, cause toothache when they are moving (*alsi roeren so swerense*)[123].

Yperman describes the dangers of tooth extraction minutely. He is more reluctant than his teacher, advising against an operative extraction even when the tooth is loose[124]. Subse-

111 Ohrt
112 Brodmann p. 26
113 Ibid. p. 46
114 Doneldey p. 9, 28—32
115 Brodmann p. 33, 8—11
116 Keil
117 Brodmann p. 17
118 van Leersum
119 See p. 91
120 Yperman IV 17 pp. 111b, 18—112a, 18
121 Lanfranchi III 3, 4 p. 201b^r, 19 f. = Yperman IV 18 p. 112a, 23—25
122 Lanfranchi III 3, 4 p. 211b^r, 28—32 = Yperman IV 18 p. 112b, 17—30
123 Yperman IV 19 p. 113b, 39 f.
124 Ibid. IV 19 p. 114a, 1—14

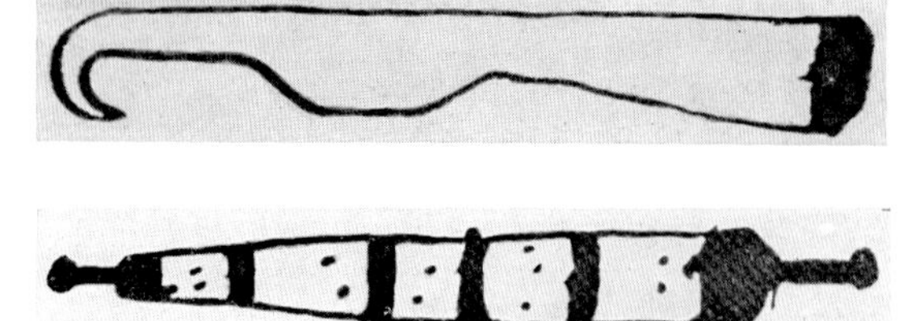

Fig. 98 *Jan Yperman: Hook-shaped instrument, about 1305*

Fig. 99 *Jan Yperman: Cautery with protective cannula, about 1305*

quently, however, referring to Lanfranchi (not by name, but by the designation "meester"), he lists the various methods of tooth removal. Initially, he speaks of cauterization with the protective cannula, using oil treated with marjoram and hemlock. For medicamentous tooth removal, as with Lanfranchi, the juice of the mulberry tree and pellitory are mixed with vinegar and laid around the root of the tooth, after *peeling off* (*ontscoyt*) the gingiva with a hook-shaped instrument, which is pictured in the manuscript just as is the cautery iron with the protective cannula (Figs. 98 and 99). The other agents listed for medicated tooth extraction also stem from Lanfranchi[125], but he, in turn, is under the influence of Roger and the Roger glosses, even if it is not expressed in the stomatological sections. Here, Yperman seems to rely above all on his "Meester's" knowledge. The Germans during the 14th century studied medicine, not surgery, in Montpellier, because in general, this university seems to have been preferred by students native to the northern regions. The German Premonstratensian monk Peter, later titular Archbishop Thomas of Sarepta, seems to have gotten his education there. Born in Silesia in 1297, he settled as a physician near Breslau in 1336. Around 1360 he began his great work, "Michi competit" (It seems to me), which contains odontological chapters. In them, he quotes the practical manuals by Constantine, Gilbertus Anglicus, and Johannes Platearius, as well as the writings of the so-called pseudo-Mesuë, Bernard Gordon, and Roger Baron, a magister of Montpellier in the 14th century and author of a widely-spread "Practica". The works of the last two particularly indicate a close relation to Montpellier.

Even in those parts where Thomas expressly relies on his own experience use of sources is sometimes apparent, such as with the regulation for setting the cupping head in the depression of the neck against toothache which is derived almost word for word from Gilbertus Anglicus[126]. Thomas frequently used his own pharmacy of antidotes, and showed through it that he had his own opinion in therapy. Thus, he lists the use of spirits of wine as a remedy against toothache, new at the time[127]. He is also critical of his authorities, as when, for example, he rejects agents which Gilbert had recommended for cleansing of the brain[128], because they do not lessen the toothache but rather increase it. For easing pain caused by toothworms, he, too, turns to the forceps as a last resort[129], yet, advised against remedial treatment with a mixture of flour and wolf's milk juice. He avoided such extreme means in order to cause no damage to a healthy neighboring tooth. He recommends on the other hand the use of mulberry tree juice with or without mixing it with a flour paste, an already ancient prescription for which he refers to Johannes Platearius, who had tested it[130]. Such observations based on personal experience are his only contributions to dental medicine. It shows the narrow limitation at this time imposed on a man of even his education, who was removed in his sphere of action far from the centers of university life.

In England, however, the situation was not to be compared with that of central Europe. Not only did Constantinus Africanus become known early, but there was also a direct contact with the second great center of adoption of Arabism, Toledo, and the medical curricula at the universities at Oxford and Cambridge were influenced by Paris from the very

[125] Lanfranchi III 3, 4 pp. 201b^{r}, 64—201a^{v}, 3 = Yperman IV 19 p. 114a, 19—114b, 11
[126] Köhler p. 6, 22—24 = Gilbertus Anglicus III p. 159b^{v}, 7—9
[127] Ibid. p. 5, 41 f.
[128] Ibid. p. 7, 25—27
[129] Ibid. p. 9, 37 f.
[130] Ibid. p. 9, 41 f.

beginning. Beyond this, there were also authentic medical studies in the English cloisters, cathedral schools, and hospitals, unlike Germany[131].

Indeed, a personage such as that of John of Gaddesden (Ioannes Anglicus), as one of the first who received his medical education in England only, does not demonstrate a particularly high level, compared with the representatives of medicine at the French and Italian universities of his time. Born in Little Gaddesden in the earldom of Buckinghamshire around 1280, he received his medical training at Oxford, where he also practiced and taught. The composition of the only book definitely written by him, the "Rosa Anglica", falls into the time around 1314. This author, praised by Chaucer and rejected by Guy de Chauliac, like all medical authors of his time, stands completely under the influence of Arabism.

In dental anatomy, John of Gaddesden, relying on Bernard Gordon, knew the designation of the incisors[132] as "anteriores"[133], as also the title of John's work "Rosa Anglica" seems to be modelled on Gordon's "Lilium medicinae." He states the number of teeth as 32, in mnemonic verses, but he also knew not only the terms "duales" and "quadrupli" for the first and the second incisors to be borrowed and translated from the Arabic into Latin[134], but also the fact that there are sometimes men with only 28 teeth[135]. Constantine had rendered the central incisors as "dentes pares"[136].

In treating toothache John of Gaddesden referred expressly to Ibn Sīnā[137], but divided his causes as Gordon did[138], into internal and external ones. This, as well as the inclusion of his observation that unilateral chewing causes damage[139], shows that John had used the "Lilium medicinae" to the same extent as the translation of the "Canon." Moreover, he even quotes Hippocratic aphorisms, such as the aphorism IV 53, whose content he condensed into a mnemonic verse:[140]

Est limus dentis morbi recedentis
Est vitae signum dens siccus maxime dignum.
(Decay in a tooth is a sign of long disease and retreating life, the most precious indication of life is a dry tooth).

In mentioning the henbane fumigation, the relevant passage from the Salernitan health rules is quoted[141]. Ideas from folk medicine are abundantly evident, as in contact with a corpse's tooth as a remedy for toothache[142], probably from the "Thesaurus pauperum."[143] Similarly, there is witness from reliable authorities that a magpie's beak bound to the neck will ease the pain[144]. An exorcism incantation written on the cheek, as in the German "Practicae Bartholomaei"[145], calling upon St. Apollonia or St. Nicasius are believed likewise to be effective as is a sign of the cross, connected with an Our Father and an Ave Maria for the salvation of St. Philip's parents to be prayed during the Gospel of the mass[146]. This mixture of the sensible and the senseless among therapies, which never provided anything really new, makes the negative judgement of a man such as Guy de Chauliac understandable.

Medicamentous tooth removal occupies a lot of space also in John of Gaddesden but is placed among his radical measures as a third alternative only. Many of these regulations are derived from the translation of the Canon, such as flour moistened in wolf's milk, enclosed furthermore in a wax casing, or hops. The raven manure from ancient times also is mentioned here again. The fat of the tree frog listed by ar-Rāzī and Ibn Sīnā is not only brought up in relation to the Qānūn passage, but also characterized as a medication that never fails[147]. The green frog, which climbs on and lives in trees, and is abundant in Provence, should be caught. His fat is to be taken and applied to the tooth which is to fall out. In reference to ar-Rāzī[148], we learn that oxen which eat such frogs with their hay lose the teeth which had come in contact with them. A tree-frog broth also is indicated for loosening the teeth as is ground cicada applied in a wax casing. For good measure partridge brain is also recommended as an effective agent[149].

131 Lauer
132 Ioannes Anglicus (a) III 4, 2 p. 152a^{r}, 39 f.
133 See p. 122
134 See p. 94
135 Ibid. III 4, 2 p. 152a^{r}, 34—42
136 See p. 111
137 Gerard of Cremona III 7, 1
138 See p. 122
139 Ioannes Anglicus (a) III 4, 2 p. 152b^{r}, 23—25
140 Ibid. III 4, 2 p. 152a^{v}, 20—29
141 Ibid. III 4, 2 p. 153a^{r}, 3—5; see p. 115
142 Ibid. III 4, 2 p. 153b^{r}, 2
143 See p. 125
144 Ibid. III 4, 2 p. 153b^{r}, 52—54
145 See p. 125
146 Ibid. III 4, 2 p. 153b^{r}, 36—39
147 Hoffmann-Axthelm. See pp. 94 and 103
148 See p. 94
149 Ibid. III 4, 7 p. 154a^{v}, 42 f.

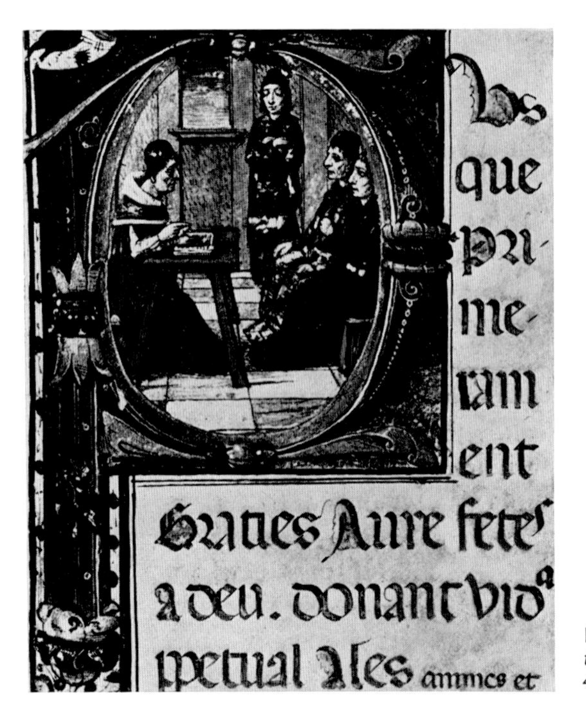

Fig. 100 *Guy de Chauliac teaching, in the initial letter of a French manuscript (Vatican Lateran Library 4804 fol. 1)*

Cauterization through 'Ali ibn al-'Abbās' protective cannula for devitalization of the painful pulp is also familiar to John, but in addition, *by excoriation of the region around the dental root* the decay of the respective tooth should be effected in single fragments, whereby, moreover, he uses ashes of nutshells and grains of incense as palliatives[150]. According to John of Gaddesden, a surgical extraction should only be undertaken in an emergency, mainly only on a loose tooth, for which he quotes Gariopont's "Passionarius Galieni" as witness. He believed it to be a true Galenic text[151]. Also, with reference to Ibn Sīnā[152], the cause of the pain must lie in the tooth itself. The detachment of the gingiva should be done first in keeping with the instruction by Constantine of Africa[153]: *The forceps should then be put to the root of the tooth, and extraction should take place straight downwards, while an assistant holds the patient's head firmly in position, so that the tooth does not break off at the root*[154]. Before the extraction, blood must be let, and the gingiva must be scarified and rubbed in with a paste of mulberry tree bark, pellitory salt, and strong vinegar[155], a prescription possibly also taken from Constantine. Thus, John of Gaddesden not only relies to a great extent on Gordon and on the translation of the "Qānūn", which he quotes 474 times in his work but also compiles from other sources of antiquity up to his own time into a colorful creation of often dubious value and without source acknowledgement. To all this he adds a variegated material from folk medicine.

According to his own statement, however, John of Gaddesden must personally have practiced tooth extraction[156], which increases the importance of a controversial passage of his. Because besides forceps, he mentions another instrument: *Take an iron, wide at the front and sharply cutting at the front* (i. e., on the inside)[157] *and force the tooth down, and it will thus fall out*[158]. Gurlt[159] wanted to interpret this instrument as a kind of punch, which is certainly in-

150 John of Gaddesden (a) III 4, 7 p. 154a^{v}, 9—11
151 Gariopontus I 17 p. 15^{v}, 11—16 = Ioannes Anglicus III 4, 7 p. 154b^{r}, 28—35
152 Gerard of Cremona III 7, 17
153 See p. 112
154 Ioannes Anglicus (a) III 4, 7 p. 154b^{r}, 38—41
155 Ibid. III 4, 7 p. 154b^{r}, 49—53
156 Ibid. III 4, 7 p. 154a^{v}, 2
157 . . . capiatur ferrum latum anterius et acutum scindens anterius et tunc compellatur dens deorsum et cum illo cadet. This second "anterius" (front) is absent in the later printings: Ioannes Anglicus (b) p. 894, 23
158 Ioannes Anglicus (a) III 4, 7 p. 154b^{r}, 43 f.
159 Gurlt II p. 161

correct, and Guerini[160] also speaks only in general terms of a lever, which should be wide at one end, and narrow and pointed at the other. Sudhoff sees in it *a kind of pelican*[161], an explanation which probably is the most probable one. In the final analysis, it must remain undecided, because, in contrast to Guy de Chauliac's mention of the pelican[162], this passage is not clear enough to allow an unequivocal judgement.

Even with such a questionable mixture of book-learning and folk medicine, of superstition and the result of his own experience John of Gaddesden clearly rises above the purely theoretical late scholastic medicine of the Paris faculty, at least insofar as dental medicine is concerned. This is because the scientific methods developed there from authoritative theology could not be of any use for an empirical science such as the healing arts. Pietro d'Abano is a typical representative of this way of thinking. This great Lombardian[163], a physician, philosopher and astronomer in one, is usually associated with the Padua school on the base of his time as a student and later as teacher in Padua (around 1308—1315). His main work, however, the "Conciliator differentiarum medicorum et philosophorum" (Advisor on the Differences between Physicians and Philosophers) with certainty originated in Paris, and presents in its scientific teachings a significant witness to the late Parisian scholasticism. The only odontological problem that Pietro discusses, however, is whether the teeth have feeling[164], which he affirms with reference to Galen and Ibn Sīnā[165]. Returning to the definition in the Aristotelian text "De generatione animalium"[166] which was again available in the second half of the 12th century in a translation directly from the Greek. Because the teeth form from bones and have the same composition he inferred further that the teeth must have sensitivity. These are conjectures, of course, which have nothing to do with practical medicine.

The situation at the universities of northern Italy was different from that in Paris. Here, for example, Sillanus de Nigris, acting at the University of Pavia, founded in 1361, criticized the 9th book of ar-Rāzī's "Liber ad Almansorem" between 1365 and 1375. He did this undoubtedly complete in the scholastic manner, but beyond that, recommended the practice in use since Hippocratic medicine[167] of firmly binding a loose tooth with wire or a linen thread, according to Abū l-Qāsim[168] *in the manner of a fence* (see Fig. 80). As a new therapy is to be found the dropping of wine spirits into the carious tooth; its distillation was known since the end of the 13th century. Thus, even this text, derived directly from a university writing of the 14th century, shows practical suggestions in its dental section which was typical of Italy.

At the scholastic universities of France and England, in contrast, progress in the practical healing arts stagnated. This had its root in the theoretical scientific controversies of that time, and even more in the class struggles of the 13th and 14th centuries, which deepened the rift between university medicine and surgery. Thereby, the representatives of the lower surgery, the barbers, became the given helpers of the physicians to an increasing degree. In the 14th century, they naturally overtook practical dentistry, which was at that time the bloody extraction consisting in general of breaking off the crown of the tooth to ease the pain.

The surgeons had their place between the academic physicians and the barbers. Their books, significantly, were absent in the Parisian faculty but were present as early as 1373 in the library of King Charles V, who was interested in the organization of the class of surgeons, even in French translation[170]. Among these translations there was even a French copy of Guy de Chauliac's "Chirurgia magna," a gift of the Duke of Anjou, the secular ruler of Avignon.

As the most important surgical author of the 14th century, Guy de Chauliac (Guido de Cauliaco) must be placed next to Montpellier. He studied medicine in Toulouse, Montpellier, and Bologna, but not in Paris. He seems to have learned surgery from Henri de Mondeville. Guy had himself taught in Montpellier at the Holy Ghost Hospital, not at the university. He was also personal physician to three popes in Avignon (Fig. 100). In 1363, he wrote his "Chirurgia magna" which was soon translated into French.

160 Guerini p. 142
161 Sudhoff (f) p. 131
162 See p. 131
163 Norpoth
164 Pietro d'Abano 43
165 Gerard of Cremona I 1,5, 1.5; III 7,1
166 Aristotle II 6 p. 745a, 19 f.
167 See pp. 60 f.
168 Albucasis XXX 2, 33 (a) p. 194, 9—28; English translation (b) pp. 292 f.
169 Chart. univ. Paris 1723
170 Seidler pp. 66 f.

In the section dealing with dental surgery Guy relies above all on the great advocators of Arabism from the second, the Toledian, period of assimilation, on Ibn Sīnā and Abū l-Qāsim. He also delved into translations from the early Middle Ages of Greek authors, such as that of the "Therapeutica" by Alexander of Tralles, or of works by earlier masters of Salerno, such as Gariopont. From among his own predecessors, the surgeons of the 13th and 14th centuries, he names most of all William of Saliceto and Lanfranchi, just as he refers to the instructional opinion of the school of Montpellier or one of its masters. Beyond these sources, Guy had only little of his own to contribute to dental medicine.

In his anatomy, Guy keeps completely to the tradition of Ibn Sīnā, from whom he even takes the differentiation of the incisors and their designation as "duales" and "quadrupli."[171] For him the teeth are by their very nature bones; he does not quote Aristotle as an authority for this, as Pietro d'Abano does, but rather refers to Galen, newly translated directly from the Greek by Niccolo da Reggio[172], that is, without the roundabout way through the Islamic physicians. The same holds true for the divided mandible[173].

As remedies against toothache Guy is familiar first of all with general prophylactic measures such as blood-letting and application of leeches, in accordance with Ibn Sīnā[174]. He puts general considerations and observations about professional history before particular therapeutic methods. With reference to Ibn Sīnā, he expressly states that physicians should leave tooth operations to the barbers and toothers *(barbitonsoribus et dentatoribus)*. *It is safer, on the other hand, if these operations are supervised by physicians*[175]. These instructions, already known to Henri de Mondeville and Arnald of Villanova from the same source, might well have prevailed at this time, since Guy seems to regard them as self-evident. We are well informed about the position in Paris of the barbers whom he discusses: since 1301, there had been a regulation requiring them to take an examination before the "maîtres du métier", before they were allowed to call themselves barber-surgeons. They were also trained, often in secret, by the faculty in order to form a team of assistants for manual performances. It is of particular importance in the light of the centuries old tension between the surgeons' guilds and the purely theoretic oriented scholastic medical faculty that this took place in Paris[176].

The existence of such "artifices" for operative dental medicine had already been observable in Salerno in the 12th century[177]. In England, in 1320, Peter de London is the first mentioned "touzdrawere," after the barbers had united to form a guild in 1308[178]. Shortly thereafter, a "tenebreker" is known in Hildesheim[179]. The report of John of Gaddesden from 1314 is indicative of the level of the barbers: he passed on to them the useless frog-fat therapy for a good sum of money, as an infallible secret remedy[180]. In Guy de Chauliac's book the "dentatores" or "dentistae" are relegated entirely to the position of physicians' helpers, because only they could really be well informed about the remedial tooth removal or about cauterization of Ibn Sīnā, expressly quoted here.

Therefore it is not surprising that Guy relies so much on his sources in his regulations for treatment of toothache whereby he even includes an instruction as questionable as the Galenic one allegedly tested by pseudo-Mesuë, that ground garlic be applied to the base of the hand on the side where toothache occurs[181]. This is, however, almost verbatim an addition of Gariopont in the "Passionarius Galieni", which he compiled. Guy lists agents for medicamentous tooth removal from *the ancients* in a merely cursory fashion, in which all that stands in Ibn Sīnā's "Qānūn" is to be found[183], including the fat of the green or tree frog[184]. The only innovation is the aqua regia (aqua fortis)[185], and the instruction that, in the case of blunted teeth, wine or wine spirits, which was then being introduced in the therapy, be held in the mouth[186]. Yet Guy states with regard to medicated tooth removal, as William of Saliceto does similarly[187],

[171] Guy (a) I 2, 2 p. 7a^r, 45
[172] Galen XVI 2 p. 381, 16 H. = Guy I 2, 2 p. 7a^r, 41 f.
[173] Galen XI 19 p. 177, 12 f. H. = Guy I 2, 2 p. 7a^r, 3 f.
[174] Gerard of Cremona III 7, 3; 7, 6
[175] Guy (a) VI 2, 2 p. 57b^r, 32 f.
[176] Seidler pp. 25 f. See p. 195
[177] See p. 115
[178] Donaldson
[179] Sudhoff (f) p. 132
[180] Ioannes Anglicus (a) III 4, 7 p. 154a^v, 24—26
[181] Guy (a) VI 2, 2 p. 57b^r, 35
[182] Ibid. p. 58a^r, 4
[183] Gerard of Cremona III 7, 17 f.
[184] Guy (a) VI 2, 2 p. 58a^r, 7 f.
[185] Ibid. p. 58a^r, 7
[186] Ibid. p. 57b^v, 54
[187] See pp. 119 f.

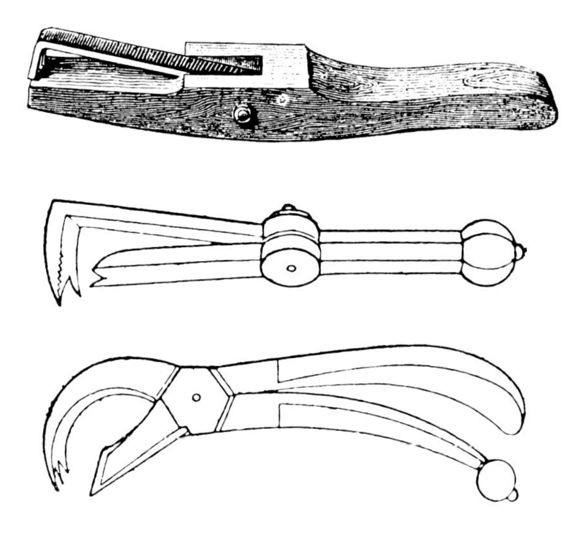

Fig. 101 *Hoop cramp (from Brockhaus dictionary, 1901); pelican and dental forceps in the translation of Guy de Chauliac of Nicaise, from a later copy*

that the ancient physicians *promise much but achieve little* with these agents[188]. Abū l-Qāsim is also frequently quoted as in the instruction to replace teeth which have fallen out with such prepared from oxbone[189].

This dependence on the Arabs[190], however, is particularly marked in dental surgical procedures. Although Guy wishes it to be understood that the "dentistae" are only assistants to physicians, they are, in any event, equipped with a good selection of instruments: razor, scraping iron, straight or bent spatulus, one- or two-armed levers, serrated forceps, probes, cannulas and also drills are listed here[191]. With regard to operative tooth extraction Guy elaborates Abū l-Qāsim's text only insignificantly: care should be taken that the correct tooth is pulled. The head of the patient should be taken between the knees, the root exposed all around the tooth, and the tooth carefully loosened. Only then is the tooth, including the root, to remove with a forceps[192]. In the same way as his informant, Guy is familiar with the one- or two-armed lever as an instrument for tooth removal. In place of the forceps shaped like a stork's beak, used by Abū l-Qāsim, he uses such *which are similar to those with which barrels are hooped*[193]. This device of the coopers, the hoop cramp, is the first description of the pelican up to this time if we disregard the unclear passage in John of Gaddesden[194] (Fig. 101). The mention of this instrument, not yet named pelican, with which human teeth and jaws were to be mishandled well into the 19th century, shows that Guy was a practitioner, because then it represented progress.

For dislocation of the mandible, Guy de Chauliac incorporates the false Hippocratic belief, with reference to Ibn Sīnā and 'Alī ibn al-'Abbās, that the patient will die of muscle stiffening on the 10th day if reduction is not carried out immediately. In therapy, however, he relies on Lanfranchi: if manual reduction fails, wedges of wood should be used[195].

These detailed observations show Guy's great experience, but leave it also uncertain whether he had undertaken all these procedures himself or with the help of assistants. His work appeared in French translation in 1478, and in the original Latin text[196] together with the surgical writings of Roger, of Roland of Parma, of Bruno da Longoburgo, and Lanfranchi and belongs into the category of early printings. It had more effect on dental surgery than on general surgery, and that well into the 18th century.

188 Ibid. p. 58a^r, 8
189 Albucasis XXX 2, 33 (a) p. 194, 2—4; English translation (b) pp. 294 f. = Guy VI 2, 2 p. 57b^v, 19—22
190 Albucasis XXX 2, 29—31; English translation (b) pp. 270 f.
191 Guy (a) VI 2, 2 p. 57b^r, 40—45
192 Ibid. p. 57b^v, 58—67
193 Ibid. VI 2, 2 p. 57b^v, 66; see v. Brunn p. 99 f.
194 See pp. 63 and 126 f.
195 Guy (a) V 2, 2 p. 42b^v, 7 f.
196 Baader (b) pp. 37 f.

In 1380, not many years after Guy de Chauliac had compiled his "Chirurgia magna," Balescon de Tarente (Valescus de Tharanta), a Portuguese, came as a professor to Montpellier, where he published his "Philonium" in 1418, a handbook of medical practice. With regard to dentistry, it represents a step backwards compared with Guy. As with him, tooth anatomy remains completely within Ibn Sīnā's concepts. Personal observations, such as that he himself had 30 teeth, namely 16 in the maxilla and 14 in the mandible, are present to a certain extent[197]. He says of the therapy of tooth complaints that he compiled it from the works of his predecessors[198]; among them he names Bernard Gordon, and particularly frequently Gerard of Cremona's translations of the "Qānūn" of Ibn Sīnā, the "Liber ad Almansorem" of ar-Rāzī, and the so-called "Brevarium" of Yūhannā ibn Sarābiyūn. He also quotes Galen mostly from the direct translation from the Greek, as Guy had already done. Regarding the prescriptions of all these authors to remedy toothache he expressly states that none helps immediately, and that their application is often in vain[199]. Even with a procedure such as tooth extraction, only to be undertaken in an extreme case, he refers solely to sources[200], failing to include an ąuthor as important as Abu l-Qāsīm. Thus, unlike his great contemporary Guy, Balescon probably neither practiced dentistry nor supervised its practice.

The 14th century had already been a time of revolutionary innovation, because at the same time when Guy de Chauliac had compiled the surgery of the Middle Ages including stomatology for the last time, a new spirit begins to stand out in the overall development of Europe. Francesco Petrarca had lived and worked in the Avignon of the papal physician Guy. From the early humanism, the ideology of the now blooming Italian city-states which they both helped to found, proceeded a whole new approach to life, rejecting the entire way of life of the Middle Ages and the accompanying feudal systems. Part of this was Petrarca's attack on Arabism and Galenism in medicine in 1352.

Little of this new spirit is perceptible, however, in actual medical literature of the 15th and the beginning of the 16th centuries. This applies to the otherwise so advanced Italian universities, and is especially true for stomatological problems. Giovanni da Concorregio (Ioannes Conregius), who was professor of medicine in Bologna, Pavia, Florence, and Milan since 1404, transmits only known material in his medical textbook "Practica nova," predominantly from the translation of Ibn Sīnā's "Qānūn." He advises in general against extraction with a forceps[201].

The situation is similar to that of the other representatives of the subject, even if it is not obvious at first[202]. The dental section of the "Sermones medicinales", by Niccolo Falcucci (Nicolaus Florentinus), who was born in Florence and died there in 1412[203], is only an excerpt from the Latin translation of Abū l-Qāsim with occasional consultation of the "Qānūn" translation as well. Falcucci had nothing new to add even in to medicated therapy against toothache. A sterile discussion about the composition of teeth takes up a great deal of space, with references to Ibn Sīnā as well as to his own predecessors Pietro d'Abano and Gentile da Foligno. Only the report that a man 70 years old grew a full new set of teeth stems from Falcucci himself[204].

This kind of relationship to practical experience remained the rule in literature on the subject until the beginning of the 16th century. Neither does Pietro d'Argellata (Petrus de Largelata), who died in 1423 as professor of medicine and philosophy in Bologna, go beyond the Persian authors. Even the stomatological part in his "Chirurgie" represents only a commentary on Ibn Sīnā's "Qānūn" in the university style. Both his own additions and the fact that he took Guy de Chauliac's opinion without mention of the source[205] as his own, that barbers should perform the tooth extraction, even though under the supervision of a physician[206], shows that he had never grained practical experience in this field. He lists only fumigation with leek seeds as a remedy against toothworm[207] as a personal contribution. He also described a horse dealer's

[197] Valescus II 71
[198] Ibid. II 72 p 105b^{r}, 34—37
[199] Ibid. II 72 p. 105b^{v}, 25—29
[200] Ibid. II 72 p. 108a^{v}, 52—108b^{v}, 3
[201] Concoregius I 93 p. 92a^{v}, 1 f.
[202] See Sudhoff (f) pp. 138 f.
[203] Nicolaus II 3, 28
[204] Ibid. VII 1, 32; see Heerklotz 14
[205] See p. 130
[206] Petrus de Largelata V 10, 1 p. 103b, 48—60
[207] Ibid. V 10, 5 p. 104a^{r}, 43—45

trick of filing the teeth of old horses to make them appear younger after the method of Abū l-Qāsim, who, however, did not mention the trick in his writings[208].

Finally, Alessandro Benedetti, the founder of the anatomical theater in Padua in 1490, discussed dental medicine in the 6th book of his medical "Encyclopedia", but also provides nothing new. True, he made frequent reference to the collected works of Galen, which had been translated directly from the Greek in the meantime, but it did not lead him any further. Thus, Benedetti warned against tooth extraction because a patient had died from it after application of an opiate[209] and did not recognize that the problem as being an overdose of opium. In another passage he reports from personal experience about loosening of teeth which was caused by the flow of humors[210].

Giovanni d'Arcoli (Ioannes Arculanus), professor in Bologna, Padua, and until his death in 1460 in Ferrara, is more receptive to practical experience, or at least to the recognition of knowledge derived from the practice of others. In his commentary on the translation of the 9th book of ar-Rāzī's "Liber ad Almansorem", he relies in tooth anatomy, in prophylaxis, and in alleviation of pain above all on Ibn Sīnā, whom he sometimes even names.

As in pseudo-Mesuë[211], d'Arcoli makes a distinction between correct and false therapy. The latter exists when the cause of the toothache is not eliminated, but rather relief is provided only with narcotics, among which henbane fumigation is foremost[212]. D'Arcoli, also, recommends the use of a drill in cauterization: *And if it is necessary, it should occur that the tooth be drilled through with a small drill (cum perforatorio minuto) so that the cautery force penetrates to the diseased site*[213]. It could almost be assumed that the author knew about inflamed pulp.

Of more importance is that d'Arcoli at the end of this chapter is the first to mention the use of gold foil for tooth conservation. At first, however, the tooth should be filled with cooling agents, when the pain is hot, or with warming ones when the pain is cold. Lest the pain be increased, this must be effected without the use of force. Then drugs are applied which—hippocratically formulated—are in contrast to the imbalanced mixture of humors in the tooth (*in contrarium discrasie dentis*). Yet, if *the deviation from a moderate degree is not too great* (i. e. probably, if the tooth does not hurt too much), *then it* (the tooth) *should be filled with gold foil (impleatur cum foliis auri)*[214].

In the subsequent chapter, d'Arcoli comments, in accord with ar-Rāzī, on tooth extraction whereby in contrast to the Persian he puts the operative extraction with the iron instrument (*cum ferro*) at the head of his list, although he takes precautions against its frivolous application. The loosening of the gingiva and the ligaments around the root must come first. He mentions the treatment with cauterization only secondarly, in which he applies boiling oil by means of cotton or, in accordance with John of Gaddesden[215], a grain of incense as a palliative. With d'Arcoli, however, the incense must be glowing. Through these procedures the pain decreases, and the tooth eventually falls out[216]. The dominant medicated tooth removal in ar-Rāzī is only the third choice for d'Arcoli. He surely replaces the former's absurd therapy with tree frog fat with the fat of the river fog, but he also includes an actually effective agent: he mixes it with the juice of wolf's milk, which we know as combined with flour from Ibn Sīnā[217]. Anyone who has felt the burning of this plant's juice on his tongue (it grows luxuriantly in the south) can well imagine that it did not remain without effect.

Dentistry occupies a great deal of space in the "Opus practicum" of d'Arcoli's contemporary Giovanni Michele Savonarola, who was acting as professor of medicine in Padua and Florence from 1434 to 1440[218]. Once again tooth anatomy is reported with reference to Ibn Sīnā, as are prophylactic measures. The numerous prescriptions taken from a great variety of authors as remedies against toothache he lists with some scepticism. *Perhaps, as is not uncommonly the case, these medications will not help, particularly if the tooth is crumbling, carious, or rotten. For this reason, as these authors attest, the last step must be taken, which involves extraction*[219]. The extraction itself, which Savo-

208 Ibid. V 10, 12 p. 105b^r, 45—48
209 Benedictus VI 13 p. 124, 31—33
210 Ibid. VI 15 p. 126, 9 f.
211 See p. 91
212 Arculanus 48 p. 194a, 37—60
213 Ibid. 48 p. 195b, 29—31
214 Ibid. 48 p. 196a, 1 f.
215 See p. 128
216 Ibid. 49 p. 196a, 30—b, 29
217 Gerard of Cremona III 7, 18 = Arculanus 49 p. 197a, 6—8
218 Lochmann p. 5
219 Savonarola VI 7, 2 p. 106a^r, 9—12

Practica in chirurgia.

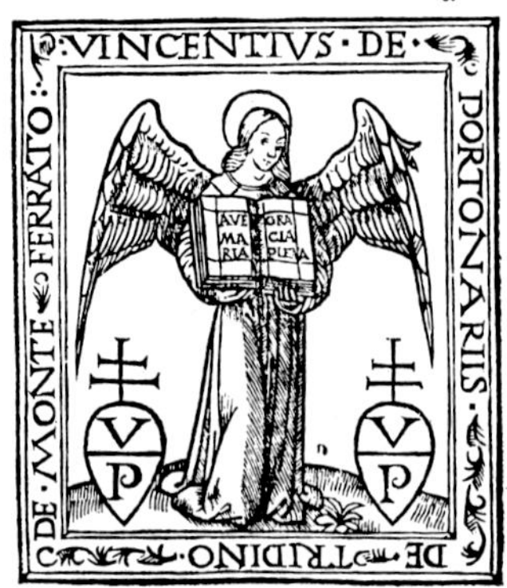

Practica in arte chirurgica copiosa Joannis de vigo Julij .ij. Pon. Max. Continēs nouē libros infrascriptos.

Primus: De anathomia chirurgo necessaria.
Secundus: De apostematibus in vniuersali et particulari.
Tertius: De vulneribus in vniuersali et particulari.
Quartus: De vlceribus in vniuersali et particulari.
Quintus: De morbo gallico: et dislocatione iuncturarum.
Sextus: De fractura et dislocatione ossium.
Septimus: De natura simplicium et posse eorum.
Octauus: De natura compositorum: et est antidotarium.
Nonus: De quibusdam additionibus totum complentibus.

Cum gratia et priuilegio.

Fig. 102 *Title page of the Giovanni da Vigo "Practica"; Leyden edition 1518*

narola describes competently on the base of his sources, particularly Abū l-Qāsim, is probably something which he had never performed himself, because he mentions as toothers those *rash and foolhardy operators who always want to pull teeth immediately*[220]. He names as their instruments the forceps, the lever, and a "caniculus"[221]. Like Guy, Savonarola did not think the medicated tooth removal was much worth: *And, though many are confident that an effect will be brought about by an extraction of them* (the teeth) *without instruments, I have never personally seen any result from it*[223]. He regards it as only a supplement to tooth extraction, and when the necessity arises to always proceed with an operation.

Giovanni da Vigo (Ioannes de Vigo), surgeon to the later Pope Julius II, was no different from Savonarola in probably never having performed tooth extraction himself, but rather leaving it to the barbers, because in his "Practica in arte chirurgica copiosa" (Exhaustive Treatise on the Art of Surgery), which appeared in Rome in 1514 (Fig. 102), he expressly states that practice is necessary in tooth extraction: *Therefore, the best physicians and surgeons have recommended, that this operation be left to experienced barber-surgeons and to the itinerant charlatans in the public market place. Hence, it is useful in pulling teeth, to visit men experienced in this operation to watch them, and to report about them*[223]. Although there is nothing precise on that subject in da Vigo, cauterization of the (as yet unknown) pulp with vitriol instead of the heated iron is included among the toothache remedies[224]. In many other passages, he is only a compiler, except that, in comparison with others, he stands at the height of the knowledge of his time. Thus, he takes the gold foil filling from d'Arcoli, but makes the indication more precise: "... *afterwards* (after re-

220 Ibid. VI 7, 2 p. 106a^r, 37—39
221 Ibid. VI 7, 2 p. 106a^r, 56 f.
222 Ibid. VI 7, 2 p. 106b^r, 9—11
223 de Vigo V 6, 5 p. 135a^r, 36—45
224 Ibid. V 6, 5 p. 135a^r, 36—40

moval of the *corrosio with drill, file, and scraper* [*cum trapano, lima, scarpo*]), *the hole should be filled with gold foil for preservation of the tooth (pro conservatione dentis foramen auri foliis impleatur)*[225]. For reducing dislocations of the mandible he prefers Lanfranchi's method with wedges and bandages[226]. All this shows a surgeon well-versed in both theory and practice, whose accomplishments provided the essential basis for the first specifically dental medical work ever, the German Artzney Buchlein of 1530[227].

In the 13th century, there had appeared a new literary form: the so-called consultation literature which, as a collection of case histories, is fundamentally rooted in practice. In this genre, however, there is at first little stomatological material to be found. A description of treatment of epulis by Ugo Benzi, the physician and professor of medicine from Siena, and finally in Ferrara, ought to be mentioned[228]. One of the two Bartolommeo Montagnana—both father and son were professors of medicine in Padua in the 15th century—used ammonium chloride for medicated tooth removal, and opium and camphor for deadening of toothaches[229]. Finally, we find a case of marginal periodontitis pointed out in connection with kidney trouble in the work of Giovanni Battista de Monte (Ioannes Baptista Montanus), professor in Ferrara and Padua[230].

This is the whole extend of literature in the 15th century on the subject of dentistry which is based on practice. In the work of the man whom we owe thanks for the most exact case histories and for overcoming the scholastic medieval thinking, to the Florentine physician Antonio Benivieni, we find nothing but superstition in regard to toothache. In his collection of case histories, under the title "De abditis morborum causis' (On the hidden Causes of Diseases), he reports the case of a country priest whose toothache made tears stream from his eyes during the celebration of the mass. A farmer helped him by pounding a stake into the earth with a hammer while repeating incantations of exorcism. After the first blow, the pain eased somewhat, after the second it was almost, and after the third completely gone. Then, however, the priest was filled with regret and prayed to God for renewed pain as penitence which promptly appeared[231].

This "staking-out", or "nailing-out" of a toothache is an ancient popular custom which is possibly practiced even today. In a similar superstition it is transmitted to animals and trees: a crust of bread, for example, is chewed and spat out into an anthill[232]. Even as late as the 18th century we can read an exact description of a "transmission" into a tree, by Valentin Kräutermann[233].

Thus elements of the medicine of the Middle Ages live on in folk medicine uninterruptedly even to the present day. In the science of medicine, on the other hand, the awakening of the natural sciences, which commenced on this subject in the 16th century, gradually put an end to them.

225 Ibid. V 6. 5 p. 133bv, 39 f.
226 Ibid. VI 6, 2 p. 142br, 40—52
227 See pp. 160 f.
228 Benzi 32
229 Montagnana 87
230 Montanus 84; see Nossol pp. 32 f.
231 Diepgen (b) p. 238
232 Wilke p. 284
233 See p. 228

What was written concerning the collaboration of Gerhard Baader, PhD, on page 87 of the Western Europe section holds without limitation for this chapter "High and Late Middle Ages in Europe", which would have remained incomplete without his expert help.
This is the point at which we should recall the medical historian Karl Sudhoff (1853—1938), who opened our eyes to the development of the field of dentistry in the European Middle Ages.

References

Albucasis
a) De Chirurgia, arabice et latine. Cura Johannis Channing, Oxonii 1778
b) On surgery and instruments. A definitive ed. of the Arabic text with English transl. and commentary by M. S. Spink; G. L. Lewis. London 1973

Ambrosius
De virginibus. Libri tres ed. Egnatius Cazzaniga. Corp. script. Lat. Paravianum, Aug. Taurinorum (1948)

Apollonia virgo martyr
In: Acta sanctorum Februarius Tomus II, col. 278—283. Antverpiae 1658.

Arculanus, Ioannes
Commentaria in nonum librum Rasis ad regem Almansorem. Venetiis 1542

Aristotle
De generatione animalium. Recogn. H. J. Drossaart Lulofs, Oxonii 1965

Arnaldus de Villanova
Breviarium practice. Mediolani 1483

Artelt, Walter
Die ältesten Nachrichten über die Sektion menschlicher Leichen im Abendland. Abh. Gesch. Med. Naturw. H. 34, Berlin 1940

Augustinus
De civitate dei. Ed. E. Hoffmann. Corp. script Lat. 40, Wien, Leipzig 1899

Baader, Gerhard
a) Zur Anatomie in Paris im 13. und 14. Jahrhundert. Med. Hist. J. 3 (1968) 40—53
b) Handschrift und Inkunabel in der Überlieferung der medizinischen Literatur. In: Buch und Wissenschaft, Technikgesch. in Einzeldarstellungen. Nr. 17, Düsseldorf 1969, pp. 15—47

Bartholomaeus
Practica. In: Collectio Salernitana. Ed. Salvatore de Renzi. Tomo IV pp. 321—406, Napoli 1856

Benedictus, Alexander
De re medica opus. Venetiis 1533

Benzi, Ugo
In: Dean Putnam Lockwood, Ugo Benzi. Medieval philosopher and physician 1376—1439. Chicago 1951

Brodmann, Karl
Deutsche Zahntexte in Handschriften des Mittelalters. Med. Diss. Leipzig 1921

Brunn, Walter von
Die Stellung des Guy de Chauliac in der Chirurgie des Mittelalters. Arch. Gesch. Med. 13 (1921) 65—106

Brunus Longoburgensis
Chirurgia magna. In: Guido de Cauliaco Cyrurgia, Venetis 1400, pp. 75r—93v

Bulk, Wilhelm
St. Apollonia. Bielefeld, Münster 1967

Bullough, Vern L.
The development of the medical university at Montpellier . . . Bull. Hist. Med. 30 (1956) 508—523

Chartularium universitatis parisiensis. Ed. Henricus Denifle et Aemilius Chatelain, 4 vols., Paris 1889/1897

Concoregius, Ioannes
Practica nova. Papie (= Pavia) 1458

Constantinus Africanus
a) Theorica. In: Ysaac Opera omnia, Lugduni 1515 pp. 1r—57v; Const. Afr. Opera, Basileae 1536, pp. 200—300
b) Viaticum. In: Ysaac Opera omnia, Lugduni 1515, pp. 144v—171r; Const. Afr. Opera, Basilleae 1536, pp. 1—167
c) Practica. In: Ysaac Opera omnia, Lugduni 1515, pp. 58r—144v

Copho
Practica. In: Collectio Salernitana. Ed. Salvatore de Renzi. Tomo IV, pp. 439—505, Napoli 1856

Creutz, Rudolf
Addimenta zu Konstantinus Africanus und seinen Schülern Joh. und Atto. Stud. Mitt. Gesch. Benediktinerordens 50 (1932) 420—442

Diepgen, Paul
a) Studien zu Arnald von Villanova. Arch. Gesch. Med. 3 (1910) 115—130; 280—296; 369—396
b) Geschichte der Medizin. Vol. I, Berlin 1949

Donaldson, J. Archie
Peter de London, Toothdrawer. Brit. Dent. J. 119 (1965) 147—148

Doneldey, Arnoldus
Das Bremer mittelniederdeutsche Arzneibuch des A. D. Ed. Ernst Windler. In: Niederdtsch. Denkmäler Vol. 7, Neumünster 1932

Eusebius
Werke. Vol. 2: Die Kirchengeschichte. Ed. Eduard Schwartz. In: Die griechischen christlichen Schriftsteller der ersten drei Jahrhunderte. Vol. 9, 1, 2, 3. Leipzig 1903/09

Fonahn, A(dolf)
Arabic and latin anatomical terminology chiefly from the middle ages. In Videnskapsselskapets skrifter II. Hist.-filos. Kl. 1921 No. 7, Kristiania 1922

Galen
De usu partium. Libri XVII. Rec. Georgius Helmreich, Vol. II, Lipsiae 1907/09

Gariopontus
Ad totius corporis aegritudinis remediorum praxeon libri V. Basileae 1531

Gerard of Cremona
Liber canonis Avicenne. Venetiis 1507

Gilbertus Anglicus
Compendium medicinae. Ed. Michael de Capella, Lugduni 1510

Glossulae quattuor magistrorum et Rolandi super chirurgiam Rogerii. In: Collectio Salernitana. Ed. Salvatore de Renzi, Tomo II, pp. 497—724, Napoli 1853

Gordon, Bernard
Lilium medicinae. Francofurti 1617

Guerini, Vincenzo
A history of dentistry. Philadelphia, New York 1909

Gurlt, Ernst
Geschichte der Chirurgie, Vols. I—III, Berlin 1898

Guy de Chauliac
a) Chirurgia magna. In: Guido de Cauliaco, Cyrurgia, pp. 1r—74r, Venetiis 1400
b) La grande Chirurgie de Guy de Chauliac . . . Trad. E. Nicaise, Paris 1890

Heerklotz, Johann-Georg Albert
Nicolo Falcucci in seinen die Zahnheilkunde berührenden Kapiteln. Med. Diss. Leipzig 1921

Hein, Wolfgang-Hagen, Kurt Sappert
Die Medizinalordnung Friedrichs II. Veröff. Internat. Ges. Gesch. Pharm. NF. Vol. XII, Eutin 1957

Henri de Mondeville
Die Chirurgie des Heinrich de Mondeville (Harmandaville) . . . Ed. Julius Leopold Pagel, Berlin 1892

Hoffmann-Axthelm, Walter
Die medikamentöse Zahnentfernung. Zahnärztl. Mitt. 60 (1970) 982—985. Idem: Atti del XXI Congresso Int. di Storia della Medicina, Siena 1968, Roma 1969, pp. 837—846

Huard, Pierre, Mirko Drazen Grmek
Mille ans de Chirurgie. Paris 1966

Ioannes Anglicus
Rosa Anglica. a) Paviae 1517 b) Augustae Vindelicorum 1595

Keil, Gundolf
Das Arzneibuch Ortolfs von Baierland. Sudhoffs Arch. Gesch. Med. Naturw. 43 (1959) 20—60

Köhler, Johannes
Zahnärztliches bei Thomas von Sarepta. Med. Diss. Leipzig 1924

Lanfranchi
Chirurgia magna. In: Guido de Cauliaco Cyrurgia. Venetiis 1400, pp. 176r—216v

Langebartels, Erich
Zahnheilkunde und Kieferchirurgie in der chirurgischen Literatur von Salerno und der weiteren Rogerglosse . . . Med. Diss. Leipzig 1919

Lauer, Hans Hugo
Zur Beurteilung des Arabismus in der Medizin des mittelalterlichen Englands. Sudhoffs Arch. Gesch. Med. Naturw. 51 (1967) 326—348

Leersum, E. C. van
Notes concerning the life of Jan Yperman. Janus 18 (1913) 1—15

Lehmann, Hermann
Die Arbeitsweise des Constantinus Africanus und des Johannes Afflicius im Verhältnis zueinander. Archeion 12 (1930) 272—283

Lochmann, Werner
Zahnheilkundiges bei Giovanni Micaele Savonarola. Med. Diss. Leipzig 1926

Löchel, Wolfgang
Die Zahnmedizin Rogers und der Rogerglossen. Pattensen (Hannover) 1976

Mansi, Joannes Dominicus (Ed.)
Sacrorum conciliorum nova et amplissima collectio. Vol. 22, Venetiis 1778

Marzell, Heinrich
Wörterbuch der deutschen Pflanzennamen. Vol. I f. Leipzig 1943 f.

Montagnana, Bartholomaeus
Consilia, Venetiis 1499

Montanus, Ioannes Baptista
Consulationes de variorum morborum curationibus. Basileae 1557

Nicolaus Florentinus
Sermones medicinales. Sermo I, II, VII, Papie 1481/84; Sermo III, Papie [c. 1487]

Nord, Karl
Zahnheilkundliches aus den Schriften Konstantins von Afrika. Med. Diss. Leipzig 1922

Norpoth, Leo
Zur Bio-, Bibliographie und Wissenschaftslehre des Pietro d'Abano. Kyklos 3 (1930) 292—353

Nossohl, Reinhard
Mund- und Zahnleiden in Consilien des Ugo Benzi, Bartolomeo Montagnana und Giambattista da Monte. Med. Diss. Leipzig 1922

Ohrt, Ferdinand
Zahnsegen. In: Handwörterbuch des deutschen Aberglaubens. Ed. Hanns Bächtold-Stäubli, Vol. 9, Berlin 1938/41, col. 877—880

Petrus Hispanus
Thesaurus pauperum, Francoforti 1578

Petrus de Largelata
Chirurgia. Venetiis 1499

Pietro d'Abano
Conciliator. Mantue 1472

Platearius, Johannes
Practica brevis. In: Johannes Serapio Practica dicta breviarium. Venetiis 1497, IV 3, pp. 176a^r f.

Rashdall, Hastings
The universities of Europe in the Middle Ages. Vol. I—III, 2nd ed., F. M. Powicke, A. B. Emden, Oxford 1936

Regimen sanitatis Salerni
a) Das medizinische Lehrgedicht der Hohen Schule zu Salerno. Übers. Paul Tesdorpf, Stuttgart 1915
b) In: Collectio Salernitana. Ed. Salvatore de Renzi. Tomo V, pp. 1—104, Napoli 1859

Rowe, Norman Lester
The history of the treatment of maxillo-facial trauma. Ann. Roy. Coll. Surg. England 49 (1975) 329—349

Savonarola, Ioannes Michael
Opus practicum. Venetiis 1497

Schipperges, Heinrich
a) Die frühen Übersetzer der arabischen Medizin in chronologischer Sicht. Sudhoffs Arch. Gesch. Med. Naturw. 39 (1955) 53—93
b) Die Assimilation der arabischen Medizin durch das Lateinische Mittelalter. Sudhoffs Arch. Add. Nr. 3, Wiesbaden 1964

Schwind, Oskar
Zahnärztliches bei den italienischen Chirurgen des 13. Jahrhunderts und bei Guy de Chauliac. Med. Diss. Leipzig 1924

Seidemann, Martin
Zahnärztliches in den Werken des Gilbertus Anglicus. Med. Diss. Leipzig 1922

Seidler, Eduard
Die Heilkunde des ausgehenden Mittelalters in Paris. Sudhoffs Arch. Add. Nr. 8, Wiesbaden 1967

Sillanus de Nigris
Exposition noni libri Almansoris. Venetiis 1490

Spink and Lewis
See Albucasis (b)

Sudhoff, Karl
a) Abermals eine neue Handschrift der anatomischen Fünfbilderserie. Arch. Gesch. Med. 3 (1910) 353—368
b) Beiträge zur Geschichte der Chirurgie im Mittelalter, 2. Teil (= Stud. Gesch. Med., Nr. 11—12) Leipzig 1918
c) Die Salernitaner Handschrift in Breslau. Arch. Gesch. Med. 12 (1920) 101—148
d) Schädigungen des Zahnfleisches durch bleihaltige Gesichtsschminken zu Anfang des 12. Jahrhunderts. Mitt. Gesch. Med. Naturw. 13 (1914) 308
e) Die kurze „Vita“ und das Verzeichnis der Arbeiten Gerhards von Cremona. Sudhoffs Arch. Gesch. Med. 8 (1914) 73—82
f) Geschichte der Zahnheilkunde. 2nd ed. Leipzig 1926

Talbot, C. H., E. A. Hammond
The medical pratitioners in medieval England. Publ. Wellcome Hist. Med. Library, London 1956

Theodoricus Cerviensis
In: Guido de Cauliaco, Cyrurgia. Venetiis 1400, pp. 97^r—134^v

Tractatus de aegritudinum curatione.
In: Collectio Salernitana. Ed. Salvatore de Renzi. Tomo II, pp. 81—368, Napoli 1853

Trotula
In: Experimentarius medicinae. Argentorati 1544

Urso
Anatomia. Ed. Karl Sudhoff. Arch. Gesch. Med. 20 (1928) 33—50

Valescus de Tharanta
Philonium. Lugduni 1526

Vigo, Ioannes de
Practica in arte chirurgica copiosa. Lugduni 1518

William of Saliceto
a) Chirurgia. In: Ars chirurgica Guidonis Chauliaci. Venetiis 1546, pp. 303—361
b) Chirurgia IV. Ed. F. Schaarschmidt, Die Anatomie des Wilhelm von Saliceto. Med. Diss. Leipzig 1919
c) Summa conservationis et curationis. Venetiis 1490

Wilke, Georg
Die Heilkunde in der europäischen Vorzeit. Leipzig 1936

Wilke, Walter
Der Arzt Petrus Hispanus und seine Bedeutung für die Zahnheilkunde. Med. Diss. Leipzig 1924

Wrede, Adam
Apollonia. In: Handwörterbuch des deutschen Aberglaubens. Ed. Hanns Bächtold-Stäubli. Vol. I, Berlin, Leipzig 1927, col. 551 f.

Yperman, Jan
Cyrurgie. Ed. E. C. van Leersum, Leiden 1912

Chapter 9

Awakening of the Natural Sciences

The 16th Century

Historians place the end of the Middle Ages, an era especially sterile for our field, in the second half of the 15th century. Emanating from Italy in the subsequent hundred years, that spiritual metamorphosis which we designate in history and art as the Renaissance, the rebirth of antiquity, took place. *It was a revival of antiquity only from one side,* says Gregorovius in his "History of the City of Rome in the Middle Ages," (it was) *in general the complete educational reform of occidental mankind.—It awakes an objective way of thinking of and treating the state, and all things of this world in general,* thus, Jakob Burckhardt defines the development of the corporately oriented man of the Middle Ages into the spiritual individual of modern times.

This new objective relation to the environment, carried into the whole world through the invention of printing about 1450, first manifested itself in medicine in the course of the 16th century. As an example of such lagging, one may recall Giovanni da Vigo, who was personal physician to the Renaissance Pope Julius II, and still strongly dependent on the ancients.

Thus, it is not too surprising that the first traces of the new spirit in medicine are to be found not in a physician but in an artist, Leonardo da Vinci. As late as 1778, when his anatomical work was discovered in the strong-box of a British royal castle, has it been known that the great anatomists of the 16th century had an adequate predecessor in this universal genius; his drawings of dissected body parts, obtained immediately from the subject, push everything else that had been done in this area to the background. The depiction of the teeth in a mouth strained open (Fig. 103) still points to physiognomic studies by a researching artist; the drawing of the skull correctly chiselled open, however, (Fig. 104) shows the purely anatomical researcher who, in 1489, completed through this preparation the discovery of the maxillary sinus, attributed later to Highmore (1651): *The eye, the instrument of sight, is concealed in the upper space, and, in the one underneath this one, there is a fluid which nourishes the roots of the teeth. The cavity of the cheek-bone (Il vacuo dell'osso della gancia) is similar in depth and width to the cavity which contains the eye in its interior, and receives veins into its interior through the holes m* [1].

Another drawing shows, in addition to the frontal view of a skull with exposed frontal and maxillary sinuses, the four types of teeth in the maxilla (Fig. 105), of which only the premolar seems incorrect. In any event, it is the first time that a differentiation is made between molars and premolars, in depiction as well as in the explanatory text, which the left-handed Leonardo, as usual, put down in mirror-image script: *the 6 upper grinding teeth (mascellari di sopra) each have 3 roots, two on the outer side, and one on the inner side of the jaw; both of these last two take two to eight years to grow in. These are followed by four grinding teeth (denti mascellari) with two roots, one inner and one outer, followed by two canines (maestre, masters) with only one root, and the four front teeth, which cut and also only have one root. The lower jaw (mascella disotta) likewise has 16 teeth, but its grinding teeth have only two roots* [2]*, the other teeth are as those of the upper jaw.*

The sum of these discoveries by an independent artist, i.e., not under the Galenic influence—which was almost greater than we can imagine today—remained unused because his presentations could hardly have reached his contemporaries among the physicians. Purging anatomy of Galenic teachings, often false because they were derived from animals, and replacing them with findings obtained by work with the human body, was reserved for the great Vesalius. Physicians had indeed already begun previously to free themselves timidly from the old conceptions, but no one had yet dared to attack Galen openly.

Andreas Vesalius was born in Brussels in 1514, the son of Karl V's personal apothecary. As the name suggests, his family came

[1] Braunfels-Esche; Tacke p. 5
[2] Huard; Sudhoff (b) p. 148

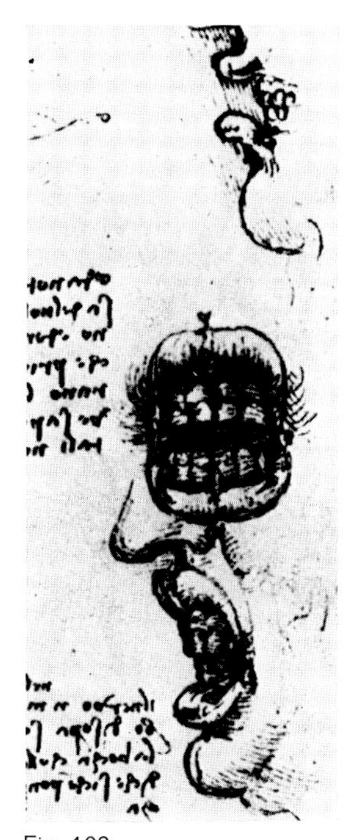

Fig. 103

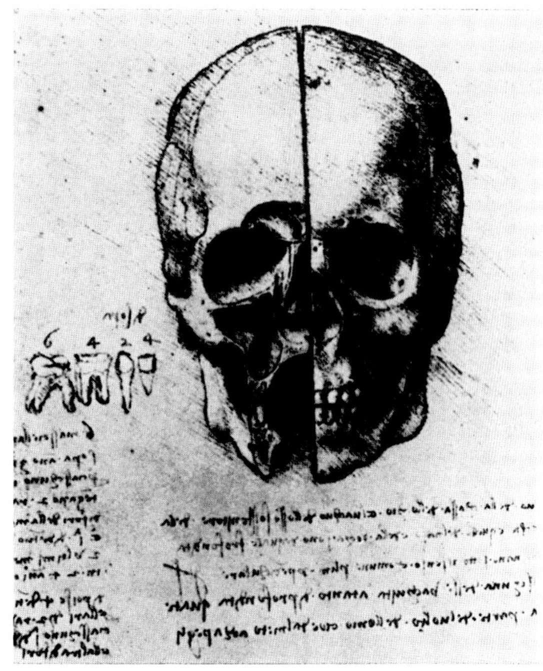

Fig. 105

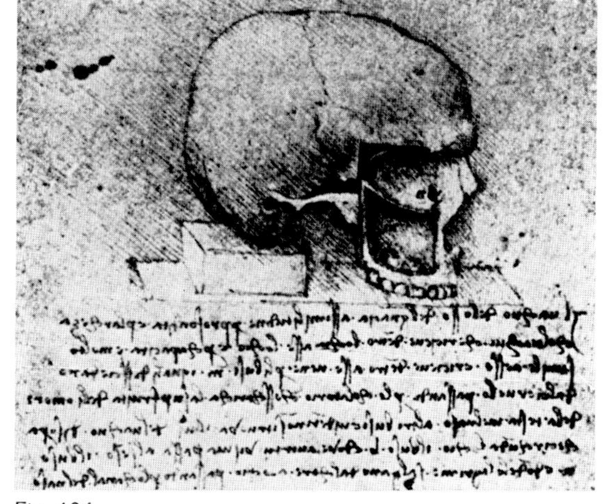

Fig. 104

Fig. 103 *Leonardo da Vinci: Studies of the mouth (Windsor, Clark 19055ᵛ)*

Fig. 104 *Leonardo da Vinci: Eye and sinus preparation (Windsor, Clark 19057ᵛ)*

Fig. 105 *Leonardo da Vinci: Skull preparation and depiction of teeth (Windsor, Clark 19058ᵛ) (Figs. 103 to 105 from Braunfels-Esche and Huard)*

from lower Rhenic Wesel. As a student in Paris (1553—1556) at the feet of Jaques Dubois (Sylvius), a disciple of Galen who was later to become his most bitter opponent, he had already determined through visual observation what 'Abd al-Latif[3] had observed some three hundred years before: the mandible is one bone ... *although I beheld mandibles elsewhere, above all in Paris at the Cemetary of the Innocents, in very large numbers (as well as other bones), I still never once found one divided into two parts* [4] (Fig. 106).

In 1534, that is, at the age of 23, Vesalius had already become a professor at the University of

[3] See p. 104
[4] Vesalius I p. 44

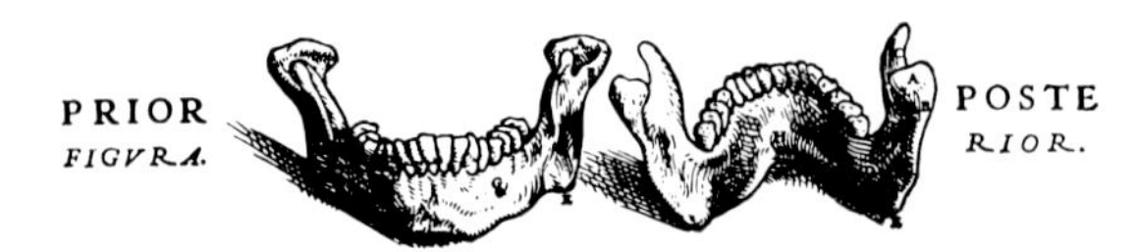

Fig. 106 *Vesalius: Mandible, 1542*

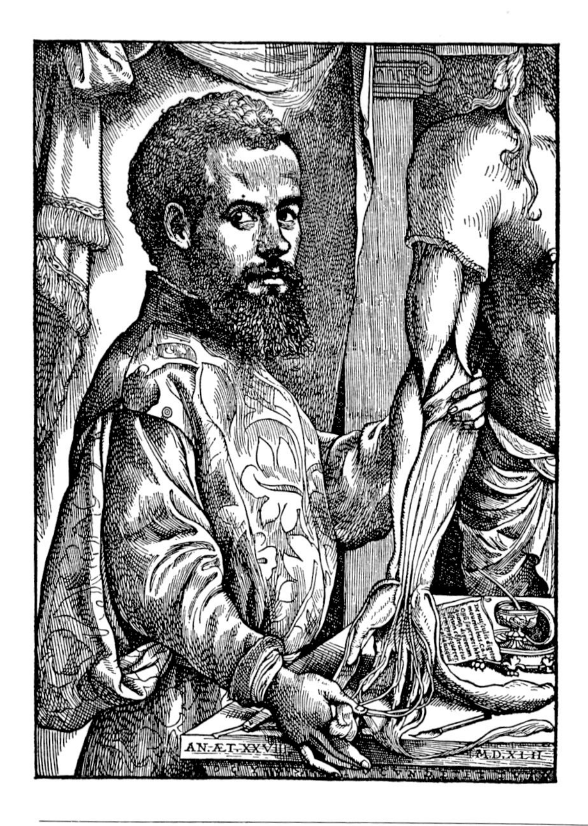

Fig. 107 *Andreas Vesalius, woodcut in the "Fabrica", 1542*

Padua (Fig. 107), where he could undertake dissections unhindered by clerical restrictions because it was part of the Venetian Republic. Here, he composed his great anatomical work, "De humani corporis fabrica," whose title presumably originated of the work of the Byzantine Theophilos[5], mentioned on page 81. It appeared in Basel in 1543, the same year in which Copernicus claimed the sun to be the center of the universe in his opus on the circular motions of the celestial bodies. The "Fabrica" was just as revolutionary for medicine as Copernicus' discoveries were for astronomy, particularly since Titian's students such as Jan Stephan van Calcar had presumably made congenial woodcuts for it. In this first realistic presentation of the rows of teeth (with the exception of Leonardo's drawing, which was unknown to his contemporaries), the only things that disturb us are the occlusion counteracted by extensive attrition, the absence of fusion in the roots of the 2nd maxillary premolar, and on the adjacent split molar the lack of the hole in the root tip (Fig. 108), with which the author was quite familar.

Only two pages of the "Fabrica" are devoted to the teeth, but they clear up many errors which had been copied repeatedly. In contrast to Ga-

[5] Schubring

DE HVMANI CORPORIS FABRICA LIBER I. 45

DE DENTIBVS, QVI ETIAM oſſium numero aſcribuntur. Caput XI.

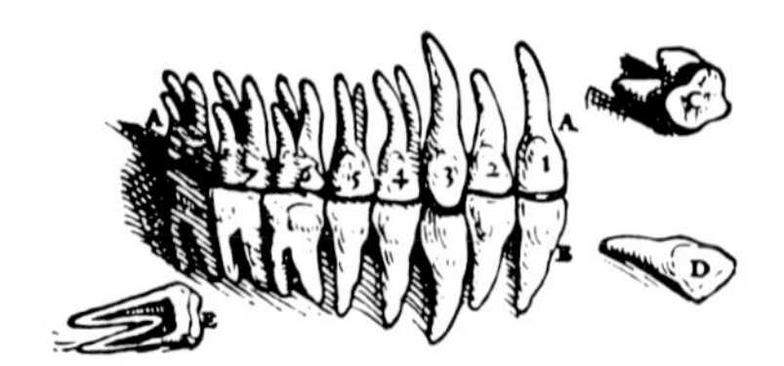

PRAESENTIS VNDECIMI CAPITIS FIGVRAE, ac ipſius characterum Index.

HAC figura tam ſuperioris maxillæ, quàm inferioris dentes, in altero latere exprimuntur. quum enim utriuſque lateris par ſit ratio, abundè eſt alterius lateris dentes ex maxillis erutos delineaſſe. Si uerò dentes maxillis adhuc infixos contemplari uiſum ſit, ſuperioris Capitis figuræ inferiorem commonſtrant ſeriem, quemadmodum tertia & quinta ſexti Capitis figuræ ſuperiorem. ubi & quarta eius Capitis figura alueolos promptè oſtendit, quibus dentes infigun tur. Quandoquidem ex caluaria, quam illa figura expreſſimus, ſtudiò ſuperioris maxillæ dentes euulſimus.

A A *Dextri lateris octo ſuperiores dentes.*
B B *Dextri lateris dentes octo inferiores.*
1, 2 *Duo dextri lateris inciſorij.* 3 *Dens caninus dexter.*
4, 5, 6, 7, 8 *Quinque molares dextri. Hunc numerum & inferiori & ſuperiori dentium claſſi accommodare integrum eſt. Nomina autem dentium, cum uarijs reliquorum oſſium nomenclaturis, ex huius libri calce ſumenda ueniūt: quòd in eum locum nomina, quæcunque mihi hactenus occurrere, duxerim reijcienda.*
C *Baſis notatur molaris dentis.* D *Acies dentis inciſorij.*
E *Media molaris dentis pars hic delineatur, ſinum in dentibus conſpicuum oſtenſura.*

EX OSSIBVS ſolos dentes ſentiendi uim obtinere, Galenus nō perfunctoriè atteſtatur, aſſerens ſe quoque dentium dolore uexatum, atque tum diligenter animum adhibuiſſe num dentes ipſi doleāt: ſenſiſſeq́ manifeſtò dentem nō modò dolere, uerùm etiam pulſare, carnibus inflammatione obſeſſis non diſſimiliter. Applantātur enim dentium radicibus molles quidam neruuli, à tertio neruorum cerebri coniugio propagati, quorum gratia dentes duntaxat euidenti inter oſſa ſentiendi facultate donatos credimus. Cæterum nonnulli Galeno haud acquieſcentes, colligunt, dentem, quum os ſit, citra dolorem affici: quemadmodum cum lima exceſſus dentium præſecare, aut ignitis ferris eos aliquando exurere cogimur. At quum in huiuſmodi artis operibus ipſos ſenſu præditos ſubinde experiamur, & à frigore potiſſimum moleſtari cognoſcamus, meritò laudandus eſt immēſus rerum Opifex, quem cæterorum oſſium ſolis duntaxat dentibus notatu dignam ſentiendi facultatē largitum arbitramur. Nouerat enim hos crebrò occurſuros ijs quæ ſecant, uel frangunt, uel rodunt, uel ualide excaleſaciunt, aut refrigerant, uel alia quauis occaſione alterant: quibus omnibus dentes multò aliter, quàm reliqua oſſa, nudi exponuntur. Quamobrem, ſi nulla ſentiendi ui pollerēt, à dolore homo neutiquam admoneretur, neque denti ſuccurreret, quod infeſtat amoturus, priuſquā moleſtati dentes uitiarentur. Porrò dentes non ſolum ſenſu, & quòd nudi ſint, ab alijs oſſibus diſtingui creduntur, uerum etiam quia hos plus cæteris oſſibus ſemper enutriri, & quouis tempore uitæ incrementum accipere, ideo præcipuè arbitramur, quod dentes illis quos eximimus oppoſiti, ſubinde in eruti dentis locū extra reliquam dentium ſeriem ſuccreſcant: ob hoc uidelicet, quod contrarijs dentibus non amplius atterantur. Reliqui enim dentes tantum augentur, quantum læuigandis cibis comminuuntur. Sunt autem plurimum dentes numero triginta duo, una ſerie in utraque maxilla ſedecim, inſtar iuſtiſſimæ choreæ ſiti. Quatuor priores aduerſiùe quia ſecant, inciſorij uocantur: ſunt enim lati & acuti, quò oblatum ipſis cibum mordendo cultri modo promptè abſcindant, diuidantq́.
Deinceps

Dentes ſentire.
Libro quinto de Medicamentorū compoſitione ſecundum locos.
2 ſi. 2 ca. li. 45 et XX.
Dentiū à cæteris oſſibus differentia.
Dentium numerus.
1, 2. D.
Inciſorij.

Fig. 108 *Vesalius: Page of text dealing with teeth*

len, Vesalius differentiates teeth from bones through numerous characteristics, but he persists in the Aristotelian error [6] that they (in contrast to bones) grow continuously. This is to be noted particularly when an antagonist is missing; if one is present, however, the growth is compensated by abrasion. For the tooth sockets, he employs the term first used by Soran, φατνίον (phatníon, or crib; in Rufus, φάτνη phátne) [7].

On the subject of the eruption of the third molar with complications, Vesalius even gives practical directions. Though in general an anatomist, he still remained a physician at all times: *The less attentive physicians either extract other teeth, or, since they are of the conviction that the patients can be suffering from a humor problem, mistreat them with drinks and similar agents, although light excoriation (scarifitio) of the gingiva above the last tooth and perforation of the bone can provide the sufferers with adequate help* [8].

Then Vesalius describes the dental pulp cavity (dentium cavitas), which serves to nourish the teeth. Naturally, there are still errors to be found. Primary teeth, which he probably only saw after or during exfoliation, are only appendages (appendices) of a soft, marrow-containing root, from which then the permanent tooth develops. Therefore, this must be protected. He remembers how, *as boys*, they had *pulled out themselves particularly the incisors with the nails or with a thread wrapped around it* [9].

In 1544, one year after the appearance of his revolutionary work, Vesalius answered the call of Emperor Charles V, and in 1559 that of Philipp II, King of Spain, as personal physician and surgeon and thus he gave up his extensive opportunity to gain further experience at the dissecting table. Therefore the second edition of the "Fabrica" contained no fundamental progress in 1555, but the author could still state with satisfaction that his students and those who emulated him were endeavoring to complete the work begun on an objective human anatomy. In 1564, the founder of modern anatomy died at the age of fifty, alone on a Greek island during his return from a pilgrimage to Jerusalem undertaken for reasons unknown to us.

In Padua, after Vesalius' death anatomy was represented for two years by Realdo Colombo (Columbus), who later taught in Pisa and Rome. In his work, which appeared in 1559, the year of his death, he did not really advance beyond his teacher. We can assume, however, that his work contains an early mention of the periodontal membrane, as he says: *These three vessels* (vein, artery, and nerve) *penetrate into those cavities* (of the dental pulp) *up to the base of the tooth, are folded together there, and form together a thin membrane, which tends periodically to become saturated with the substance which flows down from the brain (materia à cerebro defluente),* whereby the strongest toothaches arise. The latter is not to be interpreted as a festering inflammation of the periodontal membrane. It has rather to do with Hippocratic conceptions on the base of the humoral theory [10]. Vesalius' erroneous appendage hypothesis of dentition is included almost word-for-word. A case history of his family, the triple row of teeth in his son Phoebus, which is presented justifiably as a truly extraordinary phenomenon, forms the conclusion of the chapter, "On the Teeth" [11].

The second successor to Vesalius' anatomy chair in Padua, Gabriele Falloppia, definitively solved the problem of the divided mandible through his determination *that in all the corpses of children which I have disected, who had not passed their first year, I always found the mandible to consist of two bony parts, connected in the middle by cartilage mass* [12]. With persons who had died after the age of seven, however, he found it undivided. When Falloppia's "Observationes anatomicae" (Anatomical Observations) appeared in 1561, Vesalius was forced to admit, even if he did so with some hesitation, that Falloppia was right [13]. The *godly Vesalius'* theory on the exfoliation of teeth was also shaken by his successor, accompanied by expression of sincerest respect for the master's work. The permanent tooth does not develop from the soft root of the primary tooth, but from an independent soft mass, which gradually hardens during eruption [14]. The place of the permanent canine teeth, for example, is initially *under the tip of the root (sub extrema*

[6] See p. 65
[7] See p. 74
[8] Vesalius I p. 46
[9] Ibid. p. 47
[10] See pp. 60 f.
[11] Columbus I p. 33 f.
[12] Fallopius p. 36r
[13] Artelt
[14] Fallopius p. 40r

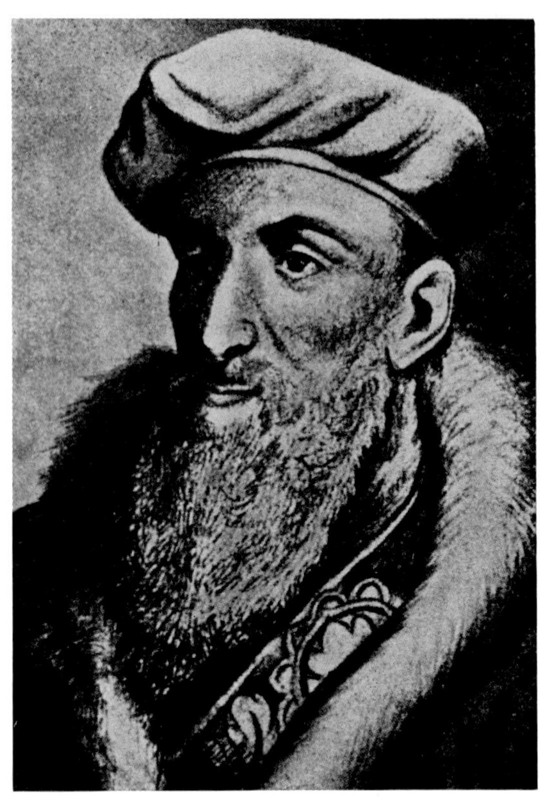

Fig. 109 *Bartolomeo Eustachi, painting by Frederigo Baroccio*

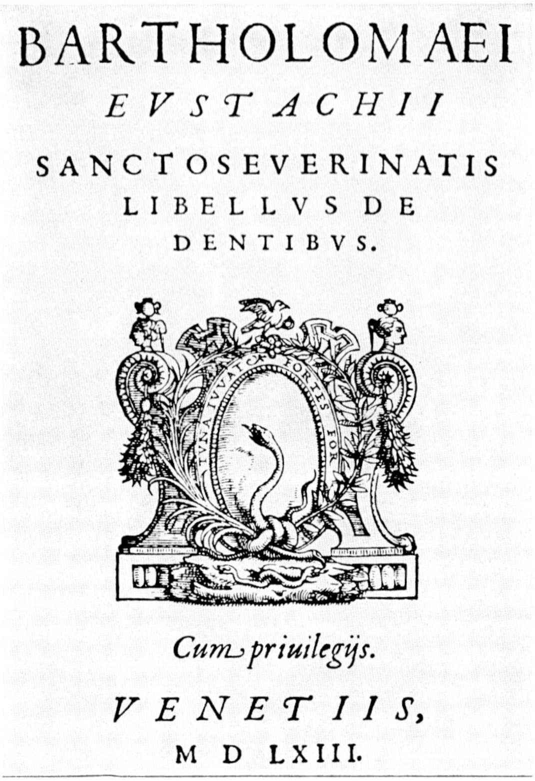

BARTHOLOMAEI
EVSTACHII
SANCTOSEVERINATIS
LIBELLVS DE
DENTIBVS.

Cum priuilegijs.

VENETIIS,
M D LXIII.

Fig. 110 *Eustachi: "Libellus de dentibus," Venice 1563*

radice) of the primary canine[15]. He clarifies tooth development at least morphologically through dissections on the products of miscarriages chiefly. Unfortunately, even this enlightened spirit also still believed in the *worms, which plague man to an amazing degree*[16].

The great progress of anatomy presented to odontology the first independent monograph on the subject, the "Libellus de dentibus" (Booklet of the Teeth) which came out in 1563 by the Roman physician Bartolomeo Eustachi (Bartholomaeus Eustachius [Figs. 109 and 110]), whose name has been carried on even to the present day by the tuba auditiva. This physician in ordinary to the pope and professor revered the ancient physicians. In contrast to Vesalius, who was constantly assaulting traditional teachings, he defended them, not only against his contemporaries, but also, necessarily, against the results of his own very thorough investigations. Thus, he clearly recognized, in contrast to Galen, the difference between teeth and bones, but protected his hero still, through the imputation that Galen was well aware, *that the teeth differ from the other bones in origin, growth, and sensitivy*[17]. Also in regard to the dental pulp cavity (concavitas) presumably unknown to Galen[18], *concerning which some newer authors* (he means Vesalius and Falloppia) *unjustly demand laurels,* he must have known, and it cannot simply be asserted, *that such a conscientious observer of nature's creatures as Galenus had no knowledge of this cavity*[19]. Like his contemporaries, Eustachi knows of the supply of the dental pulp through vessels and nerves; he can hardly imagine, however, that this takes place through an opening as small as the apical foramen. In this respect, too, we find a painful defense of Galen.

15 Ibid. p. 41^{v}
16 Ibid p. 38^{v}
17 Eustachius (a) p. 2
18 See p. 76
19 Ibid. p. 6

The fixation of teeth wedged into the jaw (gomphosis, which is correctly numbered among the synarthroses) is not effected only through the gingiva, but also through powerful ligaments (the periodontal membrane). Eustachi's familiarity with Aristotle led him to exhaustive comparative anatomical observations of the masticatory apparatus mainly in apes and fish. He is regarded as the father of that science. Enamel and dentin are differentiated, but not, however, named: *They* (the teeth) *consist ... of a dual substance, just as trees consist of the bark and the part covered by the bark*[20].

Eustachi's research in the subject of tooth development is particularly valuable; in this respect he extended his own ideas through those of Falloppia. Through methodical investigations on miscarriages, children, and young animals of every age, he identified the dental sac (folliculus) and the tooth-bud (candida squama), as well as the coalescing of this first enamel with the dentinal nucleus[21], and thus could at the same time weaken Vesalius' assertion that the second teeth form from the root of the deciduous teeth.

As a supplement to his numerous writings, Eustachi had the "Tabulae anatomicae" reproduced from his drawings in the then new engraving technique. These unfortunately disappeared for one and a half centuries after eight were printed in his lifetime. When they were rediscovered, they were published in 1714 by Lancisi, personal physician to the pope. Although they seem, in comparison to the woodcuts of Vesalius' work, to be unartistic and schematized, they still contain some advances and are correct in the essentials, even if we notice the absence of the foramen mentale on the mandible, which Vesalius had shown and even Galen had indirectly mentioned[22] (Fig. 111). It is to be noted that details in the representations are shown by a kind of coordinate system. Thus, for example, the mandibular foramen is found at point 5+28[23].

Falloppia's successor to the professorial chair in Padua was Girolamo Fabrizzi d'Acquapendente, latinized to Hieronymus Fabricius ab Aquapendente. Stomatological questions are not really treated in his anatomical work, but he devoted all the more space to them in his surgical treatise "Opera Chirurgica", which appeared in 1570 in Venice and in 1592 in Frankfurt, and was also available in several Italian, French, and German translations. Among the ancient writers he preferred the Roman Celsus, and the Alexandrian Paulos of Aigina, and he did quite well with these choices[24]. Hypertrophied gingiva is cauterized, as is still occasionally done today, and afterwards spread with honey. Epulis and parulis are cured, according to Paulos, but Fabricius indicates that he is not satisfied with an incision for opening the abscess; he rather recommends a circular excision of the gingiva, followed by application of palliatives, as systematic packing was probably not known yet[25].

Among the seven manipulations in the mouth[26], he first describes the procedures for lockjaw (constrictio dentium), whereby he quite correctly differentiates between psychic, cerebral, and inflammatory causes. Because the great power of the muscles makes nourishment difficult, the various possibilities of food intake are listed, for example, through gaps in the teeth, either present or to be made. A small tube suggested by the author for feeding through the nose is especially minutely described (see Fig. 167). The next manipulation is devoted to cleansing the mouth and removal of tartar, and the third serves the elimination of decay. For this purpose sulfuric or vitriol oil, or another strong fluid, should be dropped into the hole of the tooth with the help of a silver cone; then cauterization should be performed with a red-hot instrument, and finally, the cauterized hole can be filled preventively with gold leaf *(foramen auro foliato implere, ad praeservationem)*[27].

The fifth procedure serves the removal of teeth protruding to the outside, the sixth for the filing-down of sharp, irritating spots, and the seventh for the customary tooth extraction. The pelicans (pellicani), which were still anonymous instruments in Guy de Chauliac's time had now carried the name of this bird for a long time[28], *because they,* as Fabrizzi d'Acquapendente says, *are formed inwards, as is the beak of a pelican (quod pellicani avis rostro interius recurvo simila sint) and cling to other teeth with a base or ground*[29].

20 Ibid. p. 4
21 Ibid. p. 18
22 See p. 75
23 Eustachius (b) p. 113; Table 47
24 See pp. 70 and 81
25 Fabricius ab Aquap. (a) II p. 77; (b) II col. 450
26 Ibid. (a) II p. 33; (b) II col. 32
27 Ibid. (a) II p. 82 f.; (b) II col. 455
28 See p. 129
29 Ibid. (a) II p. 84; (b) II col. 456

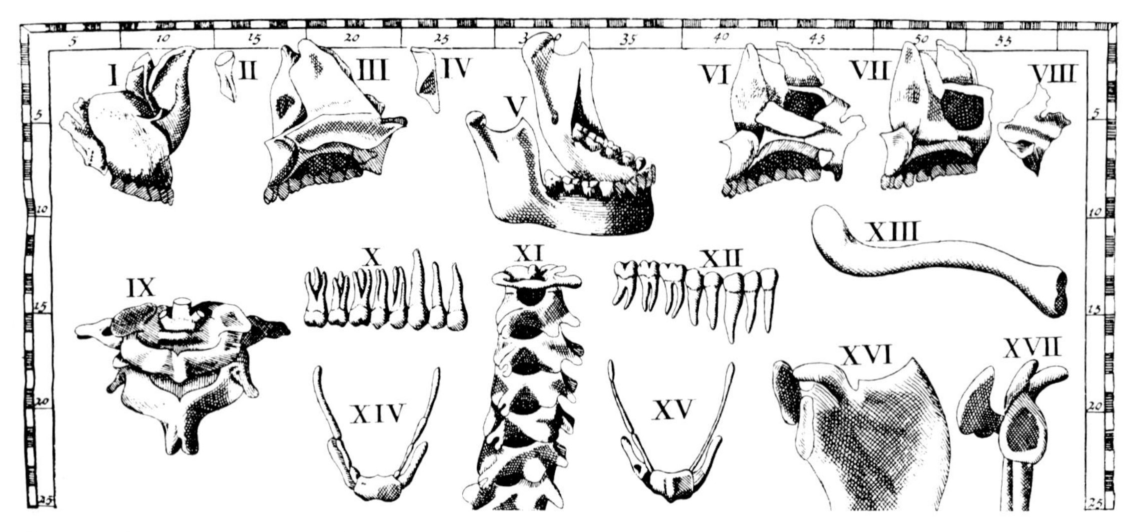

Fig. 111 *Eustachi: Illustrations of jaws and teeth in the "Tabulae anatomicae"*

Sudhoff conjectures that the *form of a wide convex support on the tooth and sharp pointed gripping supports which fit it on the inner side of the tooth led to the giving of the name, because of its similarity to the upper beak and throat pouch of the pelican* [30]. Probably, however, in light of the multiplicity of types, simply the hook laid across the tooth may have given rise to the designation, as it does bear a certain similarity to the hook on the end of the beak of this southern European aquatic bird. But how did the choice devolve specifically on the pelican? After all, numerous other types of birds show this beak formation likewise. The answer lies in a belief of the Middle Ages, which saw Christ symbolically as the "Pelican of Grace," who pierces his own breast with the hook on the beak in order to re-awaken his dead brood on the third day with the heart's blood that wells up [31]. The fable became a widely spread motif in the art of the time (Fig. 112); therefore the pelican thus popularized might have led to the instrument's name (Figs. 113 and 114).

Fabrizzi used a kind of forceps called the stork's bill (rostrum) for *lifting out the meat cutters or incisoriorum,* the crow's bill (rostrum corvinum) as it is still used today, for removal of the root. The forceps "cagnoli" follows, so called because it imitates the firm bite of a dog, and then we read in the description, which is unfortunately not illustrated, about a drill (vulgo trivellino), a three-pronged lever, a kind of raspatory, and, in conclusion, about tooth replacement according to the usual plan. Some of the instruments were later passed on in pictures by the surgeon Scultetus, than a student in Padua (see Fig. 167). One noteworthy item, which must be regarded as progress, is that we do not find a single word in this work about loosening teeth through cauterizing agents, the treatment which was so highly cultivated by the Arabs and so eagerly incorporated in the West.

With regard to defects of the palate, there is differentiation made between congenital and acquired conditions, whereby the latter are caused by the "French:" *This is now to be changed by a sponge / or cotton / or also by a sheet of silver metal / which is to be attached to the inner part of the palate / in order to cover the corroded hole* [32]. Probably, then, this is only the compiled description of a device which, as we will see later [33], had already years before been described considerably better. Cleft palate children then generally died, as our author expressly states, from the inability to nurse.

30 Sudhoff (b) p. 158 footnote
31 Vulgata psalm 122; Hoffmann-Axthelm. That is only the author's personal presumption
32 Fabricius ab Aquap. (a) II p. 85; (b) II col. 457
33 See pp. 168 f.

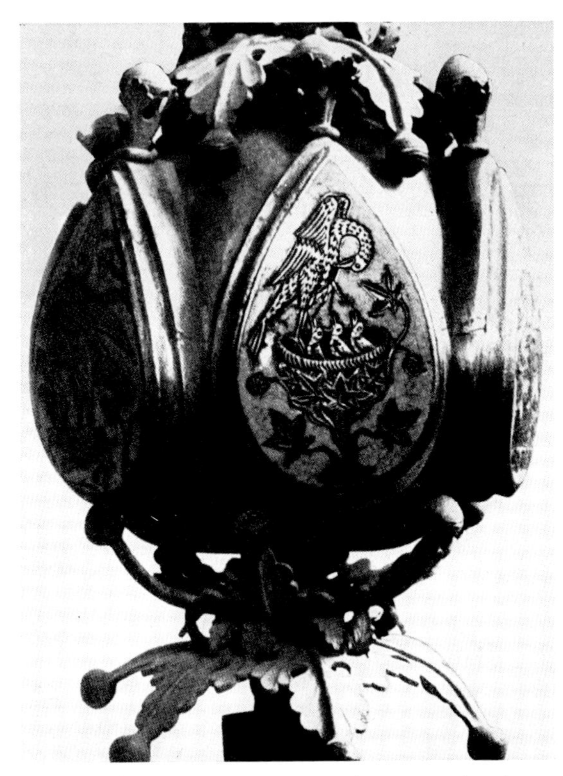

Fig. 112 *Pelican tearing open its breast, at the shrine of St. Elisabeth at the St. Elisabeth church in Marburg*

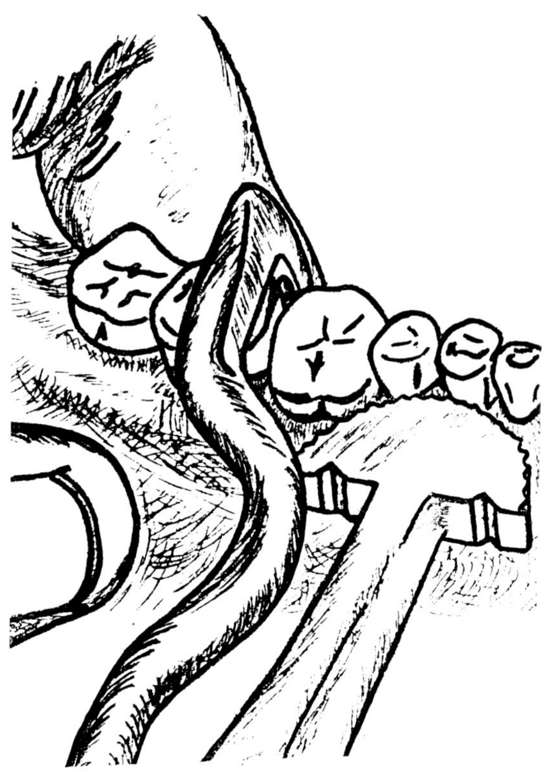

Fig. 114 *Mode of action of the pelican with support on the adjacent teeth (from Ströbel)*

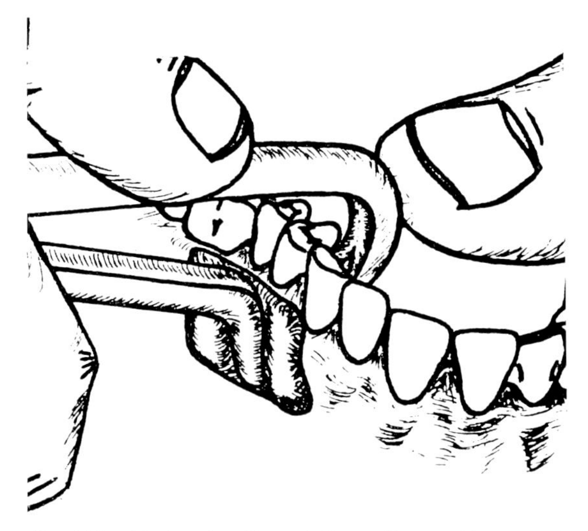

Fig. 113 *Mode of action of the pelican with support on the alveolar process (from Ströbel)*

676 IO. AND. DE CRVCE Wundtartzney/

licher Schmertzen Vrsach / zu welcher Abwendung man etwas von Bilsensamen auff glüende Kohlen zu werffen/vñ die böse Zäne durch einen Trächter darmit zu berduchern pflegt/es fallen die Würmlin also bald herauß.

Figur des Trächters.

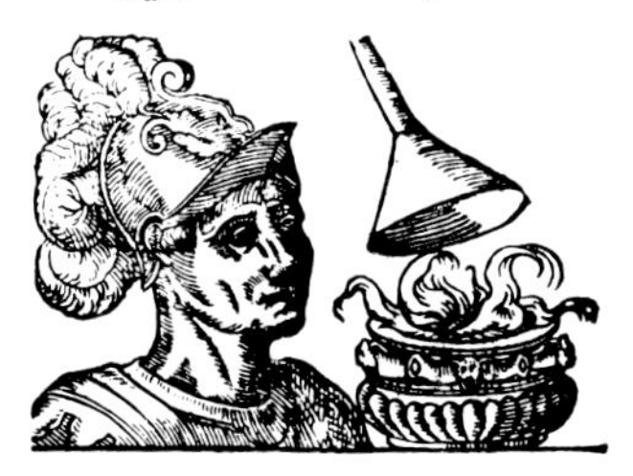

Fig. 115 *della Croce: Worm fumigation, German edition, 1607*

The necessity for constructing obturators arose in the second half of the 16th century fairly universally because of extensive localization of tertiary syphilitic symptoms of the hard palate, where they tended to leave behind a central perforation to the interior of the nose. The "morbus gallicus," the "French," as syphilis was called, was then a new disease in Europe. After the discovery of America, by Columbus' sailors, it was initially carried to Spain, and then broke out in Naples likes an eruption when the French troops occupied the city in 1495. Thereafter, it spread from there to the entire Old World. It received the name of syphilis from an instructional poem published in 1530, in which a shepherd of that name is afflicted by the plague as punishment for blasphemy against God. At first, however, it remained for a long time the French disease, or the Italian disease in French literature. Corresponding to its path from the West to the Eeast, it was known as the German disease in Poland.

Fabrizzi d'Acquapendente treats dislocations of the jaw again strictly according to Hippocrates, whom he frequently quotes. Since he proceeds more from theory than from practice, he rejects a posterior dislocation as impossible: *Wilhelmus de Saliceto*[34] *and others of his ilk / who are completely inexperienced in anatomy,* proceed in their conception *completely counter to the truth*[35].

The surgical work which appeared first in 1573 by the Venetian Giovanni Andrea dalla Croce did not contain anything new in our field. The abundant illustrations of instruments are far behind the contemporary German and French examples of ironwork, and the representation of toothworm fumigation does not appear very realistic (Fig. 115). Geronimo Mercuriale, who taught at various universities in Italy, made the resonable conclusion in the 15th chapter of his book of 1584, "De morbis puerorem" (On Children's Diseases), that teething represents not a disease, but a natural process. Then, however, follow more than eight pages with instructions taken mainly from ancient authors, and, in conclusion, the advice that a boar's tusk or a wolf's tooth be hung around the neck of the teething child. This is probably a modification of the Persian at-Tabari's hyena tooth of the 9th century[36] made necessary by the animal population of the climate.

Let us leave now the homeland of the Renaissance, torn by provincial politics, factional strife, and warlike feuds, although at the same time overflowingly fertile in culture, and turn to France, which was becoming more and more centrally consolidated.

In a book printed for the first time in 1543, that is, in the same year as Vesalius' anatomical work, the Parisian professor Jacques Houllier (Iacobus Hollerius) introduced his discussion of dental diseases with the statement that men have 32 and women 28 teeth[37]. He continues further all the way to frog-fat which forces the teeth out. The following section, however, carries the significant heading, "Contra vermes" (Against the Worms), and banishes to the realm of superstition *that which people convince themselves of and which is written of by the ancient authors about fumigation with henbane seeds . . . Because, they say, it is well-known that the worms originate from it. In truth, something akin to a small worm develops from the heated seed, even if the smoke has not touched the vermiculate tooth (vermiculosum dentem)*[38]. Houllier thus takes up a position, with the same decisiveness as his Spanish contemporary Martinez[39], against the toothworm believed in since the Assyrians. The first recorded fumigation of it appears in Scribonius Largus[40], in the first century after Christ. The final solution to this phenomenon is not given to us until the 18th century by the preacher Schaeffer[41]. After this gleam of enlightenment, however, Houllier falls once again, bound by the scholastic tradition of the Paris faculty, into the usual litany of prescriptions of antiquity and of the Middle Ages as remedies against toothache.

In France development in surgery followed the great rise of Italian anatomy by leaps and bounds. This was initiated by Ambroise Paré, who, coming from humble circumstances, rose from apprentice barber in Brittany to become the head surgeon at the Hôtel-Dieu in Paris and surgeon in ordinary to the French kings (Fig. 116). More of a practitioner than a man of letters, he became the founder of modern

[34] See p. 117
[35] Fabricius ab Aquap. (a) I p. 365
[36] Mercurialis chapter 15; see p. 91
[37] Hollerius p. 117
[38] Ibid. p. 119
[39] See pp. 153 f.
[40] See p. 73
[41] See pp. 241 f.

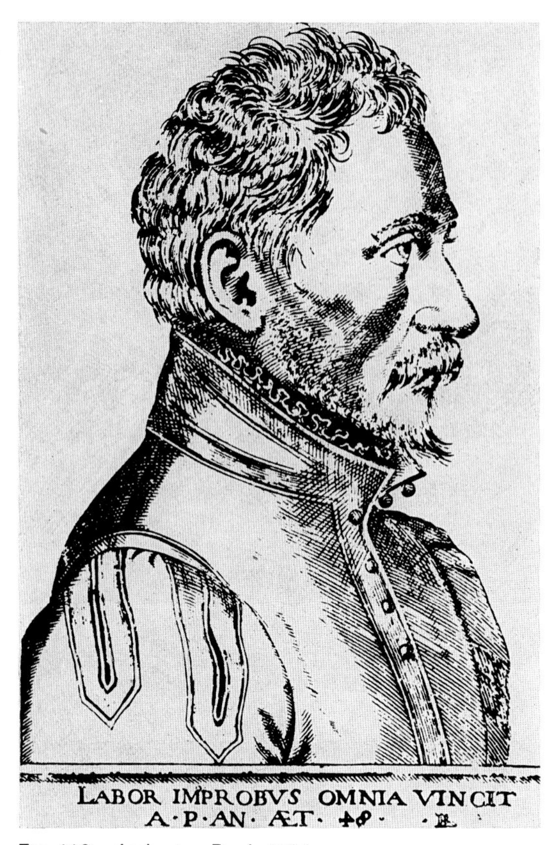

Fig. 116 *Ambroise Paré, 1564*

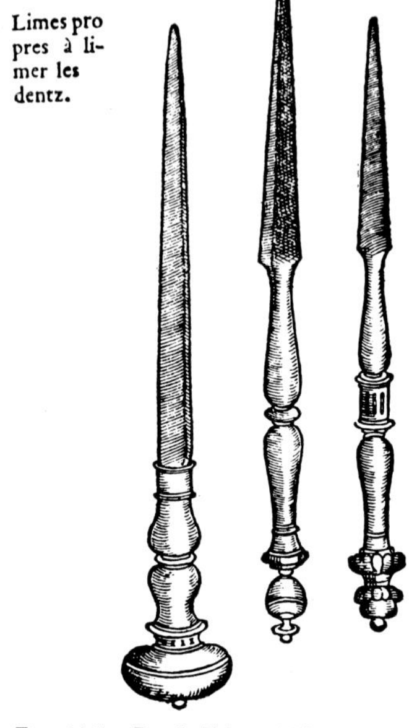

Limes pro pres à limer les dentz.

Fig. 117 *Paré: Files, 1564*

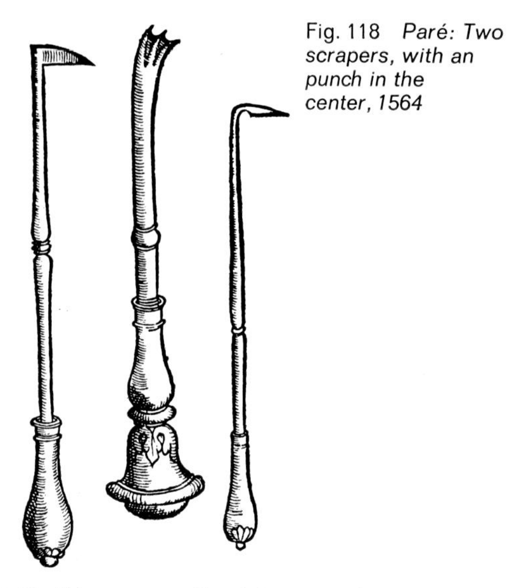

Deſchauſſoirs, auec vn pouſoir qui eſt au milieu pour pouſer & deſchauſſer les dentz.
Policantz

Fig. 118 *Paré: Two scrapers, with an punch in the center, 1564*

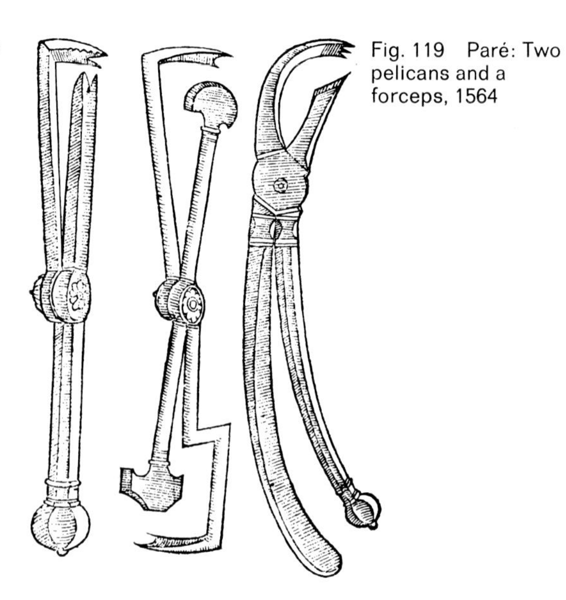

Policantz & dauiet, pour rompre & arracher les dentz.

Fig. 119 Paré: Two pelicans and a forceps, 1564

surgery, and also caused Paris to remain the unquestionable leader in it for centuries to come. Thanks to his roots in the barber-surgeon trade, he was practically able to master tooth extraction, and with it the whole dental medicine of his time. Thus, his representation of these subjects claim our particular interest. His anatomical remarks, however, provide nothing new but sensible rules are to be found periodically, such as, *Well-chewed meat is half digested.* The teeth have feeling, he asserts, referring to Falloppia, not (like bones) in the outer portions, but rather only through a membrane which they have on the inside; thus, he hints at the sensitive dental pulp[42]. Paré also claims as his own discovery without mentioning Falloppia, that the mandible is divided in small children, which is not be perceived in adults[43], and draws from this the conclusion that the mandible—*in accordance with Galen*—is formed from two bones. This concept is also implied in the chapter on fractures of the jaw[44].

The practical section is introduced with a strengthened version of an observation of Celsus[45], that toothache is the greatest and most horrifying of all pains short of death[46]. Quoting Hippocrates and Galen, the list of familiar mixtures, applications and fumigations from the Middle Ages follows. In the case of loose teeth violent chewing and extensive speaking should be avoided, and teeth torn by trauma from the alveoli should be quickly repositioned and tied firmly to the neighboring teeth. In reference to this, we hear the relevant case history of a tailor, a friend of his, whose mandible had been broken by a blow from the hilt of a dagger. He cured him by ligation of the teeth with waxed threads. This description of an actual case leads, however, to that of a successful tooth transplant, which he only knew from hearsay: a tooth was removed from a princess, and immediately replaced with the corresponding one from one of her ladies, which soon thereafter was completely functioning, ... *and if it be true, it could be good*[47].

Paré eliminates caries (erosion) which arises from caustic fluid, with acid cauterization or a small cautery which is brought into contact with the tooth by the tube known from Haly Abbas[48]. If there is crowding, then room must be made first with a file (Fig. 117). There is differentiation in tooth extraction even in the heading, between pulling out (arracher) and breaking (rompre)[49]. Breaking (off) is performed in order to drop something into the root, or to cauterize better, and thus to eliminate feeling from the nerve which is inclosed in the root.

Care must be taken during extraction, because it is possible to dislocate the mandible thereby, as well as to cause concussions to the brain and eyes. Pulling the wrong tooth must also be guarded against, since the patient himself often does not know which tooth is the painful one. Nor should one be too vigorous; otherwise it can occur that a piece of the jaw is torn off as well, as Paré had himself observed, which causes fever, festering, and bleeding, and results in death. After these personal pieces of advice, there is one taken from Celsus without mention of his name: before the extraction of a highly decayed tooth, in order that it does not break and leave the root behind, it should be filled tightly with lead or with linen. The patient should be in a low position, with his head between the knees of the tooth-drawer (dentateur). First, the alveolar process is exposed with scrapers (dechaussoirs, Fig. 118). If the tooth is loose, it is pressed out with a punch (poussoir), a kind of pes caprinus. If this is not possible, then a forceps (daviet, Fig. 119) or a pelican (polican, Figs. 119 and 120) must be employed. The manipulation with this latter device must be learned above all. Otherwise a situation can occur like the one which is quite graphically related, where a helper of a barber extracted, instead of the painful tooth which broke, three healthy ones, for which the poor farmer had to pay threefold then.—After the operation, bleeding should be performed, the alveolus should be pressed together with the fingers, and the mouth rinsed out[50].

As to general oral hygiene, the mouth should be rinsed out after meals, and the teeth must be free from calculus. Hard things should not be eaten, nor even should fruit pits or bones be cracked. Some prescriptions for tooth cleaning agents follow[51].

While personal experiences sometimes have an influence on the chapters of dentistry, Paré,

[42] Paré (b) VI 2 p. 186 f.
[43] See p. 140
[44] Ibid. VI 1 p. 185 C; XV 7 p. 536 C, B
[45] See p. 70
[46] Ibid. XVII 25 p. 619 A
[47] Ibid. XVII 26 p. 621 C
[48] See p. 95
[49] Ibid. XVII 27 p. 621 D
[50] Ibid. XVII 26, 27 p. 622 f.
[51] Ibid. XVII 28 p. 624 CD

Inftruments

Inftrument nommé Dauiet, pour arracher les dentz.

Fig. 120 *Paré: Pelican, 1564 (Error in the caption: daviet = pelican)*

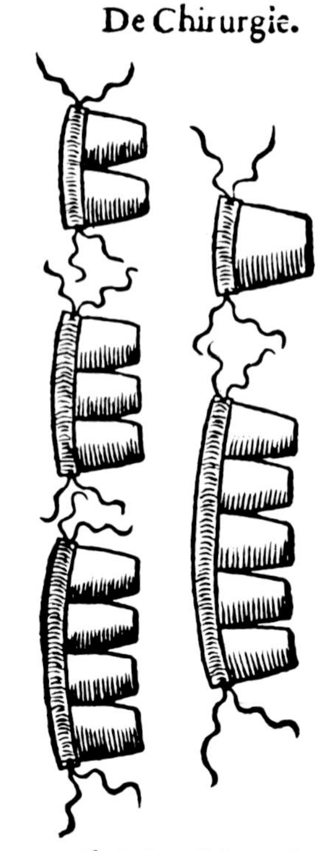

De Chirurgie.
Dentz artificielles faittes d'os, qui s'attachent par vn fil d'argent en lieu des autres qu'on aura perdues.
E ij

Fig. 121 *Paré: Dental prosthesis, 1564*

as a theoretician, refers to Hippocrates in the affixing of tooth replacements with gold or silver wire [52] (although the Greek only spoke of fixation of loose teeth) and otherwise only includes, as figure 121 shows, stale academic wisdom. Original ideas return again in the description of the palatal obturator, which was of such great importance during the epidemic of syphilis if we grant that Paré's description was in good faith, the first, (in 1561—1575): ... *with the help of our art, they* (the patients) *can regain their power of speech.* In 1561 the device still had no name, in 1564 he named it the "couvercle" and we find, from 1575 to1585, probably for the first time, the designation "obturateur" valid to the present day [53].

As a military surgeon, which he was orginally, Paré states the cause of the palatal defects initially to be musket-shots, but then adds that they primarily occur after syphilitic sores. His obturator consists of a vaulted gold or silver plate which is somewhat larger than the hole, provided with a clamp and which covers it palatally, while the apparatus is nasally affixed by a sponge clamped to it; this gradually swells (Fig. 122). Perhaps this was not very aesthetic, but the patient was able thereby to drink and speak to some extent, assuming, of course, an intact palatal velar. Only in the caption of the picture is an obturator consisting completely of metal described, the smaller plate of which is pushed through the perforation towards the nose, and twisted through the mouth *with a small crow's bill* in such a fashion that it is positioned

52 Ibid. XXIII 3 p. 909 A—C
53 Paré (a) p. 211^{v}; (b) XXIII 4 p. 909 f.; (c) p. 608

Inſtruments **De Chirurgie.**

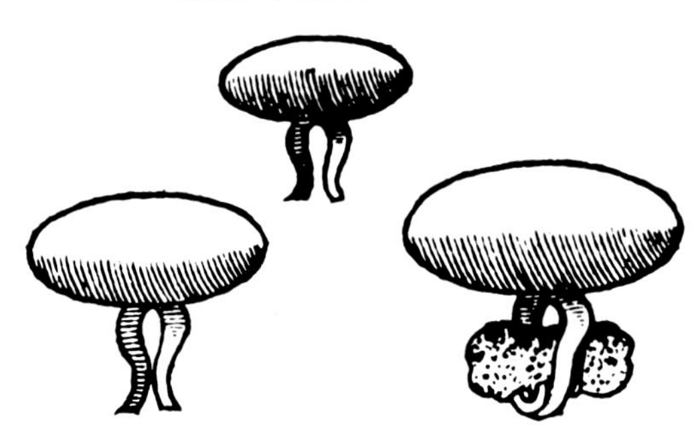

Inſtrumentz appellez couuercles, propres pour couurir & eſtouper les trouz des os perduz au palais de la bouche, ſoit de cauſe de verolle, ou autrement: & ſans iceux les patiens ne peuuent proferer leur parolles, mais parlent (comme lon dit vulgairement) regnaut. Ledit Inſtrument ſera de matiere d'or ou d'argent, & de figure courbee, & non plus eſpois qu'vn eſcu: Auquel ſera attachee vne eſponge, par laquelle eſtant appoſe ledit Inſtrumét dedans le trou, ladite eſponge bien toſt s'enflera par l'humidite contenue en la bouche, qui ſera cauſe de le faire tenir ferme : & par tel moyen le patient proferera bien ſa parolle.

Fig. 122 *Paré: Sponge obturators, 1564*

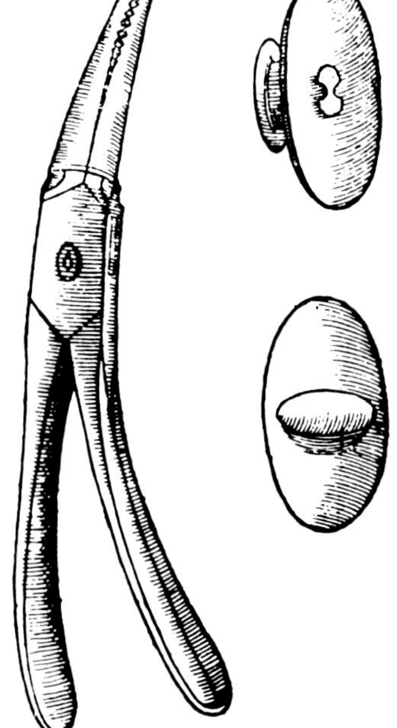

Autre inſtrumẽt pour meſme effet, ſans eſpõge, lequel a vne eminẽce par le derriere, qui ſe tourne auec vn petit bec de corbin (que tu vois en ceſte figure) lors qu'on le met dans le trou ou la perdition de l'os a eſté.

Fig. 123 *Paré: Obturator with screw closure and special forceps for placement, 1564*

with its greatest diameter adjusted to the smallest one of the defect (Fig. 123). This is well conceived, but the pressure sites might have limited its use to short periods of time only.

Paré does not provide anything new concerning fractures of the mandible, but rather proceeds no differently than Guy de Chauliac[54], and thus to Guy's Arabian authorities[55].

Dislocations of the jaw are discussed in three chapters in great detail. The symptoms, such as flattening on the luxated and bulging on the healthy side, a deviating chin position, lockjaw, tooth position, etc., are precisely described, and neither is the Hippocratic prognosis of death on the 10th day lacking, which was incorporated by and taken from Guy, if repositioning is not done *more or less* (quickly), *depending on the constitution.* A double luxation is prognostically unfavorable. Here, if the reduction does not proceed in the customary way, wedges of soft wood and a ligature must be used, as suggested by Lanfranchi[56]. The dislocation posteriorly, first described by William of Saliceto[57], was something which he himself had not yet seen, but he believed that it could be easily repositioned through a punch with the fist from below[58].

Jacques Guillemeau, Paré's successor at the Hôtel-Dieu, stands out among his students. His surgical work, printed for the first time in 1598, contains, among others, a rather

54 Guy de Chauliac V 1, 2
55 Paré (b) XV 7 pp. 536 f.; see p. 100
56 See p. 118
57 See p. 117
58 Paré (b) XVI 8—10 pp. 556 f.

Des Inſtrumens de Chirurgie

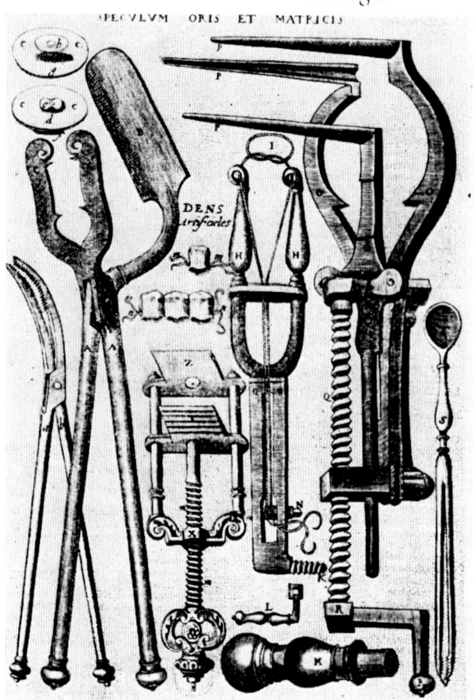

f , L'extremité de la Platine qui eſt marquee en la ſeconde Platine par h,laquelle ſe met au trou du Palais.
g , La face de la Platine qui touche contre le Palais, eſtant comme plaquee contre iceluy.
h, La petite Platine qui ſe tourne & vire , & ſe met dans le trou du Palais.
m,m,Figure d'vne Dent artificielle, faite d'iuoire ou os,laquelle s'attache par de petits filets d'or.
n,n , Trois dents artificielles ioinctes enſemble, leſquelles s'attachent par des filets d'or , aux autres dents, qui ſont proches de chaſque coſté,aux autres Dents voiſines de chaſque coſté.

Telles dents artificieles ſe font ordinairement d'Iuoire , mais d'autant que ladicte Iuoire iaunit ſoudainement pour la ſaliue & humidité qui la touche & abreuue continuellement , elles ſe feront plus commodement de quelque autre os, pourueu qu'il ſoit fort ſolide, cõme peut eſtre celuy du poiſſon nommé Rouart. Or promptement & facilement chacun peut faire des dents artificielles ,d'vne cire blanche grenee,à laquelle(eſtant fonduë auec tant ſoit peu de la gomme *Elemi*) on aura adiouſté poudres de Maſtic,Coral blanc,& perles ſubtillement pulueriſees,& telle paſte ſera gardee pour en former vne ou plusieurs dents. Ceſte paſte peut auſſi ſeruir à mettre dedans vne dent creuſe , afin d'empeſcher qu'il ne tombe & ſe cache quelque viande en mangeant, qui les pourriſt d'auantage,& excite ſouuent grande douleur.

Fig. 124 *Guillemeau: Illustration (with obturator and dental prosthesis) and text (including a description of the new material for dental prostheses) from the "Oeuvres de Chirurgie", 1598/1612*

Fig. 125 *Title page of the first French special work of Urbain Hemard, 1582*

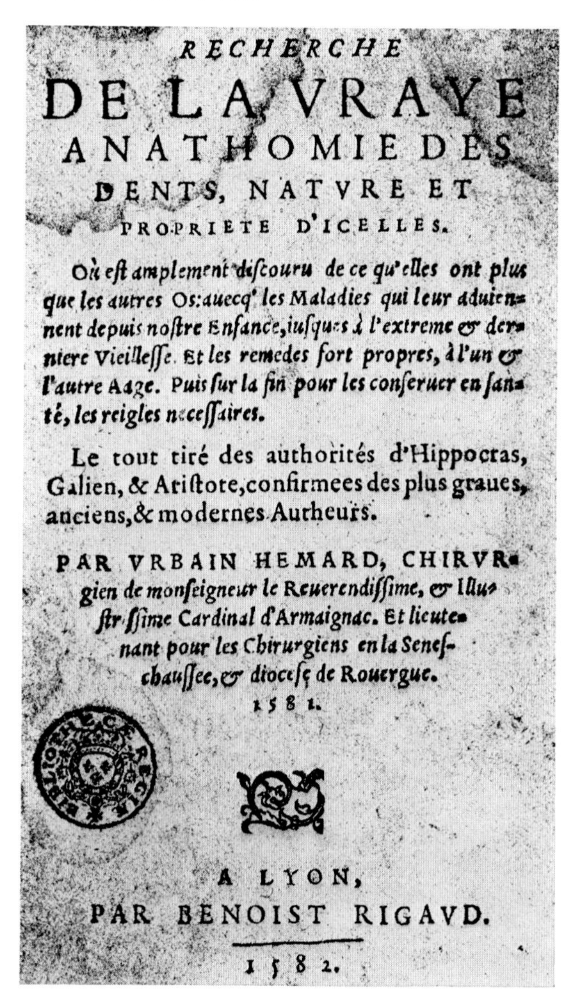

RECHERCHE
DE LA VRAYE
ANATHOMIE DES
DENTS, NATVRE ET
PROPRIETE D'ICELLES.

Où eſt amplement diſcouru de ce qu'elles ont plus que les autres Os: auecq' les Maladies qui leur aduiennent depuis noſtre Enfance, iuſques à l'extreme & derniere Vieilleſſe. Et les remedes fort propres, à l'un & l'autre Aage. Puis ſur la fin pour les conſeruer en ſanté, les reigles neceſſaires.

Le tout tiré des authorités d'Hippocras, Galien, & Ariſtote, confirmees des plus graues, anciens, & modernes Autheurs.

PAR VRBAIN HEMARD, CHIRVRgien de monſeigneur le Reuerendiſſime, & Illuſtriſſime Cardinal d'Armaignac. Et lieutenant pour les Chirurgiens en la Seneſchauſſee, & dioceſe de Rouergue.

1581.

A LYON,
PAR BENOIST RIGAVD.
1582.

unsatisfying recommendation, *from which some try to make a great secret;* namely that of cleaning the teeth with a small rod dipped in *eau forte*, acid, and rinsing out afterwards with cold water. This method, comfortable but damaging to the enamel, was later on strictly rejected by Pfaff in Berlin[59]. Only in regard to artificial teeth we learn something which goes beyond Paré, whom he follows in the essentials. Since those prepared from ivory turn yellow quickly by saliva, he recommends harder bone material, such as that of the *poisson nommé Rouart*, the walrus; he also suggests a new type of plastic material: *Artificial teeth can be made easily and quickly from white granulated wax, melted with only a little resin of the olive tree (gomme Elemi), to which are added mastix powder and finely ground white coral and pearls ... This paste can also serve to fill a hollow tooth, in order to prevent its crumbling ...*[60] (Fig. 124). It is questionable, to say the least, whether such artificial teeth with a wax-resin substance could have withstood chewing for any period of time. It is nonetheless the first known attempt to break away from bone and ivory teeth, which were susceptible to caries. As a filling material, this paste must be regarded as the first step to our current cements.

The first French publication devoted entirely to the teeth appeared in Lyon in 1582, comprising 90 pages of text; it was the "Recherche de la vraye anathomie des dents" (Investigations of the true Anatomy of the Teeth) by Urbain Hemard, physician in ordinary to the Cardinal of Armagnac (Fig. 125). The anatomical portion is essentially oriented on Eustachi's work, which had appeared 19 years before[61], and otherwise constitutes a compilation of authors from the ancients to the contemporaries, with verbose comments. In the clinical portion, his own concepts are manifested; thus, with regard to tooth extraction procedures, Hemard polemicizes against his great contemporary Paré: *Some modern physicians* (according to marginalia, this is Paré) *recommend breaking of the crown with forceps, so that the humor* (pus) *can flow out. But there are not many who wish to suffer this, because the roots which remain are soon as painful as before*[62].

Hemard believes it is necessary for a surgeon to understand the art of tooth extraction, lest he disgrace himself if there is no tooth-drawer available, *Although this part of surgery has always been left to the itinerants (coreux et passans) who are called, following the Italian example, charlatans, who did the couching of cataracts, lithotomies, and castrations. As Galen had already said, the surgeon should not follow any such example ... precisely because these operations are dangerous, they ought to be performed by an educated operator and not by an ignorant one, which is what most of the charlatans are ... In fact, people speak in general of lying like a tooth-drawer (arracheurs de dents) because they promise a successful result to all, ...*[63].

Care is to be taken of the extraction itself, *that the forceps (daviet) ... is not closed too firmly, and that the surgeon, with the great finger of one of his hands, pushes both the tooth and the iron to the outside, without ever denuding the tooth of the gingiva, and that he grasps it as deeply as possible in the alveolus ...* An additional warning against too vigorous a forceps closure ensues; otherwise it can break, *even if it is massive*, and particularly *if it is already vermiculate (vermolue)*[64]. Thus we have a quite independent description of tooth removal in which, for the first time, in contrast to Paré, the superfluous preparation of the gingiva before the operation is rejected. We can infer from the term "vermiculate" that the author still believed in the toothworm. Just as remedies for toothache were listed before, there is also now a profusion of agents to remedy loosening of the tooth. He discerns the cause in mercury, not only as a result of the massive syphilis therapy of those years, but also of the exagerrated cosmetic use of mercuric chloride[65].

In 1557 in the Spanish town of Valladolid a popular little book appeared devoted entirely to odontology, of which there are only a few known examples[66]. Its author, the baccalaureate Francisco Martinez from Castrillo, was a physician with a complete university education.

59 Guillemeau p. 689. See p. 231
60 Ibid. p. 502
61 See pp. 141 f.
62 Hemard p. 72. Film copy from the National Library of Paris
63 Ibid. p. 73
64 Ibid. p. 73
65 Ibid. pp. 82 f.
66 Film copies of the 1st and 2nd editions from the National Library of Madrid were available, with supplementation from the copy owned by the Medical Faculty of Madrid. I am extraordinarily grateful to Joachim Gantzer, D.M.D., of Bremen, for locating the originals and for providing the translation of the entire text.

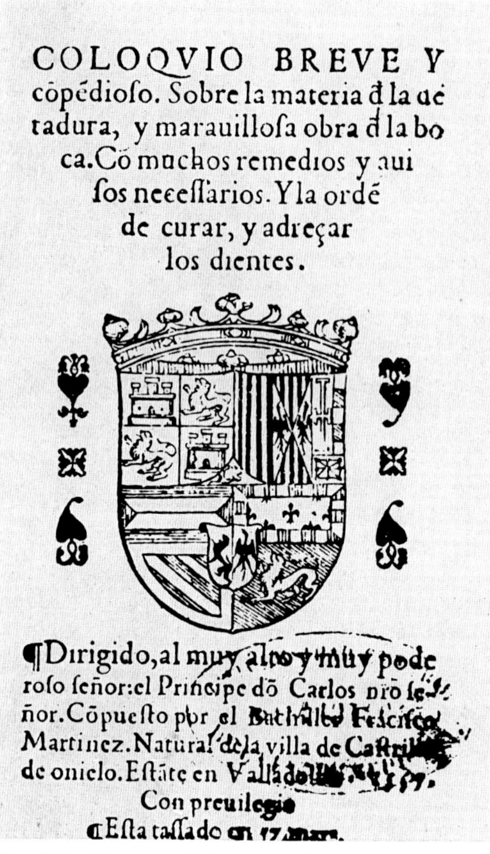

COLOQVIO BREVE Y
cōpēdioſo. Sobre la materia đ la dē-
tadura, y marauilloſa obra đ la bo
ca. Cō muchos remedios y aui
ſos neceſſarios. Y la ordē
de curar, y adreçar
los dientes.

¶Dirigido, al muy alto y muy pode
roſo ſeñor: el Principe dō Carlos nro ſeñor. Cōpueſto por el Bachiller Francisco
Martinez. Natural de la villa de Caſtrillo
de onielo. Eſtāse en Valladolid
Con preuilegio
¶Eſta taſſado en

Fig. 126 *Martinez: Title page of the first Spanish book devoted to dentistry, 1557*

TRACTADO
BREVE Y COMPENDIO-
ſo, ſobre la marauilloſa obra de la
boca y dentadura. Compueſto por el LICEN-
CIADO MARTINEZ DE CASTRILLO DE
ONIELO andante en corte, en ſeruicio de ſu
Mageſtad. De nueuo enmendado y añadido
por el miſmo Autor, donde ſe tracta la Theori
ca y Practica deſte arte, y de todas las paſsiones
que ſuelen y pueden comunicar en la boca y ſus
partes. Con los remedios de cada vna dellas
experimentados, y otras coſas muy ne-
ceſſarias no ſolamente para la dentadura, pero para la ſalud humana, co
mo veras a la buelta de la hoja.

DIRIGIDO A LA C.R.M.
de la Reyna Doña Anna de Au-
ſtria nueſtra Señora.

CON PRIVILEGIO.
Impreſſo en Madrid, en caſa de Alonſo Gomez
Impreſſor de ſu Mageſtad. 1570.
Eſta taſſado en. 48. marauedis cada volumen.

Fig. 127 *Martinez: Title page of the second edition, 1570*

Later he also belonged to the clergy, indicated by his naming himself *Chaplain to your majesty* in his dedication. He composed his "Coloquio breve y compendioso sobre la materia de la dentadura . . .", as the title suggests, in the form of an instructional dialogue which was highly regarded in the 16th century for scientific publications (Fig. 126).

In a street in Valladolid, a certain Valerio meets Ramiro on a business trip. The former was servant of his father, who had just been complaining in a monologue about the teething fever of his little son. After greetings the discussion quickly turns to the teeth, whereby examples from both families made it clear in detail, how sad the situation of toothache is. Valerio is the instructor here at all times, while Ramiro asks often quite penetrating questions. Thus we learn from Valerio that he does not believe in tooth replacement, because the existing ones are damaged by the ligation: . . . *if an artificial tooth is in place for one year, then the rest of the person's life will be spent without the natural ones* [67]. Anatomical and physiological problems are treated more from a philosophical point of view than from a medical one, always in assertion and contradiction.

In the second part, the discussing partners betake themselves to Ramiro's house, where they are joined by Ramiro's wife, Christiola. The sick child causes the discussion to turn to complications of eruption, for which application of figs and flushings with mixed decoctions are prescribed. The (rootless) primary teeth are to

[67] Martinez (b) fol. 16v

Parte. Fo. 50

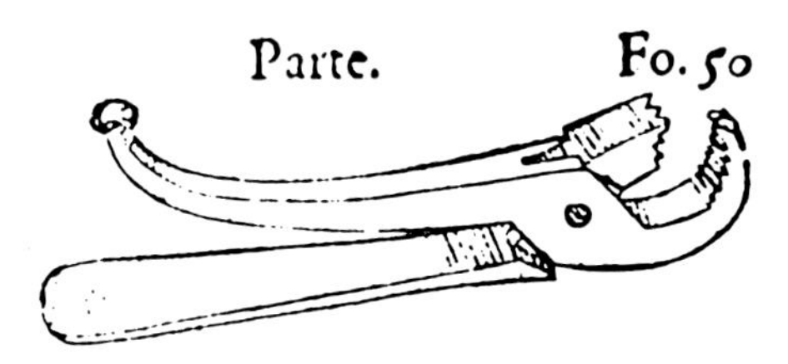

Pero ſi de la muela ſe tiene alguna ſoſpecha q̃ ſe ha de quebrar, haſe de ſacar con polican: porque ſi le ſabẽ bien exercitar aſeguran la muela, aunque eſte mas podrida que no ſe deſcabeçe. Quando ay algun peda-

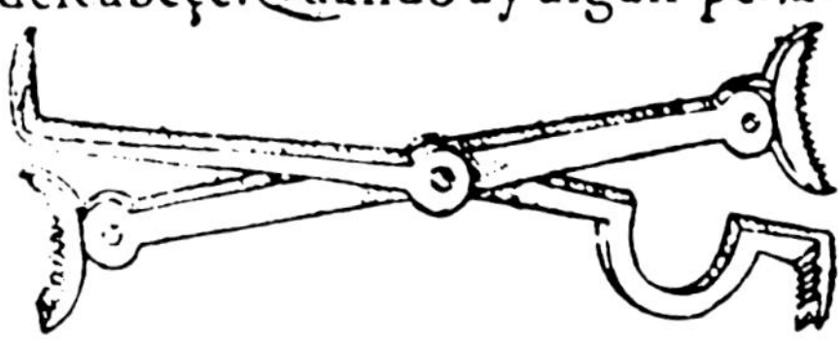

cito de muela o raygon que ſe ande haſe de quitar cõ vna deſtas dos herramientas, que tẽgan por la parte que aſen vnas raytas menudas y hõdillas como eſtas.

Gij Quan

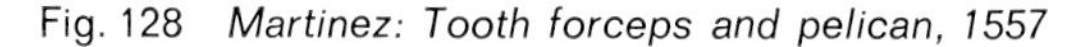

Fig. 128 *Martinez: Tooth forceps and pelican, 1557*

parte. 69

Para de parte de dentro ha de hauer vn hierro con dos puntas bueltas a manera de deſcarnador de barbero. Cõ eſte hierro han de ſaxar y cortar delicadamente la toua. Porque aconteſce por ſacarla entera ſalir con ella el diente.

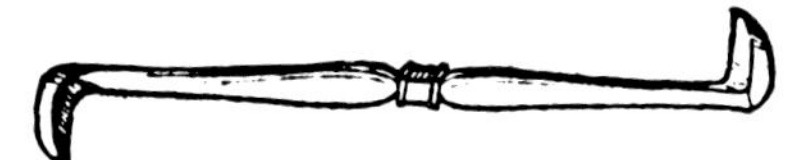

Deſpues de ſaxada ha ſe d̃ acabar de quitar con vn hierro q̃ tenga otras dos bueltas, la vna a manera de pico de perdiz, y la otra anchuela.

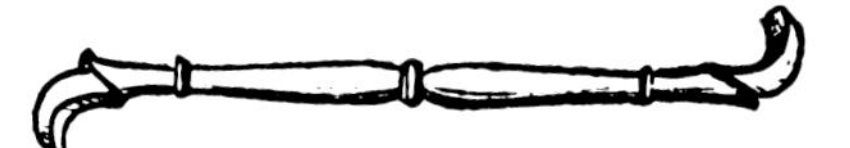

Para entre diente y diẽte ternas vn hierro llanito y delgado de bocas como eſte

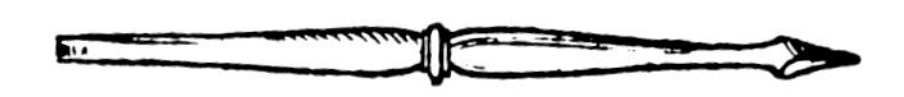

Fig. 129 *Martinez: Scalers, 1570*

be pulled at the proper time, so that the permanent ones do not grow in crookedly[68].

Now the discussion temporarily becomes almost a monologue by Valerio: before the extraction, it must be ascertained which tooth is the painful one through tapping or testing with a probe. Those which are less decayed should be pulled with the more sparing forceps (gatillo), and those which are more destroyed with the pelican (polican, Figs. 128 and 129). The baccalaureate does not engage in a closer description of the technique. He places a particular emphasis on the "age categories", which always require a specific therapy.

In the third section, Valerio lectures on tooth decay (corrupcion del dente, neguijón), in which he differentiates between a black and a white one. The first one, probably the caries sicca of today, is harmless and is caused (Hippocratically) by the flow of bile, while the white (similarly) is caused by phlegm. It is clearly established that the treatment must begin early and be carried out thorougly. But those who know how to heal it do not dare *to apply their knowledge, because if they demonstrate the necessary care and concentration, it is said they do it only to make the case more expensive*[69].

Obviously there is a position taken here, even before Houllier[70], on the issue of worms: *I say that there are no worms involved in tooth decay, but rather that is is simply corruption,* and that the fumigation with henbane constitutes

[68] Ibid. fol. 42v
[69] Ibid. fol. 67v
[70] See p. 145

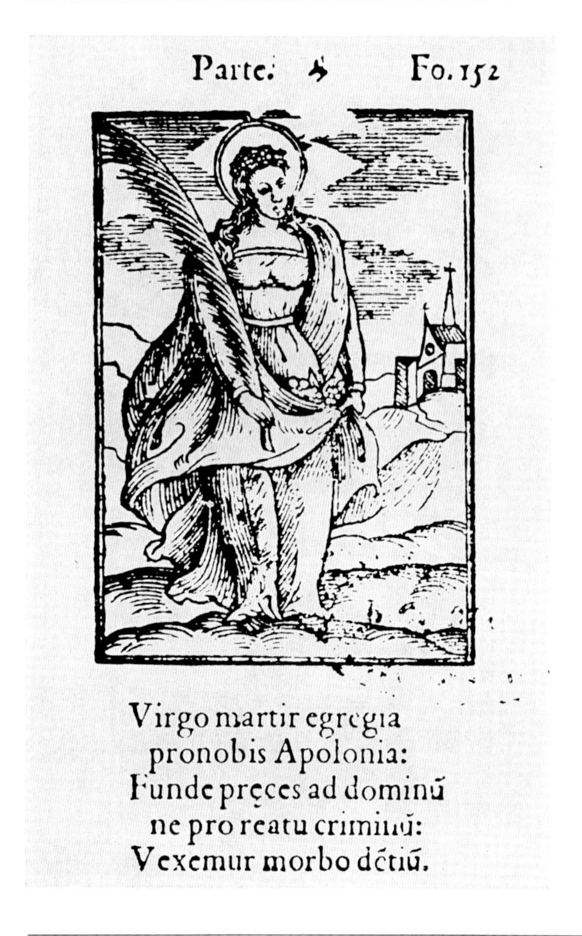
Parte. Fo. 152
Virgo martir egregia
pronobis Apolonia:
Funde pręces ad dominũ
ne pro reatu criminũ:
Vexemur morbo dẽtiũ.

Fig. 130 *Martinez: Woodcut of Apollonia as final illustration: "Illustrious Virgin and Martyr Apollonia, pray for us to the Lord so that we are not tortured for our failures through the tooth disease", 1557*

their origin and is a fraud[71]. Even the enthusiastic description of a medicated tooth removal is freed of superstition and is reduced to a reasonable measure. Some quite sophisticated remarks follow on the cause of toothache, and some critical ones on the craft of physicians. Tooth extraction and cleaning should remain barber's work, with everything else falling to physicians and surgeons.

In the fourth section, they chat about oral and dental hygiene. There are some complicated agents given, but no junk apothecary. Make-up is rejected, because its mercuric chloride content damages the teeth and the gingiva. All sweet things, including milk and milk products, are to be avoided, which refers to Galen. Less easy for us to understand is that cabbage and onions, too, are among the forbidden items. In conclusion, there is the usual collection of prescriptions; corresponding to the style of the book, however, these are particularly prescribed for the individual involved in the discussion.

We can see from the examples that Martinez has purged known material of its superstition and presented it in an easily accessible form. The text concludes—this is in Spain, after all—with a wood-cut of St. Apollonia (Fig. 130). In any event, this book, which was dedicated to Philip II's unfortunate son Don Carlos, became so popular that a second condensed edition, a "Tractado breve" followed in 1570, which the author dedicated to Anne of Austria, the fourth and last spouse of the king (Fig. 127). Among the so-called folk manuals of dentistry of the 16th century it is in quality in a leading position.

Amatus Lusitanus, as his name indicates, came from Portugal; he also was named Juan

[71] Ibid. fol. 69

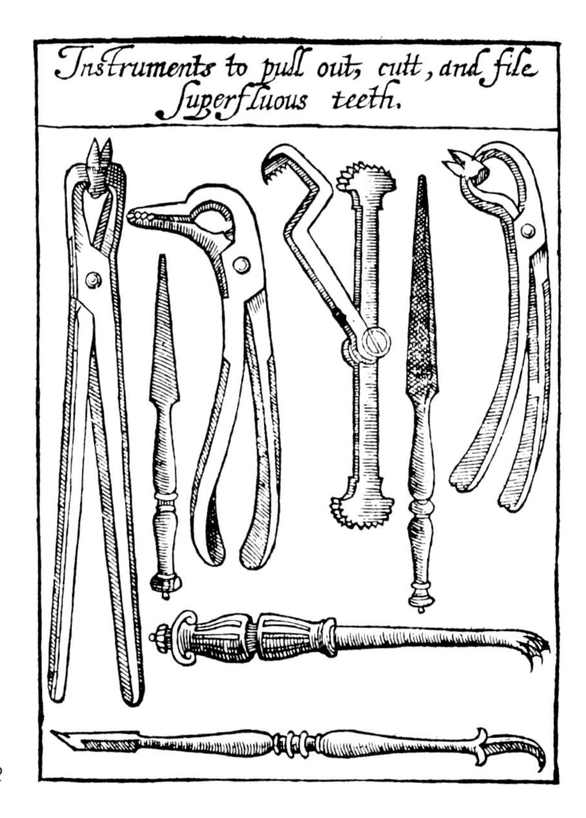

Fig. 131 *Lowe: Extraction instruments and files, 1612*

Rodriguez de Castel Branco, as a result of compulsory baptism. His Jewish heritage always made him suspect to the Inquisition, however, so that his life was a restless one, and drove him through half of Europe all the way to the Balkans, where he died in Salonica in 1568. He published his "Curationum medicinalium" in Venice. The 14th Curatio (Counsel) in the fifth Centuria (Hundred) describes his own design of a gold palatal obturator in 1560, one year before Paré illustrated it. This was comparable in principle to the great Frenchman's sponge obturator[72].

In England, in 1540 under the rule of Henry VIII, an act of parliament united the surgeons and the barber-surgeons. The former were not allowed to shave patrons any more, and barbers could not practice any other surgery, except tooth extraction according to the edict. Surgical activity was permitted, on the other hand, to the academic physicians.

Probably the first surgical book in the English language, "The whole course of chirurgie," was printed in London in 1597 and 1612. Its author was a Scot, Peter Lowe, who was educated in Paris and only returned to his homeland after 22 years of activity in France and Flanders. From 1598 on, he was the salaried municipal surgeon of Glasgow, as documented[73]. His work, which is partially written in dialogue form—son John asks and father Peter answers—corresponds to its author's education in keeping closely to the Paré school. Perhaps under the indirect influence of Houllier[74], he emphatically rejects the idea of the toothworm. In this respect, we do not discover anything new here, except, perhaps, that Lowe cauterized the painful tooth with a golden cautery in the case

[72] Christ
[73] Donaldson
[74] See p. 145

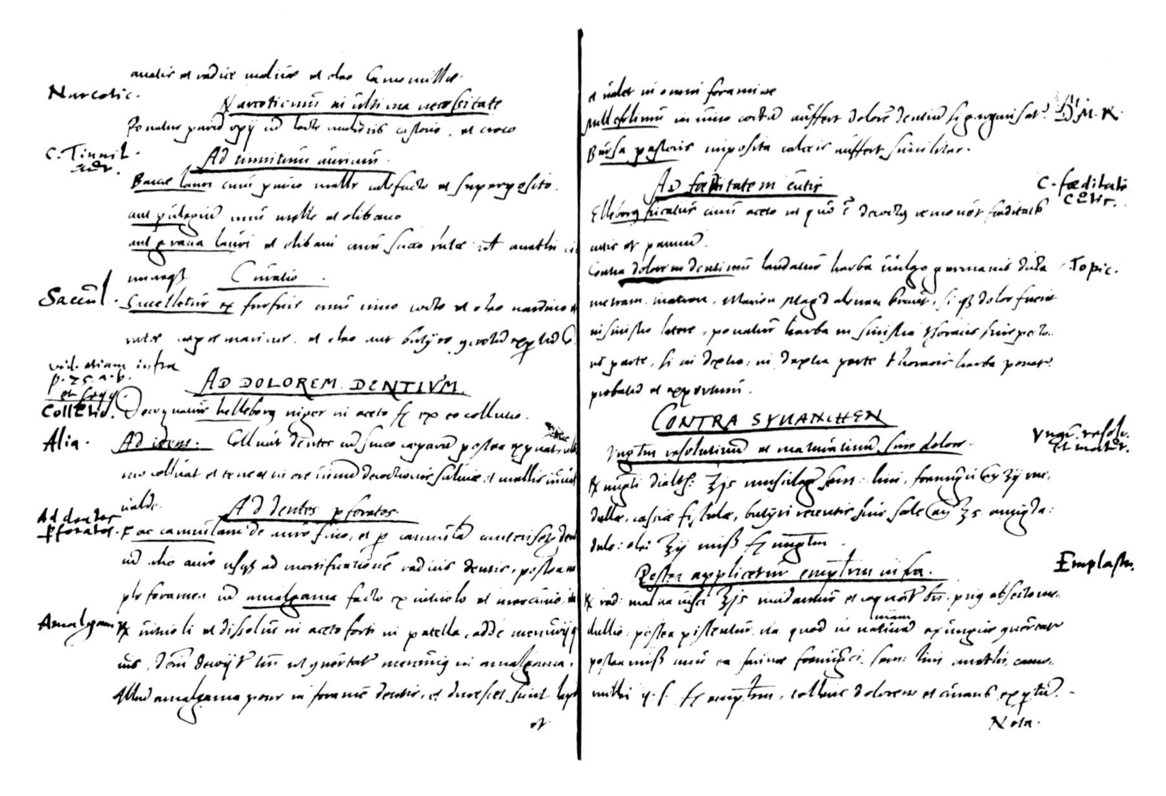

Fig. 132 *Amalgam prescription of Johannes Stockerus in the Xlyffer manuscript, fol. 75ᵛ f., 1528 (Stadtarchiv Ulm)*

of nobility. His extraction instruments, whose descriptions are quite similar to those of Paré, include forceps (turkisse or davier), the pes caprinus or punch (pufar) and the pelican (polican, Fig. 131). Artificial teeth are made from *ivory, whales bone or hounds teeth,* and fastened to the neighboring teeth *by a wyre or thread of gold*[75].

Pieter van Foreest of Alkmaar and the Leyden University professor Jan van Heurne were conspicuous among the physicians of Holland. In their works, material from ancient times and from Islam again is resurrected. In anatomy, for example in the description of tooth development in Heurne's Hippocrates-commentary, Vesalius and Eustachi do not seem to have lived yet. The author even seriously mentions the lead forceps from Erasistratos and carries out treatment with prescriptions from the ancient and Arabian dispensaries. At the same time, there is not a single word about surgical tooth removal[76].

In the southern German region, we have Johannes Stockerus to thank for the very early recommendation of an amalgam for the purpose of restorative dental medicine, a prescription which is given again in 1601 by the municipal physician of Lüneburg, Tobias Dornkreilius[77]. We know from Stocker himself, who had received his education in Bologna, that after a temporary stay in Tübingen in 1483 he entered into the service of the city of Ulm as municipal physician, where he remained until his death. In addition to the third edition of his "Praxis aurea" of 1657, used by

[75] Lowe p. 194
[76] Heurne p. 80; see p. 66
[77] Riethe (a); Baume

Artzney Buch-
lein/wider allerlei kran-
ckeyten und gebrechen der tzeen/getzogen
auss dem Galeno/Auicenna/Mesue/
Cornelio Celso und andern mehr
der Artzney Doctorn/seher
nützlich zu
lesen.
M. D. XXX.

Fig. 133 *Title page of the first edition (Leipzig, 1530) of the oldest textbook of dentistry, the "Artzney Buchlein"*

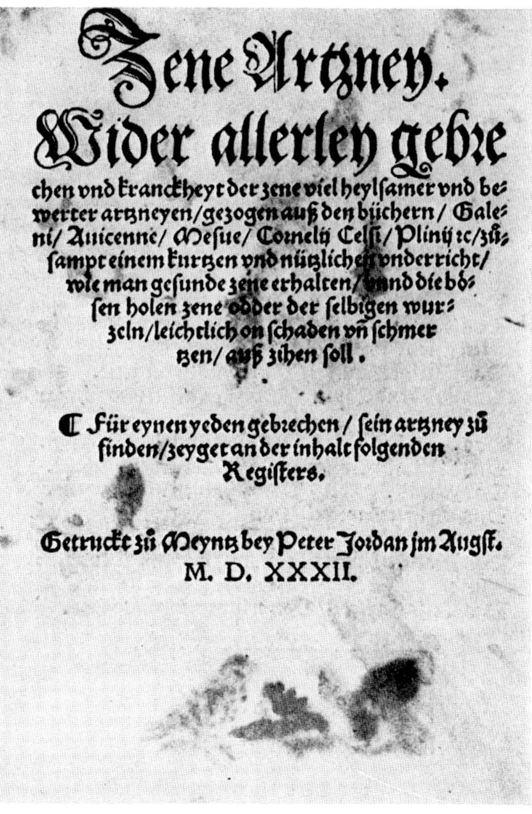
Zene Artzney.
Wider allerley gebre-
chen und kranckheyt der zene viel heylsamer und be-
werter artzneyen/gezogen auß den büchern/ Gale-
ni/ Auicenne/ Mesue/ Cornelii Celsi/ Plinii etc/zu-
sampt einem kurtzen und nützlichen underricht/
wie man gesunde zene erhalten/ unnd die bösen holen zene odder der selbigen wur-
zeln/leichtlich on schaden un schmer-
tzen/ auß zihen soll.

¶ Für eynen yeden gebrechen/ sein artzney zu
finden/zeyget an der inhalt folgenden
Registers.

Getruckt zu Meyntz bey Peter Jordan im Augst.
M. D. XXXII.

Fig. 134 *Title page of the second edition, the "Zene Artzney", Mainz, 1532*

R i e t h e and the author, the former succeeded in finding putatively older prescriptions corresponding to the 19th chapter ("On toothaches") of the first book from as early as 1528: *Remedies for holes in the teeth. Make a tube from fine gold; and the tooth should be cauterized through this with another gold* (instrument) *until the root is deadened; thereafter, fill the hole with an amalgam compounded from vitriol* (this is not specified more precisely) *and mercury, as follows: dissolve vitriol with a strong acid in a bowl, and add a sufficient amount of mercury to it. Then it should be boiled, and the mercury will transform itself to an amalgam (convertetur Mercurius in Amalgama); put this amalgam into the hole of the tooth, and it will become as hard as stone and remain firmly in any hole*[78] (Fig. 132).

Thus, for the first time in the European literature, cavity filling with amalgam is recommended here, with reference to the customary cauterization of the dental pulp through H a l y A b b a s ' tube, and three hundred years before the definitive introduction of this filling material began its rather timorous course in England and France, and about the same time as the first sure Chinese prescriptions[79].

The first academic physician who was truly caught up in the new spirit of the 16th century was the vagrant P a r a c e l s u s , who had the courage to place the observation of nature and practical experience with patients above the torpid dogmas of Greek-Arabic medicine. After his studies in Ferrara, he led an unsettled life of

[78] Stockerus pp. 132 f.
[78] Stockerus pp. 132 f. The word "amalgam" develops from the Greek málagma (soft material, padding) through the Arabic al(= article)-malagma (softening salve) into the middle Latin amalgama
[79] See pp. 43 and 289

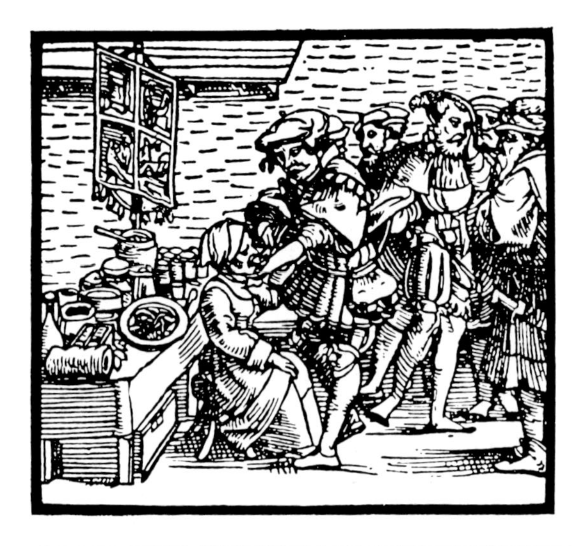

Fig. 135 *Title page of the 1563 Frankfurt printing of "Zene Artzney"*

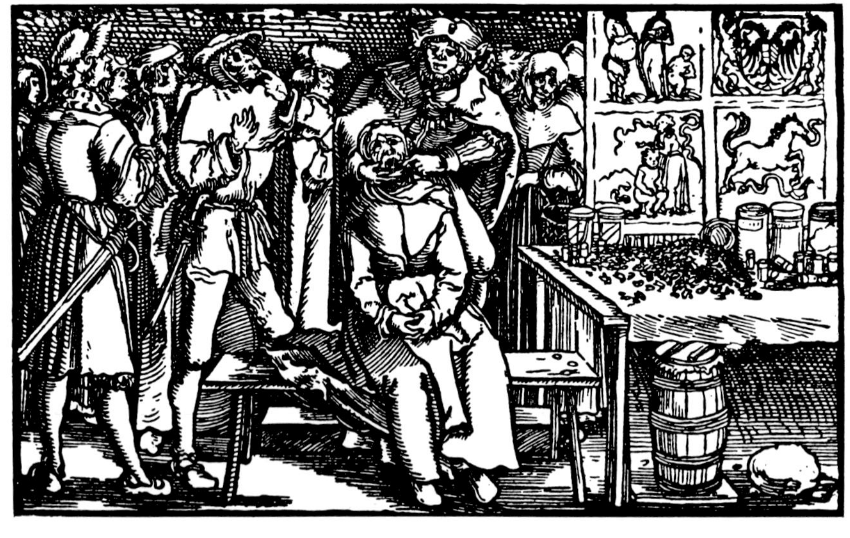

Fig. 136 *Toothbreaker, woodcut of Hans Weiditz in Petrarca's "Trostspiegel" (Mirror of Comfort), 1531*

wandering through practically all of Europe, encountering everywhere the antagonism of the prevailing scholastic medicine at the universities. He published his numerous writings in his German mother tongue, which was then extremely uncommon for a doctor. He particularly emphasized the view that the academic physician should also practice the trade of surgery. In regard to the practitioners of dentistry, Theophrastus Bombastus von Hohenheim, which was his actual name, was quite outspoken negatively in 1528: *and even if they are the best of tooth-breakers, it is true that they then break off the tooth and leave the stump inside*[80]. In his extensive works, there is only one prescription to be found to alleviate toothache: *Thus, even if there is regular toothaches present with many contingencies, with blackness, rottenness, shakiness, falling out and with great pangs, there is not much to be particularly said for observing there progress for the sake of the blackness, since powerful fluid or tooth powder can eliminate the same; thus, I will say no more on it. The rottenness, however, is to be treated thusly: it should be well washed with honey water, and afterwards, with honey and aloe-*

[80] Paracelsus VI p. 47

Der Zanbrecher.

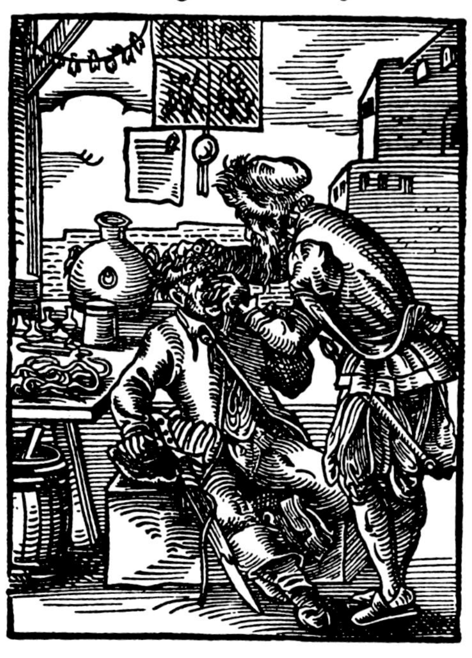

Wolher/wer hat ein böſen Zan/
Denſelben ich außbrechen kan/
On wehtagn / wie man gbiert die Kinder/
Auch hab ich Kramſchatz nicht deſtmindr/
Petrolium vnd Wurmſamen/
Thriacks vnd viel Mückenſchwañen/
Hab auch gut Salbn / für Flöhe vñ Leuß/
Auch Puluer für Ratzen vnd Meuß.

Fig. 137 *Tooth-breaker in Jost Amman's "Ständebuch" of 1568, with verses by Hans Sachs (Translation see p. 160)*

paticum (aloe hepaticum [liver aloes], desiccated aloes juice) *mixed together, it should be linimented for several days, followed by distilled and prepared with plaintain salt, consolida* (comfrey), *serpentina* (adders-word), *etc., and washed with this twice every day until the rottenness disappears* [81]. More important than this rather dubious caries theraphy is the fact that he seems to have been familiar with the painful inflammation of the gingiva resulting from treatment with quicksilver, mercurial stomatitis, because he repeatedly mentions that there is, among other things, tooth pain connected with working with heated "mercuris" [82].—Thus, in general, we see that dental medicine does not have much to thank Paracelsus for directly; nonetheless, this great progressive physician in clinical therapy remains significant for every area of practical medicine.

The first book ever devoted completely and exclusively to dental medicine is also written in the German language. The "Artzney Buchlein (Little Medicine Book) for all kinds of diseases and defects of the teeth...", which was first published in Leipzig in 1530, written by an anonymous author (Fig. 133), later became more

[81] Ibid. IX p. 540
[82] Ibid. IX p. 241; X pp. 187 and 240

widely known under the title "Zene Artzney" in later editions (Fig. 134). Until 1576, there were actually around 10 to 19 new editions and reprints, however, all of which can be definitely documented[83]. Only two years after the first Leipzig edition, the "Zene Artzney" came out in a reworked print by a publisher in Mainz, in which form the book then proceeded, to the Frankfurt printer Egenolff starting in 1536. Reprinting of both the Leipzig and the Mainz editions followed, not only in Frankfurt and in Leipzig itself, but also in Speyer, Königsberg, Nürnberg, and Erfurt, as well as in other places as there were no copyrights then. It was also included in popular health manuals, such as the "Haus Apoteck oder Artzneybuch" (House Apothecary or Medicine Book) of 1565. The uncommonly great number of editions for this era of a little book of only 44 pages is an indication of its popularity and marketability.

The only documentury facts about the author are from the scanty references to him in the text of the first edition. We know that he grew up in Mittweida, a little town in Saxony, and also practiced there as a surgeon, and perhaps also as a physician. The way in which the authors cited are documented in marginalia implies a university education (Fig. 140), but this is just as speculative as the assumption that he had himself portrayed in the title picture[84]. This initial representation is still interesting, as it does not show the patient in the position directed since ancient times, between the knees of the operator, but rather on an armchair fitted with massive braces, while the operator, standing behind him and bending over him, immobilizes the chin with his left hand and manipulates the forceps with the right. Moreover in such a manner that the forceps are grasped only with the fingers and only on the outermost ends of the handles, in a way that certainly no barber of that period would have used.

Another operating scene is to be found on the title page of the edition printed in Frankfurt in 1563 and 1576 (Fig. 135). Noteworthy is that the operator stands here in front of a female victim, surrounded by patients, among whom there is a richly dressed one who is holding his cheeks. The signboard of the town crier is decorated with a trophy necklace of strung molars in a line.

A similar board, also divided into quarters, on which, among others, a female patient is represented with a gigantic toothworm, can be seen in the wood-cut "On the Aching of Teeth," by Hans Weiditz in the German edition of Petrarca's "Mirror of Comfort" from 1531 (Fig. 136). Here again, the patient, surrounded by a pile of extracted teeth, is a woman, sitting on a bench. The same theme is found in the 1568 edition of a German "Ständebuch" (Professional Register, Fig. 137). The accompanying verses by Hans Sachs, which also exist in Latin, give the best description of the status of practical dental medicine at that time[85]:

Well then, who has an evil tooth,
Which I can break out without pain,
Like somebody bears children.
I also have much groceries,
Petroleum, and seeds for worms,
Theriacs and sponges for gnats,
Good ointments against fleas and lice,
Also powders against rats and mice.

The wood-cut from an edition of Galen from 1550 (Fig. 138) shows an ancient scene, appropriate to the contents of the book, of the somewhat more elevated activities of a barber's shop, in which a patient sits in what is already a kind of operating chair with head supports, and in which there is no evidence about the kind of stomatological procedure being undertaken. The suffering peasant represented in the engraving by Lucas van Leyden in 1523 (Fig. 139), on the contrary, is standing. The tooth breaker imperturbably probes the painful tooth, holding the head with the left hand, while his female assistant, with an apparently very sympathetic expression on her face, empties the purse of the victim, who is distracted with pain. Under the signboard, which is only suggested, there hangs a sealed certificate, for effect, and the charlatan's beret is decorated with single-rooted teeth.

Now, let us examine the contents of the "Zene Artzney": The author lets it be known immediately in the heading that his opus is based on the work of Galen, Avicenna, (the false) Mesuë, and Celsus; Pliny, who is also mentioned in the text of the first edition, is included in the title of the second revised edition of Mainz (Fig. 134). All those ancient authors, with the exception of Celsus and Pliny, are only indirectly quoted through Giovanni

[83] Benzing; Budjuhn; Weinberger (b) p. 257 f.
[84] Aupperle
[85] Ammann. Hans Sachs, shoemaker and poet, was one of the "Meistersinger" of Nürnberg

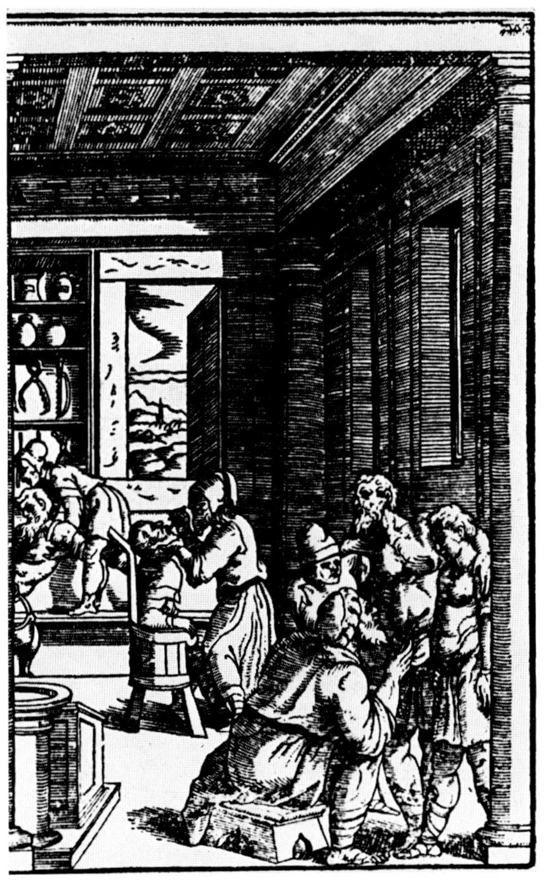

Fig. 138 *Treatment in a barber's shop. Woodcut from a Galen edition, 1550*

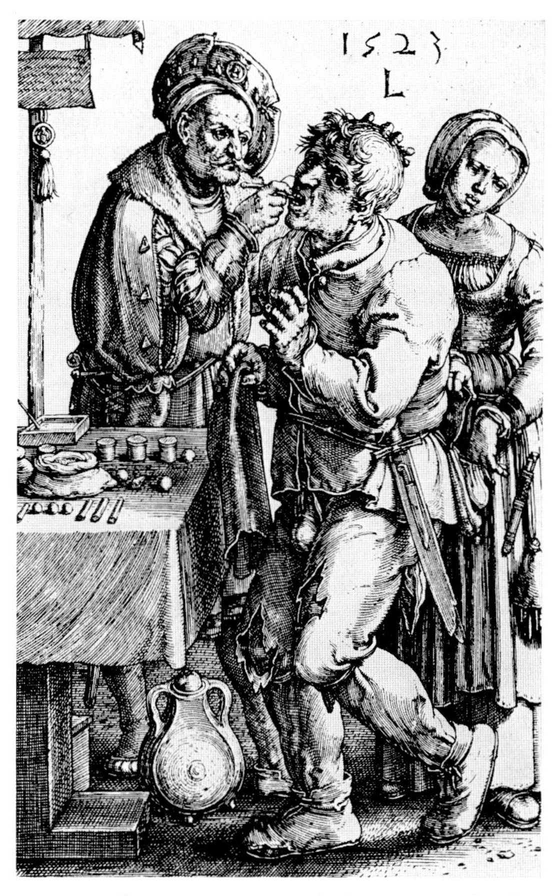

Fig. 139 *Copper-engraving of Lucas van Leyden, 1523*

da Vigo[86], whose "Practica copiosa", which having come out in print in 1514, is also recognizable in the division of material.
The first chapter of this unpaginated little book, which was printed 13 years before Vesalius' "Fabrica," is devoted to anatomy, and consists essentially of anecdotes and cases taken from Pliny. In the second chapter the author discusses tooth decay, and derives from this the customary, quite sensible rules of oral hygiene, such as rinsing after meals and avoiding tidbits such as hard nuts and fruits pits, as well as hot and cold foods; also, *all foods which are viscous, sticky, and fat* (should) *be shunned / because they remain adhering to the teeth / not without damaging them.* Nor are the old prescriptions withheld from us, as in the marginal note from Avicenna: *frogs boiled with water and vinegar are very good for the teeth, when the broth is held in the mouth* (chapter 4). In the fifth chapter, "On perforated and hollow teeth," decay (corrosio) is described as a disease which causes holes and makes the teeth hollow, particularly the molars. According to the legendary Mesuë this can be cured in three ways: through purging, through all sorts of instructions for magic agents, or through scraping away of the corrosion with a fine chisel or small knife, *as the practitioners well know,* and, according to Vigo, *filling the hollow part of the tooth with gold leaf to preserve the other parts.—For worms of the teeth, take henbane seeds / leek seeds / onion seeds / and boil them together in vinegar, / hold it in the mouth and rinse it well throughout.* Alter-

[85] See pp. 132 f.; Budjuhn pp. 42 f.

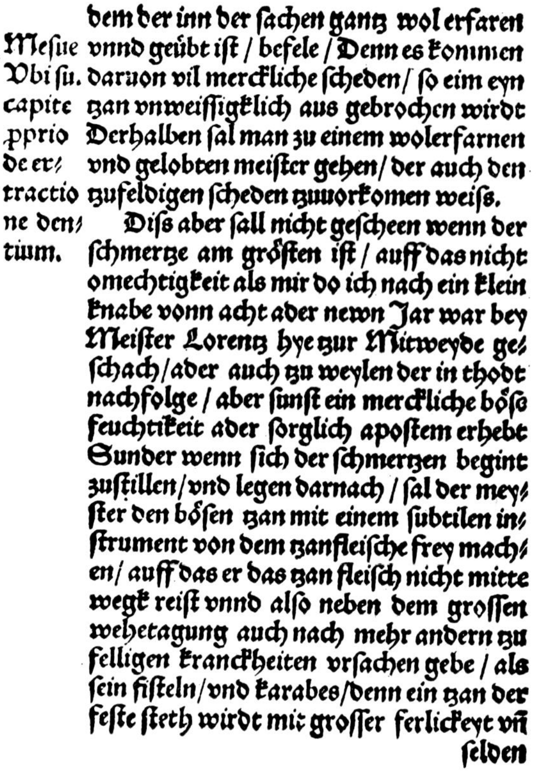

Mesue Vbi su. capite pprio de ex⸗tractione den⸗tium.

dem der inn der ſachen gantʒ wol erfaren vnnd geübt iſt / befele / Denn es kommen daruon vil mercklíche ſcheden / ſo eim eyn ʒan vnweiſſigklich aus gebrochen wirdt Derhalben ſal man ʒu einem wolerfarnen vnd gelobten meiſter gehen / der auch den ʒufeldigen ſcheden ʒuuorkomen weiſs.
Diſs aber ſall nicht geſcheen wenn der ſchmertʒe am gröſten iſt / auff das nicht omechtigkeit als mir do ich nach ein klein knabe vonn acht ader newn Jar war bey Meiſter Lorentʒ hye ʒur Mitweyde ge⸗ſchach / ader auch ʒu weylen der in thodt nachfolge / aber ſunſt ein mercklíche böſe feuchtikeit ader ſorglich apoſtem erhebt Sunder wenn ſich der ſchmertʒen begint ʒuſtillen / vnd legen darnach / ſal der mey⸗ſter den böſen ʒan mit einem ſubtilen in⸗ſtrument von dem ʒanfleiſche frey mach⸗en / auff das er das ʒan fleiſch nicht mitte wegk reiſt vnnd alſo neben dem groſſen wehetagung auch nach mehr andern ʒu felligen kranckheiten vrſachen gebe / als ſein fiſteln / vnd karabes / denn ein ʒan der feſte ſteth wirdt mit groſſer ferlickeyt vñ ſelden

Fig. 140 *Text page (unpaginated) from the "Artzney Buchlein" of 1530*

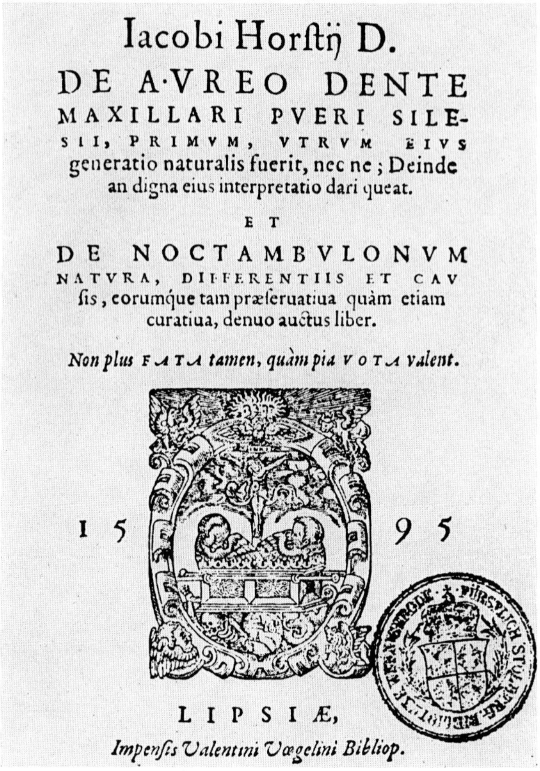

Iacobi Horſtij D.
DE A·VREO DENTE MAXILLARI PVERI SILESII, PRIMVM, VTRVM EIVS generatio naturalis fuerit, nec ne; Deinde an digna eius interpretatio dari queat.
ET
DE NOCTAMBVLONVM NATVRA, DIFFERENTIIS ET CAVſis, eorumque tam præſeruatiua quàm etiam curatiua, denuo auctus liber.
Non plus FATA *tamen, quàm pia* VOTA *valent.*
1595
LIPSIÆ,
Impenſis Valentini Vœgelini Bibliop.

Fig. 141 *The "Book of the Golden Tooth", 1595*

natively, these three agents should be rolled into little balls the size of beans, with the fat of a goat's kidney, and laid on hot coals; the smoke should be directed at the bad tooth through a small cone, so that it will *kill the worms which are within.*

The title of the 12th chapter is "How to break out bad teeth" (Fig. 140). Here, a personal experience comes to light, after the recommendation that in such a dangerous matter, only *a well-experienced and respected master* should be consulted, and not *when the pain is at its worst.* With regard to these, the anonymous author reports that *no one should be more conscious of these than I, still a small boy of eight or nine years, who was treated by Master Lorentz here in Mitweyde* (Mittweida in Saxony). Only when the pain has subsided should the master (surgeon, not physician) remove the bad tooth in the customary fashion (according to Celsus): the gingiva should be freed, the tooth loosened, and filled with lead, tin, silver, or iron, if it is hollow, and then *the master* (should) *pull straight out / and not bend it much to the side* (not luxate it too much) / *whereupon the root of the tooth is to be broken without bending / so that the cheeks are not damaged. Thus, when the tooth is broken out, and no further damage appears,* cold vinegar, which has been boiled previously together with gall-nuts and pomegranate flowers, should be held in the mouth. *Our barbers, however, simply take a bit of salt and press it in there where the tooth had been.* If the patient is too afraid of this, he can be helped with the cautery and a tube, here iron, by thus deadening the dental pulp.

After all this has been brought forth quite reasonably, there is a serious lapse in the conclusion of the chapter: *Take the fats from the green frog which lives in the trees / and spread the tooth*

with it to break it and make it fall out without causing any pain.
The "Final Chapter" repeats the good suggestions for care of the teeth, and is then followed by the impressum: *Printed in Leyptzigk by Michael Blum. In the year A.D. XXX* (1530). Of the printer it is transmitted that he had distributed reformation writings, and had initially been persecuted for it, but then had turned a good profit from them[87].
It is no wonder that a book as successful as this one soon had successors. As early as 1531, the likewise anonymous "Pestregiment" (Plague instruction) was printed by Wolffgang Resch, Formschneyder (form cutter) in Nürnberg, in which a section "On the teeth" was included; this section, one and a half pages long, constitutes about a fourth of the whole pamphlet, which was only five pages long. Only three original examples of this opus are known to survive, although it has now been reprinted twice. It contains a few worthless prescriptions which are essentially based on henbane seeds, but also an old Roman suggestion for eliminating an aching tooth: *of raven manure: put it in the hollow tooth / it crushes.* The well known recommendation first mentioned by Pliny[88].
The "Nützliche Bericht" (Useful Report) printed without a date sometime after 1554 in Würzburg, proceeds in a similar direction, without, however, plagiarizing directly. Its author, the compiler and prolific writer Walther Hermann Ryff (Rivius), includes discussion of the eyes, the teeth (16 pages), and teething of unweaned children (2 pages)[89]. In this text, which is basically oriented around d'Arcoli's commentary about Rhazes[90] his ten rules for care of the teeth and the plethora of prescriptive remedies for toothache are repeated, indeed, but the essential things, such as the perforation of the painful tooth with a drill and filling it with gold are left out. Ryff did not succeed in replacing the popular "Zene Artzney".
Even more worthless is the essay by Iohannes Digitius, a medical student from Franconian Hopferstadt in 1587, on "Useful and valuable / medications for all kinds of toothaches / ...". Of the total 22 pages, six are used for title and the dedications, which are as detailed as they are unusual. For example, there is one from the author to the printer, Dalbin of Speyer, and also one from the printer to the Mayor and the councillors of that city. The contents include a collection of quotations from the Middle Ages and ancient times, partially in Latin; we are not even spared *the suet of green tree frog*[91].
Also belonging to this era of folk manuals of dental medicine is the tale of the golden tooth in the left side of the mandible of a Silesian youth, seven years of age, who began exhibiting himself at yearly fairs in 1593. Behind the story was a gold crown prepared for fraudulent purposes, which was gradually bitten through, so that after three years the deception was obvious. What is interesting for the development of dental medicine in this really not so unimportant episode is the response it aroused. Learned professors and physicians produced essays and counter-essays which debated, in a scholastic manner, the issues of whether the gold tooth was attributable to mysterious forces of nature or astrological influences, whether it was a miracle from God or deception from Satan, whether it was a good or a bad omen, unfavorable impressions upon the mother during pregnancy, or perhaps a result of the gold content of the waters and mountains of Silesia. Among those who supported concepts of this kind was the professor of medicine in Helmstedt, Jakob Horst, who did so in a Latin book of 145 pages which appeared in 1595 (Fig. 141), to be followed in the next year by a German translation[92].
Even in the 17th century, J. J. Rousseau satirically mentions this miracle, and, presumably motivated by him, Frederick the Great, King of Prussia, in 1779 instituted research *into the legend of the Silesian boy with a golden tooth*[93]. The court dentist in Paris, Mouton, also quoted *la Dent molaire d'or de l'Enfant de Silesie* in 1746 and subsequently gave the first description of a gold crown[94].
In 1630, that is, eighty years later, in Vilna another gold tooth, this time a deciduous molar, was spoken of. The man who described it, the Jesuit priest Adalbert Tylkowski, was honest enough, after thorough consideration of all possible physical and metaphysical causes, to admit in a postscript that the tooth, which he had personally seen to be golden, had lost this color

[87] Budjuhn pp. 50 f.
[88] Proskauer (a); Schöppler; see p. 73
[89] Ryff (a)
[90] See p. 131
[91] Digitius p. 21
[92] Horstius
[93] Tylkowki p. 34
[94] See p. 209 f.

wol vnd glich vnnd eben stant mit
den gesunden zennen vnnd dan so
nym ein gütten fyer oder seß feltigē
starcken siden fadem der wol gewe
schet sy oder ein silberin drat oder
ein messin drat der geglüwet ist ge,
wechsen vnnd flicht im die zen also

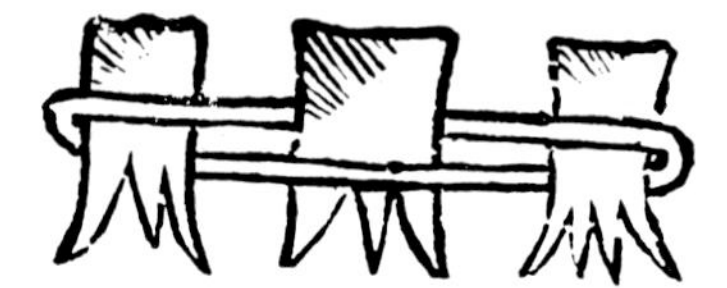

in ein ander glich eim zün vnd so dz
geschicht so nym diß puluer ver//
mengt mit eyerwiß vnd vff ein düch
gestrichen wie ein plaster vnd gebū
dē alß ich gelert hab im capittel vō
den wunden der kind backen im dri
ten dractat oder leg im dar vff pul
sterlin von duoch das mengfeltig sy
vnd dar nach schiennen von leder

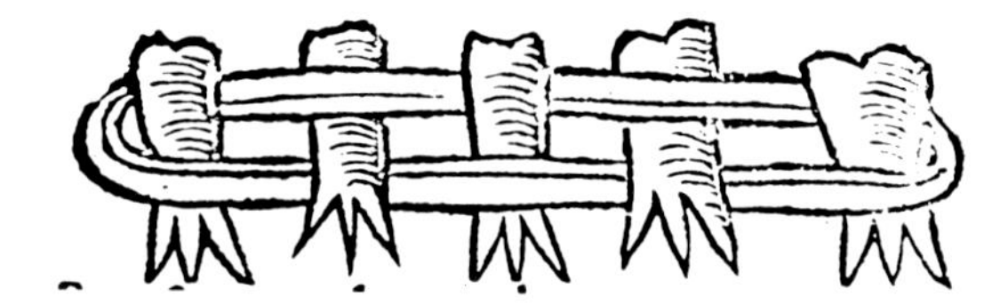

Fig. 142 *Brunschwig: Woodcut of a mandibular fracture splinting, in the "Buch der Cirurgia" (Book of Surgery), 1497 printing; below: the picture in the 1518 edition*

during an attack of fever and resumed its normal bony appearance[95].

Odontological problems also appear sometimes in German surgical books. Thus, in one of the oldest of these, the hand-written "Bündt-Ertzney" (Dressing-Medicine) of 1460 by a Knight of the Teutonic Order, Heinrich von Pfalzpeint, an untaught practitioner, a powder is recommended *for the aching of the teeth,* consisting of pulverized stalactites or rock-crystal or sandstone with pounded pepper. This is a remedy thus directed more towards inflamed gingiva (*if a person's gingiva is very red, and if it itches*) than against actual toothache[96].

A little later, the "Buch der Cirurgia" (Book of Surgery) by Hieronymus Brunschwig of Strassburg was printed in 1497. In its chapter on wounds of the mouth, where he discusses only fractures of the jaw, the author's preferred traumatological orientation comes into play in a way that brings William of Saliceto to mind: if the chin has been broken through, so that the jaw is apart, it should be straightened *and the teeth simply laced together like a hurdle with soft silver wire.* Then, a wooden chin should

[95] Ibid. pp. 56 f.
[96] Pfolsprundt pp. 46 f.

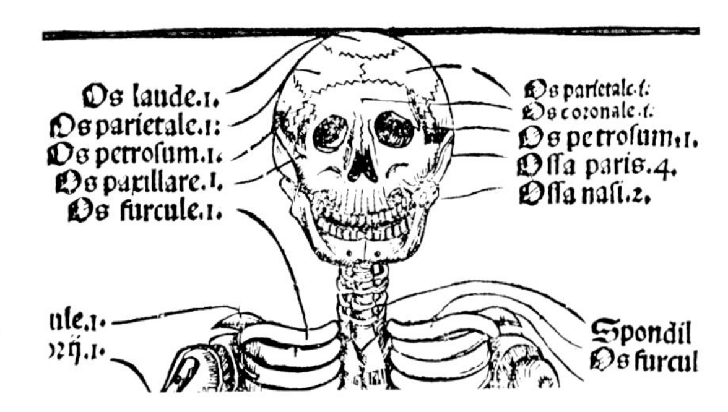

Fig. 143 *Brunschwig: Section of a representation of a skeleton with separated mandible, 1497*

be formed, and a cloth sewn over it and three or four cloths should be glued to it with bread flour. When it has hardened, the result is a hollow form which is cut to size and attached with ties fastened around the head. Thus, this is the chin cup made today with plaster bandages, which supports without compressing the fragments [97]. In the tract on fractures, there is found a second description, which deviates somewhat, and a wood-cut (Fig. 142). The dislocation of the mandible is treated, according to Lanfranchi, with a protective wrap [98]. In an anatomical section, which is not appended to all examples, a skeleton is shown, the mandible of which is naturally still divided [99] (Fig. 143), since this was in 1497, almost half a century before Vesalius' "Fabrica". The book underwent numerous editions, and was translated into English, Dutch, and Bohemian. In 1518 a low German edition also appeared in Rostock [100]. In it, there is a description of jaw fracture treatment, on folio 100 b^{v}, which is similar in principle, except that here leather, in accordance with Hippocrates, is recommended for the capistrum.

The "Feldtbuch der Wundtarzney" (Field-Book of Wound Medicine) which appeared in 1517, by Hans von Gerssdorff, who was likewise active in Strassburg, contains in its anatomical section the statement that the teeth are by nature bones, even though they do have feeling, as Galen says. There are usually 32 of them, *although persons are sometimes to be discovered with no more than 28* [101]. With this, the author's stock of stomatological instruction is exhausted.

Of greater interest ist the "Gross Chirurgei" (Great Surgery) by Walther Ryff, who is also from Strassburg and whom we already mentioned. This was first printed in 1545, like the late "Zene Artzney" by Egenolff in Frankfurt. In any event, its importance lies less in the text than in the illustrations of the instruments. The scalers presented in figure 144, which the Welsh were more enthusiastic in using than the Germans, correspond to those of Abulcasim (see Figs. 76 and 77). The third and next-to-last instruments of figure 145 are termed as "Überwürfe" in the text, a device which now appears close to the pelican. This lever is essentially differentiated from the latter by the fact that instead of a serrated support surface, it has a kind of fork which serves as a fulcrum. Paré indeed depicted a corresponding instrument 20 years after Ryff, but he called it, a "polican" too (see Fig. 119). Later, it was called a "levier" in France by, for example, Fauchard, and "lever" in England, The pelican's serration, which seems particularly fierce here, was tempered somewhat by the fact that the whole supporting section was wrapped during use with a patch of leather [102].

Figure 146 shows a "Geissfuss" (pes caprinus or punch), still used in our century for expressing roots which are not too firmly fastenened, as well as a pushing iron and a hook, two primitive instruments known as "poussoir" and "crochet" in France, which were still in use even in the 19th century. The punch is also a modified pushing iron. Figure 147 shows an executed wire splinting of a jaw fracture as part of an instruction for the preparation of skeletons [103].

97 Brunschwig (a) fol. 59 b^{v}—100 b^{r}; see p. 117
98 Ibid. fol. 100 b^{r}—100 a^{v}; see p. 118
99 Ibid. fol. 112 a^{v}—113 a^{r}
100 Brunschwig (b)
101 Gerssdorf p. 6
102 Kieser
103 Ryff (b) fol. 38^{r}

Teutschen Chirurgei. XXXVIII

hůt den mund fein gemach vnnd seuberlich damit auffzuschrauben/ nit allein dem Patienten lufft vnd labung zugeben/ sonder jm auch vnderweilen mit bequemer artznei zuhelffen ꝛc.

So wir nun des munds gedencken / kommen vns auch die zän für / welche mit jrem scharpffen vnleidlichen schmertzē trefflich vil Instrument durch die notturfft erfunden haben.

Vnd seind alle dise Instrumentlin so hernach verzeychnet stehn/ nicht anders geordnet/ dann allein die zän damit zuseubern / reinigen/ vnnd schaben/ Werden von den alten Dentrificia genant welche diser zeit bei den Walhen/ die sich leibliches schmuckens vil mehr wann wir Teutschen gebrauchen/ noch im brauch/ die zän damit frisch vnd sauber zubehalten.

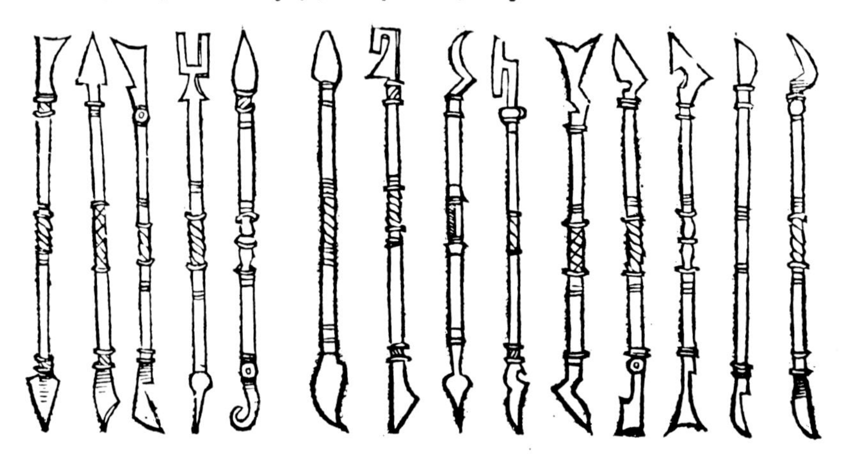

Dise hernachfolgende Instrument/ wie du sie nach einander fürgemalt sihest/ Als nemlich/ Entenschnabel/ Pellican/ Zänzangen/ Vberwürff/ Geyßfüßlin vnd dergleichen/ wie sie genant werden mögen/ seind mancherley art vnd gestalt geformiert/ nach dem sie ein jeder Meyster nach seiner hand weyß zubrauchen vnnd regieren. Deren hab ich dir die aller gemeynesten vnnd gebreuchlichsten fürreissen oder malen lassen. Wie sie aber zugebrauchen seind/ sampt der gantzen zänartznei/ findest du hernach in folgender Chirurgei weitern bericht in einem besondern Capitel/ in dem letzsten Theyl. Wiewol wir auch kurtz verschinener zeit ein besonder Büchlin haben außgehn lassen / darinnen alle fehl vnd gebrechen der augen vnnd zän gnůgsamlichen beschriben vnd angezeygt werden.

Entenschnabel zu den stümpffen:

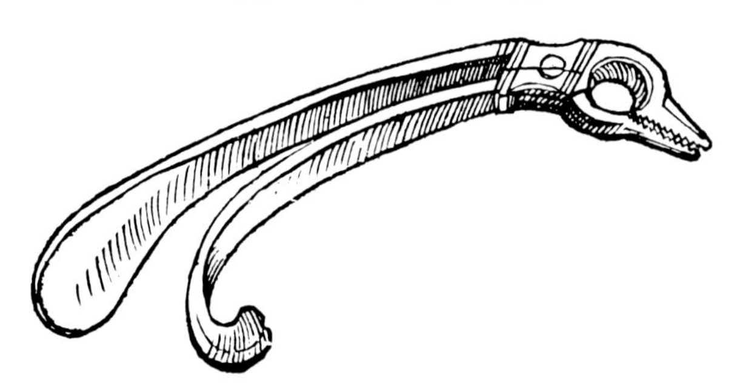

Fig. 144 *Ryff: Scalers and root forceps in the "Gross Chirurgei" (Great Surgery), 1559 edition (Announcement of eye and tooth booklets, in the last sentence)*

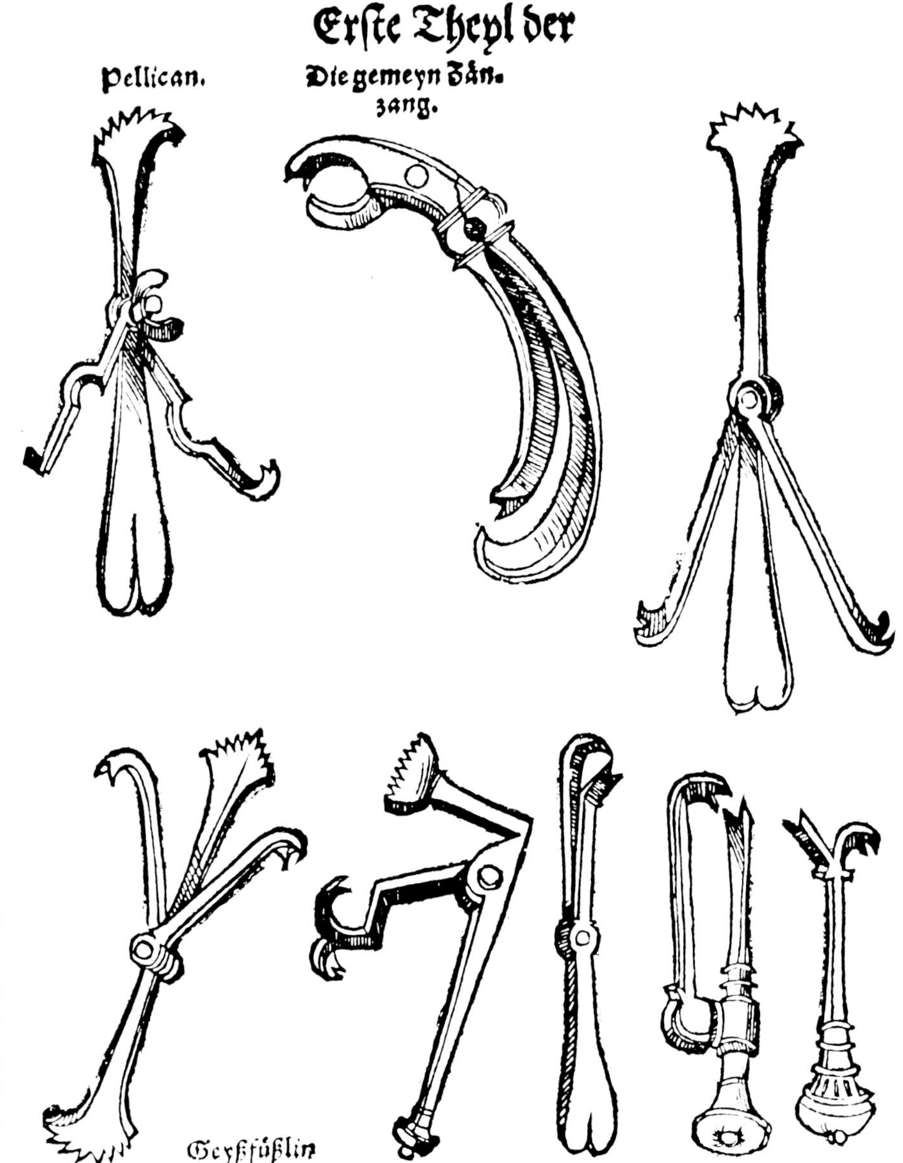

Fig. 145 *Ryff: Extraction instruments: top the first and third instruments and bottom first and second — pelicans of various types; bottom third and fourth — "Überwürfe" (a variation of pelicans), and a combination of hook and punch as last*

Furthermore, we find tongue-scraper, calculus instruments, and mouth spatulas in forms that are in part still customary today. We also know of an "Anatomie" (Anatomy) by this author who, already condemned by Albrecht von Haller as a poor compiler and scribler, wrote about medicine just as he had written about mathematics, architecture, and cookery[104]. In any case, the mandible in this small anatomical book printed in 1541, that is even before Vesalius' rectification, is already represented as undivided (Fig. 147; see also Fig. 143)[105].

The surgeon Franz Renner, like Ryff, was municipal surgeon of Nürnberg; he was the one who provided us with the first description known up to this point of an obturator in his "haylsam

[104] Gurlt III p. 42
[105] Ryff (c) unpaginated

Geyßfüßlin mancherley form vnd geſtalt / brüchlin vonn zänen damit außzuſtechen.

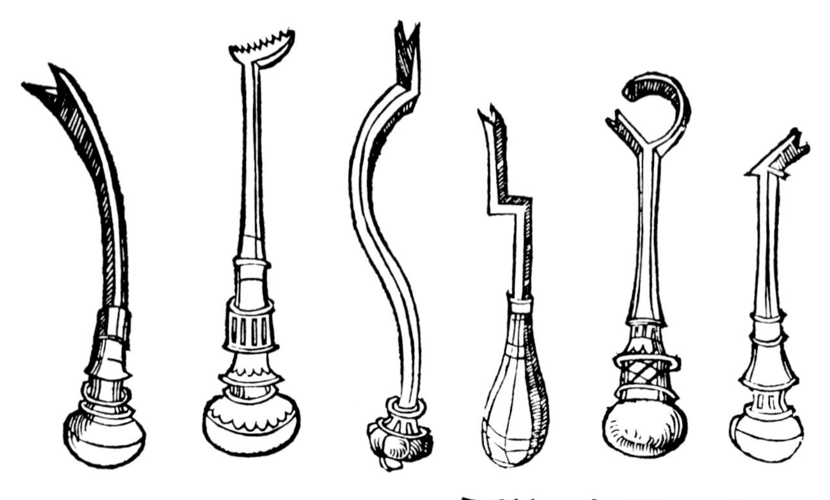

Fig. 146 *Ryff: "Geißfüsse" (Pedes caprini, second and last instrument), punches and a hook (penultimate), 1559*

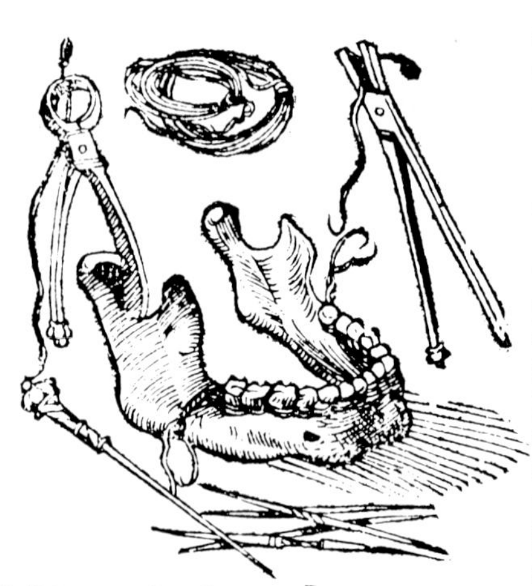

Zu ſolcher arbeyt dienen dir mancherley alē / eiſen ſo die Schůchmacher brauchen / die bein damit zuboren / wie du ſolchen zeug hie bei einander ſiheſt ligen / als nemlich / die pfetzzang / die drätlin darmit abzupfetzen. Die biegzang ſolche in einander mit flechten zubiegen / ſampt dem gebendlin kleiner vnd groſſer drät / welche du vorhin ſolt erglüen laſſen / damit ſie zehe werden / vnd nit brechen. Zu vnderſt ligt die ale / ſampt vilen aleiſen / damit kleine vnnd groſſe löchlin zuboren. Aber der kyfel oder vnderſt kinback mit ſolchen drätlin vmbzeunet vmb die zän / bedeut die befeſtigūg der zän / wie mann ſie in verwundung des kyfels oder bruch des ſelbigen an einander verzeunen ſol / daß ſie ſtedt vñ feſt bleiben / ꝛc. Wie dir dann hernach in folgender Chirurgei / in zweyen beſondern Capiteln vom bruch vnd verwundung ſolches kyfels / gnůgſamlicher bericht geſetzt wirt.

Fig. 147 *Ryff: Splinting of a jaw fracture*

Handtbüchlein" (Little Handbook of Healing ... against the terrible, repulsive disease of the French), an early work on syphilis, of course[106]. His palatal obturator described in 1557, that is, several years before Amatus Lusitanus, Paré, and Fabrizzi d'Acquapendente, was manufactured from sheets of leather, softened and glued one on top of another like an hour-glass. The original page is shown in figure 148.

According to Renner, these obturators can also be prepared from ivory or gold and silver, but he does not find these as satisfactory, because they are painful when put in; for this reason a simple correctly cut sponge or the type prepared from leather is to be preferred[107]. The progress in the later devices by Amatus Lu-

[106] Sudhoff (a)
[107] Renner p. 86 f.

LXXXVI.

men zeucht/aus füllen/(so die hailung gar volbracht ist) mit eim lucken schwemlein/nach grösse der öff- nung geschnitten/vnd als dann mit zugestopfft/ da- von die red widerumb gescherpfft vnnd zu recht ge- bracht wirdt/einer nicht mer so nüselt vnd durch die nasen redt/wie sunst geschicht/deshalb wol etlich ge dulden/das man solche löcher mit erwaichtem leder aus fült/der gestalt/man nimbt zwey oder drey leder die ründ oder scheiblecht/nach art des lochs formirt seindt/die hefft man mit eim hafft auff einander/das die diesen form bekommen ▬ wie dann die grösse des orts sein sol / solche leder werden also zugericht/ damit das obertheil innwendig des verborgnens Gomens einwartz ein hab vber kom/das ander vn- ten am sichtbarn Gomen stehe/ so kan also eins das ander halten / vnnd die offnung bedecken vnnd zu dempffen / das also die sprach vnuerhindert bleibt/ etlich lassen solche muster von helffenbain dreen / od von gold od silber formirn/wie vngefer obens bezei- chnet vñ fürgerissen ist zu einē muster / die man auch also in solche öffnung dreet/od ein vnd aus thut/wie die not einen selbs lernet/ aber dises von bain/ gold oder silber/seint nit so leidlich/als die vō schwamen oder leder gemacht / gefallen mir auch dieser vrsach nicht / dieweil die schmertzlich auß vnd eingehoben/ vnnd doch etwo von jhn selbs bald auß fallen/

Y ij wo

Fig. 148 *Renner: Page of text with description and depiction of the obturator, 1557*

sitanus and Paré consisted fundamentally in combining metal obturation and nasal sponge retention.

The widely-read municipal physician of Freiburg im Breisgau, Johann Schenck von Grafenberg, shows himself to be a pure man of letters on the subject of dental medicine in his "Observationes medicae de capite humano" (Medical Observations on the Human Head), which appeared in 1584. Even if there is hardly anything original to be found, we must acknowledge his constant efforts to be unbiased. The problems are mostly treated as thesis and antithesis: thus, for example, with regard to the toothworm[108]. Schenck placed the correct conception of his Parisian contemporary Houllier, that the so-called toothworms develop from henbane seeds[109] in immediate opposition to that of Benedetti, already mentioned, who firmly believed in the beasts[110], and was here still completely rooted in the ancient ideas. Similarly, Schenck contrasted the outdated notion of the divided mandible with the correct one of Colombo, a successor to Vesalius[111], although only the chapter heading allows the inference that Schenck himself probably adhered to the latter view. Replacement and also transplantation of teeth[112] are discussed with quotations from Paré, and with regard to the palatal obturator, Renner and Lusitanus are mentioned as well. While surgical tooth extraction is completely absent, the remedial method is exhaustively described, whereby the whole nonsense of the junk apothecary, including the tree frog fat, is brought to light[113]. As a child of his

108 Schenckius Obs. 390
109 See p. 145
110 See p. 131
111 Schenckius Obs. 406; Columbus I p. 32
112 Schenckius Obs. 401
113 Ibid. Obs. 396; 397

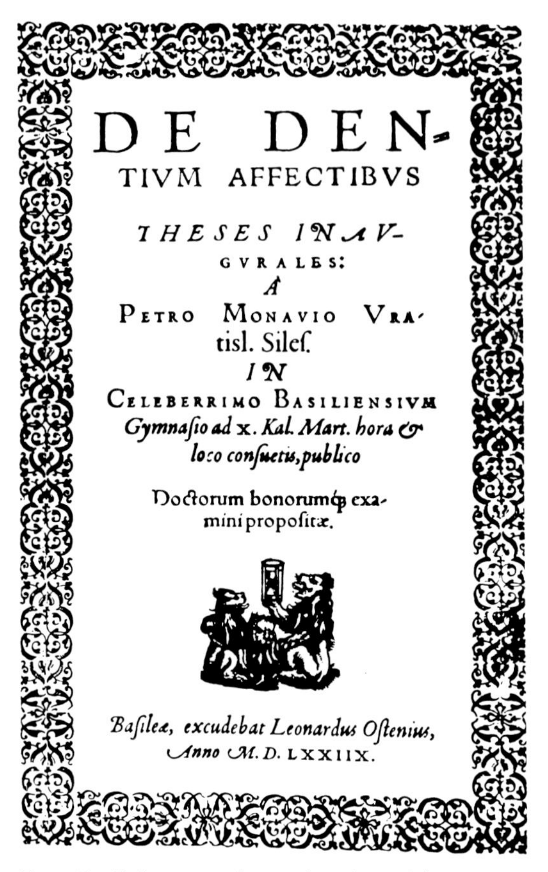

DE DENTIVM AFFECTIBVS

THESES INAVGVRALES:

A

PETRO MONAVIO VRAtisl. Sileſ.

IN

CELEBERRIMO BASILIENSIVM Gymnaſio ad x. Kal. Mart. hora & loco conſuetis, publico

Doctorum bonorumque examini propoſitæ.

Baſileæ, excudebat Leonardus Oſtenius, Anno M. D. LXXIIX.

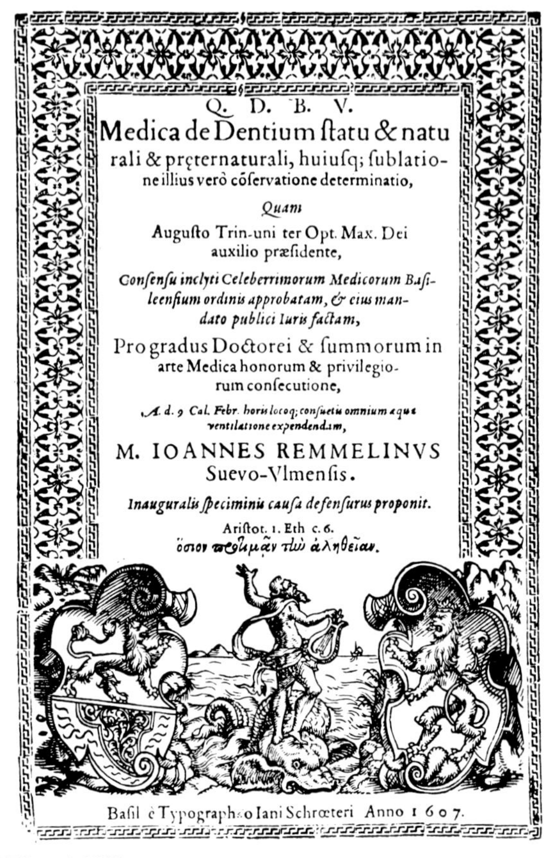

Q. D. B. V.

Medica de Dentium ſtatu & naturali & prçternaturali, huiuſq; ſublatione illius verò cõſervatione determinatio,

Quam

Auguſto Trin-uni ter Opt. Max. Dei auxilio præſidente,

Conſenſu inclyti Celeberrimorum Medicorum Baſileenſium ordinis approbatam, & eius mandato publici Iuris factam,

Pro gradus Doctorei & ſummorum in arte Medica honorum & privilegiorum conſecutione,

A. d. 9 Cal. Febr. horis locoq; conſuetis omnium æque ventilatione expendendam,

M. IOANNES REMMELINVS Suevo-Vlmenſis.

Inauguralis ſpeciminis cauſa defenſurus proponit.

Ariſtot. 1. Eth c. 6.

ὅσιον προτιμᾶν τὴν ἀλήθειαν.

Baſil. è Typographeo Iani Schrœteri Anno 1607.

Fig. 149 *Title pages of two odontological dissertations, 1578 and 1607*

age, Schenck is not free from superstition himself, as is seen by the quotation from the Italian scholar Gerolamo Cardano: *After he had written a few mysterious signs on a piece of wood with a nail, he touched the tooth three times, and not only freed it immediately* (of pain), *but after he had held the nail, which he had fastened in the wood, against it, promised him permanent unipairment of that tooth, which also took place* [114]. The fixation of the toothache in a piece of wood brings to mind the similar description of the "staking-out" in Benivieni [115].

All in all, Schenck von Grafenberg, as a physician between the old and the new times provides within his "Observationes" nothing more than a theoretical summary of dentistry as it presented itself to a well-educated doctor of this transition period.

The first doctoral dissertations on odontological themes, all examples of which were equally sterile, already had been submitted at the universities; for instance, that of the Breslau physician Peter Monau (Monavius) [116] in 1578 in Basel, and that of Johannes Rümelin (Remmelinus) from Ulm, in 1607 in Tübingen (Fig. 149). Thomas Erast, a professor at the universities of Heidelberg and Basel, wrote a disputation on the teeth, which were called, he points out, ὀδόντες (odóntes) by the Greeks and dentes by the Latin-speakers, almost as if they wanted to say edentes (eaters) [117]. This paragram, however, is already to be found in Eustachi and Hemard.

[114] Ibid. Obs. 394
[115] See p. 133
[116] Monavius; he died as physician in ordinary to Emperor Rudolf II in Prague in 1588
[117] Lorber (a)

The 17th Century

In the 17th century, the era of the beginning of absolutist states, England and France stepped forth on the path to world power and forced Spain and Portugal, and later the Netherlands, into the background. Germany, too, lost importance through the affliction of the Thirty Years' War. Meanwhile, to the North, Sweden grew powerful for a time, as did Russia, finally in the East.

If, in the Arts of the 16th century, the great sceptics Erasmus, Montaigne, and Rabelais effected a turning away from the scholastic methods of the Middle Ages, in a positive manner in the 17th century a reestablishment of the theoretical disciplines followed. Francis Bacon, the many-faceted philosopher and shadowy British statesman, shrewd and influential, elevated experience above speculation. In accordance with his motto, "Knowledge is power", he discerned the successful path in medicine in epicritical thinking, pathological and anatomical research, and in the evaluation of animal experimentation. He and the French mathematician René Descartes (Cartesius) taught an inductive-empirical and analytic approach, which resulted in a blossoming in physics and chemistry.

Art at this time did not merely loll in voluptuous forms and colors, it also produced above all in paintings of masters of the Netherlands, Gerhard van Honthorst and Theodor Rombouts, Adriaen Brouwer and David Teniers, Adriaen van Ostade and Jan Steen, contributions to the history of dentistry through a rich assortment of true-to-life representations of toothdrawers, shown with their instruments, pain-relieving tinctures and at the yearly fair, in the barber's shop or in the inn, during or after their painful work. The practical side of the discipline is put before our eyes with an unsurpassable realism (Figs. 150 and 151).

In the field of medicine, the great Englishman William Harvey led the way to a new epoch of physiology with his discovery, published in 1628, of the circulation of the blood. His countryman Nathanael Highmore in 1651 described the maxillary sinus, which bore his name from then until into our own century, although it had already been described by numerous anatomists after Leonardo da Vinci[118], and in 1660, the Dane Niels Stensen (Nicolaus Stenonius) ascertained the secretory duct of the parotid gland. In 1685, the important Italian physician and physicist Giovanni Alfonso Borelli published, in "De motu animalium" (On the Movement of Animals), investigations into the mechanics of the muscles, among which are the probably first measurements of the masticatory force[119] (Fig. 152).

The construction of the first microscope, probably around 1590 by the Dutch Zacharias Janssen, made further discoveries possible in the 2nd half of the 17th century: in 1661, Marcello Malpighi, the founder of microanatomy, through the discovery of the capillaries closed the remaining gap in the theory of blood circulation and in 1675, compared enamel and dentin with the bark and core of trees in his plant anatomy: *Because they* (the teeth) *are put together in two layers, of which the outer is reticular and fibrous, since it constitutes a protruding section of the skin or at least its fibers. The filaments leading from the root forward to the base of the teeth are bent in different ways, and become curly, so that an elegant weave appears, which is finally covered by a supervening ossification, caused by a fluid poured on it*[120] (Fig. 153).

These researches were completed by the Dutch Anthony van Leeuwenhoek, who was not a physician; he was a draper and minor official of Delft, but an important proponent of microscopy as a lay researcher into nature. He gave a description of tooth canals to a gathering of the Royal Society in 1678 in London, where it was published in the same year in the "Philosophical Transactions." In this, it is asserted that the tooth is formed from very narrow, transparent tubes. *Six or seven hundred of these Pipes put together, I judg(e) exceed not the thickness of one Hair of a Man's Beard. In the Teeth of a Cow, the same Pipes appear somewhat bigger and in those of a Haddock somewhat less*[121]. It remains uncertain whether the preparation described and depicted here was a model for a piece of enamel or, as is more probable, of dentin, as the author could not have been able

[118] See p. 136
[119] Borellus pp. 127—129
[120] Malpighius (a and b) I p. 4; a detailed anatomy of teeth is to be found in Malpighius (c) pp. 51—56
[121] Leeuwenhoek (a); Cohen (a)

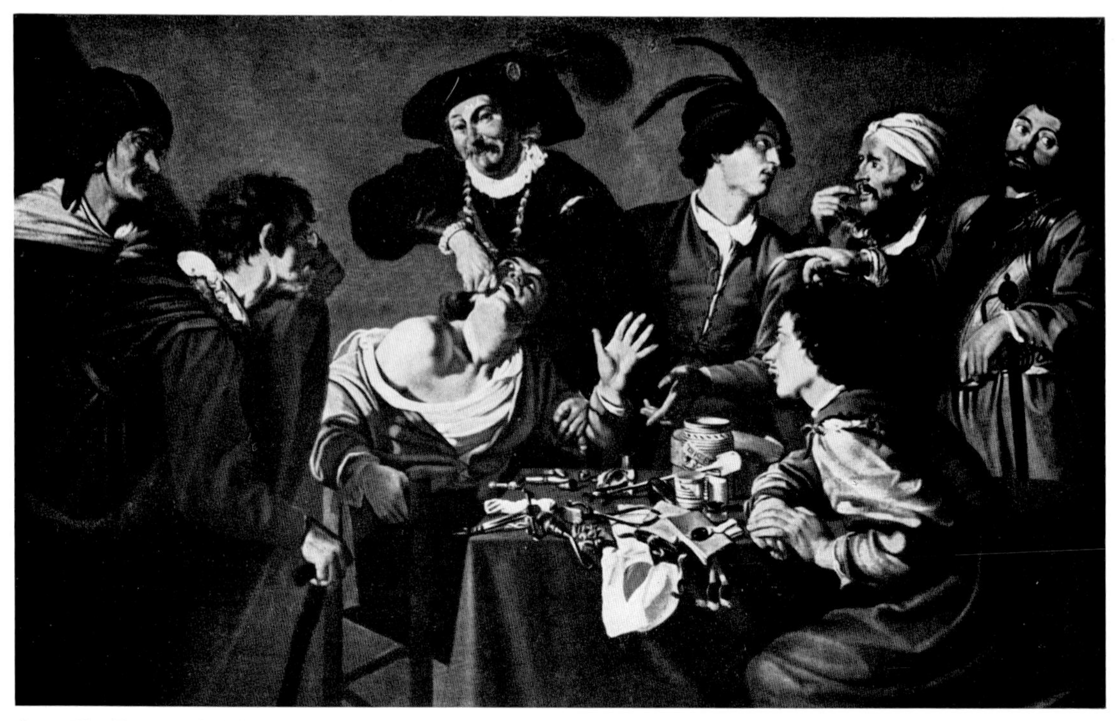

Fig. 150 *Painting by Theodor Rombouts (Prado, Madrid)*

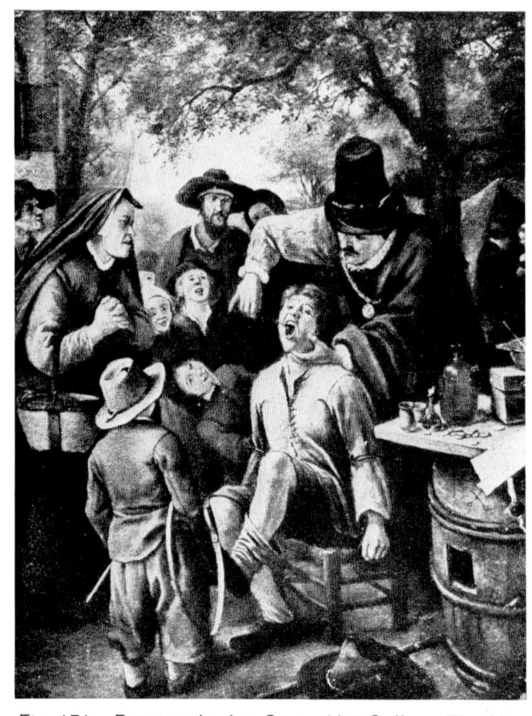

Fig. 151 *Painting by Jan Steen (Art Gallery, The Hague)*

Fig. 152 *Borelli: Measuring masticatory force in "De motu animalium", 1685*

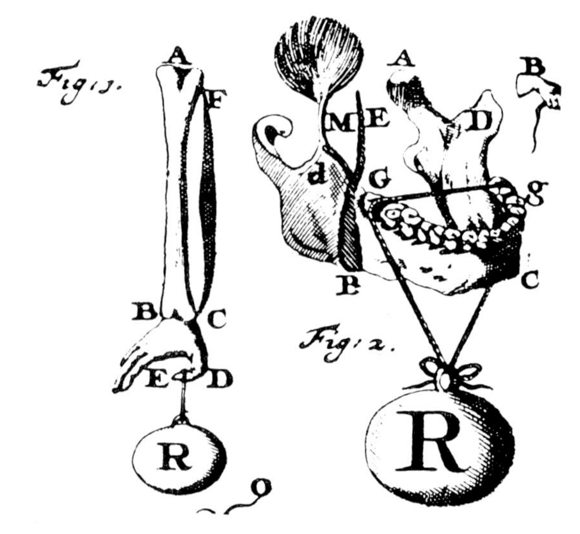

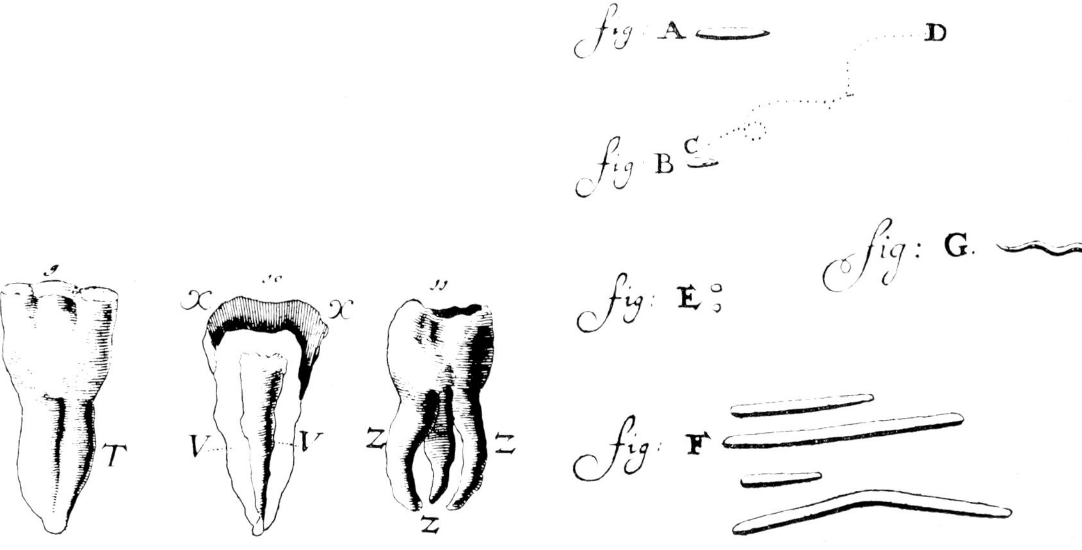

Fig. 153 *Malpighi: Depictions of teeth in "Anatomes plantorum idea", 1686*

Fig. 155 *Leeuwenhoek: Little salivary animals, 1683*

Microſcopical Obſervations of the Structure of Teeth and other Bones: Made and Communicated, in a Letter by Mr. Anthony Leeuwenhoeck.

I Have ſome time ſince applyed a Glaſs, (eſteemed by ſeveral Gentlemen, who had try'd it, a very good one) to obſerve the Structure of the Teeth, and other Bones. Which both to them and my ſelf alſo, then ſeemed to conſiſt of *Globules*. But ſince then, having drawn out one of my Teeth, and for further Obſervation, applyed better Glaſſes than the former; the ſame Gentlemen, with my ſelf, agreed, from what we plainly ſaw, That the whole Tooth was made up of very ſmall ſtrait and tranſparent Pipes. Six or ſeven hundred of theſe Pipes put together, I judg exceed not the thickneſs of one Hair of a Mans Beard. In the Teeth of a Cow, the ſame Pipes appear ſomewhat bigger and in thoſe of a Haddock ſomewhat leſs.

Fig. 1. *Fig.* 2.

B
A C
D
E

Fig. 1. *A. B. C. D. E.* is a Square piece of a Bone, whereto, although you apply a good *Microſcope*, yet at the end *A. B. C.* it will ſeem as if compoſed of *Globules*. Nor will the Pipes diſtinctly appear on the ſides *A. C. D. E.* by reaſon of the thickneſs of the Bone, and thereby the trajection of leſs light.

Fig. 2. Is a flat piece of a Bone, in which the aforeſaid Pipes may be ſeen.

Fig. 154 *Leeuwenhoek: Description of dentinal tubules, 1678*

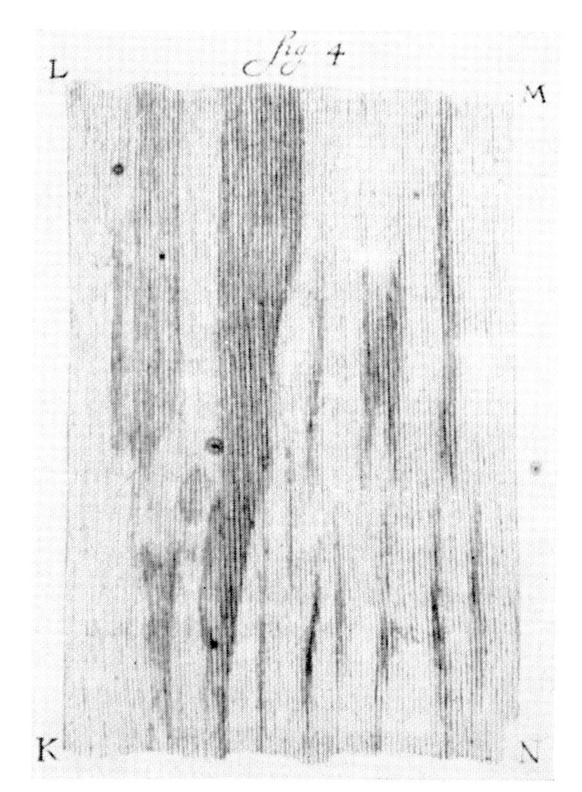

Fig. 156 *Leeuwenhoek: First illustration of human dentin fibers, 1696 (from Cohen a)*

then to differentiate these tissues (Fig. 154). In 1683, with the help of a microscope he had built himself, he recognized little animals (animalcula) in saliva and tooth plaque [122] (Fig. 155), and he published the first representation of the dentin fibres in 1696 (Fig. 156).

Little significant progress was made in the development of the profession. The academic physicians occupied themselves periodically with a scholarly monograph or dissertation on odontological questions, but these represented in general only compilations of anatomical and physiological knowledge, and limited themselves to quotations, mostly from Arab authors. With regard to therapy, surgeons discussed dental medicine peripherally, of course, in their already quite pragmatic writings; the actual practice of the field, as usual, was in the hands of the toothdrawers (or toothers in England, arracheurs de dents in France, Zahnbrecher in Germany, cavadenti in Italy) and barbers, as well as in those of quacks and charlatans. Toward the end of the century, the sovereign national governments issued medical regulations, much as they had previously existed, for example, in independent cities. They arranged the development of the practice of medicine, and established the base for a dentist class by mentioning dental practitioners, but these measures began to have an effect only in the subsequent century [123].

With regard to publications of the 17th century, let us turn first to the academicians. The "Institutiones chirurgicae" (1601), by Johann Jessenius, professor in both Wittenberg and Prague, represents almost exclusively an anthology of earlier writers on the subject of dental medicine. Unfortunately for him, he became involved in politics, so that at the beginning of the Thirty Years' War the Habsburgs had him beheaded and quartered [124].

The Imperial physician in ordinary in Karlsbad, and physician in Augsburg when the Emperor was absent, Johann Stephan Strobelberger (Fig. 157) was a much more adept tactician. He was educated in Montpellier and although Protestant, was spared by both the Counter-Reformation and the iniquity of war [125]. His work "De dentium podagra" (On Toothache), which appeared in 1630, the year of his death, represents a clear retrogression, compared with the "Zene Artzney", which had been printed exactly one hundred years before. Once again, the therapy here is dominated by tortoise blood and frog broth, also a lion's tooth hung about the neck as a remedy against toothache, which immediately reminds us of at-Tabari's hyena tooth or Mercuriale's wolf's tooth, both for the same purpose [126]. The whole 10th chapter is devoted to the fat of the tree frog as an infallible means of making teeth fall out, while Strobelberger adheres to John of Gaddesden, and even reports of whose sale of this prescription to barbers. Going beyond his authority figure, who after all only quoted Rhazes and Avicenna on his part [127], Strobelberger relates that not only cows lost hair and teeth when they inadvertently ate a tree frog, but Indian elephants did so, too. Indeed, Andreas Libavius [128] questioned this because many people ate frogs cooked in vinegar and oil without losing their teeth, and also because he himself had extracted this frog fat and applied it without success. The good doctor was not to be convinced, however, by such practical experiments. Libavius ought to have distilled the fat in the summer, and the animals should have come from Provence, where it is warm. The sceptic should have journeyed there first [129].

Nothing but rehashed ancient wisdom is to be found in the four dissertations by Melchior Sebizius, a professor in Strassburg in 1645, and the mandible still consisted of two bones in the surgical work by Johannes von Beverwyck, a physician and professor in Dordrecht in 1651 100 years after Vesalius; the halves of the mandible are not firmly coalesced in children, *but in adults, they are so close together / that is seems as though there is only one bone* [130]. The dental anatomy here is likewise full of stories from the ancients, but on the other hand, there is not a single word said from practical experience.

The often-used term "junk apothecary" probably derives from a work of Christian Franz Paul(l)ini, the literarily extreme fertile court and municipal physician who was active in his

[122] Leeuwenhoek (b) p. 42 f.
[123] See pp. 195 f.
[124] Höser
[125] Wilker
[126] See pp. 91 and 145
[127] See pp. 94 and 125
[128] Andreas Libavius, physician and chemist, worked as a physician and teacher, later as director of the Classical high school in Ilmenau, Jena, Rothenburg and Coburg. Author of the first significant textbook of chemistry (1595)
[129] Strobelbergerus 10
[130] Sebizius; Beverwyck p. 158

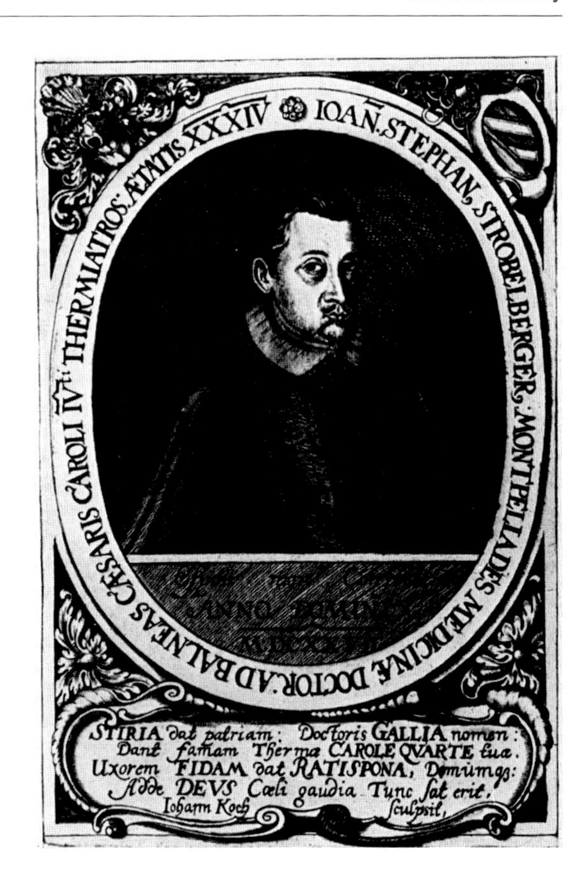
IOAN. STEPHAN. STROBELBERGER, MONTPELLIADES. MEDICINÆ DOCTOR. AD BALNEAS CÆSARIS CAROLI IV: THERMIATROS: ÆTATIS XXXIV
STIRIA dat patriam: Doctoris GALLIA nomen:
Dant famam Therma CAROLE QVARTE tua.
Uxorem FIDAM dat RATISPONA; Domumq:
Adde DEVS Cœli gaudia. Tunc sat erit.
Iohann Koch sculpsit.

Fig. 157 *Johann Stephan Strobelberger, 1627*

native city of Eisenach until his death, after long travels throughout almost all of Europe [131]. In his "Heilsame Dreck-Apotheke" (Healing Junk Apothecary, Fig. 158) dental and oral therapy are carried out with excrements whose contributors are almost all types of creatures. In each of these disgusting recommendations, he conscientiously acknowledges the source of the prescription, but does not seem to report from personal experience at all. Thus, according to a pastor on the Danish isle of Moen, Norwegian pitch should be applied to the painful molar with raven or mouse manure, or the ancient method of putting raven manure into the hollow tooth *makes it, so that it falls out.* A Jew recommends that pulverized sparrow manure with sweet almond oil be dropped into *the ear on the same side,* while a Danish sailor steeped fresh sage in his urine and rubbed the tooth with it, which had as good an effect against scurvy as the suggestion of a friend in Frankfurt, to spread every morning and evening a salve on the gingiva, made from honey with pulverized white dog manure, to be collected in March, and a little pounded nutmeg. It continues in this way, page after page, with fatiguing repetition. This book, which appeared in five editions from 1696 to 1734, and was reprinted as late as 1847, forms the literary high point of the manure medications we have encountered constantly since ancient times [132].

Toward the end of the century, in 1699, there is found among the reports of the Paris Academy of the Sciences one of two pages called "Sur les dents" (On the Teeth), by its member Gabriel Philippe de la Hire, which was quoted (inaccurately) 29 years later by Fauchard. In it the author determines that the enamel (l'émail) is composed of innumer-

131 Köhler
132 Paulini (a) pp. 68—72. In the posthumous "new, enlarged" edition of 1734, the author's name is written with a single "l"

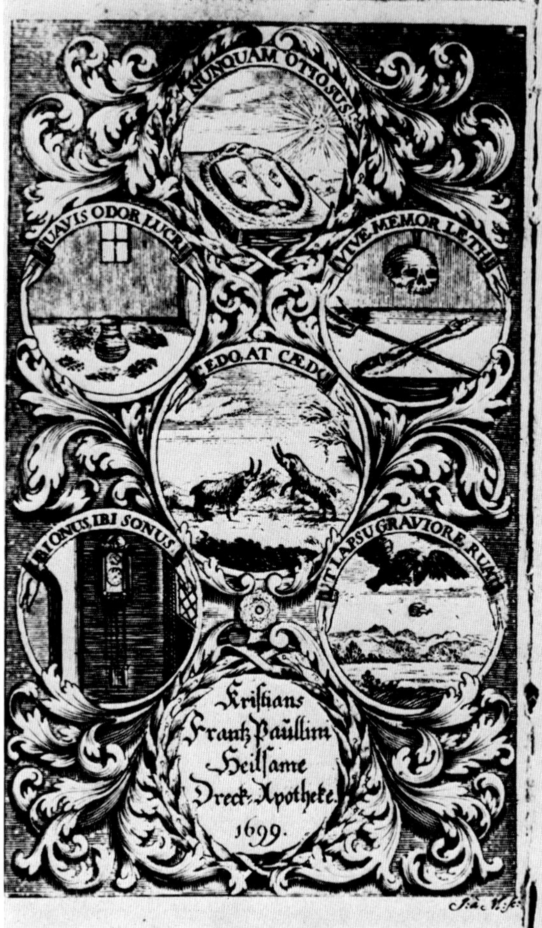
NUNQUAM OTIOSUS
SUAVIS ODOR LUCRI
VIVE MEMOR LETHI
CEDO AT CÆDO
UBI ONUS IBI SONUS
UT LAPSU GRAVIORE RUANT
Kristians
Frantz Paullini
Heilsame
Dreck-Apotheke.
1699.

Neu-Vermehrte/
Heylsame
Dreck-Apotheke,
Wie nemlich mit
Koth und Urin
Fast alle/ ja auch die schwerste/
gifftigste Kranckheiten, und bezauberte
Schäden vom Haupt biß zun Füssen, inn-
und äusserlich, glücklich curiret worden;
Mit allerhand raren, so wohl nütz-
als ergötzlichen
Historien und Anmerckungen/
Auch andern
Feinen Denckwürdigkeiten,
Nochmahls bewährt, nun zum vierdten mahl
um ein merckliches verbessert,
Und mit dem
Andern Theil
vermehrt
Von
Kristian Frantz Paulini.
Franckfurt am Mayn,
In Verlegung Friederich Daniel Knochen.
MDCCXXXIV.

Fig. 158 *Title page of Paul(l)ini's "Junk (excrement) Apothecary", 1734 printing, with 1699 frontispiece*

DES SCIENCES. 43

D L E I I A C F H E G M M N N

La ligne *AC FH.* marque l'extremité des deux tables osseuses qui enferment les dents, & qui font la mâchoire.

Les parties *AEC.* & *FGH.* sont les racines des dents qui sont enfermées dans les tables osseuses.

Les parties *ADCB.* & *FLHII.* representent l'émail, composé de petits filets rangés les uns à côté des autres, qui couvre toute la partie de la dent qui est hors de la mâchoire.

II. Montrent plusieurs filets qui font l'émail, joints par la partie superieure, & éloignés par la partie inferieure.

M, M. Trous par où les nerfs entrent dans les racines des dents.

N, N. Dent fermée.

Fig. 159 *de la Hire: Depiction of the Hunter-Schreger stripes in enamel, 1699*

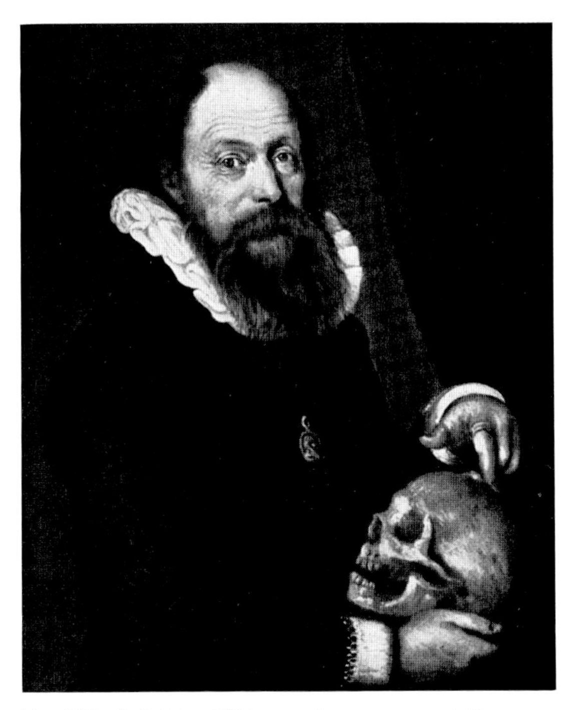

Fig. 160 *Fabricius Hildanus: Anonymous painting (Medical Faculty of Bern)*

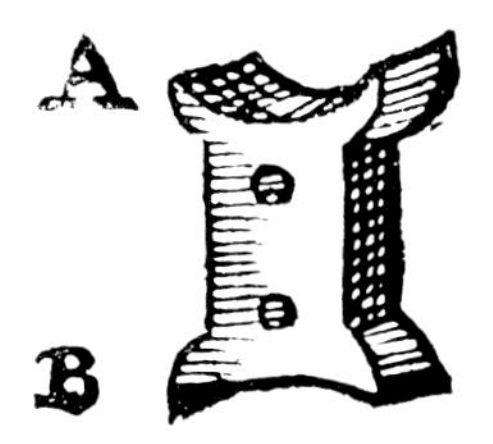

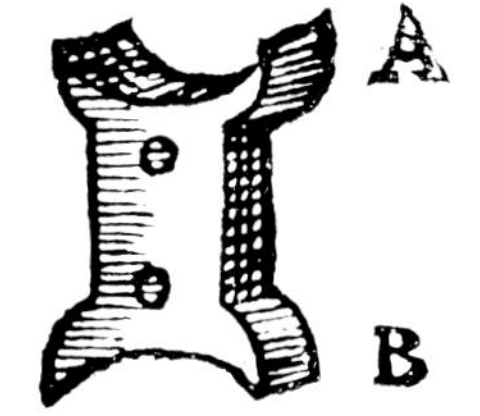

Fig. 161 *Fabricius Hildanus: Wooden wedge as a mouth prop*

able small filaments (filets), which are affixed to the dentin (l'os) much as nails or horns are, and which originate in the region of the cervix of the tooth. He is misguided in believing that the root passages close in old age and thereby cut off nervous connection to the dental pulp (Fig. 159). There is also a new caries theory: occasionally, the bundle of filaments which form the enamel are not firmly attached to the dentin. If then the outside of the enamel wears away, a small opening forms, the dentin is laid bare, and the tooth as a result becomes rotten. *This minor damage can be cured through plugging the hole with lead, . . .*[133].

As soon as we turn from the compiling academicians to the surgeons who set down their own practical experiences, we immediately find ourselves on much more sound therapeutic ground. The most important of these practitioners north of the Alps after Paré was unquestionably Guilhelmus Fabricius Hildanus, more simply Wilhelm Fabry of Hilden, near Düsseldorf. After learning a craft in the lower Rhine region and in Switzerland, and following extensive travels, he was able to practice for the last 20 years of his life as municipal physician for the Council of Bern, undisturbed by the tumult of the Thirty Years' War (Fig. 160). As an educated man, the son of a clerk of the court and former classical high school student in Cologne[134], he set down his experiences in 1606 in Latin. His "Observationes et curationes" (Observations and Counsels) were, in the style of the era, a collection of case histories. They constitute a colorful menage of experiences which, in contrast to Schenck, are mostly real personal perceptions. They are available to us also in a German translation of 1652.

If we skim through the book from front to back, we read in the 38th of the first Centuria (Hundred) "Observation or Perception" about a tumor removal *on the seam of the right jaw* with cauterization and corrosive agents, after thorough Hippocratic preparation through purging, bloodletting, and diet. In order to facilitate the wound's healing through immobilization, Fabry placed two wooden wedges between the dental arches

[133] de la Hire
[134] Mentler

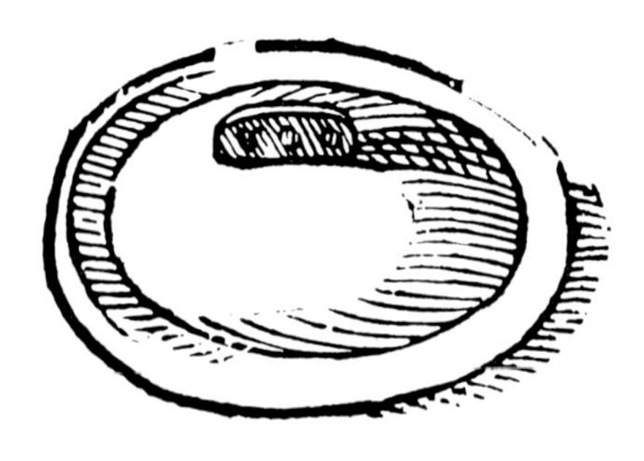

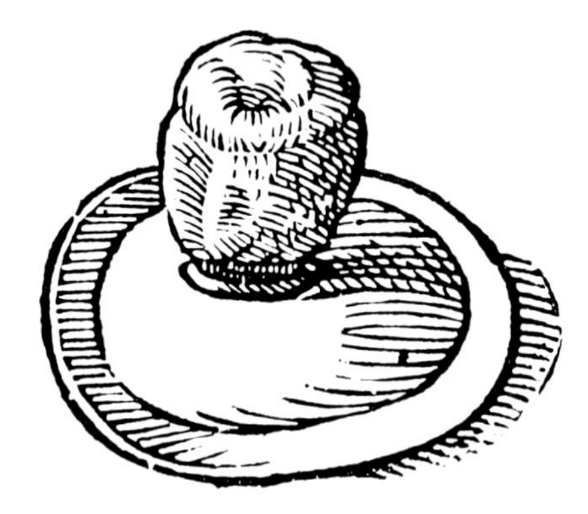

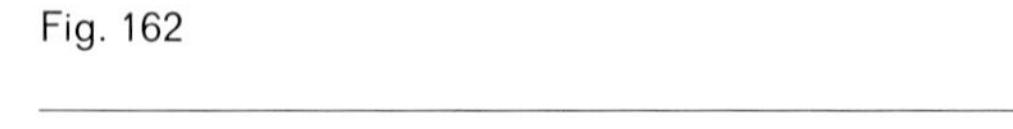

Fig. 162

ΧΕΙΡΟΠΛΟΘΗΚΗ,
Seu
D. JOANNIS SCULTETI,
Physici & Chirurgi apud Ulmenses
olim felicissimi,
ARMAMENTARIUM
CHIRURGICUM XLIII. TA
BVLIS ÆRI ELEGANTISSIME INCISIS,
nec ante hac visis, exornatum.
OPUS POSTHUMUM,
Medicinæ pariter ac Chirurgiæ Studiosis perutile
& necessarium,
IN QUO TOT, TAM VETERUM
AC RECENTIORVM INSTRVMENTA AB AU-
thore correcta, quàm noviter ab ipso inventa, quot ferè hodiè ad usitatas
operationes manuales feliciter peragendas requiruntur, justa & hactenus semper desiderata ma-
gnitudine & applicandi modo, depicta reperiuntur, cum annexa brevi Tabularum descriptione,
& sequentibus cautionibus ac curationibus Chirurgico-Medicis per omnes ferè
corporis humani partes externas observatis.
Nunc primum in lucem editum,
Studio et Opera
JOANNIS SCULTETI, Authoris ex fratre Nepotis,
Philosophiæ & Medicinæ Doctoris,
Cum triplici Instrumentorum, Curationum, rerumque
memorabilium Indice.
VLMÆ SVEVORVM,
Typis & impensis Balthasari Kühnen / Reipubl. Ulmens. Typographi
& Bibliopolæ, Anno M. DC. LV.

Fig. 163

and fastened them to the teeth with brass wire[135] (Fig. 161).

In the 10th observation of the second Hundred, he freed a noblewoman in Lausanne from headaches which had recurred for years, through the removal of four decayed teeth from the maxilla, prescribing at the same time, however, numerous additional purgatives, one of which alone contained 25 herbal drugs. He reports on the following page[136] that a woman from Cologne who had refused to have a completely decayed molar tooth extracted had lost her eyesight through *cataract and blinding,* whereby it was still uncertain whether this was a result of the inflammation or of the cooling medications. We also find a constant striving for a causal therapy, even if it was sometimes based on errors.

The 22nd observation, which is composed in epistolary form, describes a (syphilitic) sore on the palate, which led to perforation in spite of all possible medications, including "French wood" (from the guaiac tree), an anti-syphilitic agent as beloved as it was useless. Afterwards it was covered by the customary sponge obturator (Fig. 162). He proceeded in the case of a noblewoman in a convent *with unbearable implacable toothache,* menstrual problems, and constipation essentially through medicational means and bleeding. This poor woman had undergone formerly an intraoral preparatory treatment with nitric acid, with the gruesome result that her entire maxilla and mandible regions were etched away[137]. In his consultation letter, F a b r y forbade any further cauterization treatment and recommended flushings with volatile oils without, however, advising removal of the original problem teeth after the acute symptoms had subsided, as would have been expected. Immediately thereafter it is shown through five further examples that skin fistulas in the jaw region will heal after extraction of the teeth causing the problems[138].

In the 27th and 28th observations of the 5th Hundred, we must defend G a l e n against the

135 Fabricius Hildanus (a) I 38
136 Ibid. II 12
137 Ibid. IV 21
138 Ibid. III 32—33

Fig. 162 *Fabricius Hildanus: Sponge obturator*

Figs. 163—166 *Scultetus (Schultheiss): Armamentarium chirurgicum (Wund-Artzneyisches Zeug-Hauss), Latin edition (Ulm, 1655), French edition (Lyon, 1672), English edition (London, 1674), Dutch edition (Amsterdam, 1748)*

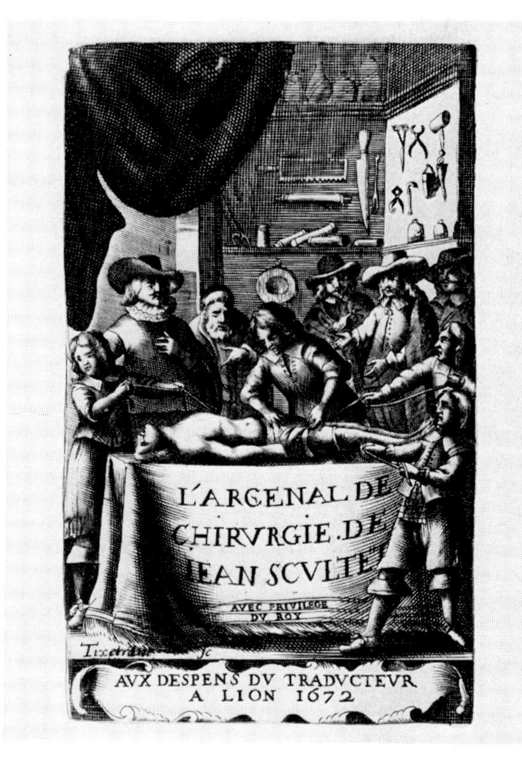

Fig. 164

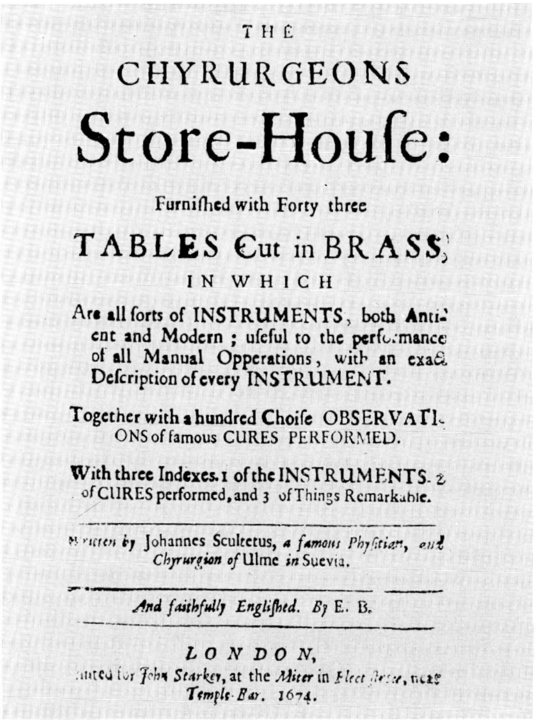

THE

CHYRURGEONS

Store-Houſe:

Furniſhed with Forty three

TABLES Cut in BRASS;

IN WHICH

Are all ſorts of INSTRUMENTS, both Antient and Modern; uſeful to the performance of all Manual Opperations, with an exact Deſcription of every INSTRUMENT.

Together with a hundred Choiſe OBSERVATIONS of famous CURES PERFORMED.

With three Indexes. 1 of the INSTRUMENTS. 2 of CURES performed, and 3 of Things Remarkable.

Written by Johannes Scultetus, *a famous Phyſitian, and Chyrurgion of* Ulme *in* Suevia.

And faithfully Engliſhed. By E. B.

LONDON,

Printed for John Starker, at the *Miter* in *Fleet ſtreet*, near *Temple-Bar*. 1674.

Fig. 165

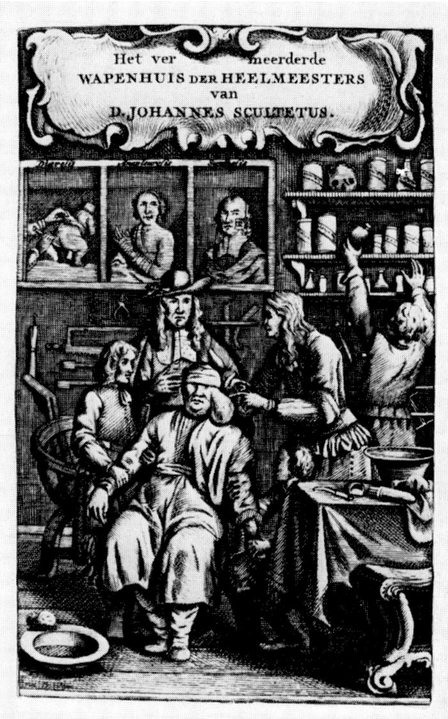

Fig. 166

author: Fabry reproaches him for having claimed that cancer of the pharynx is incurable. In the mouth, at least, once on the gingiva and another time on the cheek, he had clasped the tumor with a thread and then extirpated it with a knife without a recurrence. Without doubt, they were benign growths in both cases.

In his book "Von der Fürtrefflichkeit und Nutz der Anatomy" (On the Applicability and Usefulness of Anatomy), Fabricius states a therapy for toothache from the Middle Ages: in front of the auricle, more precisely in front of the antitragus, is the path of an artery, through *which flows a thin and sharp materia to the teeth; it awakens an extremely intense raging and pounding pain, dolorem pulsatium, which can well extend through the entirety of the cheeks and into all the teeth, so that finally the patient cannot tell which tooth is the damaged one.* As therapy he interrupts this flow at the ear, with a red-hot cautery (*cum cauterio actuali*) like the masters of the 12th century[139]. As illustration of this, the case of a woman from Bern, naturally genteel, is cited who after this treatment *experienced noticeable improvement*[140]. We can discern absurdities in Wilhelm Fabry but it is still positively satisfying to see an individual ever making effort, in contrast to the stale wisdom of the academicians.

We notice this particularly in the illustrations in the "Armamentarium chirurgicum" by the municipal physician of Ulm, Johannes Scultetus (Johannes Schultheiss), which first appeared posthumously in Latin in 1655, and again later in several other languages (in English "The chyrurgeous Store-House", in 1674; Figs. 163 to 166)[141]. He received his education primarily from the anatomist and surgeon Adriaan van den Spieghel (Spigelius), the second successor of Fabricius ab Aquapendente to the professorial chair in Padua, who became acquainted with the able young man, son of a Danube shipper and working in the same profession. Spieghel met him on a trip to Vienna and took him along to Italy. He may possibly have been an adherent of the then already aged Fabricius as he quotes him frequently. Thus, we also find in Scultetus, in table XXXIII, *the funnel or pipe of silver* mentioned by this teacher[142] (Fig. 167) for the purpose of feeding through the nose in cases of lockjaw. Scultetus, however, recommends its use *between the outmost gum of the patient,* behind the wisdom teeth. Figure III presents a doubled pelican, as also shown by Paré. Figure IV shows *a common pair of pincers for the teeth (forceps dentaria communis),* called "cagnolo" by the Italians, i. e., by his teacher, because they resemble the jaws of a dog, and figure V presents *a crow's bill, with which the roots of the teeth are drawn forth (rostrum corvinum).* Figures VI and VII obviously depict two levers already introduced to us by Ryff[143], but according to Scultetus, in the English edition, *they are the patterns of toothed pincers that serve to pull out teeth which neither the Pelican nor common pincers can draw forth.* These inconsistencies in nomenclature are probably an indication that the author himself had not used these beautiful baroque instruments. In figures VIII and IX, there are the *Levitors divided in three parts* (vectes trifidi) from Acquapendente, while figure X shows an angled raspatory (dentiscalpium), *a tooth-picker with which the gum is separated from the teeth, that they may be pulled out with less danger and trouble.* After describing the technique, however, Scultetus admits that he would wish for himself a *toothdrawer (dentispicum)* who was *very expert and eager* in the use of these dental forceps.

In plate XXXVI (Fig. 168), some procedures are demonstrated for us. Figure I shows the cauterization of a carious tooth with a red-hot cautery, in figure II we see the removal of a tooth incorrectly erupted which has wounded the cheek, and in figure III the already familiar silver funnel for feeding in situ in the case of trismus. Figure IV presents a perforation ex lue gallica (syphilitic lesion) of the palate, with the corresponding obturator next to it, ready to be inserted with the forceps. Figure VI shows the use of a mouth gag with a screw thread. Figure VII shows the use of an oral speculum for examination of the pharynx, and in figure VIII the detachment of a frenulum which is too short is minutely illustrated, so that the procedure is not as bloody and painful as with the "beard-shavers" (barbitonsores). The tongue is held with a cloth, and the child is wrapped in the same way as infants are occasionally wrapped when a cleft lip is to be corrected. In figure IX, a foreign body is removed from the pharynx.

139 See p. 113 and Fig. 87
140 Fabricius Hildanus (b) p. 127
141 Scultetus
142 See p. 142
143 See p. 165

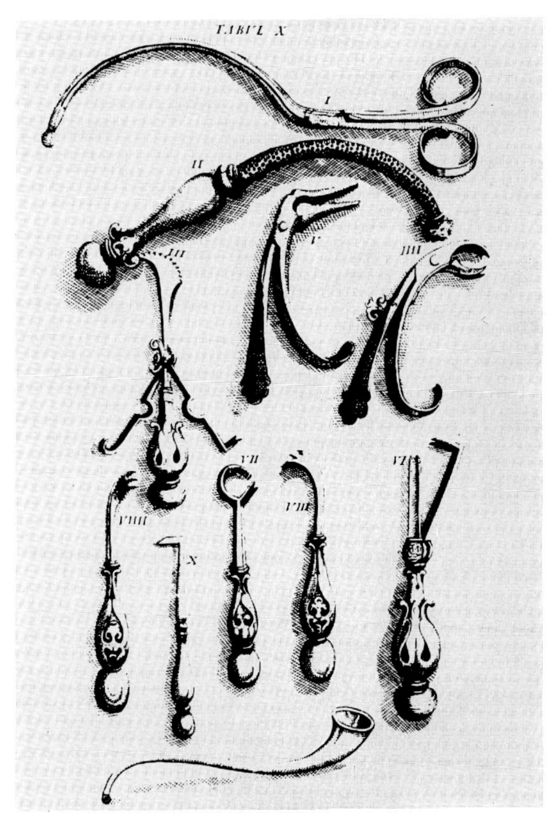

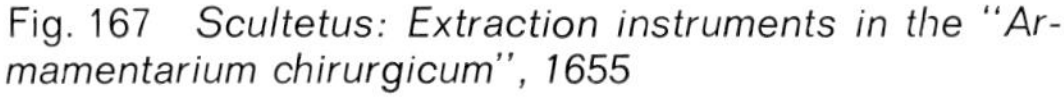

Fig. 167 *Scultetus: Extraction instruments in the "Armamentarium chirurgicum", 1655*

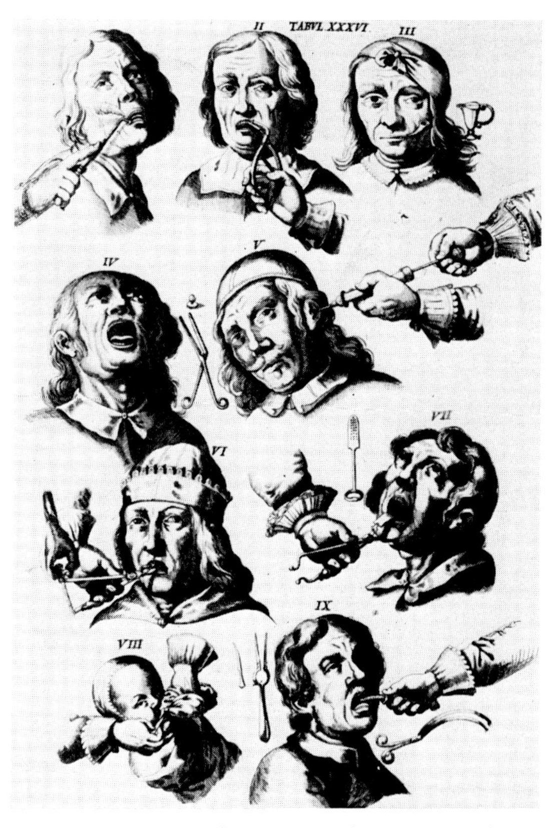

Fig. 168 *Scultetus: Stomatological operations, 1655*

In accordance with the custom of the time, a few more observations follow the pictorial section, among which is perhaps the first description of a cyst operation in the maxilla. This *Tumour* was initially treated in the Galenic manner, with bleeding, purging, sweating, drawing liniments, and many various herbs and mixtures, in order to dry out the moist head. When a recurrence set in, though, after an apparent improvement, an operation had to be performed: *We placed the Lady in her bed, tieing her hands to her side.* At first, Scultetus tried in vain to scrape out the visible *bag*, then he cut it in two, and there *flowed out a thick yellow matter like honey, and the Tumour subsided.* The cavity was kept open for two months, cauterized with a decoction of sarsaparilla root (containing saponin), *till the bone might skale.* Some days later, a sequestrum was removed and the wound healed. With this quite thorough postoperative treatment, the surgeon presumably achieved a healing free of recurrence of the cyst[144].

The list of German-speaking surgeons of the 17th century who were literarily active is completed by the municipal physician of Breslau, Matthaeus Gottfried Purmann, whose life history is available in detail in one of his books[145]. After completing the customary years of study and travel, Purmann was able, as a regimental-surgeon (Feldscher) of Brandenburg to collect rich experience in military surgery in the campaigns of the Great Electors against Sweden. In 1678 he departed, to settle seven years later in Breslau, where he became municipal physician in 1690 and as such was clinically active at the hospital there. From his first book, "Der rechte und wahrhaftige Feld-

[144] Scultetus (b) pp. 271 f.
[145] Proskauer (b)

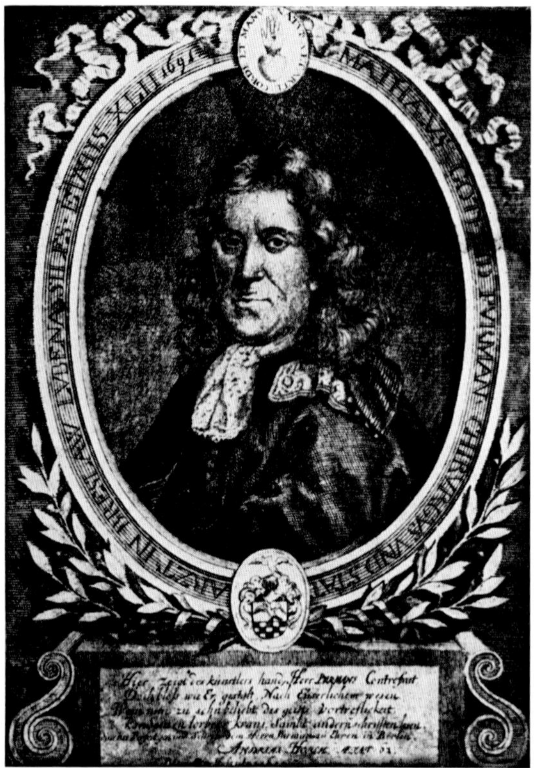

Fig. 169

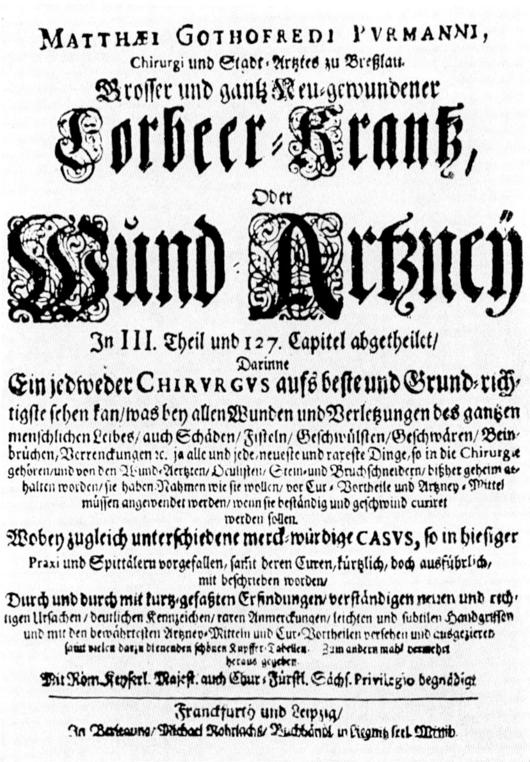

MATTHÆI GOTHOFREDI PURMANNI,
Chirurgi und Stadt-Arztes zu Breßlau.
Grosser und gantz Neu-gewundener
Lorbeer-Krantz,
Oder
Wund-Artzney
In III. Theil und 127. Capitel abgetheilet/
Darinne
Ein jedweder CHIRURGUS aufs beste und Grund-richtigste sehen kan/ was bey allen Wunden und Verletzungen des gantzen menschlichen Leibes/ auch Schäden/ Fisteln/ Geschwülsten/ Geschwären/ Bein-brüchen/ Verrenckungen rc. ja alle und jede/ neueste und rareste Dinge/ so in die Chirurgie gehören/ und von den Wund-Aertzten/ Oculisten/ Stein- und Bruchschneidern/ bißher geheim gehalten worden/ sie haben Nahmen wie sie wollen/ vor Cur-Vortheile und Artzney-Mittel müssen angewendet werden/ wenn sie beständig und geschwind curiret werden sollen.
Wobey zugleich unterschiedene merck-würdige CASUS, so in hiesiger Praxi und Spittälern vorgefallen/ samt deren Curen/ kürtzlich/ doch ausführlich/ mit beschrieben worden/
Durch und durch mit kurtz-gefaßten Erfindungen/ verständigen neuen und richtigen Ursachen/ deutlichen Kennzeichen/ raren Anmerckungen/ leichten und subtilen Handgriffen und mit den bewährtesten Artzney-Mitteln und Cur-Vortheilen versehen und ausgezieret/ samt vielen darzu dienenden schönen Kupffer-Tabellen. Zum andern mahl vermehret heraus gegeben.
Mit Röm. Kayserl. Majest. auch Chur-Fürstl. Sächs. Privilegio begnädigt.
Franckfurth und Leipzig/
In Verlegung Michael Rohrlachs/ Buchhändl. in Liegnitz seel. Wittib.

Fig. 170

Figs. 169 and 170 *Frontispiece (1691) and title page (1722) of the „Lorbeer-Krantz" (Laurel wreath) of Matthäus Gottfried Purmann, municipal physician of Breslau*

scher" (The correct and true Regimental surgeon) which appeared in 1680, he developed three very different books which underwent numerous editions, including some posthumous ones. In his main work, "Grosser and gantz neugewundener Lorbeer-Krantz, oder Wund-Artzney" (Great and completely rewoven Laurel Wreath, or Wound Medicine) which first appeared in 1684, the number of teeth is stated, somewhat offhandedly, as *34 or 36*[146]. Nonetheless, he was familiar with the contemporary anatomists: the Dane Bartholin is mentioned by name, and the formation of teeth is correctly described[147] (Figs. 169 and 170). Purmann believed in the toothworm, not as a cause of cavities, but as a cause of toothache: ... *small worms sometimes grow within, which cause men great pains and annoyance*[148]. Caries, the *corruption of the teeth,* arise from a rapid alternation of hot and cold foods, and *if one frequently bites very hard things on them, and eats too much sugar and sweet things, then they quickly turn into an acidic fermentation, and decay the teeth, whereby they can then become even more corrupted, if ... knives and needles and other pointed things are always being poked about, disturbing the interior*[149]. As is the case everywhere in these centuries of transition to scientific thinking, we can see in Purmann as well the confrontation of thoroughly modern views with those of ancient times.

Within the framework of the case history of a gunshot injury, we find Purmann's familiar contribution to prosthetics: *Have another* (tooth) *made from a servicable bone or elephant tooth, corresponding in extensiveness, size, and pro-*

146 Purmann (a) p. 3
147 Ibid. p. 46
148 Ibid. p. 280
149 Ibid. p. 281

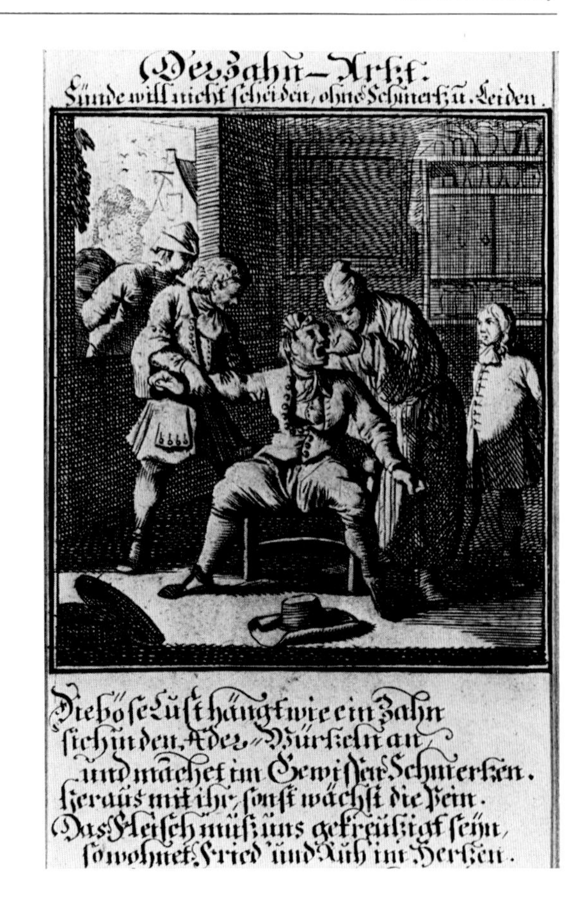
Der Zahn-Artzt.
Sünde will nicht scheiden, ohne Schmertz zu Leiden.
Die böse Lust hängt wie ein Zahn
und machet im Gewissen Schmertzen.
heraus mit ihr, sonst wächst die Pein.
so wohnet Fried und Ruh im Hertzen.

Fig. 171 *"Der Zahn-Artzt" (The dentist), engraving by Georg Weigel, Nürnberg, from the painting by Kaspar Luyken, Amsterdam, with verses by Abraham a Santa Clara, Regensburg, 1698*

portion to the former one, for which you can prepare a wax model beforehand, in accordance with conditions and composition of the teeth and mandible, with everything to be made and adjusted exactly from it, and if afterwards its lower part fits well into the jaw, on both sides, both on the part of this new one and of the natural ones, then small holes should be drilled; thus, slide it into the gaps between the neighboring healthy (teeth), *and make it fast with a silver wire and a small pincer, as outwardly subtile as is at all possible* [150].

Purmann thus had not yet reached the point of taking a wax impression of the jaw, but rather modelled in the mouth a freehand imitation of the replacement to be made, which was then carved according to this model by a craftsman. Drilling holes through the neighboring teeth is not something we would approve, but the author could hardly be speaking here from personal experience, particularly since he also always left tooth removal to a "Zahn-Arzt" (dentist). We find in his writings that there were at least three of these residing in Breslau, an item quite significant for the history of the profession. We also learn about the death of an apothecary, *which was an accident caused by our Zahn-Arzt, who not only clumsily pulled out a tooth, but also split and splintered the mandible at the same place* [151]. Things went better for an illustrious duchess, from whom the dentist of Breslau Adam Plahnen did remove the tooth, but only *after two very hard attempts,* and not without great pains [152].

In the "Chirurgia curiosa", we are provided with a large number of remedies for oral decay and

150 Ibid. p. 219
151 Ibid. p. 239
152 Purmann (b) p. 248

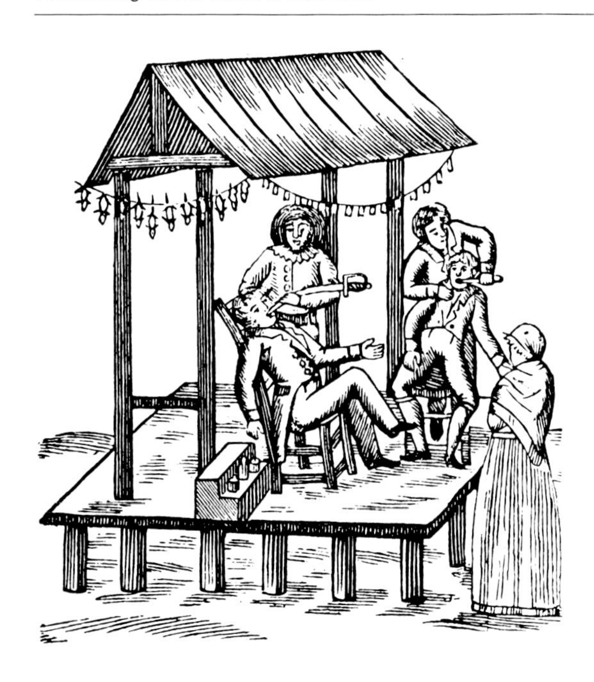

Fig. 172 *Luxation of a tooth with the tip of a dagger, woodcut from the 18th century (Klein Collection, Utrecht)*

toothache, mainly listed under the name of an author; none of them, however, had helped him when he was afflicted with unbearable toothache for 12 days, with the exception of *oleum origani* (marjoram oil) *packed in the hollow tooth* [153]. Presumably the dental pulp was mortified precisely at that time. Purmann prepared the obturator *according to the teaching of Paraei* (Paré) [154] from sheets of gold, silver or copper, combined with a sponge, which was to assure that the moisture can *not drip down from the brain through the mouth and throat* [155]. Thus, the Hippocratic doctrine of mucus which separates from the brain, lived on into the beginning of the 18th century.

In Amsterdam the anatomist Nicolaas Tulp, with whom we are quite familiar through Rembrandt's famous anatomy picture, published clinical experiences too in his "Observationes medicae". He begins, like Paré, by emphasizing what a serious matter toothaches are, and then relates the case of the physician Gosvinus Hallius, whose gingiva was split to accelerate the eruption of the third molars, and who then, tortured by the most terrible pains, ran back and forth in his room day and night until his death [156].

In the essay, "Procedures in Wound Medicine" by Tulp's countryman Cornelis Solingen, Surgeon and Doctor of Medicine in The Hague, which appeared in Dutch in 1684, and in German in 1693 and 1712, it is immediately evident that this man had actually practiced dental medicine, when he recommends that the removal of calculus, *this disgusting operation,* which is furthermore poorly paid, be left to the tooth-drawers and barber-surgeons [157]. Hollow teeth should be cauterized and filled afterwards with gold, silver, or lead; he himself preferred iron wire for this, but since moisture still penetrated, and resulted in decay and pain, he turned to a filling with mastix and turpentine. He rejected vitriol because it destroyed the tooth and often attacked the jaw as well. Once, when he was to file smooth the teeth of a lawyer, the seed of the idea of using drills occurred to him by chance in this workshops: *and* (I) *filed / by constantly turning this elongated little ball around with my thumb and fingers / and these angular hooks, which were cutting and pricking, were gradually and quickly smooth* [158]. Thus, we have here a precursor to the hand drill,

153 Ibid. p. 198
154 See p. 148
155 Purmann (a) p. 222
156 Tulpius I 36
157 Solingen p. 119
158 Ibid. p. 122

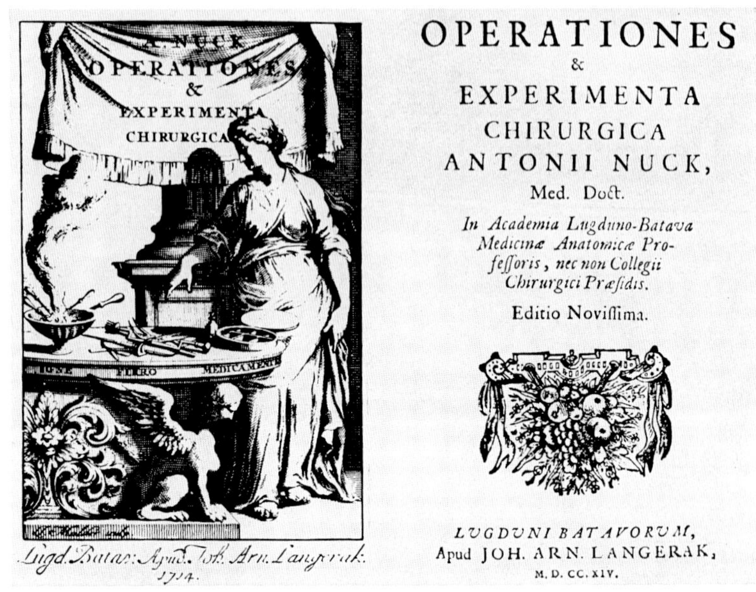
A. NUCK
OPERATIONES
&
EXPERIMENTA
CHIRURGICA

Lugd. Batav: Apud Joh. Arn. Langerak.
1714.

OPERATIONES
&
EXPERIMENTA
CHIRURGICA
ANTONII NUCK,
Med. Doct.
In Academia Lugduno-Batava Medicinæ Anatomicæ Professoris, nec non Collegii Chirurgici Præsidis.
Editio Novissima.

LUGDUNI BATAVORUM,
Apud JOH. ARN. LANGERAK,
M. D. CC. XIV.

Fig. 173 *Frontispiece and title page of Anton Nuck's surgery book, 1714 edition*

which we are to encounter again in the 19th century.

The following seven pages are devoted to tooth extraction. Every circumstance is taken into consideration: not only the degree of preservation of the tooth itself, but also that of the antagonist must be noticed. Likewise, it must be observed *whether the patients cannot suffer / the teeth to be pressed against one another,* i. e. whether they are sensitive to pressure as a result of a periodontal inflammation, and whether the teeth are crooked or have been loosened by scurvy. The procedure itself is precisely described for both maxilla and mandible, using forceps, the pelican, and the pes caprinus. When using the latter, the finger of the other hand must be placed against it, so that if it slips out of place, the tongue will not be injured. If the neighboring tooth, during the removal of a root, is firm, the "little outbreaker", a kind of lever pressed between it and the root, is turned and thereby lifts the object out; this is a technique which we still employ today. Otherwise, it can be done *like the quacks or toothdrawers* (do) */ to pull the teeth out with the point of a dagger / which works for these gentlemen / even if they do not understand any proportion of it / still successfully all the time*[159]. This trick of lifting out the painful tooth with the point of a dagger was then a favorite and enticing attraction at the annual fairs, and is confirmed many times over in pictures (Fig. 172).

It is precisely through these minute descriptions of technique that we recognize that Solingen speaks not as a compiler, but as a practitioner of dentistry as well. On the other hand, he discusses tooth replacement with a brevity which does not indicate any personal experience.

Prominent in this area is Anton Nuck, the respected professor in Leiden, who did research as an anatomist, especially on the lymphatic vessels. In his "Operationes et experimenta chirurgica" of 1692, he is noted for his suggestion that hippopotamus teeth, above all their outside parts, be used for preparation of dentures instead of ivory, which yellows quickly through saliva and food. This is the first mention of a material which was the leading base material for prostheses until its replacement by India rubber in the second half of the 19th century.

If all the teeth are missing in the mandible, a one-piece row of teeth should be carved and inserted in such a fashion that it moves together with movements of the mandible, and thus grinds the size of food in the mouth. Here, we

[159] Ibid. pp. 127 f.

THE

OPERATOR

For the

TEETH,

Shewing how to preſerve the *TEETH* and *GUMS* from all the Accidents they are ſubject to.

By CHARLES ALLEN *Profeſſor of the ſame.*

Entered according to Order.

YORK,
Printed by *John White* for the *Author*, and are to be ſold by himſelf at his own Lodging, at Mr. *Galloway's* Apothecary in *Stone-gate*, Anno Dom. 1685.

THE

OPERATOR

For The

TEETH:

SHEWING
How to Preſerve the Teeth and Gums from all the Accidents they are ſubject to: With particular Directions for Childrens Teeth.
As alſo the Deſcription and Uſe of the *POLICAN*, Never Publiſhed before.

By *CHARLES ALLEN*; Profeſſor of the ſame.

To which is Annexed
A Phyſical Diſcourſe, wherein the reaſons of the Beating of the *Pulſe*, or *Pulſation* of the *Arteries*, together with thoſe of the circulation of the *Blood*, are mechanically Explained; which was never done before.

By an Unknown Hand.

DUBLIN, Printed by *Andrew Crook* and *Samuel Helſham* for the Author, and are to be Sold by *Robert Thornton* Bookſeller, at the *Leather-Bottel* in *Skinner-Row*, and by the Author at his own Lodging at Mr. *Bauiſter's* at the *Smiths-Arms* in *Eſſex-ſtreet*.

Figs. 174 and 175 *Allen: Title page of the 1st and 2nd editions, 1685 and 1686*

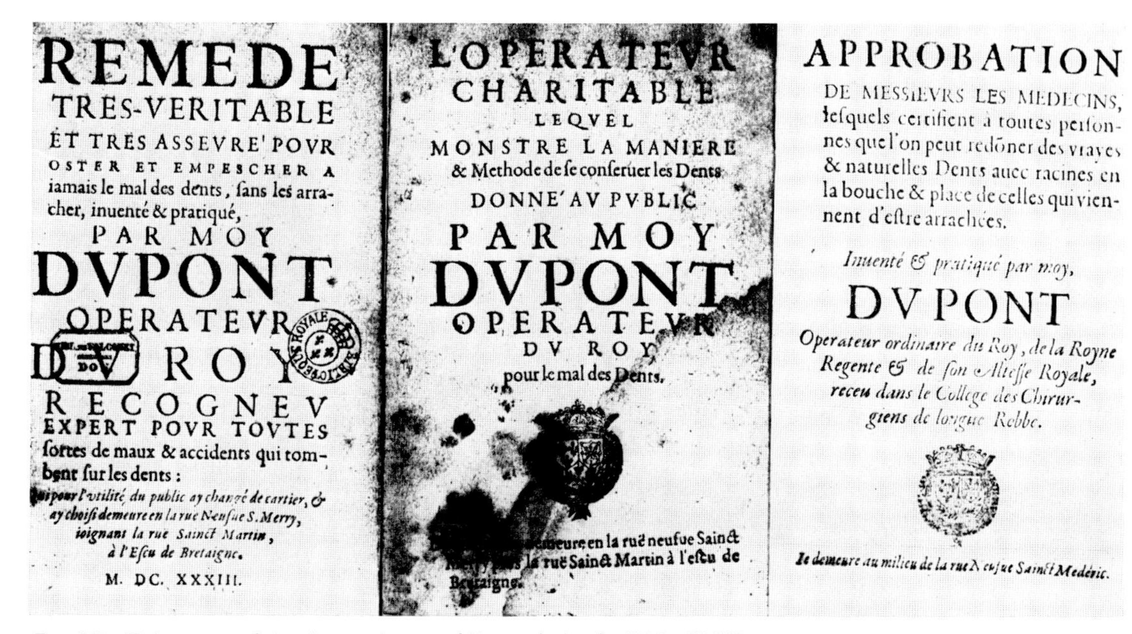
REMEDE
TRES-VERITABLE
ET TRES ASSEVRE' POVR
OSTER ET EMPESCHER A
iamais le mal des dents, ſans les arracher, inuenté & pratiqué,
PAR MOY
DVPONT
OPERATEVR
DV ROY
RECOGNEV
EXPERT POVR TOVTES
ſortes de maux & accidents qui tombent ſur les dents:
qui pour l'vtilité du public ay changé de cartier, & ay choiſi demeure en la rue Neufue S. Merry, ioignant la rue Sainct Martin, à l'Eſcu de Bretaigne.
M. DC. XXXIII.

L'OPERATEVR
CHARITABLE
LEQVEL
MONSTRE LA MANIERE
& Methode de ſe conſeruer les Dents
DONNE' AV PVBLIC
PAR MOY
DVPONT
OPERATEVR
DV ROY
pour le mal des Dents.
...demeure en la ruë neufue Sainct ... la ruë Sainct Martin à l'eſcu de Bretaigne.

APPROBATION
DE MESSIEVRS LES MEDECINS,
leſquels certifient à toutes perſonnes que l'on peut redõner des vrayes & naturelles Dents auec racines en la bouche & place de celles qui viennent d'eſtre arrachées.
Inuenté & pratiqué par moy,
DV PONT
Operateur ordinaire du Roy, de la Royne Regente & de ſon Alteſſe Royale, receu dans le College des Chirurgiens de longue Robbe.
Ie demeure au milieu de la rue Neufue Sainct Medéric.

Fig. 176 *Title pages of the three editions of Dupont's book, 1633—1647?*

finally find the function of chewing considered[160]. Nuck also combats toothache with the cautery, not at the site, but rather, like Fabricius Hildanus, at the auricle, on the antitragus. On the title page, which is shown as a witness to the baroque art of printing in figure 173, there is, among other things a representation of the heating of a "cauterium actuale"[161].

Nuck differentiates the teeth according to their shape: the smallest are the incisors (incisores), the longest are the canines (oculares et canini), and the thickest are the molars. Each of these teeth must be removed with a particular instrument. For this purpose, punches (Pedes Caprini), crow's bills (Rostrum Corvinum), various forceps, pelicans, dental scalpels (Dentiscalpium, for loosening the gingiva), and rinsing basins (Trulla) are required. In this regard, he refers in a marginal note to the depictions in Scultetus' "Armamentarium" (see Fig. 167). One should never pull teeth from pregnant women, particularly not the eye teeth, because the child could suffer eye damage from this, a widely spread superstition only cleared up in the middle of the following (18th) century by Bunon[162].

The first specialized book of dental medicine in the English language was "The Operator for the Teeth", which originally appeared in York in 1685, then in Dublin in 1686, and in London in 1687; thus, it was issued three times, one shortly after another. The 2nd and 3rd editions differed only in the title pages, since the last edition appeared under an altered title[163] (Figs. 174 and 175). The "Operator" completes the list of the popular dental books: the German "Zene Artzney" of 1530, the Spanish book by Martinez in 1557, and the French by Hemard in 1582. It ranks lowest among these, however. The only thing we know about the author, Charles Allen, who provides himself with the title of professor in both of the first editions, is that he was active first with a master in York, and then in Dublin. Thus, the writer is no academician, but rather a barber-surgeon who had read some things without always completely understanding them. Nevertheless, he does differentiate enamel from a softer, darker substance, which is again harder than bone[164]. Otherwise, there are some statements quite peculiar indeed. He takes a stand in Section III in favor of preservation of the teeth, removes decay with a particular instrument, and fills teeth with ingredients which are neither corrosive nor bad-tasting, but he does not supply anything further on either the instrument or the filling material. The pelican is not described until in the second edition, and only in the one after that there is some mention about the extraction instruments of his own design, although the last two are practically the same. In the *Inoculation of the teeth,* he rejects transplantation from one man to another for humanitarian reasons (*robbing Peter to pay Paul*), and advises instead that the patient's teeth be replaced by teeth from dogs, sheep, goats, or baboons. He extolls this idea of his as *a natural restoration or renovation of human teeth*[165]. To us, however, it has finally become clear that the only reality in this book consists in "Professor" Allen's wishful thinking.

In general popular medical treatises, as, for example, in the booklet "The poor-man's physician and chyrurgion", a kind of "Thesaurus pauperum" by a *Student in Physik and Astrology,* Lancelot Coelson, which appeared in London in 1656, is found a *method of drawing teeth,* for which he recommends the pelican after the hollow tooth has been plugged with lint. In order to avoid breaking the jawbone, extraction must be performed carefully. If there is bleeding afterwards, lint saturated with lemon juice is to be applied. In the following section of prescriptions it is recommended that essence of clove be put in the cavity; also, *the root of a crowfoot* can be laid in or on the painful tooth. *Powder of red coral* placed in the tooth will cause it to fall out. This is probably a fundamental misunderstanding of some source, possibly Guillemeau[166].

In Paris of the 17th century, we encounter three essays of eight pages each from a certain Dupont, some aspects of whose professional career can be derived from the title pages (Fig. 176). In probably the oldest of the essays, from 1633, he calls himself the *Operating Surgeon to the King* (Louis XIII) *for all Cases of Suffering and Misfortune in the Teeth,* and in the next one, which is undated, but probably prior to 1643, the year when Louis XIII died, he is the *Operating Surgeon to the King for Den-*

160 Nuck pp. 68 f.
161 See p. 180
162 See p. 207
163 Weinberger (a); (b) p. 291; Cohen (b)
164 Allen Sect. I
165 Ibid. Sect. IV
166 Coelson pp. 15 f., 44, 150

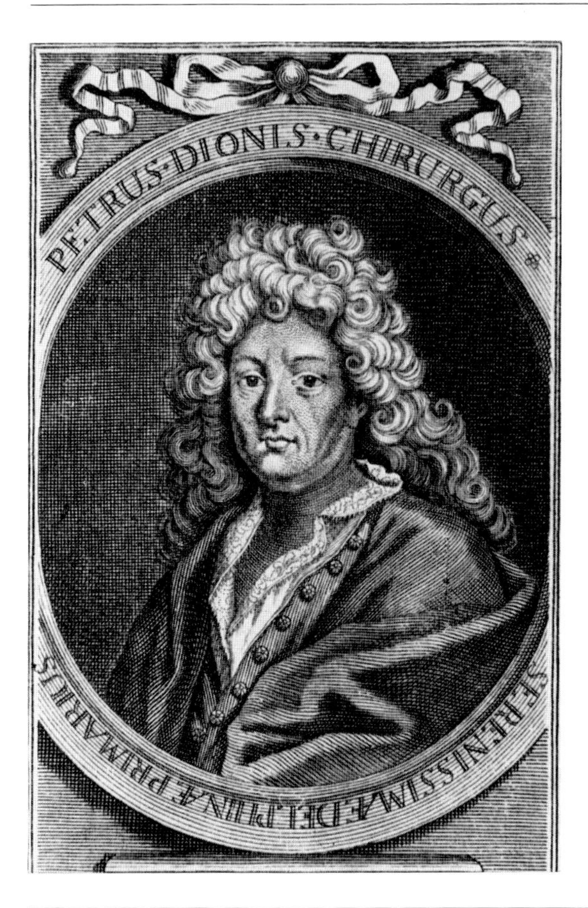

Fig. 177 *Pierre Dionis: Frontispiece of the 4th edition of the "Cours d'Operations", 1746*

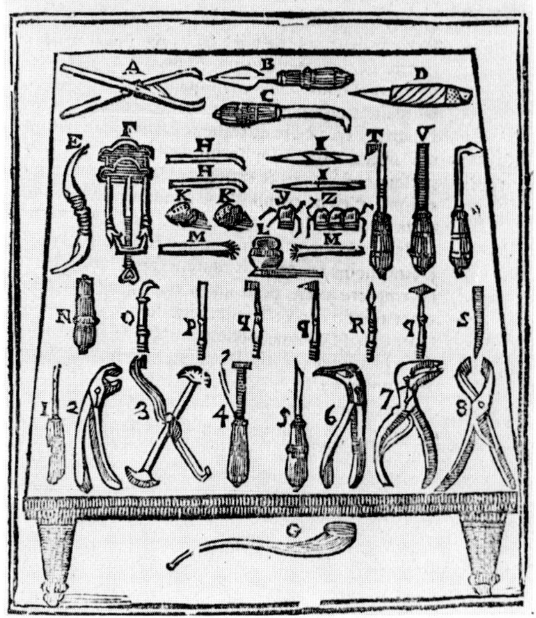

Fig. 178 *Dionis: Oral surgical instrument set, 1746 edition*

tal Suffering, while in the third, probably composed in 1647, he asserts himself as general operating surgeon to the king (the then nine-year-old Louis XIV), the royal dowager regent (the Queen-mother Anna of Austria), and of a royal highness, as well as member of the Surgeons' Guild of the Long Robe [167]. The booklet itself is nothing more than advertisements in which Dupont recommends himself for tooth extraction, bleaching of the teeth, and for preparation of artificial teeth which cannot be told from natural ones and which can be used without stuttering [168]. In both of the first essays, he emphasizes with the pride of a parvenu that he had moved away from the Pont Neuf area, the charlatan quarter, *because it is often said that bad company spoils good morals* [169]. With regard to dental care it is best to take a leaf of sage in the mouth for a while in the morning; tobacco has the same effect, but it is stronger. A ruined tooth should be cleaned of caries (*netoyer la carie et corruption*) and filled with gold or lead [170]. In the third edition he informs *all peoples, nations, and languages, and above all the inhabitants of this great and royal city of Paris,* as well as others, that he extracts painful teeth *with great expertise and little pain,* and puts them back in immediately, whereupon they once again become firm, and *are never again subject to pains, flows, and catarrhs, through the loss* (tearing-off) *of their sensitive nerve* [171]; he also claims that he can extract diseased teeth with the greatest ease and immediately implant natural teeth from dead or living men. Moreover, he published a testimonial from the medical faculty of 1647, signed by 18 physicians, among them the dean and four court physicians.

167 The masters accepted in the St. Côme Guild wore a long jacket; the barber-surgeons a short one
168 Dupont (a) p. 3
169 Dupont (b) p. 8
170 Ibid. p. 6
171 Dupont (c) pp. 6 f.

In conclusion, he recommended his nephew, who represented him when he was absent [172]. All in all, Dupont is nothing more than one of the tooth-drawer types common to the era, simply on a higher social plane. Instead of a crier, he used advertisements, and instead of tambourines and trumpets, he used the medical faculty.

On a higher level, still without constituting an advance, however, is the "Dissertation sur les dents" of 1679, by Barthélemy Martin, a member of the faculty. Like Vesalius, he rejected the notion of primary teeth having roots, firstly because otherwise they would not be able to make room for the permanent ones, and secondly because the permanent ones *would grow in crooked (elles sortiroient tortuës)* if there were roots in the alveolus. Thirdly, because it would be dangerous for the tender jaws of children to pull primary teeth with roots [173]. Avoiding diseases during the deciduous dentition depends above all on a proper nursemaid, her temperament, her hair color (blonde is preferred), and her qualities of character. If the eruption of the teeth is difficult, it should be facilitated with a golden needle, and under no circumstances with a nail, because poison can thus be introduced into the gingiva [174]. Methods for care of the teeth which are described somewhat abstractly, include gargling in the morning with one's own urine, which had already been praised by Catullus, or cleaning of the teeth with dung of wild cats. These are both useful agents, because they contain salts which are *opponents of decay and corruption* [175]. For extraction, the pelican is used, or, if the tooth is already loose, the forceps. There is nothing on the subject of tooth replacement.

Among the French surgeons, Lazare Rivière (Lazarus Riverius), a professor at Montpellier University, devoted the sixth book of his ten-volume "Praxis medica cum theoria", which first came out in Latin in Paris in 1640, to stomatological problems. He places the blame for toothache, on one hand, on the humors which flow specially into the carious tooth, and on the other hand, on the worm which originates in them. The different causes are to be recognized by the symptoms: with the worm, for example, the pain appears at intervals [176]. Noticeable among the profusion of prescriptions is the medieval recommendation that almond oil be dripped into the ear on the painful side with vapors of vinegar in which pulegium (pennyroyal) and origanum (marjoram) has been boiled, *because the small veins which bring nutriment to the teeth pass through those parts* (of the body) [177]. If none of this helps, the tooth must be pulled with the utmost care, and the usual advice is given that the wound should afterwards be compressed with the fingers. *Tobacco ash* (*cinis tabaci,* mentioned here for the first time) *is also amazingly effective in wiping off the teeth and making them white* [178].

The surgeon in ordinary to the royal family (of Louis XIV), Pierre Dionis (Fig. 177), was equally outstanding as both anatomist and surgeon. Before being called into court service, he had represented both of these subjects at the Jardin Royal, an educational institution in addition to the medical faculty in Paris, where botany was formerly taught. In his "Cours d'opérations de chirurgie" of 1707 we find numerous diagramatic pictures of instrument tables for the various procedures, just as in a modern manual for surgical nurses. The work was translated into many languages, the second German edition presented in 1734 by the famous surgeon Lorenz Heister [179].

In the dental medicine section, Dionis adhered closely to Fabrizzi d'Acquapendente, both in the division into seven groups of manipulations as in those offered, although not mentioning him. He writes in his introduction that *it must be confessed that these persons (ces MM.) who call themselves operators for the teeth (Operateurs pour les dents) and have a sphere of activity limited only to these areas, can distinguish themselves more in them than the surgeon, whose branch of knowledge is almost without limit* [180]. *In the case of trismus,* the mouth gag F in figure 178 and the small funnel G, with which we are familiar from Fabrizzi for nourishment, are recommended. The teeth are cleaned with a *curedent* H or a feather I. The instruments are usually made of iron, but in the case of princes and kings, of gold: *and if there were a more costly metal, then it would be used, because they remunerate*

172 Ibid. p. 8
173 Martin p. 25
174 Ibid. pp. 17 f.
175 Ibid. pp. 64 and 66 f.; see p. 69
176 Riverius pp. 362 f.
177 Ibid. p. 365
178 Ibid. p. 374
179 See pp. 142 f.
180 Dionis (a) p. 608

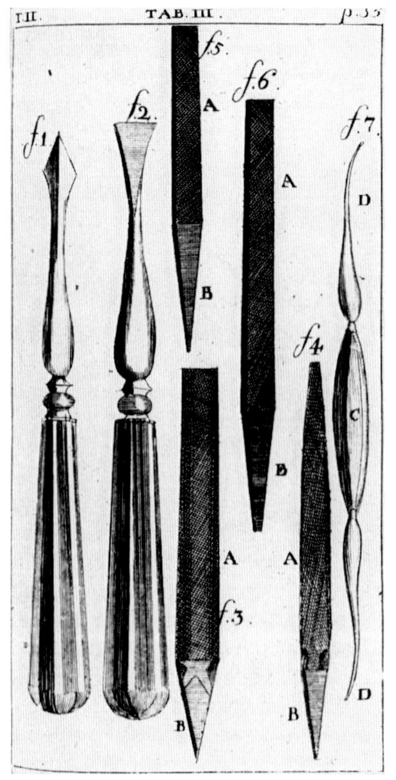

Fig. 179

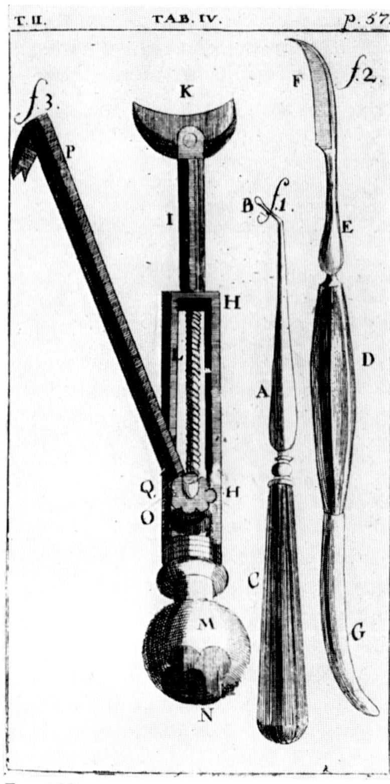

Fig. 180

Fig. 179 *Garengeot: "Serpent's tongue" for the removal of calculus and caries (F. 1), chisel (F. 2), files (F. 3—6), bent probe (F. 7), German edition, 1719*

Fig. 180 *Garengeot: Plugger to close cavities with pieces of lead (F. 1, bourroir), knife to separate gingiva (F. 2), pelican (F. 3), 1719*

so generously[181]. In reference to these court devices of Dionis, Fauchard remarked 20 years later that they had the appearance of having only gold handles, and not gold blades[182].

Dionis believed that caries arose through a caustic fluid, such as aqua fortis, flowing through the periodontal membrane, that means he believed caries to be an endogenic ailment. The teeth can be saved only if this flow can be redirected. Otherwise, he recommends burning or etching with vitriol, a therapy he is criticised for as early as Fauchard[183]; and extraction, if these do not help. He undertakes filling of teeth not to preserve them, but because the holes are annoying. He used appropriately small pieces of gold or silver, because foil is not durable. Some practitioners also used the softer lead or wax, which offers the same advantage of denying food to stick in the teeth.

Filing is described as fifth procedure on the list, and the most useful, the extraction (arracher), comes sixth. Firstly he lays out the indications: *It is a very poor principle to proceed immediately as a tooth-drawer.* It is ridiculous to do as most *opérateurs* do and promise painlessness; that only confirms the proverb: *He lies like a tooth-drawer (arracheur)*[184]. Urbain Hemard made the same remark, but not in such pithy way[185]. Dionis advises surgeons against performing the operation, although he devotes more than six pages to it, because they thereby put themselves in the same class with a charlatan and conjurer (bâteleur). *In fact, most tooth-drawers use their talents to deceive the public, by making them believe they need only their fingers or the point of a dagger in order to remove the most deeply rooted tooth*[186]. Thus, we hear again the undoubtedly impressive dagger trick of the annual fairs, of which we have already read in Solingen (see Fig. 172).

181 Ibid. p. 611
182 Fauchard II p. 5
183 Fauchard I pp. 161 f.
184 Dionis p. 617
185 See p. 151
186 Ibid. pp. 620 f.

The seventh and last arrangement has to do with tooth replacement, which is described for cosmetic and speech reasons, and not because of chewing functions. *Old women are known of who carry complete sets of dentures (rateliers), and never dare open their mouths for fear that the forgery will be recognized.* Subsequently, he quotes Guillemeau's mineral paste, in his almost word-for-word description [187].

René Jacques Croissant de Garengeot, the surgeon, already belongs chiefly to the 18th century. We discuss him here, however, as the last remaining Parisian surgeon in the tradition of Paré. Just as did Paré, he came from Brittany, taught at the Ecole de médecine, and published, among other things, an instrument manual in 1723: "Nouveau traité des instruments de chirurgie les plus utiles" (New Treatise on the most useful Surgical Instruments). We are taking as a basis here the translation which appeared in Berlin in 1729. In it, we learn a few things from this able surgeon which are important for dentistry: caries must be discovered as early as possible with a steel probe (Fig. 179, F 7). This is removed with an instrument designated as a "langue de serpent" (serpent's tongue) (Fig. 179, F 1). The cavity is dried with cotton, and then plugged with one piece of lead after another in all angles and corners, with a device called a "bourroir", after which the excess is taken away with a rasp. If the tooth is painful at this point, the lead is touching the nerve, and must be removed immediately. After this, *in the language of the market-criers and of the masses,* the nerve must be killed off through insertion of clove or cinnamon oil, or aqua regia, and the cavity sealed with cotton. If the pain has subsided, then renewed filling with lead is to be done (without treatment of the dental pulp tissue) [188]. Garengeot recommends above all his own pelican as an extraction instrument; it possesses a concave support surface instead of the customary convex one (Fig. 180, F 3). However, there was nothing to be found concerning the instrument he had developed from the English key according to Lecluse's statement, and, as early as 1803, the same fate befell the dentist from Berlin, Serre [189].

Garengeot particularly advised young surgeons who had settled in the province and small cities to concern themselves with this segment of surgery, since they are alone there and must rely on themselves. He himself had made this effort and recognized that even *the most minor things* (i. e. dental medical procedures) required *expertise, industry, and no small understanding.* Beginners especially could obtain benefits from this, before they reach the point of more complex cures [190].

Among the French surgeons, Garengeot's knowledge of dentistry seems to be based most firmly on personal experience, for he provides the most precise description of the practice of tooth preservation. It is not to be said against him that there is no mention of the manufacture of tooth replacements, because this cannot be expected from the title of his work. A regimental physician from 1742 on, this respected surgeon died in Cologne during the Seven Years' War, in 1759.

In 1728, five years after the printing of Garengeot's instrument manual, the work of the dental expert Pierre Fauchard was edited in Paris which initiated the awakening of an independent dentistry, not only in France, but rather far beyond its borders in the Old and New Worlds.

[187] Ibid. pp. 621 f.; see p. 151
[188] Garengeot (a) pp. 36 f.; (b) pp. 30 f.
[189] Ibid. (a) pp. 53 f.; (b) pp. 44 f. According to Gurlt (Biographisches Lexikon der hervorragenden Ärzte, ed. 2, 1929 printing, vol. I pp. 368 f.), Jean Baseilhac, a surgeon who worked benefically as a monk, Frère Côme of St. Bernhard, in Paris in the 18th century, improved Garengeot's key to the extent that the instrument as we know it today (see Fig. 235) perhaps may be ascribed to this extraordinary surgeon. Only Serre refers to him in 1803 (see pp. 212 f., 221 f., and 240 f.; Riethe b)
[190] Garengeot (a) p. 17; (b) p. 15

References

Allen, Charles
a) The operator for the teeth, . . . York 1685. Reprint ed. R. A. Cohen, London 1969
b) Curious observations . . . relating to the teeth. London 1687. Reprint ed. Lilian Lindsay, London 1924

Amman, Jost; Hans Sachs
Das Ständebuch. Reprint Leipzig 1960

Artelt, Walter
"Ossa mandibulae inferiores duo". Sudhoffs Arch. Gesch. Med. Naturw. 39 (1955) 193—215

Artzney Buchlein/wider allerlei kranckheyten und gebrechen der tzeen . . . Leyptzigk 1530 (see Zene Artzney)

Aupperle, Hermann
Bisher Unbeachtetes über den Drucker, den Verfasser und das Titelbild der Zene-Artzney vom Jahr 1530. Zahnärztl. Mitt. 47 (1959) 865—867

Baume, L.-J.
Amalgamfüllung anno 1601. Österr. Zschr. Stomat. 55 (1958) 188—193

Benzing, J.; P(eter) Riethe
Zur Bibliographie der "Zene Artzney" unter besonderer Berücksichtigung des Mainzer Drucks von 1532. Zahnärztl. Reform 56 (1955) 82—87

Beverwyck, Johannes von
Allgemeine Artzney. Part 3: Von der Wund-Artzney. Franckfurt am Mayn 1674

Borellus, Joh(annes) Alphonsus
De motu animalium. Partes II, Lugduni in Batavis (Leyden) 1685

Boyde, A(lan)
The history of 'enamel fibres'. Brit. Dent. J. 121 (1966) 85—89

Braunfels-Esche, Sigrid
Leonardo da Vinci, das anatomische Werk. Stuttgart 1961

Brunschwig, Hieronymus
a) Dis ist das Buch der Cirurgia. Handwirckung der Wundartzny. Strassburg 1497
b) idem Rostock 1518

Budjuhn, Gustav
Die Zene Arznei 1530. Berlin 1921

Choulant, Ludwig
Geschichte und Bibliographie der anatomischen Abbildung . . . Leipzig 1852

Christ, J.
Geschichtliches zur Behandlung der Gaumendefecte. Janus 6 (1901) 531—539, 587—591

Coelson, Lancelot
The poor-mans physician and chyrurgion, . . . with a method of drawing teeth. London 1656

Cohen, R. A.
a) The development of dental histology in Britain. Brit. Dent. J. 121 (1966) 59—71
b) Rare books in the B.D.A. Library. Brit. Dent. J. 118 (1965) 280—281

Columbus, Realdus
De re anatomica libri XV. Venetiis 1559

Cruce, Ioannes Andreas de
Güldene Werckstatt der Chirurgy oder Wundt-Artzney . . . Franckfort 1607

Diepgen, Paul
Krankengeschichten aus dem Mittelalter und der Renaissance als Quellen zur Kulturgeschichte. Festschr. G. Leyh 70. Geb., Zschr. Bücherkd., Add. 75, Leipzig 1950

Digitius, Johannes
Nutzliche und bewerte/Artzneyen für allerhand zanwehe/. . . Speyer 1587

Dionis, (Pierre)
a) Cours d'opérations de chirurgie. 4th ed., Paris 1746
b) Chirurgie, oder Chirurgische Operationes. 2nd ed., transl. Lorentz Heister, Augspurg 1734

Donaldson, J. Archie
Peter Lowe. Zahnärztl. Mitt. 53 (1963) 1062—1065

Driak, Fritz
Des Bartholomäus Eustachius Libellus de dentibus. Wien 1951

Dupont
a) Remede tres-veritable et tres asseuré pour oster et empescher a jamais le mal des dents,. . . Paris 1633
b) L'operateur charitable . . . Paris
c) Approbation des messieurs les medecins, . . . que l'on peut redonner des vrayes et naturelles dents . . . Paris (1647?)

Endelman, Julio
A dental book of the sixteenth century. Dent. Cosmos 45 (1903) 39—43

Eustachius, Bartholomaeus
a) Libellus de dentibus. Venetiis 1563
b) Tabulae anatomicae. Ed. Io(hannes) Maria Lancisius, Amstelaedami 1722

Fabricius ab Aquapendente, Hieronymus
a) Wund-Arznei. Franckfurt 1684
b) Opera chirurgica. Lugduni batavorum 1723

Fabricius Hildanus, Guilhelmus
a) Wundt-Artzney. Transl. Friedrich Greiff, Franckfurth am Mayn 1652
b) Von der fürtrefflichkeit und Nutz der Anatomy. 2nd ed. Aarau, Leipzig 1936

Falloppius, Gabriele
Observationes anatomicae. Venetiis 1562

Fauchard, Pierre
Le Chirurgien Dentiste. Tomes I and II, 2nd ed., Paris 1746

Garengeot, René Jacques Croissant de
a) Nouveau traité des instruments de chirurgie les plus utiles. 2. éd., Paris 1727
b) Abhandlung von denen gebräuchlichsten Instrumenten der Chirurgie, . . . Transl. J. A. Michel, Berlin/Potsdam 1729

Gerßdorf, Hans von
Feldtbuch der wundtartzney. Strassburg 1517

Guerini, Vincenzo
A history of dentistry. Philadelphia, New York 1909

Guillemeau, Jacques
Les œuvres de chiurgie. Paris 1612

Gurlt, Ernst
Geschichte der Chirurgie. Vols. I and III, Berlin 1898

Guy de Chauliac
In: Guido de Cauliaco, Cyrurgia. Venetiis 1400, pp. 1ʳ—74ʳ

Hallerus, Albertus
a) Disputationes chirurgicae selectae. Tomus I, Venetiis 1755
b) Collection de Thèses medico-chirurgicales. Tome I, Paris 1757

Hemard, Urbain
Recherche de la vraye anathomie des dents, nature et propriete d'icelles. Lyon 1582

Heurnius, Ioannes (Jan van Heurne)
a) De morbis oculorum, aurium, nasi, dentium . . . Ed. Otho Heurnius, Lugduni Batavorum 1602
b) In Hippocratis . . . commentarius. Ed. Otho Heurnius (Leyden) 1609

Hire, (Gabriel Philippe) de la
Sur les dents. Histoire de l'Academie Royale des Sciences, Année 1699, 41—43, Paris 1702

Höser, Arno
Die Zahnheilkunde bei Johannes Jessenius von Jessen. Med. Diss. Leipzig 1924

Hoffmann-Axthelm, Walter
Warum heißt der Pelikan "Pelikan"? Zahnärztl. Mitt. 62 (1972) 1174—1177

Hollerius, Iacobus
Omnia opera practica, Periocharum Holleri ad libros Galeni de compos. pharm., Lib. V. Genf 1635

Horstius, Iacobus
De aureo dente maxillari pueri silesii . . . Lipsiae 1595

Huard, Pierre
Léonard da Vinci, dessins anatomiques, Paris 1961

Kieser, R. A.
Het oude extractie-instrumentarium. Ned. Tijdschr. Tandheelkd. 66 (1959) 279—287

Leeuwenhoek, Antonius van (Anthony)
a) Microscopical observations of the structure of teeth and other bones. Phil. trans. 140 (1678) 1002—1003
b) Arcana naturae. Delphis batavorum 1695

Libavius, Andreas
Singularium, Pars II, Francofurti 1599

Lorber, Curt Gerhard
a) Thomas Erasts Disposition über die Zähne. Ruperto-Carola 34, 200—205

b) Peter Monaus Doktordissertation "Über die Erkrankungen der Zähne" aus dem Jahre 1578. Zahnärztl. Mitt. 53 (1963) 764—765
c) Ärztliche Anschauungen über Zähne und Zahnleiden im 16. Jahrhundert. Verh. XX. Kongreß Gesch. Med. Berlin 1966. Hildesheim 1968, pp. 542—552

Lowe, Peter
A discourse of the whole art of chyrurgerie. London 1612

Malpighius, Marcellus
Anatomes plantorum idea. In: Opera omnia.
a) Londini 1686, Magnae societate regiae anglicanae
b) Lugduni batavorum 1687, Pars prima
c) Opera posthuma. Londini 1694

Martin, B(arthélemy)
Dissertation sur les dents. Paris 1697

Martinez, Francisco
a) Coloquio breve y compendioso. Sobre la materia de la dentadura, . . . Valladolid 1557
b) Tractado breve y compendioso, sobre la maravillosa obra de la boca y dentadura. Madrid 1570

Mentler, Erich
Die Zahn-, Mund- und Kieferchirurgie des Fabricius Hildanus. Med. Diss. Leipzig 1922

Mercuralis, Hieronymus
De morbis puerorum. Basileae 1584

Monavius, Petrus
De dentibus affectibus. Med. Diss. Basileae 1578. Ed. and transl. Curt Gerhard Lorber. Private print Bayer, Leverkusen (1971)

Nuck, Antonius
Operationes et experimenta chirurgica. Lugduni Batavorum 1714

Paracelsus, Theophrast von Hohenheim
Complete works. Ed. Sudhoff and Mathiessen. Vol. VI, München 1922. Vol. IX, München 1928, Vol. X, München, Berlin 1928

Paré, Ambroise
a) Dix livres de la chirurgie . . . Paris 1564. Engl. transl. by Robert White Linker and Nathan Womade, Athens 1969
b) Les oeuvres . . . en vingt huit livres. 4th ed., Paris 1585
c) Oeuvres complètes. Ed. Joseph François Malgaigne, vol. 2, Paris 1840

Paul(l)ini, Kristian Frantz
a) Neu-vermehrte heylsame Dreck-Apotheke . . . Franckfurt am Mayn 1734
b) heilsame Dreck-Apotheke, . . . Stuttgart 1847

Pfolsprundt, Heinrich von
Buch der Bündth-Ertznei, 1460. Ed. Heinrich Haeser and Albrecht Middeldorp, Berlin 1868

Proskauer, Curt
a) Pestregiment und Artzney zu den bösen Zähnen of the year 1531. Bull. Hist. Med. 12 (1943) 83—95
b) Matthäus Gottfried Purmann (1648—1721 recte 1711). Dtsch. zahnärztl. Wschr. 19 (1916) 13—44

Purmannus, Matthaeus Gothofredus
a) Großer und gantz neu-gewundener Lorbeer-Krantz oder Wund-Artzney. Frankfurt and Leipzig 1722
b) Chirurgia curiosa. Frankfurt and Leipzig 1699
c) Funfftzig sonder- und wunderbahre Schuß-Wunden-Curen. Frankfurt und Leipzig 1703

Remmelinus, Ioannes
Medica de dentium statu et naturali et preternaturali, . . . Med. Diss. Tübingensium 1606, Typ. Basileae 1607

Renner, Franz
Ein new wol gegründes nützliches und haylsams Handtbüchlein . . . wider die erschröckliche, abscheuliche Kranckheit der Frantzosen . . . Nürnberg 1557

Riethe, P(eter)
a) Amalgamfüllung Anno Domini 1528. Dtsch. zahnärztl. Zschr. 21 (1966) 301—307
b) Die Zahnschlüssel der Tübinger Sammlung. Zahnärztl. Welt 84 (1975) 66—71

Riverius, Lazarus
Praxis medica cum theorica. Ed. ultima, Lugdini 1660

Ryff (Rivius), Walter Hermann
a) Nützlicher Bericht, . . . wie man die Augen und . . . den Mundt, die Zähn und Biller . . . erhalten . . . Wurtzburg
b) Die große Chirurgie, oder vollkommene Wundtartzeney . . . Franckfurt 1559
c) Des allerfürtrefflichsten . . . Menschen . . . warhafftige Beschreibung oder Anatomi, . . . Strassburg 1541

Schenckius de Grafenberg, Iohannes
Observationes medicae de capite humano. Basileae 1584

Schöppler, Hermann
Ein Arzneibuch über böse Zähne aus dem 16. Jahrhundert. Dtsch. zahnärztl. Zschr. 9 (1910) H. 18, 6—7

Schubring, Konrad
Der Titel von Vesals Hauptwerk. Med. Hist. J. 1 (1966) 149

Scultetus, Joannes
a) Armamentarium chirurgicum, Ulmae suevorum 1655; idem Venetiis 1665
b) The chyrurgeous store-house. Transl. by E. B., London 1674

Sebizius, Melchior
Disputationes de dentibus quatuor. Argentorati (Strassburg) 1645

Solingen, Cornelis
Handgriffe der Wund-Artzney. Franckfurt/Oder 1693

Stockerus, Ioannes
Praxis aurea, . . . 3rd ed., Lugdunum Batavorum 1657

Strobelbergerus, Joh. Stephanus
De dentium podagra. Lipsiae 1630

Ströbel, Hans Georg
Bau und Wirkung der Extraktionsinstrumente sowie ihre Entwicklung. Med. Diss. Düsseldorf 1961

Sudhoff, Karl
a) Vom Alter des Gaumenobturators, eine Feststellung. Janus 28 (1924) 451—454
b) Geschichte der Zahnheilkunde. 2nd ed., Leipzig 1926

Tacke, Walter
Zur Vorgeschichte der "Highmore's Höhle" vor Highmore. Med. Diss. Leipzig 1923

Tulpius, Nicolaus
Observationes medicae. Amsterdami 1672

Tylkowski, Adalbert
Disquisitio physica über den Wilnaer Knaben mit dem goldenen Zahn 1674. Transl. Paul Fuhrmann, Berlin 1921

Vesalius, Andreas
De humani corporis fabrica libri septem. Basileae 1543

Weinberger, Bernhard Wolf
a) Charles Allen's "The Operator for the Teeth." York 1685. J. Am. Dent. Ass. 18 (1931) 67—76
b) An introduction to the history of dentistry. Vol. I, St. Louis 1948

Wilker, Hermann Heinrich
Der Arzt Joh. Stephan Strobelberger mit besonderer Berücksichtigung seines Werkes "De dentium podagra", 1630. Med. Diss. Leipzig 1923

Zene Artzney. Meyntz 1532; Franckfort 1536 (see Artzney Buchlein)

Chapter 10

The 18th Century – Dentistry becomes Independent

Age of Enlightenment

With the death of Louis XIV (1715) in the 18th century France's position of world power yielded to that of England. Within the confusion of the German provincial states Austria and Prussia developed into great European powers, while the bond of the Holy Roman Empire finally broke. In the East, however, important monarchs were constantly strengthening the Russian Empire. Towards the end of the century, the French people reacted to the surviving absolutism with the great Revolution, and from the chaos arose the dictatorship of Napoleon. His coming released a flood of wars which overwhelmed all of Europe until 1815. In the meantime, England's North American colonies had fought for their national independence under Washington, and proclaimed it in 1776.
Intellectual life was shaped to a great extent by the movement of the "Enlightenment" which had received its essential impulse from English philosophers, particularly John Locke. His thoughts, which were spread by Voltaire in France, had a revolutionary effect there, while they became influential only later in Germany which was then still backward in industrial development. The philosopher Immanuel Kant explained the concept in 1784: *Enlightenment is man's departure from his self-imposed immaturity.* This signifies the rational self-determination of the individual through the use of his reason, and his last protest against medieval scholastic science and belief in authority.

For medicine in general this era was mostly a phase of waiting, of marking time before the great advance of the 19th century: the circulation of the blood and the microscope had already been discovered, the great anatomists, physiologists and surgeons had already lived, and now speculative theories determined the progress of the time, perhaps as a reaction to the preceding period of the natural sciences, or perhaps resulting from the influence of the philosopher Leibniz and his student Christian Wolff. Men such as the opposing professors Friedrich Hoffmann and Ernst Stahl in Halle, and François de Sauvages in Montpellier created and defended theories of disease in disputes which were mostly sterile. To be sure, the great clinician Herman Boerhaave of Leyden opposed these dogmatists his "Simplex veri sigillum!" (Simple Things are the Seals of Truth), and influenced with his more eclectic orientation almost all the clinics of Europe, even including some in North America, such as Philadelphia. Nonetheless, in comparison with the forward-surging 16th and 17th centuries, abounding in great names and discoveries, a perceptible lull had set in. Not even such significant personalities as the innovator of experimental physiology, Albrecht von Haller, Boerhaave's greatest student who worked predominantly in Göttingen, and Giovanni Battista Morgagni of Padua, the creator of the field of pathological anatomy, were able to overcome this standstill.
A completely different development showed in dental medicine: the furious toothache could hardly be forced into any system, and the disfiguring anterior diastema of a Rococo beauty could not simply be discussed out of existence. Therefore, in dentistry, advances in the natural sciences and in technology, even if they were somewhat late in comparison with the rest of medicine, were put to practical use to an extent never before achieved. After centuries of coexistence, an autonomous dentistry materialized surgeons, obtained in actual practice, and from the accumulated specialized knowledge of the surgeons, obtained in actual practice, and from the techniques of the itinerant toothdrawers and industrious craftsmen, as well as from the academically educated anatomists. It was a new branch, free of both surgery and of lesser crafts.
Furthermore, through the formation of strictly governed state structures, under sometimes outstanding rulers, the basis was provided for the social classification of the medical professions, including the dental practitioners, and with it was laid the foundation for the modern licensed dentist's duties and education.

Governmental Recognition

The first step in the direction of governmental recognition of the practitioners of dentistry, regardless of the regulations of cities and guilds, had already been made in the 17th century in Berlin. The Great Elector, Frederick William of Brandenburg, issued an edict on medicine on the 12th of November 1685, the basic outline of which, mentioned and expanded by his personal physicians, had been submitted as early as 1661 [1]. The fundamental "Edict concerning the Collegium Medicum established in Berlin and what Physicians as well as Apothecaries and Surgeons are to observe" contains the stipulation that an examination be taken before a government commission for the actual practice of dentistry. It reads: *When oculists, operators, lithotomists, hernia operators, toothdrawers (Zahnbrecher), etc. wish to advertise themselves and wish publicly to practice and offer for sale their art and science, then they should be inhibited by this Collegio no less than by the magistrate, in submitting to their examinations, whereupon depending on the result they should be permitted or forbidden to do so.* There is a sharp distinction made of the group of *meddlers, frauds, and quacks, etc., of all of whom not one belongs to the medical world.* These persons should be *tolerated nowhere,* and suppressed *with unrelenting harsh punishment* [2]. In the French wording appended for the Huguenot colony in Brandenburg we find the familiar designation "arracheur de dents" [3]. It may be concluded from the fact that the edict had to be restated, *re-enjoined* repeatedly in the following decades, that its practical enforcement was far behind.

A fundamental reworking and expansion is found in 1725, in the edict effective from then on in the kingdom of Prussia, under the government of the "Soldier-King," Frederick William I, who was exceptionally open with regard to problems of sanitation. This "General and Restrengthened" medical edict already established the present-day standards of governmental health management, and therefore was adopted in the course of the century by almost all the German and many European states, with locally adjusted modifications. In the official language appeared the term "Zahn-Aertzte" (Tooth-physicians; dentists) in an order of the king on October 9, 1713 for the first time as *Tooth-,* (bladder-) *Stone-, and Hernia-Physicians* [4]. They are not permitted *to publicly set up or offer for sale in Our cities, if We have not specifically given them that privilege* [5].

It is singular that these government edicts of Berlin are hardly mentioned in the historical literature of our profession, while the Paris guild statutes, which were directed at a similar group of persons, are valued in every history of dentistry of the Old and New World as milestones in the development of a dental professional class, even though they were issued 14 years later and limited only to the city of Paris and its vicinity. In 1699 in this city then leading in surgery, practice in the field of dentistry was made dependent on passing an examination as a result of the efforts of the surgeons who wanted to take minor surgery out of the hand of the market hawkers and bring it under their own control. These Parisian surgeons of the respected Collège de St. Côme [6] had just succeeded in the task of establishing their independence from the patronizing academic physicians, who still persisted largely in medieval concepts. Next to the church of St. Côme, they built a splendid anatomical theatre and an examining hall, and dared to slam the door in the faces of the high faculty when in 1725, led by Deacon Andry, its members appeared in full dress in the Rue des Cordelliers to demonstrate their claim to leadership. They even refused to open the door after the doorknocker was used forty times. In 1731 the Cosmas Guild assumed the character of a royal academy, whereby the leading position of French surgery was further confirmed. Not until 1743, however, did the Collegium forbid the practice of the barber trade by the last of its members [7].

The statute of May 11, 1699 declared that specialists such as hernia-operators, truss-makers, oculists, dental experts ("Experts pour les dents"), and bone resetters had to submit to theoretical and practical examinations before the First Royal Surgeon, his deputy, four provosts, and — still — the deacon of the medical faculty; otherwise any activity in Paris and its suburbs was forbidden to them. This did not prevent, however, market hawker types such as Jean Thomas (le Grand Thomas), even though

[1] Artelt p. 22 f.
[2] Mylius col. 21
[3] Ibid. col. 22
[4] Ibid. col. 73
[5] Medicinal-Edict p. 37
[6] See p. 117
[7] Besombes pp. 73 f.

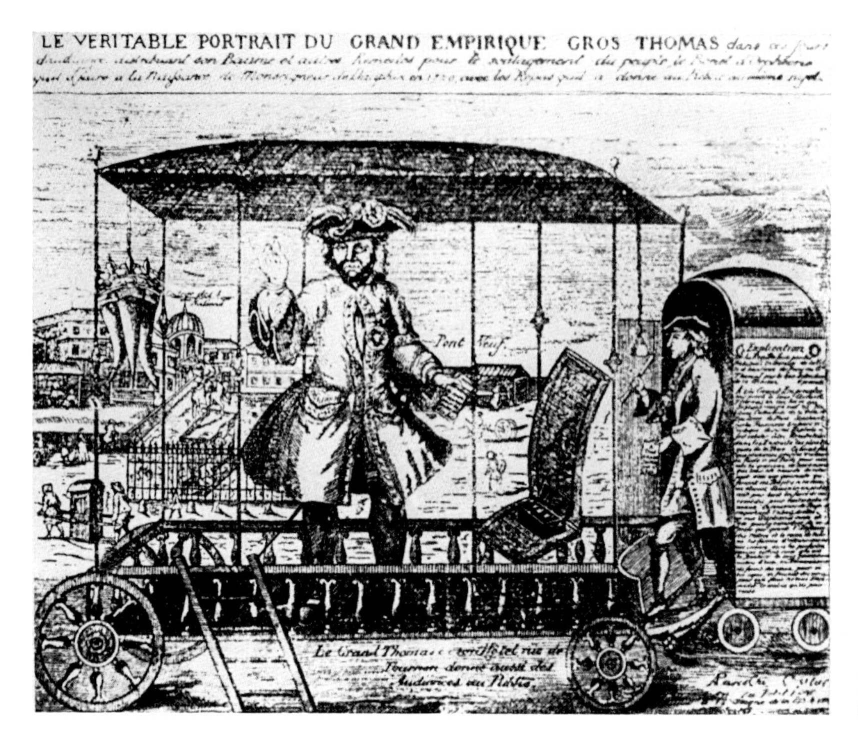

LE VERITABLE PORTRAIT DU GRAND EMPIRIQUE GROS THOMAS
Pont Neuf

Fig. 181 *The Great Thomas; anonymous flyer*

reçue à St. Côme—today we would say "governmentally certified"—from doing their mischief at the Pont Neuf, literally with tambourines and trumpets (Fig. 181). A report of Berlin's *Vossische Zeitung* from 1729 (No. 102) gives us a description of the activities there: *Paris, Aug. 15: Today, several students played a humorous practical joke on the familiar toothbreaker named the Great Thomas, who has his shop standing only on wheels at the Pont Neuf; they bound four large rockets to the underside of his little house, and ignited these at exactly the time when he was in the middle of extracting a tooth from a patient, whereupon the latter fell to the ground, and the Great Thomas fell on him, which caused a great deal of laughter from the crowd of people gathered around him*[8].

Even if the new regulation and its supervision by the police department constituted a significant advance, Pierre Fauchard justifiably criticised that the examination commission lacked *a skillful and experienced dentist (un Dentiste habile et experimenté).—From this it can be seen that the majority of the dental experts (experts pour les dents) are only equipped with less than average knowledge*[9]. This completely justified requirement is heard from the man who is regarded everywhere as the father of scientific dentistry. He was not, however. Fauchard was essentially an empiricist. His lasting merit lies in his having compiled for the first time all the contemporary knowledge of his field, enriched with a profusion of his own ideas, in a single work, a work which determined our field, at least for the century in which it was written. With it he became the initiator of independent dentistry.

France — Pierre Fauchard

All we know of Pierre Fauchard's youth is that he was born in 1678, probably in Brittany, that he began his training with a surgeon in the royal navy, and that, after residing in Angers and Nantes and in Rennes and Tours, he settled in Paris in 1719 (Fig. 182). He remained faithful to this city for the rest of his 83 years. In 1729 he married into a respected family of

[8] Buchner p. 93
[9] Fauchard (a) I p. XII; (b) I p. 8; (c) I p. VIII

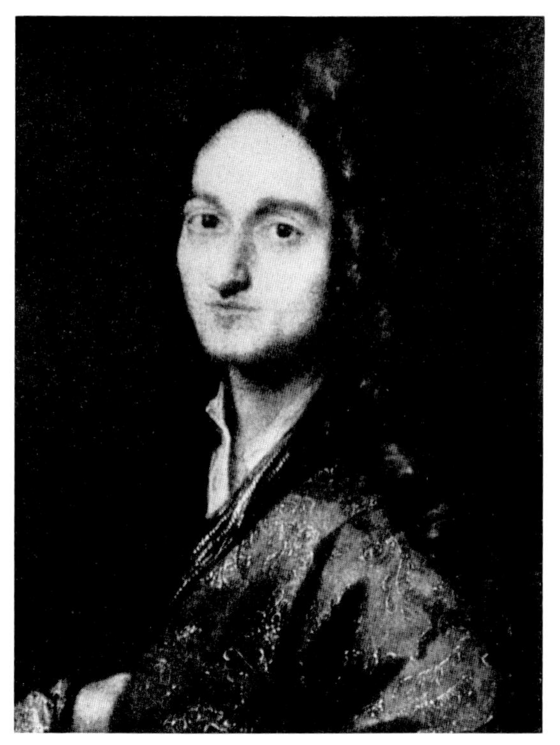

Fig. 182 *Pierre Fauchard, around 1726; anonymous painting (Bibl. École Dentaire, Paris)*

Des Herrn PIERRE FAUCHARD
Frantzösischer
Zahn-Artzt,
Oder Tractat
Von den Zähnen:
Worinnen die Mittel,
selbige sauber und gesund zu erhalten, sie schöner zu machen, die verlohrne wieder zu ersetzen, und die ungesunden, wie auch die Kranckheiten des Zahnfleisches, und die Zufälle, welche anderen nahe bey den Zähnen liegenden Theilen zustossen können, zu heilen, gelehret werden;
Samt Observationen und Betrachtungen über viele besondere Fälle;
Mit viertzig Kupffer-Tafeln ausgezieret.
Mit einer Vorrede
Herrn D. Augustini Buddei,
Königl. Hof-Raths und Leib-Medici, des Ober-Collegii Medici Assessoris, Directoris classis Physico-Medicæ bey der Königl. Societät der Wissenschafften, Professoris Anatomiæ und Physices bey dem Collegio Medico-Chirurgico, wie auch der Römis. Kayserl. Academie Mitgliedes.
Der Erste Theil.

BERLIN,
Zu finden bey Joh. Andreas Rüdigern. 1733.

Fig. 183 *Pierre Fauchard: Title page of the German edition, 1733*

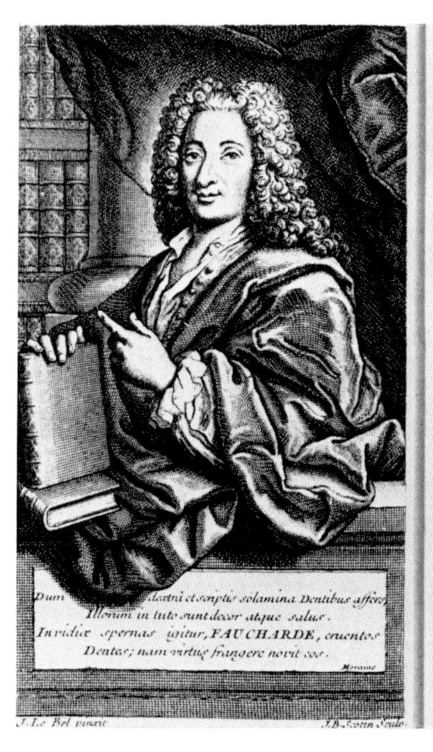
Dum dextrâ et scriptis solamina Dentibus affers;
Illorum in tuto sunt decor atque salus.
Invidiæ spernas igitur, FAUCHARDE, cruentos
Dentes; nam virtus frangere novit eos.
J. Le Bel pinxit
J.B. Scotin Sculp.

LE CHIRURGIEN
DENTISTE,
OU
TRAITE' DES DENTS,
OU L'ON ENSEIGNE LES MOYENS
de les entretenir propres & saines, de les embellir, d'en réparer la perte & de remédier à leurs maladies, à celles des Gencives & aux accidens qui peuvent survenir aux autres parties voisines des Dents.
Avec des Observations & des Réflexions sur plusieurs cas singuliers.
Ouvrage enrichi de quarante-deux Planches en taille douce.
Par PIERRE FAUCHARD, Chirurgien Dentiste à Paris.
Deuxiéme Edition revûë, corrigée & considérablement augmentée.
TOME PREMIER.

A PARIS,
Chez PIERRE-JEAN MARIETTE, ruë S. Jacques aux Colonnes d'Hercule.
Et chez l'Auteur, ruë des grands Cordeliers.

M. DCC. XLVI.
Avec Approbations & Privilége du Roi.

Fig. 184 *Frontispiece and title page of the second edition of "Chirurgien Dentiste," 1746*

actors, a profession which his son, too, was to enter. In 1734 he was in a position to acquire the castle and domains of Grand Mesnil. Now he was a seigneur and magistrate, to whom it might have been somewhat embarrasing that his partner in practice, Gaulard, was hanged on the gallows in the Place de Greve for a theft in 1740. His two volume work, "Le Chirurgien Dentiste, ou traité des dents," had already come out in 1728, and was followed in 1746 by a second considerably enlarged edition which is generally taken as a source here. Their effect was so great that a third edition followed in 1786, 25 years after the author's death. Herewith we have the publication of the first useful textbook devoted entirely to dentistry and *to the other parts in their vicinity (aux autres parties voisines des dents).* This work combined all the era's knowledge on the subject, based on the publications of both surgeons and anatomists and on the practical knowledge of the tooth-drawers. It presented furthermore a great many of this manually adept and intellectually keen man's personal experiences, designs, and case histories.

The impression which this work made on the professional world was uncommonly strong, as documented by the fact, among others, that already in 1733, that is five years after the first printing, a German translation was published in Berlin by the scholarly physician, Georg Matthiae, who worked there from 1732 to 1734 and later in Hamburg. The preface was written by an anatomist also in Berlin, the Privy Councillor August Buddeus[10] (Fig. 183). Translation into English was not done until 1946[11].

As was customary, "Le Chirurgien Dentiste" commences with a detailed anatomy of the teeth and their environment in which function, development, and eruption are treated elaborately. When Fauchard ventures into an area where he feels unsure of himself, such as that of the histology of dental tissue, he inserts quotations, in this case a slightly edited one from de la Hire, a member of the Academy[12], while he allows the Danish anatomist Jacob Benignus Winslow, also a member of the Parisian Academy, to speak concerning tooth development[13]. Winslow's anatomical work from 1733 contained an excellent description of the teeth with early histological findings[14].

The copper engraving of normal anatomy of teeth included in the first chapter of this work is obviously lacking all the finer elaborations. However, the remaining 41 plates of the second edition—the first had only forty—represent partly small works of art, in particular the frontispiece of the author: dignified, with a stately full-bottomed periwig, his work in his right hand, with the index finger of his left pointing to the library in the background, as if he wished to indicate modestly whom he had to thank for his wisdom (Fig. 184).

In the 38 chapters of the first, and the 26 of the second volume, on a total of 919 pages, every category of the subject is included with astounding thoroughness, in a conception which is clear throughout and which is even often in correspondence with present-day conditions. Among them are surgical, preventive, and prosthetic dental medicine, orthodontics and instructions with regard to instruments, but again, suddenly a piece of the Middle Ages is interspersed. Fauchard shocks us, thus, with the prescription of rinsing the mouth mornings and evenings with a few spoonfuls of one's own fresh urine for the prevention of caries. He is himself not completely comfortable with this medication but, he asks, what won't one do for tranquillity and health? This age-old advice, possibly taken from Martin, is in any case a quotation found in the second edition for the first time[15]. On the other hand, he decisively rejects the toothworm. He himself had examined both cavities on extracted teeth as well as the tartar adhering to them often enough through an excellent microscope without ever having discovered any worms at all, in contrast to Andry, who had seen these creatures and described them with precision. Fauchard seems to have derived particular pleasure from this statement, because it had been Nicolas Andry, known as the quarrelsome pioneer in the field of orthopedics, who had then, as deacon of the medical faculty, instituted the demonstration against the surgeons, among whom Fauchard felt he belonged[16]. He himself regarded caries

[10] Meusel p. 535; Jöcher coll. 997—998; Fauchard (b)
[11] Fauchard (c); (c) I p. 11. See p. 218
[12] See pp. 175 f.
[13] Fauchard (a) I p. 29; (c) I p. 11
[14] Winslow p. 42
[15] Fauchard (a) I p. 167; (c) I p. 61. See p. 189
[16] Ibid. (a) I pp. 151 f.; (b) I pp. 138 f.; (c) I p. 56. See p. 185

fundamentally, like the Hippocratics, as the result of a humoral imbalance [17].

Fauchard characterized enamel hypoplasia as *erosion of the surface of the enamel,* which is to be eliminated through smoothing with a file [18]. Only in the second edition he expressly takes a stand on this problem beginning in the appended second chapter on children's diseases during teething [19]. An interesting item is the first description of tooth dysplasia, which we call today opalescent dentin or dentinogenesis imperfecta: *sometimes the teeth look transparent and translucent,* a congenital systemic disease which he incorrectly blames on rickets [20].

For every procedure, the position of the therapist in relation to the patient is described in detail. The latter must be seated *in an arm chair (fauteuil) which is steady and firm, suitable and comfortable, the back of which should be of horsehair or with a soft pillow raised more or less according to the stature of the patient and particularly to that of the dentist* [21], already the principle of our contemporary treatment. As to tooth extraction he decisively rejects the low position, in which the patient sits on the ground, and cannot understand why certain authors were still teaching it [22]. The primary teeth are to be retained as long as possible, just as the indications for extraction should always be carefully weighed. The epulis should be excised, and the parulis and abscess split which is explained, in principle according to Paulos of Aigina, with all possible precision and a bit circumstantially. He requires an early incision at the deepest point, for packing was still unknown. The culpable tooth should then be removed as quickly as possible. He always attacks the quacks and hawkers in the market (*empiriques, charlatans*) and advises to consult a physician or surgeon in serious cases [23].

The disease of marginal periodontitis is found for the first time in the second edition (of 1746), and described with great precision initially as *a kind of scurvy.* Later, however, Fauchard disavows this etiology and determines that it is more of a local circulatory or humoral problem. He is the first to describe it, a fact which he emphasizes, as a problem which manifests itself on the sockets and the teeth, or, in modern terms, on the periodontium. If the mandible is rubbed from below, and the maxilla conversely from above, then the pus which has collected is emptied. This pus collects in the space between the gingiva and the alveolus, and sometimes between the alveolus and the root of the tooth, in greater quantity on the outside than on the inside. Since internal medications including remedies for scurvy are of no avail, he recommends cleansing the teeth, rinsing the mouth and massage of the gingiva with the fingers [24].

The first volume is concluded by a list of disease aspects, as usual in the form of "Observations" which are succeeded in every case by a sound "Reflexion," an epicrisis. Even today we can agree very often with the correctness of the author's therapeutic advice. As an "Observation" he describes the succesful transplantation he performed on a captain with a tooth from a soldier of his company, without, unfortunately, recording in his "Reflexion" any thoughts he might have had on the possibility of transmitting veneral disease or even on the morality of the procedure [25].

In two further case histories, we find the unequivocal description of cysts, which Fauchard correctly regarded as the products of carious teeth or roots. After extraction he widely opened a hollow tumor that extended as far as the base of the mandible. *To prevent the opening of the wound to close too soon,* he packed it for four days and sprayed the cavity *until* (the) *twenty-fifth day when the disease was perfectly cured.* Another cyst, of the maxilla, which extended up to the orbital cavity, discharged after extraction *a considerable quantity of serous and yellow matter.* He reduced the external swelling through compression so that this disease, too, was cured after a few days. In contrast to Scultetus' more thorough treatment, a permanent cure was probably not achieved in either case [26]. The tumorous nature of cysts, however, still remained unknown until the 19th century.

The practical measures follow in the second volume, mostly proceeding from the instrumentarium which is described and illustrated in detail. In this manner first scaling is dis-

[17] Ibid. (a) I pp. 142 f.; (b) I pp. 131 f.; (c) I p. 53
[18] Ibid. (a) I p. 127; (b) I p. 117; (c) I pp. 46 f.
[19] Ibid. (a) I pp. 58 f.; (c) I pp. 20 f. See pp. 207 f.
[20] Ibid. (a) I p. 129; (b) I p. 118; (c) I p. 47. The first more recent description comes from C. W. Stainton (see p. 276) in Dent. Cosmos 24 (1892) 978—981
[21] Ibid. (a) I p. 189; (b) I p. 165; (c) I p. 70
[22] Ibid. (a) I p. 193; (b) I p. 170; (c) I p. 70
[23] Ibid. (a) I p. 200; (b) I p. 177; (c) I p. 74
[24] Ibid. (a) I p. 275 f.; (c) I p. 102 f.
[25] Ibid. (a) I pp. 383 f.; (b) I pp. 354 f.; (c) I pp. 142 f.
[26] Ibid. (a) I pp. 433 f. and 438 f.; (b) I pp. 405 f. and 409 f.; (c) I pp. 162 f. and 164. See p. 181

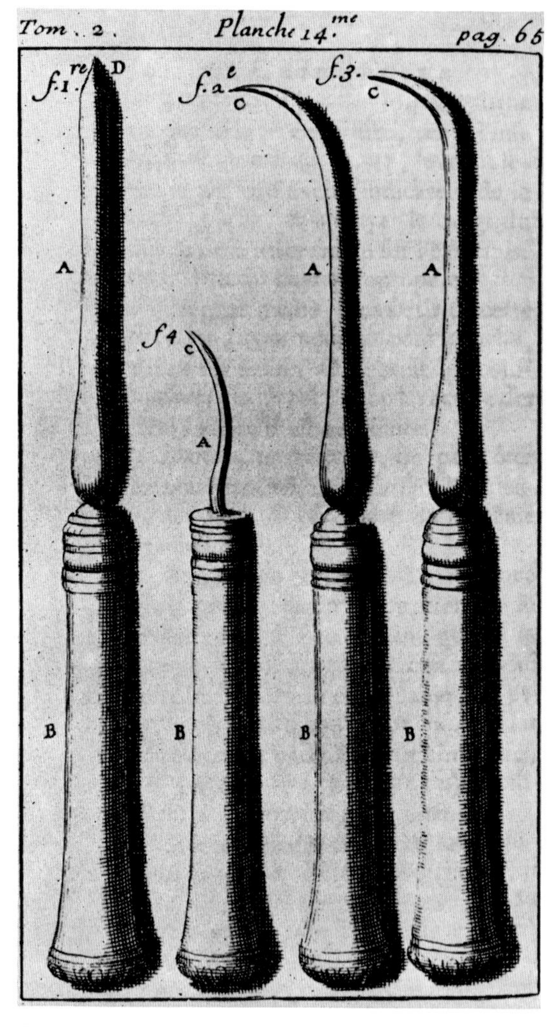

Fig. 185 *Fauchard: Instruments to treat caries*

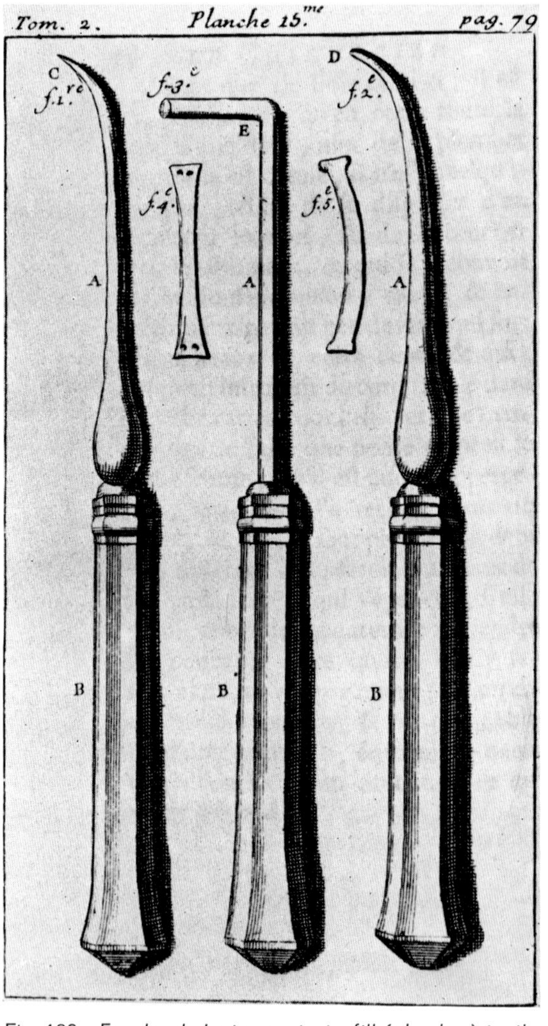

Fig. 186 *Fauchard: Instruments to fill (plomber) teeth (F. 1—3); metal strips to arrange single teeth in the dental arches*

cussed, and then the preventive care of the teeth: the carious substance is removed as completely as possible with pointed awl-like instruments (Fig. 185), and then moisture and the loose remains of the caries are removed by blotting with a cotton compress [27]. The cavity then is stuffed with lead with a sturdy instrument, because the procedure requires strength (Fig. 186, F. 1—3). Tin is even better but he regards gold foil as a superfluous luxury. He describes the filling process minutely for the various sites on the individual teeth. Toothache is eliminated in the traditional manner with the cautery [28].

The eighth chapter of the second volume is devoted to orthodontic problems. Teeth deviating from the arch are rearranged with silk ligatures; those which are more radically out of place are corrected with a perforated metal strip of gold or silver, which is fastened on the inside or the outside to the straight adjoining teeth in such a way that it pushes the tooth

[27] Ibid. (a) II p. 64; (b) II p. 62; (c) II p. 25
[28] Ibid. (a) II pp. 80 f.; (b) II pp. 76 f.; (c) II p. 31

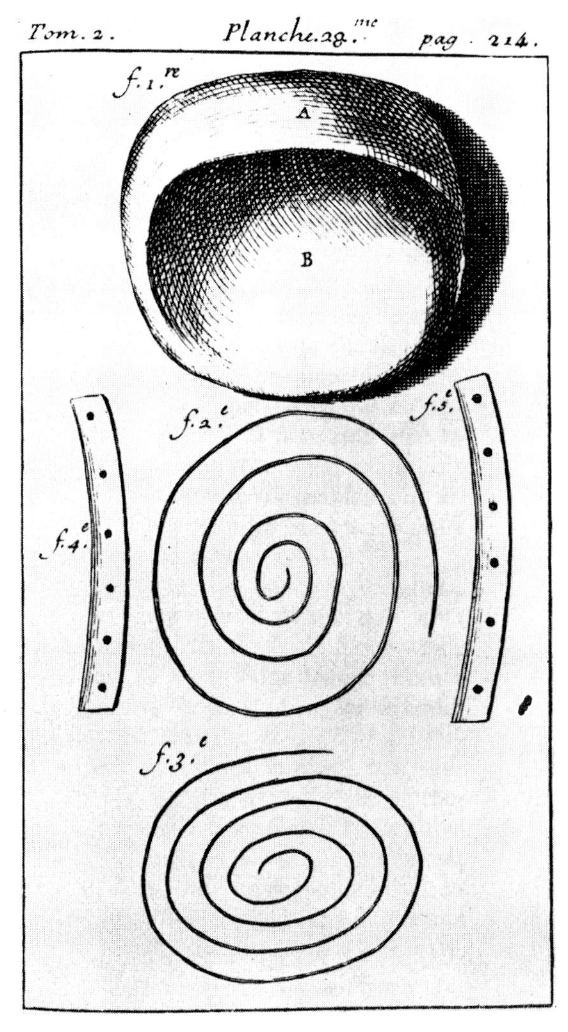

Fig. 187 *Fauchard: Lead piece to loosen teeth to be removed with the punch (F. 1), gold wires (F. 2 and 3), and lead strips (F. 4 and 5) to splint loosened teeth*

Fig. 188 *Fauchard: Raspatory (déchaussoir, F. 1), punch (poussoir, F. 2), and hook (crochet, F. 3)*

between them in or out (Fig. 186, F. 4,5). In the case of older persons with inverted teeth Fauchard recommends adjustment by force (redresser) with forceps or, allegedly his own idea, with the pelican[29]. This method is somewhat problematic, but is still occasionally used even today.

In the same chapter the splinting of teeth which have been knocked out and replanted is described with a perforated strip of lead fitted to the inside and outside of the dental arch (Fig. 187, F. 4,5). Loose teeth are fixed with drawn gold wire, whereby the figure-of-eight ligature is pushed to the edge of the gingiva with a blunt probe, just as we still do it today. Fauchard expressly claimed the priority to this method too, known to us from Abulcasim[30].

Many pages are devoted to the extraction of teeth[31]. The instruments are, in principle, the same as those from Paré. Fauchard also does not yet forgo the use of the raspatory

[29] Ibid. (a) II p. 113; (b) II pp. 95 f.; (c) II p. 43
[30] Ibid. (a) II p. 116; (b) II p. 105; (c) II p. 44; see p. 99
[31] Ibid. (a) II pp. 130 f.; (b) II pp. 121 f.; (c) II pp. 49 f.

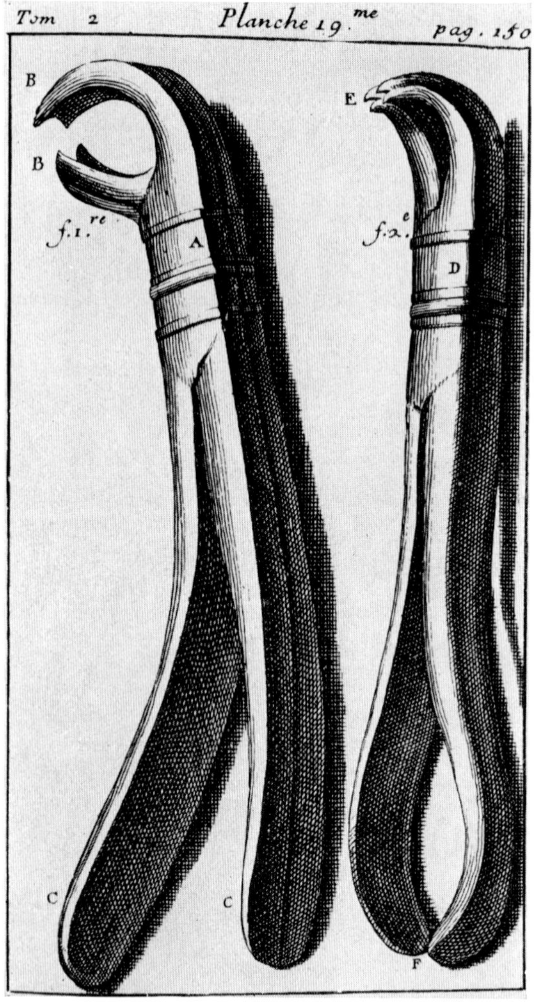

Fig. 189 *Tooth forceps (daviers)*

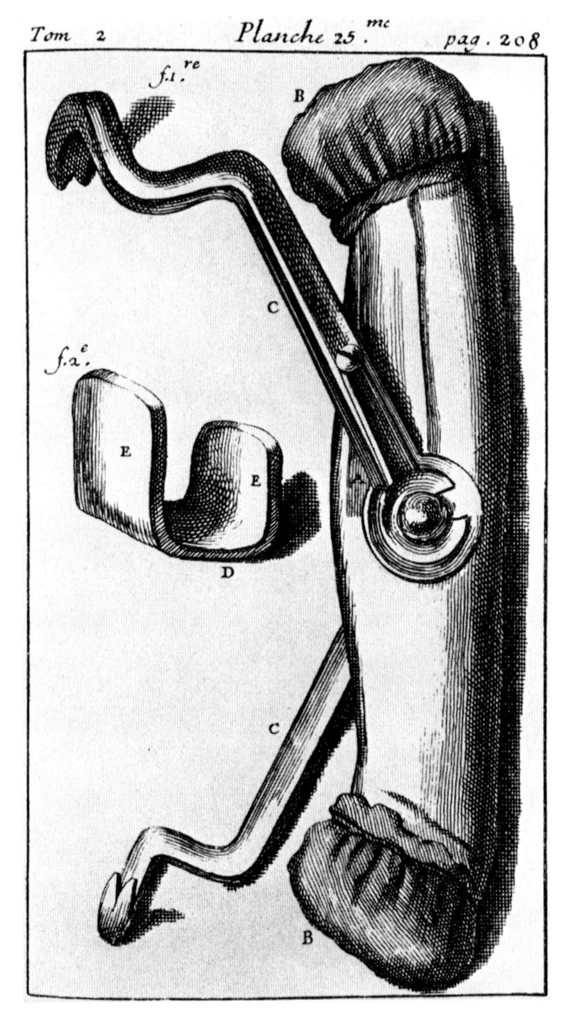

Fig. 190 *Fauchard: Pelican (pélican F. 1), lead plate for compression in post-extraction bleeding (plaque de plombe, F. 2)*

(déchaussoir, Fig. 188, F. 1) for detaching the gingiva before the extraction. The punch (poussoir, Fig. 188, F. 2) forces the tooth inwards and out of the socket. If brachial power is not enough, then a one pound lump of lead is struck against it (Fig. 187, F. 1), quite a robust procedure which was already criticised by his younger contemporary B o u r d e t[32]. With the hook (crochet, Fig. 188, F. 3), however, the tooth is luxated from the inside. The forceps (davier, pincettes, Fig. 189) still possess the traditional shapes. F a u c h a r d devotes a special chapter (the eleventh) to his improved pelican (pélican, Fig. 190), which he regards as the most useful, but also the most dangerous instrument for tooth extraction[33]. He describes four different constructions with well-padded support surfaces, but also shows a lever (levier, Fig. 191, F. 1).

F a u c h a r d ' s most fruitful activity was in the area of prosthetics, simply because in contrast to all his predecessors, he described every

32 Ibid. (a) II pp. 139 f.; (b) II p. 131; (c) II p. 52; see p. 210
33 Ibid. (a) II pp. 152 f.; (b) II p. 163; (c) II pp. 56 f.

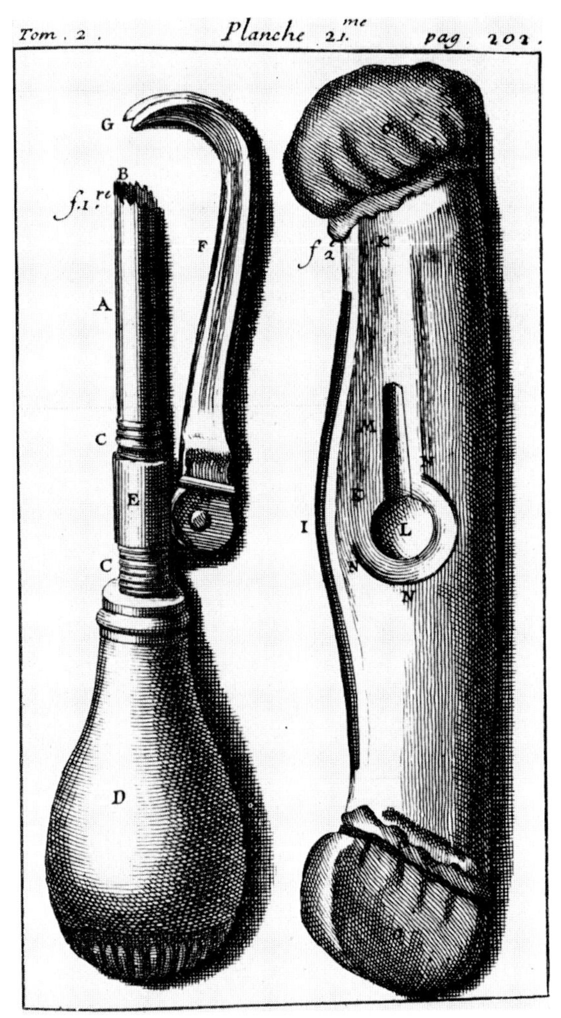

Fig. 191 *Fauchard: Lever (levier, F. 1), grasp for the pelican*

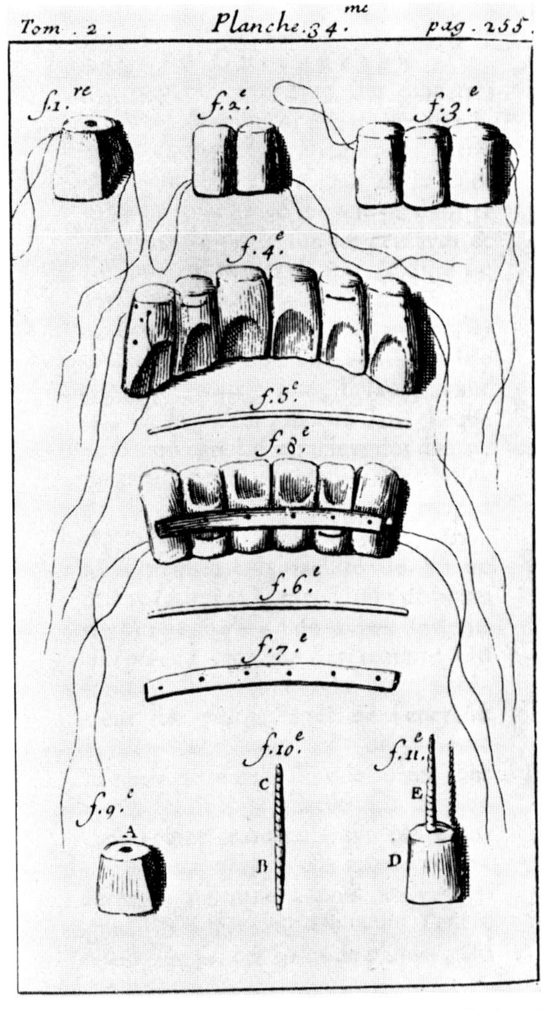

Fig. 192 *Fauchard: Dental prostheses and dowel crown fixed in place with threads*

detail of the technical method. He also declared in the preface that by doing so he was prejudicing his own interests [34]. With this sacrifice, however, he delivered dental prosthetics from the province of handicrafts to that of dentistry in the modern age.

The best materials are, now as before, human teeth, ivory, hippopotamus bone, and walrus tusks (cheval marin), which were then coming into fashion [35]. For the replacement of individual teeth with human teeth the root is filed off, and the dental pulp cavity filled with lead. Then the crown is drilled through, threaded with twine or silk, and made fast to the neighboring teeth (Fig. 192, F. 1—4). For several teeth, they are riveted to a gold or silver splint (Fig. 192, F. 6—8). To prepare a dowel crown (dent à tenon) the crown of the replacing tooth is ground to the root, from which all carious material has previously been removed and replaced with lead. Then the notched dowel is joined with

[34] Ibid. (a) I p. XIX; (b) I p. 14; (c) I p. IX
[35] Ibid. (a) II p. 215; (b) II p. 190; (c) II p. 75

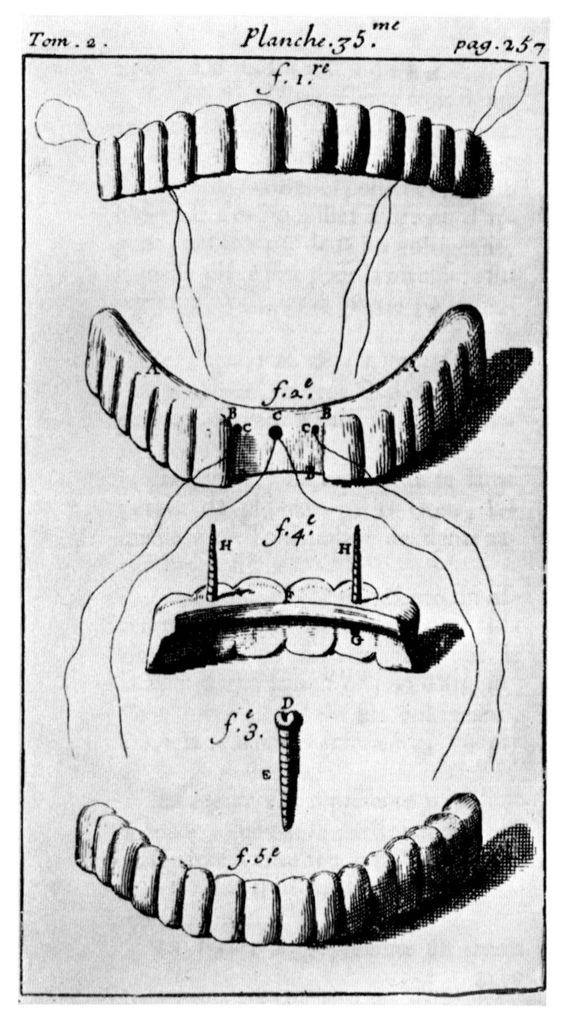

Fig. 193 *Fauchard: Post crown bridge and complete dentures*

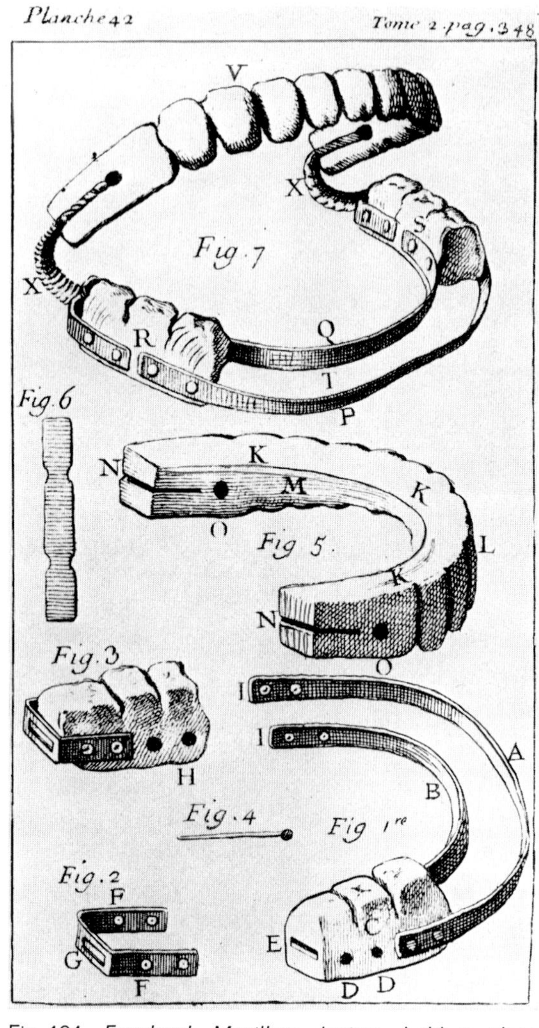

Fig. 194 *Fauchard: Maxillary denture, held in place with whalebone springs covered with a spiral wire (Fig. 7)*

the drilled crown with a rubber cement (Fig. 193, F. 9—11), the composition of which is explained in the most minute manner just as is every other detail. Only if necessary is the dowel wedged tight into the root canal with wrappings of hemp, flax, or a thread.

Teeth such as these last in some cases 15 to 20 years or more [36]. Furthermore, a kind of bridge replacement is carved from walrus bone or hippopotamus with dowels set in two roots (pièce ou dentier à tenon, Fig. 193, F. 3,4), probably the first construction since Roman times which is anchored by abutments and spans gaps in the arch [37].

Complete lower dentures, turned on a lathe in one piece from bone, rest by their own weight on the arch of the jaw (pièce dentière ou dentier artificiel, Fig. 193, F. 5). Upper dentures, on the other hand, are held by flat springs, which support themselves on the mandible (Fig. 194), according to the same principle applied even today for fastening obturating prostheses

[36] Ibid. (a) II pp. 224 f.; (b) II pp. 198 f.; (c) II pp. 78 f.
[37] Ibid. (a) II pp. 252 f.; (b) II pp. 224 f.; (c) II pp. 86 f.

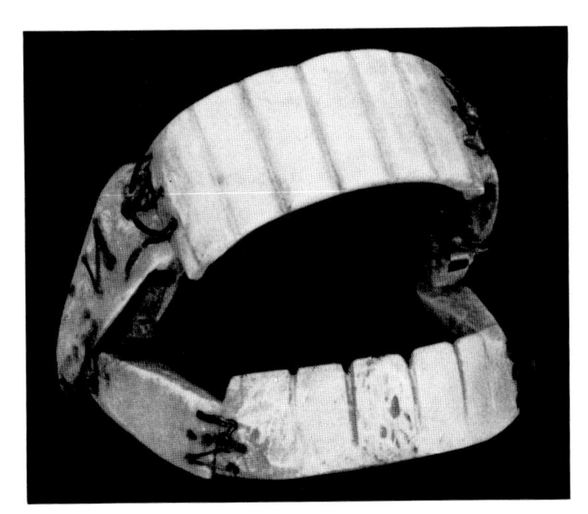

Fig. 195 *Denture of oxbone with spring joint, about 1500 (Forschungsinstitut für Geschichte der Zahnheilkunde, Cologne)*

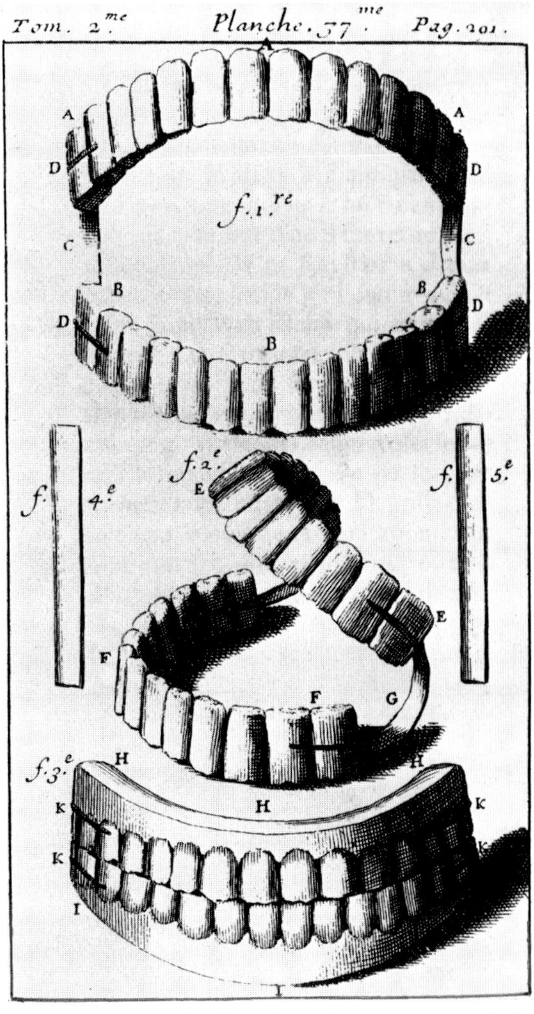

Fig. 196 *Fauchard: Complete denture, retained by steel band springs, F. 3 with enamelled metal base*

to replace a surgically resected maxilla. Also, complete upper dental arches can be fastened in this manner to complete lower arches. The steel springs (ressorts d'acier)—he writes that only very fragile springs of fishbone were known previously—are claimed by him expressly as his own invention [38], yet we find a similar principle applied in the prosthesis shown in figure 195 from a 16th century grave in the vicinity of Basel. These crude dentures carved from oxbone are connected by two strips of metal, which surely allowed a certain degree of mobility, and, perhaps, (though this is no longer demonstrable today) even possessed a light spring effect. Fauchard also used the fishbone springs (ressorts de baleine) criticized before, but fortifies them with wire wrappings (Fig. 193, F. 7).

Fauchard's artifical teeth possessed no cusps yet, and the denture (ratelier, dentier) did not lie flat on the profile of the jaw. Nor did this author devote any thought to the vertical dimen-

[38] Ibid. (a) II pp. 262 f. and 343; (b) II pp. 229 f. and 293 f.; (c) II pp. 89 f.

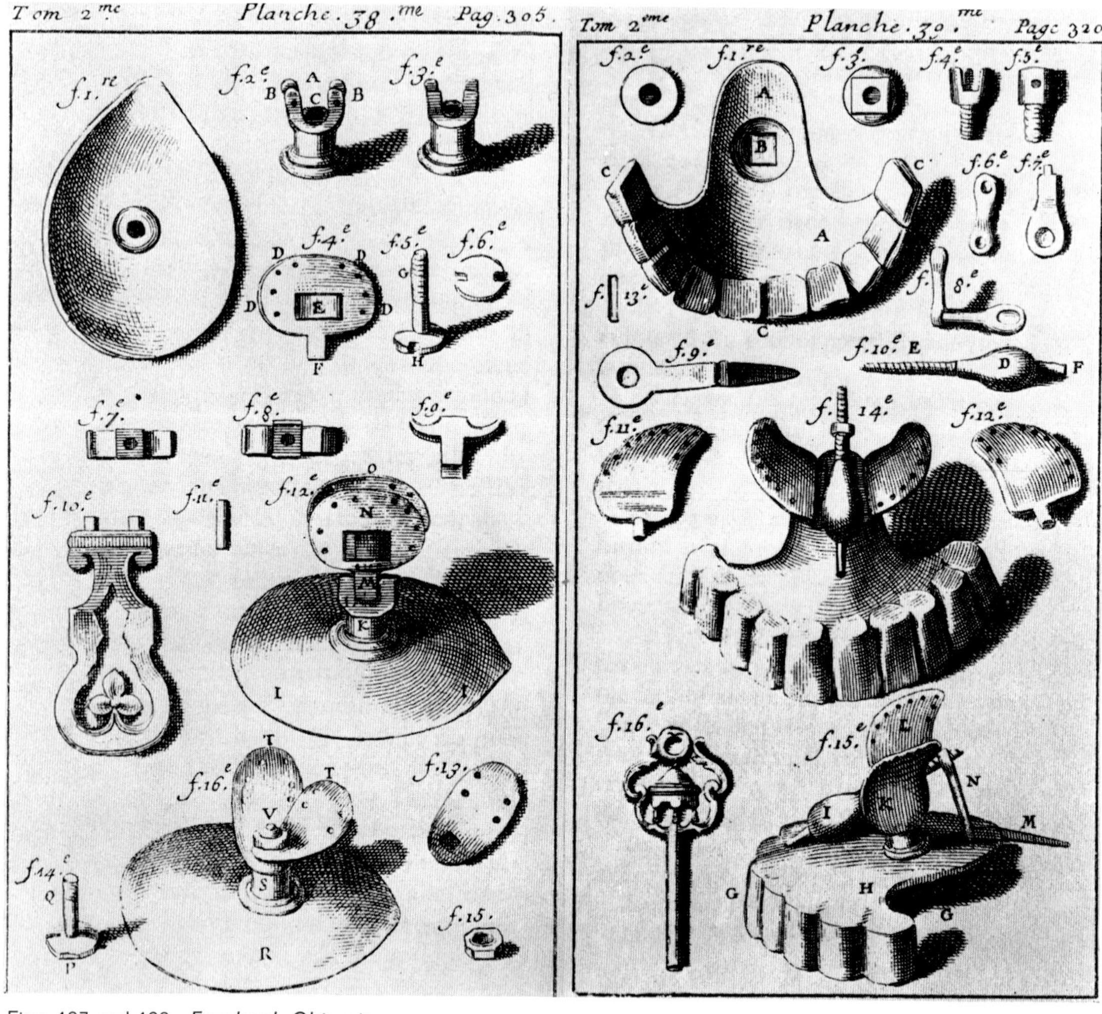

Figs. 197 and 198 *Fauchard: Obturators*

sion still, however, the first attempt, if we disregard Guillemeau's unusable paste[39], to use an inorganic material for artificial teeth comes from him, a step which was, surely, undertaken chiefly for cosmetic reasons. He covered a bone prosthesis with sheets of gold or silver, gave the metal housing thus formed to a skillful enameller, and had teeth and gingiva fired onto it after his markings and a model tooth (Fig. 196, F. 3). The advantages of pieces prepared in this manner are not limited, in his opinion, to better appearance; they are also particularly durable[40]. Fauchard used the drilling engine shown in figure 324 to make dentures, but exclusively for this purpose.

The master also took an interest in the palatal obturator. Since the usual metal plate, fastened by means of a sponge which quickly became fetid considerably and by swelling widened the opening in the course of time, he provided his device with two wings which were inserted through the perforation in a vertically upright position and then brought to a horizontal position by means of a threaded screw. In this manner the apparatus was anchored on the nasal side of the palatal arch, an additional development of the metal obturator of Paré (see Fig. 123). Furthermore, he combined this apparatus, al-

[39] See p. 151
[40] Ibid. (a) II pp. 283 f.; (b) II pp. 248 f.; (c) II pp. 96 f.

ready quite heavy by itself, with a denture (Figs. 197 and 198). Although this was an excellent example of watchmaker's handiwork, it represented no real advance because all physiological factors were disregarded.
In any case, it must be acknowledged that Fauchard, in contrast to the contemporary customs of dentists, did not keep even this complicated construction secret. Rather he published them with drawings that made it possible for anyone to copy his inventions [41].
As Fauchard himself writes in the last chapter he completed the manuscript in 1723 but did not find time to publish it until in 1728. He was accused of having it revised in the meantime by colleagues. Corrections by a Paris surgeon also were found in it, and fault was found for having ended the second edition, in keeping with the times, with a recommendation of his own services. Be that as it may, it is uncontested that this man, highly respected and well-to-do when he died on the 21st of March 1761 in his house in the Rue des Cordeliers, had laid the cornerstone for an independent dentistry, that is, dentistry freed from surgery and from the crowd of quacks and hawkers, even if it was still predominantly empirical. With proud self-assurance, he had two Latin distichs placed under the portrait in his books:
Since Monsieur Fauchard has tried to save the Charm
And Health of Teeth with Wisdom and with Skill,
Mad Fangs of Envy cannot do him Harm,
For his noble Mind has Cures for them as well.
Fauchard's title of dental surgeon ("Chirurgien dentiste"), which he possibly conferred on himself [42], and which is today the customary title for French dentists, may characterize him as a surgeon who, not certified as such by St. Côme, had turned to dentistry. It is therefore that he figures in a register of Parisian dental workers from 1761 handed down to us only as an "Expert," while three stomatologically oriented members of the Cosmas fraternity, that are fullfledged surgeons, were listed as "Maistres en chirurgie" (Fig. 199). In all, there were 30 dental experts in the city, including two women about whom more will be said later.
Fauchard's epochal work initiated a comprehensive body of literature in Paris which then was France. His colleagues suddenly began to reveal their knowledge which until then had been so carefully guarded. Claude Geraudly led this dance of disclosure in 1737 with his little book "L'Art de conserver les dents" (The Art of Conserving Teeth), which was addressed to novices, chiefly to laymen. There is not much that is new to be learned from it. He goes beyond Fauchard when he stipulates that for tooth transplants from man to man both teeth including the one to be removed must still be vital, and that the donor must be between 12 and 15 years old [43]. Unfortunately, we find the customary relapse into the charlatan past at the conclusion of the small volume, where secret medications, elixirs for strengthening and bleaching the teeth are offered for sale with a price list. Nonetheless, his reputation spread as far as the Russian court, whence he was expressly summoned in 1737. *This Empress* (Anna) *had 3000 pounds paid to him for this journey,* reported the *Vossische Zeitung* in Berlin [44].
More important from a scientific viewpoint was Robert Bunon, who settled in Paris after years of travel in the northern part of the country and Flanders. In 1741 he was the first to publish a "Lettre sur la prétendue dent d'œillère" (Letter concerning the so-called eyetooth) in a newspaper in which he contested the connection between the eye and the canine traditional since ancient times. In the subsequent "Dissertation sur un préjugé très pernicieux concernant les maux de dents qui surviennent les femmes grosses" (Discussion of a very damaging Preconception with Regard to Dental Problems of Pregnant Women) he also broke with the superstition that the teeth of pregnant women must not be touched, and thus not treated. It is precisely then that it is often necessary, he states, and Fauchard agrees with him appreciating in the second edition of his work (1746) [45]. Bunon published a compilation of his research in 1743 as "Essay sur les maladies des dents" (An Essay on Dental Diseases), encouraged by the example of two famous "Dentistes" [46], and in 1746 in enlarged edition under the title "Expériences et démonstrations faites à l'Hôpital de la Salpêtrière, et à S. Côme en présence de l'Académie Royale de Chirurgie" (Experiences and Demonstrations in the Hospital of Salpêtrière and St. Côme in the Presence of

[41] Ibid. (a) II pp. 292 f.; (b) II pp. 257 f.; (c) II pp. 99 f.
[42] Ibid. (a) II p. 201; (b) II pp. 188 f.; (c) II pp. 73 f.
[43] Geraudly p. 118
[44] Buchner p. 93; Kowarski p. 8
[45] Fauchard (a) I pp. 59 f.; (c) I p. 21
[46] Bunon (a) p. VI, footnote "MM Fauchard et Geraudly"

6 *Dentistes.*

DENTISTES.

MAISTRES EN CHIRURGIE

Messieurs, BEaupreau, *rue Dauphine.* Dupouy, *rue S. Roch, près celle des P. Champs.* Garre, *rue des Cordeliers.*

EXPERTS.

Messieurs,

Barusseau, *rue de la Jouaillerie.*
Barraud, *rue S. Honoré.*
Bourdet, *rue de l'Arbre-sec.*
Brocart, *près la Barriere des Sergens S. Honoré.*
Chardon, *rue de la Draperie.*
Courtois, Duchemin, *rue des Fossés S. Germain.*
Dumas, *pres la rue des Fondeurs.*
Duverdier, *rue S. André des Arts.*
Fauchard, *rue des Cordeliers.*
Flamand, *rue Dauphine.*
Fontaine, *rue des Fossés Saint Germain.*
Foucou, *rue Ste Marguerite.*
Gaillard, *rue des Fossés Saint Germain.*
Garde, *rue Comtesse d'Artois.*
Hallé de la Touche, *Quai de l'Ecole.*
Herbert, *rue des Fossés Saint Germain.*
Jourdain, *Pont S. Michel*
Laudumiay, *Quai Pelletier.*
Laverne, *Cloitre S. Germain l'Auxerrois.*
Le Monier, *rue Fromenteau.*
Le Roy, *rue de Grenelle Saint Honoré.*
2 Leroux, *Cimétiere S. Jean.*
Mouton, Dentiste du Roi, *rue d'Orléans S. Honoré.*
Quétissant, Perria, *rue du Four S. Germain.*
Senequier, *rue de la Harpe.*
Tubeuf, *Pont Marie.*

Mlles. Calais, *rue de Grenelle S. Honoré.* Hervieux, *rue Geoffroi-l'Asnier.*

Fig. 199 *Register of Parisian "Dentistes" (from Dagen)*

EXPERIENCES ET DEMONSTRATIONS

Faites à l'Hôpital de la Salpêtriere, & à S. Côme en présence de l'Académie Royale de Chirurgie.

Pour servir de suite & de preuves

A L'ESSAI SUR LES MALADIES DES DENTS, &c.

ET UNE

PHARMACIE ODONTALGIQUE, ou Traité des Médicamens, simples & composés propres aux maladies des Dents, & des différentes parties de la bouche, à l'usage des Dentistes.

Par M. BUNON, *Chirurgien Dentiste à Paris.*

A PARIS,

Chez Briasson, rue S. Jacque, à la Science. Chaubert, à l'entrée du Quai des Augustins du côté du Pont S. Michel, à la Renommée & à la Prudence. La Veuve Pissot, à la descente du Pont-Neuf, à la Croix d'or.

M. DCC. XLVI.

Avec Approbation & Privilege du Roi.

Fig. 200 *Bunon: Title page of "Expériences et démonstrations . . . ," 1746*

the Royal Academy of Surgery; Fig. 200), a book of 410 pages [47].

In this latter work Bunon is concerned mainly with the question how tooth decay could be prevented *at the source. . . . I never undertook the extraction of a tooth without regretting the loss of such a useful device (un meuble si utile)* [48]. He recognized enamel hypoplasia as a factor in susceptibility which he designates in accordance with Fauchard as *érosions,* but indicated that he was dissatisfied that the great man had not thought about their origin. Actually, though, in the second edition of his work, which came out simultaneously with Bunon's "Expériences," Fauchard put the blame on measles, smallpox, and malignant fever and quoted the famous surgeon Jean Louis Petit, according to whom *rickets in children (rakitis des enfants),* described by the London physician Francis Glisson in 1650, caused enamel hypoplasia [49].

Petit had also deduced intensified teething problems in children with rickets from the fact that these teeth *with many small points* tear the gingiva which is particularly firm in such children [50].

47 Hoffmann-Axthelm
48 Bunon (b) p. 9
49 Fauchard (a) I pp. 58 f.; (c) I pp. 20 f.
50 Petit (b) pp. 357 f.

In order to clarify this, Bunon conducted a series of researches on the great pool of subjects at the Hôpital général, and then at the Sapêtrière, the hospital for women in Paris, with the support of the First Surgeon to the King, La Peyronie, to whom both books are dedicated. These investigations met with unexpected difficulties on the part of the patients, who feared that their teeth were to be transplanted to rich people or that they had been selected for the colonies. Dental examinations were simply something completely out of the ordinary then. He reported his results before the Surgeons' College of St. Côme and also demonstrated on corpses that children who had suffered from rickets, scurvy, measles, smallpox, and other diseases had erosions on teeth which were still unerupted. Bunon's standing was enhanced by these experiments to such an extent that the royal dentist (to Louis XV), Caperon, recommended him as his successor in this lucrative position in 1748 but Bunon died at the age of 42 in the same year.

In his place, Claude Mouton became the "Dentiste du Roi" in 1757. His "Essay d'Odontotechnie", which was published in 1746, represented the first specialized work on prosthetics. Interesting from the historical perspective of the profession is his long description of a visit to a young, beautiful and aristocratic woman, whose hesitation to have two artificial upper incisors he destroyed. Since similar situations recur not infrequently in contemporary case histories, it can be inferred that the dental practitioners who had become permanent residents pursued their calling in general in the houses of their usually well-to-do patients. Interestingly, these authors seldom neglected to note that they provided their services to the poor free of charge [51].

For Mouton, the dentist is the *Architect of the Mouth,* who ought to pay particular attention to decorative effect, comfort, and durability in his artificial teeth. He especially advocates the use of a dowel crown (*Dent à tenon,* or *pivot*), which requires, however, the highest technical skill for its preparation [52]. The crown of a tooth from a corpse — those from sudden death or accidents are the best — is fitted with a gold pin with a thread wrapped around it; this is inserted into the appropriately prepared root, and held in place by the swelling thread [53]. A short section is devoted to the *inserted tooth,* to the *Dent à coulisse* [54]. This is a false tooth inserted in a gap, where the neighboring teeth are tipped with the cutting edges against each other. It *fits a small spring (un petit ressort) on each side, to hold it firmly.* This might well represent the first mention of a kind of clasp attachment.

Mouton regarded the use of gold as the extravagant luxury of a Midas. Nor does he assume that still so many people would believe today in the golden molar of the Silesian child [55]: *It is known that this skillfull deception was the work of a goldsmith, who wanted to test the sagacity of the curious with a sample of his talent. Here it is suited to recommend a useful procedure, which, although it might be believed to have arisen from these false conceptions, has come to me only after rational consideration* [56].

Even if Mouton denies it, it is not to be ruled out that the knowledge of this miraculous tooth stimulated him to the construction of the first gold crown in the modern sense, and that this object of deception was not quite as lacking in significance for practical dentistry as was partly assumed. Mouton writes as follows about his own design: *I do not believe . . . that there is a more certain means of protecting them* (the teeth) *from this affliction* (abrasion) *than that which I invented and with which I have had complete success. The abraded tooth must be covered with a gold cap (recouvrir . . . d'une calotte d'or), covers the entire surface, and is applied in such a manner that no bits of food can be cought. This method is very advantageous for the great teeth or molars, because they give rise to very intense pain when the tooth is worn away to a point near the nerve, and there is no other means to eliminate these pains outside of sacrificing the tooth* [57]. Its preservation can be assured, however, if it is covered at an early time. The only thing that disturbs him is the golden color, but it is possible to enamel the surface of the premolars (petits molaires) and incisors in natural tooth hues. We learn nothing of a binder of the type of our cements, as yet. — It is to be regretted that

[51] Geraudly p. 159, for example
[52] Mouton p. 42
[53] Ibid. p. 79 f.
[54] Ibid. pp. 107 f
[55] See p. 163
[56] Ibid. pp. 131 f.
[57] Ibid. pp. 137 f.

this book, written for laymen, has no illustrations.

Louis Lecluse (also L'Ecluze and Lecluze)[58] was a scintillating personality, whose activity was divided his entire life between dentistry, the theater, and poetry. In Paris for a decade, until 1747, he was equally successful in acting at the Opera Comique and in working as a dentist; he then accompanied the Marshall of Saxony in this double capacity on five campaigns, practiced and acted in Geneva, from where, in Fernay, he came also in both functions, close to Voltaire who mentioned him in his letters[59]. We find him in Paris again in 1772, where he purchased a theater and became so indebted thereby that he died, it seems, a poor man during the years of the Revolution[60].

He published a summary of his writings devoted to dentistry in 1754 as a book "Nouveaux éléments d'odontologie" (New Elements of Odontology), although *the famous M. Fauchard and the sainted Bunon, as well as others,* (have) *almost exhausted the material*[61]. This book contains an anatomical section, a practical section, and a section devoted to the deciduous teeth. The special oral anatomy, which first came out in 1752, is divided, just as our modern textbooks, into osteological, myological, angiological, neurological, and sarcological parts. More interesting are the anatomical observations in the part entitled "Pratique abrégée du Chirurgien Dentiste" (Abridged Practice . . .), in which he antagonized justifiably Barthélemy Martin, who had maintained that primary teeth had no roots. He then attacks the theories of Geraudly, Bunon, and Fauchard concerning the disappearance of the roots of the deciduous teeth[62], and finally argued with Mouton about the physiology of the digestive process in the mouth.

On the practical side, Lecluse mentions some new tooth removers, for example a *pelican, which M. Garengeot fashioned from the English key (Clef Angloise), and which was improved by me 12 years ago*[63]. Mainly he mentions his own specialized instrument for luxation of the mandibular third molar (he also used it for the maxillary counterparts). This instrument which is adjusted with a bayonet-shaped bending joint is still used today as the "Lecluse," and numerous modern levers operate on its principle (Fig. 201). Point A is applied diagonally between the two last molars, and levers the third molar out when turned with the next-to last tooth as a fulcrum (assuming a relatively normal root configuration). The third section, which was in fact Lecluse's first work in 1750[64], concerns itself with generalities (Traité utile au public . . .), with a wide variety of good suggestions for preservation of the primary teeth, but unfortunately also with high praise for an elixir.

Etienne Bourdet, probably the most significant author after Fauchard, came from Agen in southern France. In Paris he married the daughter of a colleague, and succeeded Mouton as Dentiste du Roi in 1760[65]. His two-volume work, "Recherches et observations sur toutes les parties de l'art du dentiste" (Investigations and Observations on all parts of Dentistry), appeared for the first time in 1757. Numerous editions were printed including some in foreign languages. For example, it was translated into Russian in 1790, constituting the first dental textbook in that tongue. Furthermore, he published several short essays, of which the most well known, "Soins faciles pour la propreté de la bouche . . ." (Easy Means of Keeping the Mouth Clean . . ., of 1759, in German in 1762, and Italian in 1773), was addressed like the small book by Geraudly more to the public than to the specialist[66].

His main work, which Bourdet dedicated to the Academy for Surgery (the Royal Academy, since 1731), is oriented to a great extent in partition and contents to Fauchard, *who had broken the ground so well,* and of whom he says that he was his leader[67]. The whole preface, however, is a defense against the expected reproach *of copying him*[68]. Here we are compelled to take Bourdet's side, because he frequently goes beyond his great model. For example, he justifiably rejects striking the punch with a lead bar, and suggests that a cerebral concussion could be the result[69]. He also believed he could reveal some mistakes of Bunon's with regard to enamel hypoplasia although not in its etiology[70].

[58] See Besombes p. 90; Lecluse pp. 44 f.
[59] Dagen p. 152
[60] Besombes and Dagen pp. 91 f.; Dagen p. 168
[61] Lecluse p. III
[62] Ibid. pp. 101 f. See p. 189
[63] Ibid. p. 139. See p. 191
[64] Böhmecke p. 7
[65] Besombes p. 95
[66] Bourdet (a); (b)
[67] Bourdet (c) I p. VIII
[68] Ibid. I p. XI
[69] Ibid. II pp. 116 f.
[70] Ibid. I p. 84

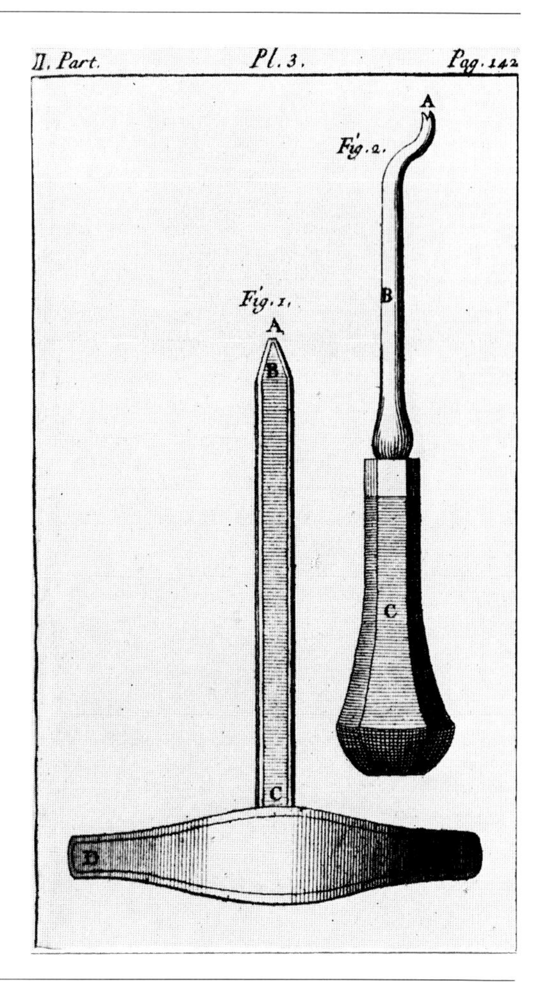

Fig. 201 *Lecluse: Lever (Fig. 1), 1754*

In connection with the origin of caries he is like Fauchard an adherent of the humoral theory: *If the humors which the vessels carry are too thick, they become dammed up and decompose during this stop; soon they attack the tooth*[71]. The formation of abscesses (no longer parulis) is very clearly explained as the result of caries, inflammation of the dental pulp and the periodontal membrane (*perioste qui révête la racine et l'alvéole*)[72]. Contrary to Fauchard, whom he quotes for pages, Bourdet does not regard scurvy as a cause of marginal periodontitis which he unfortunately named *gingival festering (suppuration des gencives)*, but rather as a congestion of the humors which become acidic and corrosive thereby and attack the bones. The therapy consists in minor cases of cleansing and scarification of the gingiva, and in serious ones of inserting a flat cautery *all the way to the bottom of the hollow space between the gingiva and the root of the tooth.* If this is also of no help, then *the gingiva is cut away in a triangular shape on both sides to the depth of the pocket (on coupe la gencive des deux côtés de la poche dans toute son étendue . . . en triangle),* and the root is cleansed which anticipates our contemporary gingivectomy[73].
In the orthodontic chapter, too, which introduces the second volume, Bourdet follows essentially Fauchard's course, which he expands and improves. If the anterior teeth are crowded so that they overlap each other, the first premolars are to be extracted. Then the canines and the incisors are shifted distally,

[71] Ibid. I pp. 95 f.
[72] Ibid. I pp. 249 f.
[73] Ibid. I pp. 288 f.

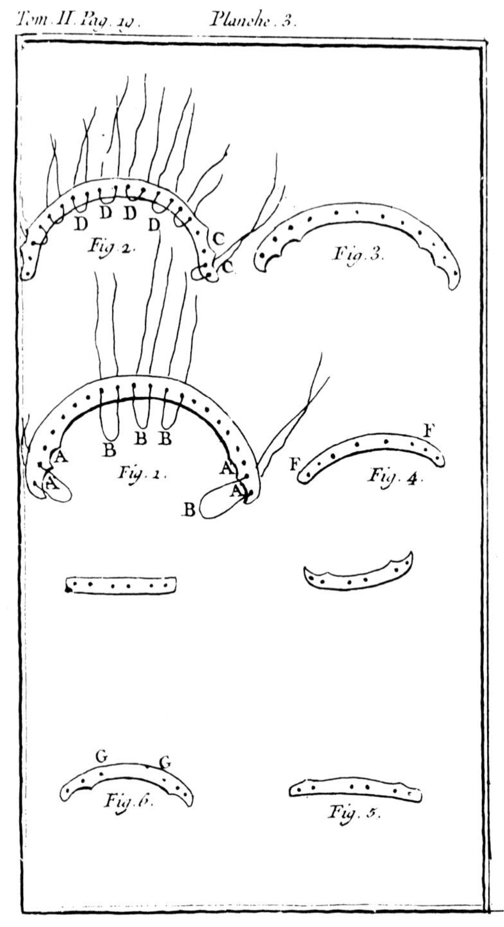

Fig. 202 *Bourdet: Orthodontic devices, 1757*

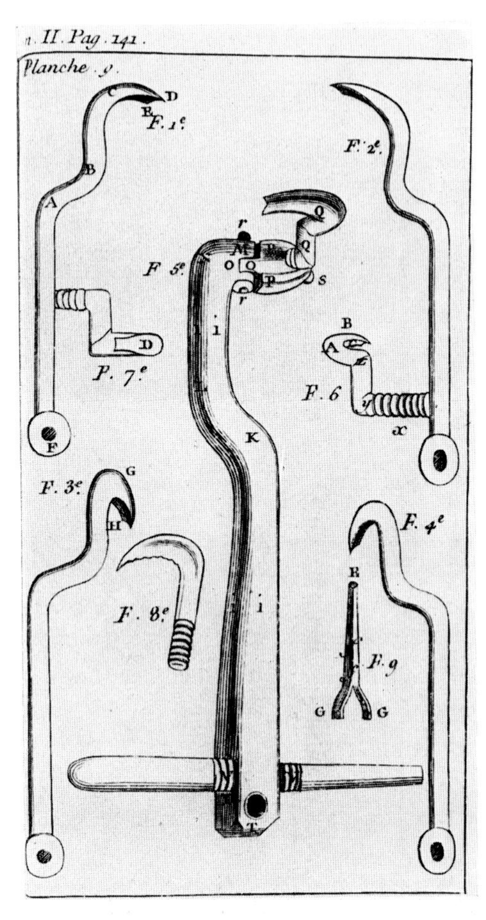

Fig. 203 *Bourdet: Key, "pelican for the upper wisdom teeth," 1757*

one by one, by threads anchored on the first molar and second premolar, and thus rearranged. The bands must not be of silver because it blackens the teeth, but rather of gold. If he used a clasp made of walrus bone, both correctly and incorrectly placed teeth are fastened to it with threads drawn through its holes, and the deviating ones are pulled towards the splint and therewith brought in proper alignment by tightening of the threads twice a week [74].

In this manner he tries to eliminate prognathism: A splint is tied labially to the maxilla and lingually to the mandible which extends to the premolars and fits close to them, while an intermediate space is left in the region of the anterior teeth. Now the maxillary anteriors are systematically pulled towards the lips, and the mandibular teeth toward the tongue until the overbite is corrected [75] (Fig. 202, F. 2).

For Bourdet, too, the "redressement" with the pelican, of course with his own, is the quickest and most reliable means for which room must be made first through filing of the adjoining teeth, actually quite a heroic method. Also noteworthy is his report on a serial extraction in a ten-year-old: of four carious molars two occasionally caused trouble. The parents wanted to have the two painfree teeth filled (plomber), but he recommended the extraction of all four. He was justified by the successful result: the

[74] Ibid. II pp. 6 f.
[75] Ibid. II pp. 15 f.

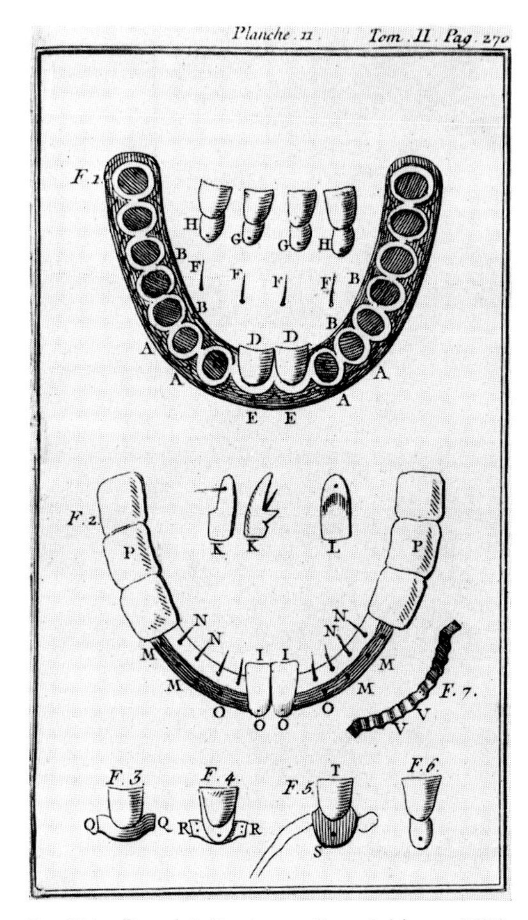

Fig. 204 *Bourdet: Denture with metal base, 1757*

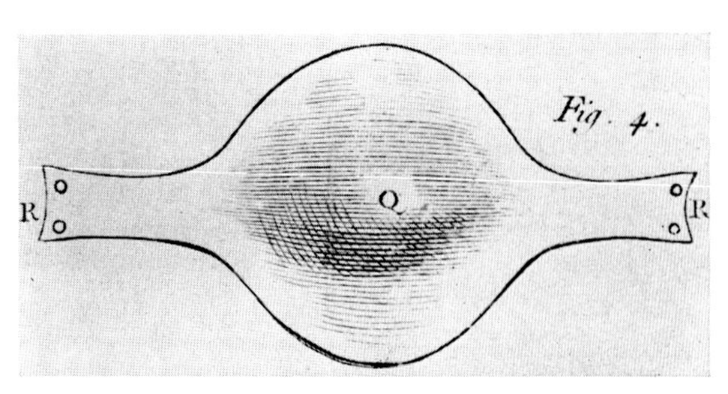

Fig. 205 *Bourdet: Obturator, 1757*

gaps were closed by the second *great molars* [76].

We do not find much that is new in the field of preventive dentistry.—Tooth extraction can be either easy or difficult, depending on the condition of the roots. His specialized pelican for the upper third molars represents an instrument which Lecluse had already mentioned as the English key and which is here given as a picture for the first time [77] (Fig. 203). Bourdet called it variously as "pélican" and "levier." [78]

Unfortunately Bourdet also shows us the complete lack of thought with which tooth transplants were then performed from one person to another. This is seen in his suggestion that, because of the difference in size of the roots, *you should make sure you have several subjects, Savoyards or others, namely, if the tooth of one does not fit, it can be put back in, so that he be not deprived of it, and several others could be tried* [79].

Bourdet's greatest importance is also in the field of prosthetics. Just as Fauchard and Mouton did, he regarded the dowel crown as the best replacement. If there were no more roots available, and if the jaw was extensively

[76] Ibid. II pp. 26 f.
[77] In contrast to Weinberger (p. 320), this is not Bourdet's special pelican, about which he provides a certificate from the Royal Academy for Surgery dated 18. 5. 1753 (Bourdet [c] II p. 137)
[78] Bourdet (c) II pp. 118 f. and p. 141
[79] Ibid. II p. 194; see p. 222

resorbed, he would have a goldsmith make a base of gold (une espèce calotte d'or) with two holes on each end through which the silk customarily used for fastening to the neighboring teeth, can be threaded. In this base, there are small chambers (chatons) like the sockets, into which the shortened roots of the corpse's teeth are inserted. They are here either fastened with a pin (Fig. 204) or cemented with Fauchard's mastix. The finished piece is then enameled, *more or less red, according to the direction given by the Dentiste* [80]. It is noteworthy that the goldsmith prepares the base after a wax model (modèle en cire) as already recommended in the 17th century by Purmann, while the impression method, after a plaster model, published at about the same time (1756) by Pfaff [81] in Berlin, was still unknown in Paris, and remained so for decades. Bourdet correctly believed that his gold base was an improvement over Fauchard's metal capsule. Moreover, he used gold for the springs supporting the upper prosthesis, instead of the steel used by his precursor which was prone to rust [82]. As in other instances he had improved on the model, too.

In the construction of obturators Bourdet went his own way. He was well aware that the complicated apparatuses placed in the nose only widen the defect through pressure on the tissue, and that, on the other hand, without this disturbing factor a certain spontaneous healing occurs after the tertiary syphilitic phase has subsided. Therefore he covered the central perforation orally with a plate that was only slightly larger than the defect. He fitted this with two arms which were fastened by gold threads to two teeth [83] (Fig. 205). So much, then, from the two-volume work which can deservedly take a place alongside Fauchard's, but only for not having come first.

A publication is found in the *Journal de Médecine, Chirurgie, Pharmacie* of 1770 which is probably the first one entirely devoted to periodontal pathosis. It was compiled by the certified Parisian dentist (dentiste reçue à St. Côme) Botot and was entitled "Observations sur la suppuration des gencives" (Observations on Festering of the Gingiva). In it the author differentiates between three forms: suppuration of the gingiva, of the edge of the alveolus, and of the alveolus itself. Etiologically he holds *scurvy and generally all other special maladies* responsible, although *a modern author* — Bourdet is probably meant here — rejects scurvy. Botot regards this, as he takes it, infectious disease as the chief culprit.

In therapy Botot is gratifyingly conservative when he recommends that only hypertrophied and necrotic parts of the gingiva be debrided. Otherwise, he advises that cauterization and incision be foregone, and in their place oral flushing and above all thorough removal of calculus followed by long-term rubbing of the pocket with camphor oil be undertaken. In one of the case histories, we find an interesting observation from a historical point of view, to the effect that Botot was not allowed as dentist to perform bleeding. In another he shows himself still obliged to Galenic terminology when the medial portion of the mandible is spoken of as the *symphysis of the chin* [84]. This does not detract, however, by any means from the importance of the publication. Its therapeutic recommendations are to be evaluated throughout as progressive.

On the other hand, there is hardly anything new brought forth in the book from 1775 by the "Expert-Dentiste à Paris" (again a different title) Honoré-Gaillard Courtois. According to his own statement he wrote it only because of his new pelican (which was completely superfluous) since Fauchard had already presented everything. Nevertheless, he manages to fill 343 pages.

Anselme Jourdain, a native Parisian, was both a brilliant technical writer and also a man of letters, but he too brought little that was new to dental practice. According to a biography of Duval in 1816, Jourdain turned to surgery for philanthropic reasons [85]. After six years of training at the Hôtel Dieu he changed to dentistry and became a student of the multifaceted Lecluse. He devoted himself to anatomical investigations of tooth development, and wrote two essays on the treatment of the maxillary sinuses (in 1761 and 1765). In 1778, his comprehensive "Traité des maladies et des opérations réellement chirurgicales de la bouche..." (Treatise on the Diseases and Surgical Operations of the Mouth ...) came out in two volumes.

80 Ibid. II pp. 233 f.
81 See p. 231
82 Ibid. II pp. 255 f.
83 Ibid. II pp. 278 f.; see Fig. 295
84 Botot
85 Duval

A German translation was printed in Nürnberg in 1784, an English one in Baltimore in 1849, and in Philadelphia in 1851. The first volume of the work of this "Dentiste reçue au Collège de Chirurgie" is devoted to the diseases of the maxilla and the second to those of the mandible. It represents a specialized surgical textbook of the jaw according to the author's education. His often quoted mentor was the surgeon at the Jardin du roi, Antoine Petit.

In the first volume a great deal of space is occupied by the author's specialty, the maxillary sinus, which in his opinion had been therapeutically neglected by surgeons in spite of Heister's admonition[86]. In hundreds of pages all forms of inflammation, cystic and tumorous alterations of the sinuses are presented, but the therapeutic efforts are unsatisfactory for the most part. Still, the classic maxillary sinus operation according to Caldwell and Luc was not known until 1893 and 1894. In the case of a maxillary cyst, which he, like Fauchard, had not yet recognized as a tumor, and therefore identified with the sinus, he ascertained *a kind of crackling (une espèce de craquement)*[86a] which he compared elsewhere with the cracking of eggshells being broken between the fingers. Problems which are purely oral surgical in nature are treated in an appendix as miscellaneous observations, but here Jourdain for the first time quotes the case histories of other physicians, such as those of Fabricius Hildanus, among others. A surprisingly large number of these case histories deal with treatments for toothworm, so that the impression is unavoidable that even the well-read M. Jourdain himself was not completely free of this superstition.

In the second volume, chapter 17, dealing with complications of the eruption of the mandibular third molars is particularly interesting. The author correctly recognizes the cause in a disproportion in size between the teeth and the jaw[87]. We cannot agree, however, with his extracting a third molar from a young girl, using Lecluse's lever (levier de M. Lecluze), in an acute stage, even if the success of the treatment justified him. In another case, during the course of a wisdom tooth extraction, he came upon a large suppurating cyst which was brought to healing in three months with his therapy of packing and cauterizing with different means[88]. M. Jourdain completes the list of French authors of the 18th century. As already mentioned, two female "Experts" are found in the roster of Parisian practitioners from the year 1761 (Fig. 199), in last place. Marie-Madeleine Calais had to fight a hard struggle for recognition: after eight years as a student and an assistant under Geraudly, which incidentally gave her an excuse not to publish his secret medications[89], she passed a brilliant examination before the board of examiners of St. Côme. However, because the surgeons protested the precedent of admitting a woman, La Peyronie, as First Surgeon to the King and also Head Master of the surgeons, supported her with a recommendation with the approval of Parliament. Thus, the first certified female dentist in France was allowed to open a practice in Paris, which she shared, ten years later with a colleague and spouse.

Two Italians, then unregistered, who were working in Paris also had difficulties with the authorities. Of one of these two, Giovanni Batista Ricci, the father of a recognized Parisian dentist, it is recorded that in 1751 on the Pont Neuf he put out for show a calf with five feet and two tails[90]. Otherwise, there is nothing outstanding from their mother country to report about in this century from the Italy once so exciting in medicine. The book of the Florentine dentist Antonio Campani, "Odontologia, ossia trattado sopra i denti" (Odontology, or Treatise on the Teeth), which appeared in 1786, remains the only significant contribution from an Italian pen if we disregard Ruspini in London. Still, not even this beautifully printed work illustrated luxuriously with copper engravings represented any real progress.

In 1782, outside of the French metropolis, even a physician as prominent as Jean-Baptiste Timothée Baumès, then a practitioner in Nîmes and later professor in Montpellier, devoted no less than 350 pages to odontology in his "Traité de la première dentition et des maladies souvent très graves qui en dépendent" (Treatise on first Dentition and the frequently serious Disorders which depend upon it). In this work, which was first printed in Paris in 1806 and translated in New York in 1841, with an abundant knowledge of literature the dental

[85] Jourdain (a) I p. 18; (b) I p. 18
[86a] Ibid. (a) I p. 107
[87] Jourdain (a) II pp. 613 f.; (b) II p. 618
[88] Ibid. (a) II pp. 625 f.; (b) II pp. 655 f.
[89] Geraudly pp. 157 f.
[90] Besombes and Dagen pp. 100 f.; p. 74; p. 81; Guerini

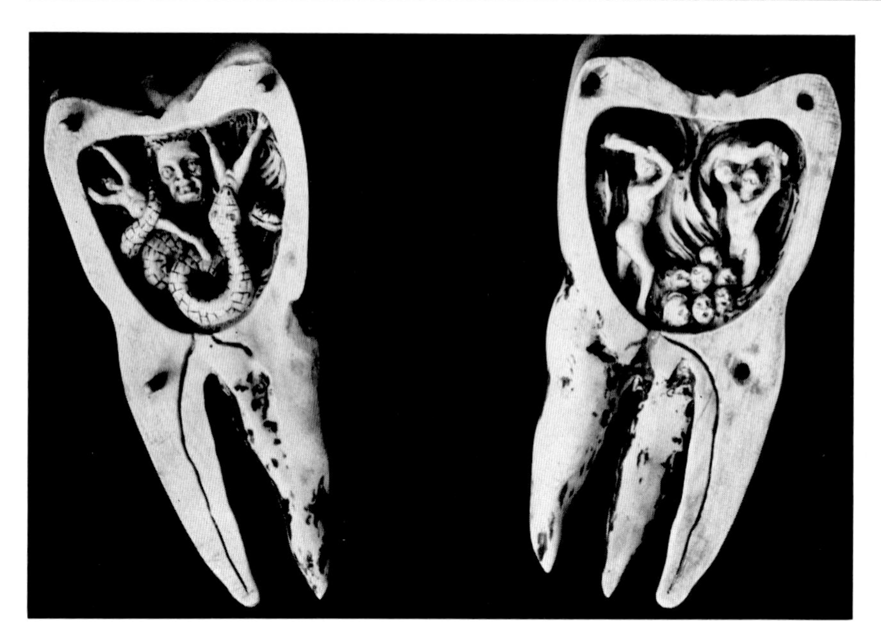

Fig. 206 *The toothworm as tormentor of Hell; ivory carving from the south of France in the 18th century (Forschungsinstitut für Geschichte der Zahnheilkunde, Cologne)*

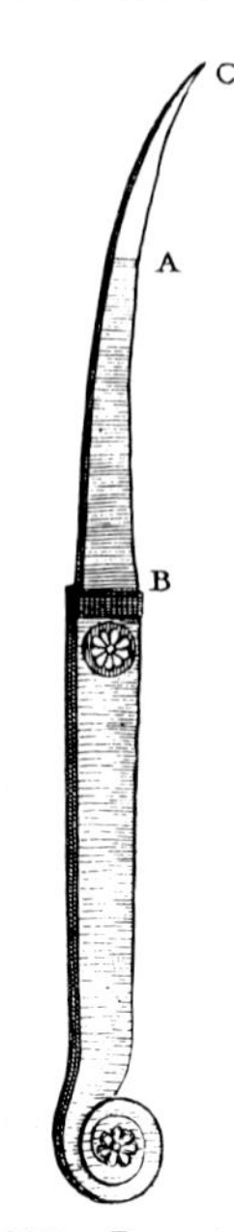

Fig. 207 *Baumès: New scalpel for incising the gingiva, 1782/1806*

authors are singled out for particular attack. Still in the introduction he assails Laforgue as *a man who calls himself an expert-dentiste, certified by the Paris College of Surgery,* for the reason that he rejected eruption as the cause of infant diseases. His Parisian colleague Hébert and even the later member of the academy Duval also receive strong criticism. Baumès perceived the causes of teething trouble as a "mobilité" of the child connected with irritability, salivary flow, and accelerated digestion, among others. Furthermore the incorrect rearing of infants, who are, for example, fed with various broths and mashes instead of being nursed by the mother and, finally, constitutional and nosological factors. He takes van Swieten in Vienna and the surgeon Le Camus sharply to task for not believing in eruption as the cause of cramps and for rejecting splitting of the gingiva with an x-shaped incision to facilitate eruption, inasmuch as Le Camus listed Nicolaas Tulp's irrelevant case as proof of the opposite this attack is justified. Baumès presents comprehensive case histories of incisions, and the only illustration in the book shows a special scalpel for this procedure, which was especially popular in England [90a] (Fig. 207). Thus there is a colorful mixture of the reasonable and the irrelevant in this work which was awarded a prize by the Parisian "Societé royale de Médecine." It is still slightly fettered by the medieval university style, and practical knowledge tends to recede all too often behind theory and quotations.

Great Britain — John Hunter

The emanation from the works originated in Paris by Fauchard and Bourdet very quickly influenced France's European neighbors, particularly the Germans, but also the English, even if it was later and somewhat less obvious.

Joseph Hurlock, a London surgeon, broke the ground for an independent literature in 1742 with quite a misleading opus, "A Practical Treatise upon Dentition; or, the Breeding of Teeth in Children." To establish the necessity for his book, he gave statistical figures on mortality in children, in the introduction with the causes of death allotted to cramps, smallpox, and teeth [91]. In the remaining of the total 285 pages

[90a] Baumès pp. 316 f.; p. 338. See p. 217
[91] Hurlock pp. XV f.

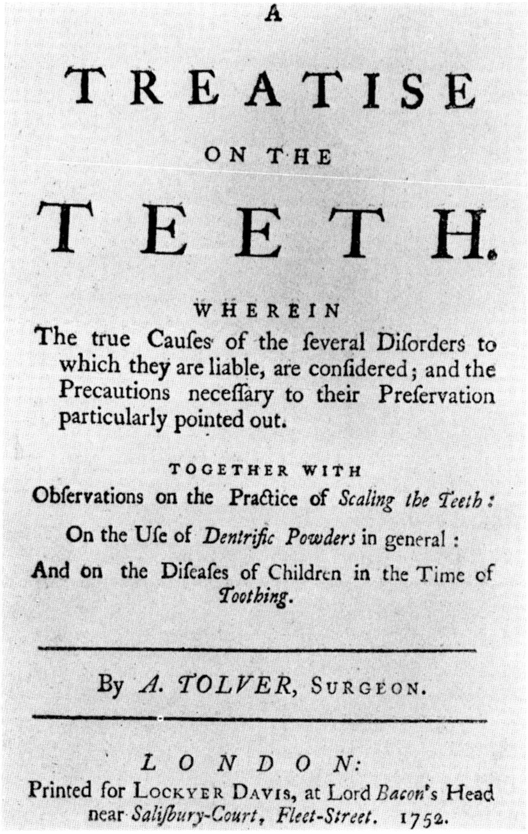

A
TREATISE
ON THE
TEETH.
WHEREIN
The true Caufes of the feveral Diforders to which they are liable, are confidered; and the Precautions neceffary to their Prefervation particularly pointed out.
TOGETHER WITH
Obfervations on the Practice of *Scaling the Teeth*:
On the Ufe of *Dentrific Powders* in general:
And on the Difeafes of Children in the Time of *Toothing*.

By *A. TOLVER*, SURGEON.

LONDON:
Printed for LOCKYER DAVIS, at Lord *Bacon*'s Head near *Salifbury-Court*, *Fleet-Street*. 1752.

Fig. 208 *Title page of Tolver's "Treatise on the teeth," 1752*

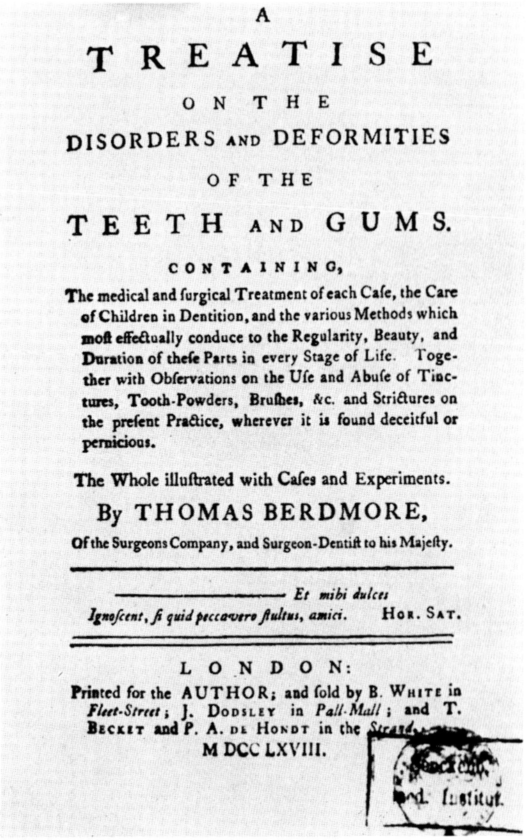

A
TREATISE
ON THE
DISORDERS AND DEFORMITIES
OF THE
TEETH AND GUMS.
CONTAINING,
The medical and furgical Treatment of each Cafe, the Care of Children in Dentition, and the various Methods which moft effectually conduce to the Regularity, Beauty, and Duration of thefe Parts in every Stage of Life. Together with Obfervations on the Ufe and Abufe of Tinctures, Tooth-Powders, Brufhes, &c. and Strictures on the prefent Practice, wherever it is found deceitful or pernicious.
The Whole illuftrated with Cafes and Experiments.
By THOMAS BERDMORE,
Of the Surgeons Company, and Surgeon-Dentift to his Majefty.

Et mihi dulces
Ignofcent, fi quid peccavero ftultus, amici. HOR. SAT.

LONDON:
Printed for the AUTHOR; and fold by B. WHITE in *Fleet-Street*; J. DODSLEY in *Pall-Mall*; and T. BECKET and P. A. DE HONDT in the *Strand*.
M DCC LXVIII.

Fig. 209 *Title page of Berdmore's "Treatise," 1768*

he tries to prove through quotations ranging from Hippocrates to Mercuriale and to his contemporaries Boerhaave and Friedrich Hoffmann, and chiefly from his own case histories, that incising the gingiva above the erupting primary tooth is the only true lifesaving treatment. Presumably as a result of this book, "lancing the gum" remained a typical British specialty until far into the 19th century. Not even the great John Tomes could completely free himself from this prejudice in his textbook which was published in 1859.

The surgeon A. Tolver to the contrary believed, according to his small "Treatise on the Teeth" which appeared in 1752, that healthy children would overcome teething (Fig. 208), and moreover he gave the regulations of Hippocrates which were not quite up-to-date any more [92], and advised the services of an experienced surgeon only for serious cases [93]. He considered tartar a good protection of the cervix of the tooth, a support for the teeth, and therefore recommended maintaining it. Tolver did not believe in the toothworm and suggested, like Fauchard, that doubters take a glance through a microscope. He does not seem to have known the great Frenchman. Apart from the ancient authors Urbain Hemard is the only continental one cited.

The first British dentist to make a significant literary contribution was the court dentist Thomas Berdmore, "Surgeon-Dentist to his Majesty" (Fig. 209), in the 1770 edition "Dentist in ordinary to his Majesty (George III)." This work, which first appeared in 1768 as

[92] See p. 62
[93] Tolver pp. 48 f.

"Treatise on the Disorders and Deformities of the Teeth and the Gums," came out in many editions, and had already been translated into Dutch in 1769, and into German in 1771; it was reprinted in the United States as late as 1844.

We learn from the title page that Berdmore, beside his court duties, was a member of the surgeons' guild. The "Surgeons Company" had annulled the unification with the barbers in 1745 which had been effected under the government of Henry VIII [94]. His predecessor in court office, Samuel Green, had still been a member of the barbers' guild, and had carried the title of "Operator for the teeth," which, as we know from Charles Allen's book, corresponded about to the French "Arracheur de dents," or the German "Zahnbrecher," or the Italian "Cavadenti." [95] The professional designation "dentist" was imported from France, and Berdmore absolutely refused to be categorized as such in the same class with every *Tooth-drawing Barber and itinerant Mountebank.*

Berdmore's presumptuousness is seen in his statement in the preface, that he was not able to list any quotations because he did not know of anyone but a couple of Frenchmen who had only written to make themselves famous, and one or two Englishmen, who had done some highly incomprehensible translations. We know for a fact that the first assertion was not true, but the reason for this attitude may well have been the almost permanent state of war between France and England, which also may explain why hardly any English translations of the great French dentists are known. Thus, Fauchard for example, was first translated into English in 1946, by Lilian Lindsay, the first examined and licensed female dentist (1895) in the British United Kingdom, for historical interest.

From a professional point of view, Berdmore's book is nothing more than a practitioner's essay, setting down his experiences. Toothache is remedied by bleeding and purging [96] and by application of medications such as for example camphor and poppy juice. The painful tooth can also be extracted, cleaned outside of the oral cavity, filled with gold or lead, and re-implanted, although this method can fail [97]. Probably the best method is then still the cautery [98]. In the case of a destroyed crown, a corresponding human tooth should be placed on top of the root. It is important that the "nerve" be destroyed previously and that the post be screwed in, as Bourdet did [99]. He recognizes his limits in serious cases, and advises referral to a surgeon. The toothworm is strictly rejected. Four methods of straightening irregular teeth are given: gold or silk threads attached to the neighboring teeth, a resilient leaf of gold forced adjustment, and filing down, this latter, however, only for aged persons. He regards the first method as the best, carried out between the ages of 7 and 12 years, *whilst the Teeth are growing, and the sockets in a condition to yield by degrees to any constant pressure* [100].

The last chapter is devoted completely to artificial teeth which, when made of bone or ivory, quickly discolor, but which can be made of more durable material. We do not learn what this is. Presumably it is hippopotamus tusk. Otherwise Berdmore also seems consciously to avoid going into detail in this area, including his intimation of knowledge about springs as retainers for complete upper dentures. Thus, this book too, in spite of all the strong words against tooth-drawers and quacks, ends with a relapse into the charlatan past. Here especially, we learn to appreciate Fauchard's openness. On the other hand, it should be noted on the positive side that Berdmore strictly rejects tooth transplants [101].

In 1768, the same year when Berdmore's book came out, an Italian working in London, Bartholomew Ruspini, published his "Treatise on the Teeth." He was born in Bergamo, trained there as a surgeon and in Paris under the court dentist Caperon, came to Bath in Britain in 1759, and settled in London in 1766. There he maintained a brilliant practice, played a highly respected social role as a freemason, and became the founder of a Masonic orphanage that still exists [102] (Fig. 210). Although there is hardly a single new idea to be found in it his work underwent another edition in the same year it came out. Eleven others followed during the years until 1797. It should be mentioned that Ruspini regarded periodontal atrophy as a caries of the socket, which destroys it much like the roots of the primary teeth. The causes lie in congestion of humors in the gums

[94] See p. 155
[95] Lindsay; Matheson
[96] Berdmore (a) p. 40; (b) p. 28
[97] Ibid. (a) pp. 98 f.; (b) pp. 68 f.
[98] Ibid. (a) p. 152; (b) p. 104
[99] Ibid. (a) p. 154 f.; (b) p. 105
[100] Ibid. (a) pp. 217 f.; (b) p. 146 f.
[101] Ibid. (a) pp. 101 f.; (b) pp. 70 f.
[102] Campell pp. 51 f.

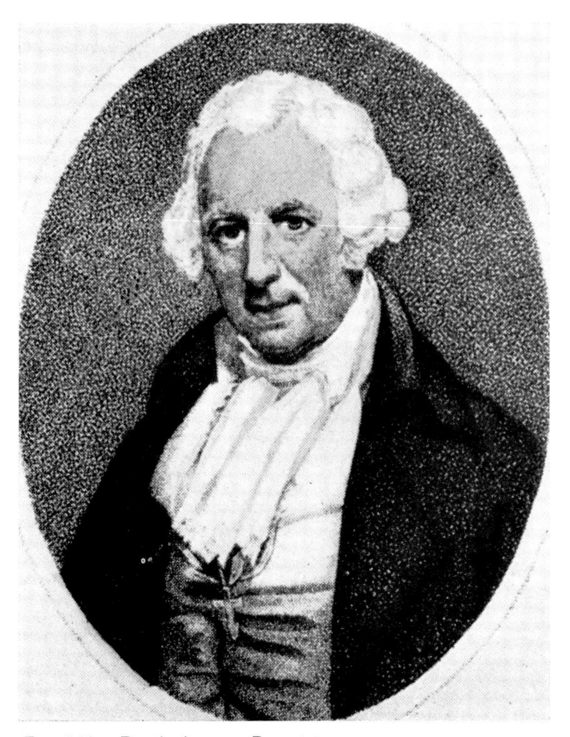

Fig. 210 *Bartholomew Ruspini*

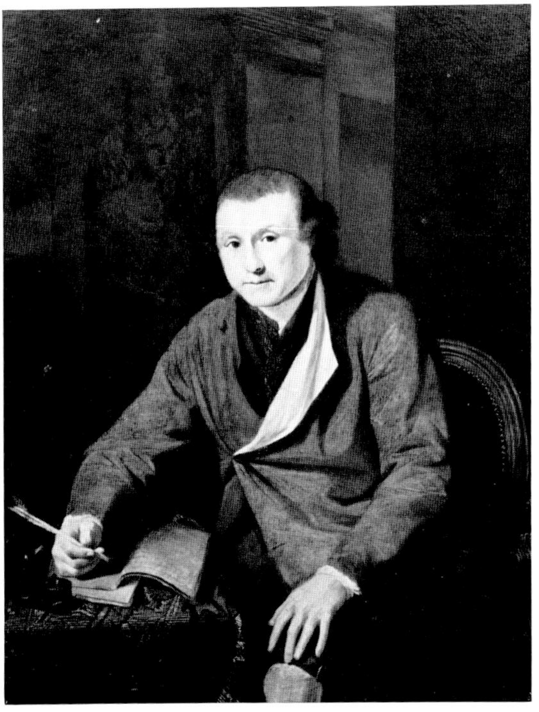

Fig. 211 *John Hunter, oil painting, approximately 1771, the year of publication of "Natural History of Teeth" and of his marriage to Ann Home; painted by his brother-in-law, Robert Home (Royal College of Surgeons, London)*

and in precipitating caustic particles which penetrate into it[103]. Six additional case histories were appended to later editions (we refer here to the second one from 1768)[104].

In the *Medizinisch-chirurgische Zeitung* from 1804, which came out in Salzburg, we find an anonymous report on the invention of a dental mirror, a double mirror which seems to have had little similarity to its modern descendant, particularly since it was intended for the patient only: *The Chevalier Ruspini, dentist to the Prince of Wales, has invented an instrument, by means of which every person can see his own teeth, inside and out, as well as a dentist can . . . The so-called instrument consists of two small elliptical mirrors. One is held between the teeth, and the other in front of them . . . The item is completely new, and therefore the price is as yet unknown . . .*

While the 18th century saw significant advances in France and in German-speaking areas in the fields of dental surgery and prosthetics, England provided a highly important contribution to anatomy through John Hunter's "The Natural History of the Human Teeth." It was by this work that the great anatomist and surgeon based his fame. When he came as a twenty-year-old from his native Scotland to London, he was initiated into anatomy by his already respected brother William and taught himself surgery, which he elevated, as he rose to a position of high honor, from a trade in England to a discipline on a par with internal medicine (Fig. 211).

Hunter's first work appeared in 1771 and was repeatedly reprinted until 1841 in almost all European languages. In it he created a modern anatomy of the teeth and jaws with which

103 Ruspini pp. 83 f.
104 Smitt

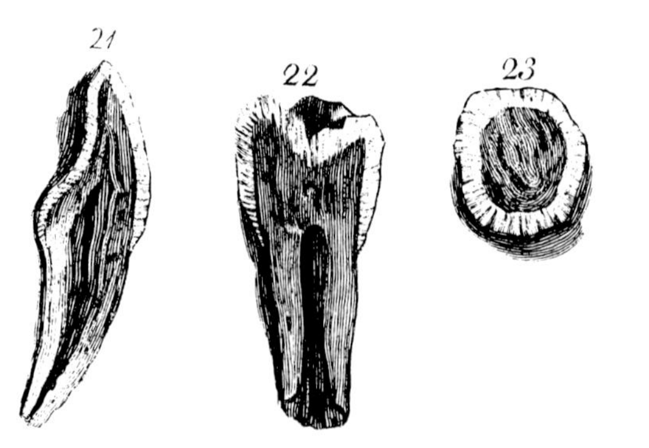

Fig. 212 *Hunter: Tooth sections with exposition of the Hunter-Schreger bands, 1771*

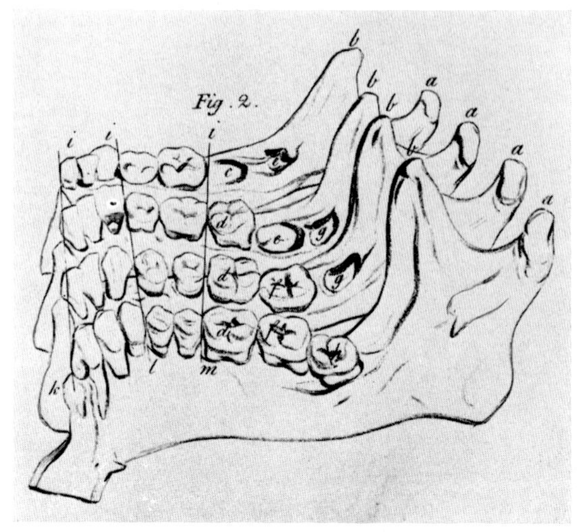

Fig. 213 *Hunter: The growth of the mandible in relation to the size of the teeth*

he opened a scientific path to the previously empirically oriented dentistry, even if his own involvement with the subject was only an episode. The new designations "Cuspidati" and "Bicuspidati" are introduced for the canines and the premolars. Enamel and dentin are described of course, but are not yet differentiated from cement; as are the Hunter-Schreger bands in the enamel, named after the author, which are caused by enamel prisms (as yet unknown) but had already been recognized by others [105] and made pictures of (Fig. 212). Vessels he did not find in the enamel.

Hunter takes a stand against the old concept of constant growth of the teeth and explained the apparent increase in width by tooth migration to which he devoted a great deal of thought. Also, knowledge of the curve of Spee of the mandibular teeth, which was first described in 1890, is indicated [106]. The growth of the mandible in relation to the teeth is demonstrated very clearly through four jaw specimens of different ages side by side (Fig. 213).

The "Practical Treatise on the Diseases of the Teeth," which followed in 1778, and in which he unfortunately supports incision of the gingiva when there are complications in eruption *as far as my experience has taught me* [107], is not as significant as the anatomical work. John Hunter was still a general surgeon and had to obtain his specialized knowledge from the London dentist James Spence, for which his critics reproached him. Later he assisted Spence to the position of personal dentist to George III [108]. For this reason we also learn little that is new about preservation of the teeth. If toothache is to be eliminated while the tooth is to be preserved, then cauterizing agents, an acid or an alkali, must be applied as far as into the tip of the root in order to destroy the soft portions in which the pain lodges. But that is very difficult [109]. We do not learn anything about the fate of the mortified tissue. He observed on removed roots *a pulpy substance,* that is granuloma, which he interpreted as the beginning of dental abscesses [110].

Periodontal infections are minutely described in two chapters of which one is devoted to diseases of the alveolar process and the other one to those of the gingiva. The symptoms of periodontal atrophy and marginal periodontitis, as well as those of gingival inflammation, which was regarded as scurvy, were surely described in

[105] Hunter (a) p. 23; (c) p. 37. See Figs. 153, 159, and 495
[106] Hunter (a) p. 111; (c) pp. 117 f. See p. 271
[107] Ibid. (b) pp. 121 f.; (c) pp. 266 f.
[108] Campbell p. 91
[109] Hunter (b) pp. 17 f.; (c) pp. 162 f.
[110] Ibid. p. 23; (c) p. 168

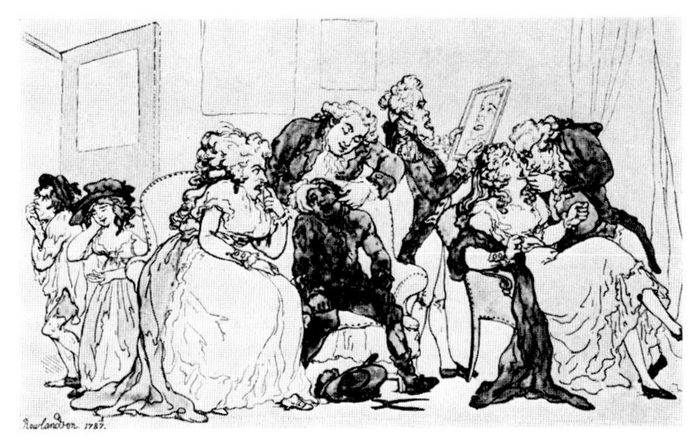

Fig. 214 *"Transplanting of Teeth," engraving by Thomas Rowlandson, 1787*

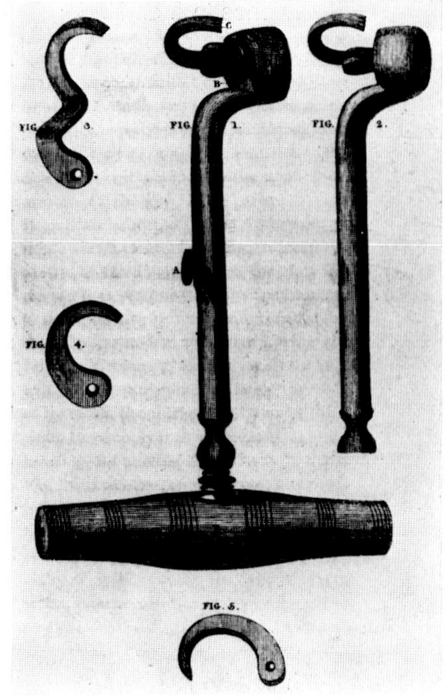

Fig. 215 *Bell: Keys, 1786*

detail but were not clearly differentiated. Hunter suspects that the alveolar abscess is the result of lack of a *perfect harmony* [111] between tooth and alveolar process, which causes an irritation similar to that which makes the tooth fall out. The solution is to eliminate this irritation, which he attempted to do, allegedly with success, through extraction of a loosening tooth and implantation of another tooth. He considers as further causes of alveolar abscesses inflammation and scurvy: *This is most remarkable in the scurvy of sea . . . How far these diseases can be prevented and cured, is, I believe, not known* [112]. His therapeutic suggestions are scarification, shortening with a file of teeth which have become too long, and rinsing with tinctures of myrrh and cinchona bark, as also with seawater.

According to the rather unclear description, various things can be meant by a *thickening of the gum . . . of a hard callous nature:* an epulis (because it recurrs easily and bleeds massively), fibromatosis of the gingiva, or *they really have a cancerous disposition; . . . But here the skill of the surgeon, rather than that of Dentist is required* [113].

Hunter pays special attention to malocclusion, the theoretical base of which he clearly recognizes: *This principle, is the power which many parts (especially bones) have of mouving out of the way of mechanical pressure* [114]. Accordingly, it probably would be possible to shift a tooth to any desired position in the mouth. This works best, however, at a young age. Clear guidelines are given for extraction therapy, but the mechanical measures, on the other hand, which were probably taken from Fauchard (plates of silver), are described in such a hazy fashion that they seem to have no base in practical experience. The recommendation that a cross-bar be applied between the canines for expansion of the maxilla might also be a mere intellectual play of ideas. On the other hand, the positioning of the upper front teeth

[111] Ibid. (b) pp. 49 f.; (c) pp. 193 f.
[112] Ibid. (b) p. 51; (c) pp. 195 f.
[113] Ibid. (b) pp. 59 f.; (c) pp. 202 f.
[114] Ibid. (b) p. 75; (c) p. 218

over the lower ones in a small degree of mesial occlusion through the application on an *inclined plane* fastened to the mandibular incisors is very clearly described in the subsequent chapter 8.
Hunter, the general surgeon, does not regard tooth extraction as a particularly difficult procedure. Just as we are to read in Heister he justifiably advised against extraction during the acute stage [115]. He also dismissed the customary separation of the gingiva as superfluous, but otherwise does not discuss the technique.
A great deal of space is reserved for the transplantation of teeth (Scion tooth) from one person to another as this poor method of tooth replacement was still customary in England in the 18th century. Later critics justifiably take exception to the fact of Hunter's assertion that it would be impossible *to transplant an infection of any kind from the circulating juices,* a dangerous error with regard to the transmission of syphilis. Actually he forbids the procedure to patients who have been treated with mercury, but only as a precaution against the gingival affections which can be induced thereby. Because of possible differences in the length of the roots Hunter imperturbably gives the same advice as Bourdet: *The best remedy is to have several people ready whose teeth in appearance are fit, for if the first will not answer the second may.* — The execution of the operation he leaves to the dentist, but he advises him [116]. The fact that Rowlandson, with whom we are already familiar, had recorded this operation in a picture, also speaks for the popularity of tooth transplants in England (Fig. 214). We can recognize the well-to-do recipient in the bright light, while the poor victim suffers in the shadows.
Benjamin Bell, an important surgeon who like Hunter came from Scotland, practiced until his death in his native Edinburgh. He broadened his education at numerous continental universities, chiefly in Paris. His major work, the six-volume "System of Surgery," was printed in seven editions and was translated into German and French. In the fourth volume, which came out in 1786, far more than a hundred pages and many illustrations were devoted to dental problems; these, however, in contrast to Hunter, are discussed on the base of his own wide personal experience. Bell, too, recommends the splitting of the gingiva to the tooth-bud, which was so intensively propagated by Hurlock for complications of eruption [117]. With regard to epulis he observes the different consistencies and also describes the pedicled fibroma. Like the ancient Paulos of Aigina [118], he elevates tumors with a (double tined) hook and separates them sharply [119].
In Benjamin Bell we find the first British description of the key, which he claims as being English [120]. The claw is placed over the tooth, and the heel, wrapped in linen, is supported on the gingiva (Fig. 215). With this arrangement firmly rooted teeth are luxated alternately to the outside and to the inside, which naturally never ensues without contusions. In principle the claw should be applied to the spot where the tooth is the least destroyed [121]. Roots, on the other hand, are removed with forceps or a lever. With regard to tooth transplants, of which he speaks with enthusiasm, Bell is not as unconcerned about the transmission of disease as Hunter whom he criticizes here: *I am not, however, of opinion with those who think that diseases cannot be communicated in this manner.* Teeth should not, therefore, be taken from persons who appear to be sick. *And . . . every risk of infection being conveyed in this manner, the tooth to be transplanted should be immersed in lukewarm water and should afterwards be entirely cleared of any blood or matter that may adheare to it, by rubbing it gently between the plies* (sic) *of a piece of soft old linen* [122].

Germany — Philipp Pfaff

The beginning of the real history of dentistry came, as we have stated in Paris of the 18th century, at least from a literary perspective. In German-speaking areas, in the theoretically still existing Holy Roman Empire of the German Nation, the starting point was about the same as in France. Indeed, the first book at all devoted especially to the subject, the "Artzney Buchlein" of 1530, was printed in German. Otherwise, however, the actual practice was as usual the concern of itinerant tooth-breakers and the surgeons.
The most popular of these travelling surgeons, both then and now, is Johann Andreas

[115] Ibid. (b) pp. 87 f.; (c) pp. 231 f.
[116] Ibid. (b) pp. 94 f.; (c) pp. 238 f. See p. 213
[117] Bell p. 192
[118] See p. 81
[119] Ibid. p. 228
[120] See pp. 191 and 240 f.
[121] Ibid. pp. 276 f.
[122] Ibid. pp. 323 f.

Eisenbart, who was not unimportant from a professional point of view. He roamed through the German countries for 40 years with a retinue of assistants, conjurors, comedians, and *servants in red livery, adorned with silver.* His residence was in Magdeburg, where, as a Prussian citizen, he possessed a stately patrician house. Moreover, he was among other things a royal Court Councillor which was certainly more a question to King Frederick's II thrifty father of the required payment of 200 Taler than of scientific merit[123]. In an "Announcement" which is handed down he also recommends himself for *an immediate end to wobbly teeth / and toothache as well / and for insertion and removal of artificial teeth.* He probably left this area in general to a tooth-drawer in his retinue, while he devoted himself, not without success, to operations for cataracts, hernias, and bladder stones. The surgeon Heister quotes these procedures repeatedly in his "Wahrnehmungen" (Perceptions)[124].

In Germany, as in England, the fledgling dentistry was not able to detach itself very quickly in literature from its mother, surgery. Thus for the first half of the century, it was represented chiefly by the most important German surgeon of his time, the physician Lorenz Heister, in the special chapters of his surgery books.

As the son of a wealthy wine merchant and tavern-keeper in Frankfurt am Main, Heister was raised carefully, and had early opportunities in that city of commerce and fairs to observe the travelling surgeons performing their cures. Even the famous Eisenbart stayed at his father's tavern twice, in 1701 and 1702 as is traceable. After his studies in Giessen Heister went to Holland, where he came into contact with the clinician Boerhaave in Leyden, and in Amsterdam he worked with Frederik Ruysch, the anatomist and surgeon, and also with the surgeon Johann Jacob Rau.

Both were concerned with odontological problems: Ruysch published results of research on senile atrophy of the ridge of the jaw in 1691, and ascertained that the loosening of the teeth which results from it is not alleviated by any remedies for scurvy[125] (Fig. 216). Rau, the other teacher, was awarded his degree in 1694 in Leyden on the thesis, "De ortu et regeneratione dentium" (On the Origin and Regeneration of the Teeth). In this dissertation, the so-called secretion theory of tooth formation (which appeared later in Raschkow and Magitot)[126] is mentioned: a fluid secreted by the glands which form the teeth (succus dentificus) flows between the lamellae of the (tooth-)membrane, and coagulates there in the directed form[127].

In 1709, Heister followed the Dutch banner as Senior Medical Officer into the War of the Spanish Succession, and had sufficient opportunity to put his surgical knowledge to work in the greatest battle of the century, at Malplaquet. In 1710, after a journey to England for study, he answered a call to the Nürnberg Altdorf University, where he acted for a decade as an academic physician, anatomist, and surgeon. In 1720 he went to the then important Helmstedt University, and died there at the age of 75 as a highly respected man (Fig. 217).

Heister's most important works had already been written when he left Altdorf. The title of his first, "Dissertatio anatomico-physiologica de masticatione" (Anatomical-physiological Dissertation on Mastication), which was completed in 1711, proves his interest in stomatology. The anatomy and particularly the physiology of the masticatory musculature are thoroughly discussed in 36 pages, and explained by diagrams (Fig. 218). Figure 2, for example, shows how the digastric muscle functions: E is the origin at the mastoid process, H the loop round the hyoid bone, and F the insertion at the mandible. The plate AA symbolizes the body of the mandible, with the articular processes BB and the cheeks CC as ropes.

The description of the dental system in the "Compendium anatomicum," which first appeared in 1717, provides little new material. More important to us is the "Chirurgie," printed in the following year, reissued again and again, and translated into almost all European languages. In the second part of this work, which comprises 856 pages, seven chapters describe "Operations on the teeth," and three others present "Operations which involve the gingiva." If there is trismus, Heister advises that the causative wound be treated first, and, if necessary, even that the injured arm or leg be amputated. As a military surgeon he thinks essentially of a tetanus

[123] Buchner p. 10
[124] Brethauer
[125] Ruyschius 87, pp. 104 f.
[126] See pp. 393 f.
[127] Rau Thes. 15 and 16

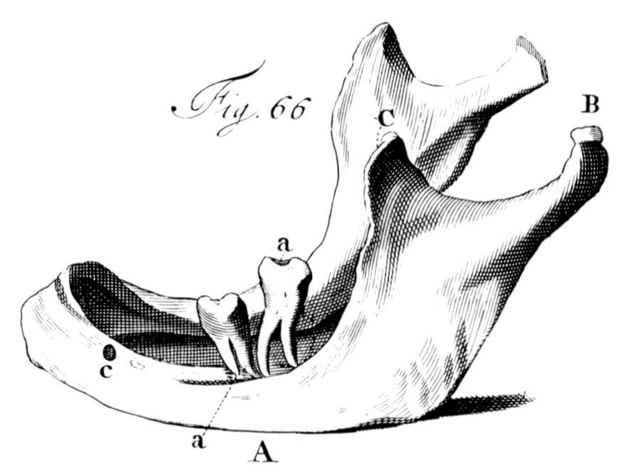

Fig. 216 *Ruysch: Senile atrophy of the mandible, 1694*

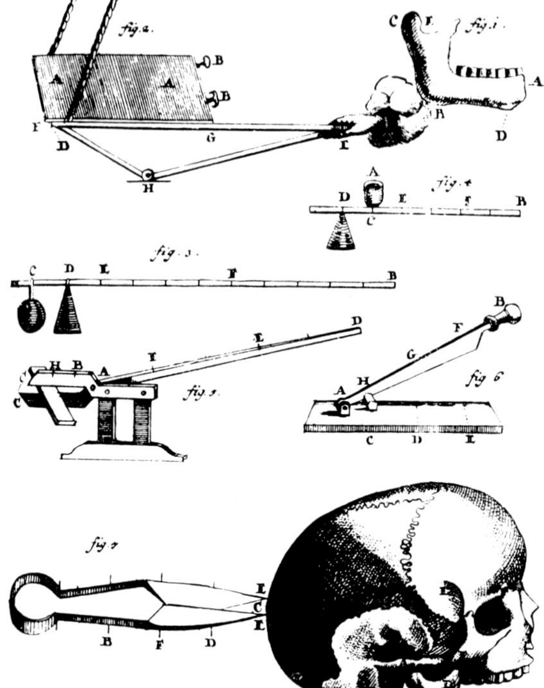

Fig. 218 *Heister: Schematic drawing of the mode of action of the chewing muscles, 1711*

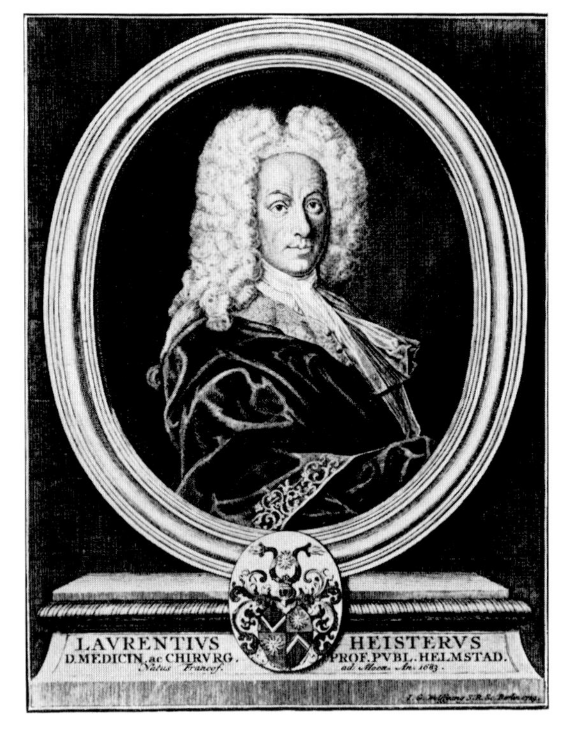
LAVRENTIVS HEISTERVS
D.MEDICIN. ac CHIRVRG. PROF.PVBL.HELMSTAD.
Natus Francof. ad Moen. An. 1683.

Fig. 217 *Lorenz Heister, 1729 (copper plate etching by J. G. Wolfgang in "Institutiones chirurgicae," 1750*

infection, not of the most frequent cause, complications in the eruption of the mandibular third molar. In this case the teeth should not, as Dionis writes, be struck out, or *the teeth forced apart with special instruments,* in order to feed the patient. He can, which is actually true, suck broth between the teeth. *Such instruments tend to be called mouth screws, many types of which are described and illustrated by the Autoribus.* The mouth-opener shown in figure 219 corresponds to the eponymic instrument which is still present nowadays in many instrument cabinets and anesthetic sets. It is especially interesting to us that Heister did not claim the authorship for it, and also advises against vigorous use of Heister's mouth gag: *I maintain,*

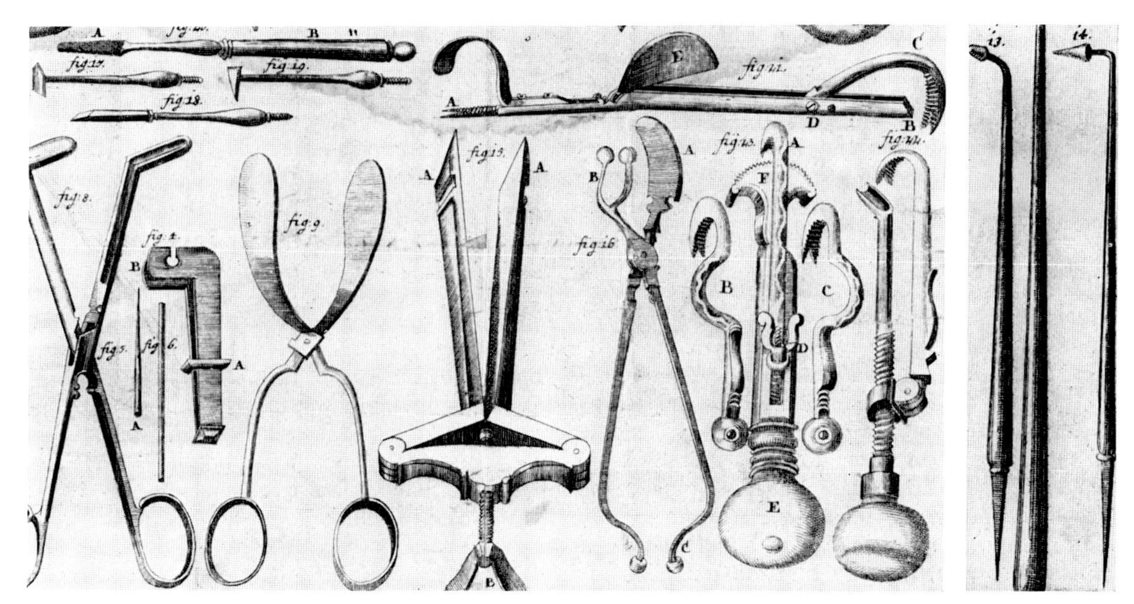

Fig. 219 *Heister: Jaw screw (Fig. 15), calculus remover (Figs. 17-19), dental file (Fig. 20), pelicans (Figs. 21-23), 1724*

Fig. 220 *Heister: Cautery, 1724*

however, that through the great power of this screw great pain must necessarily be caused when there is inflammation or cramps of the muscles, and subsequently even more intense cramps or inflammation must be the result[128]. The instrument is advised for procedures within the oral cavity, for which a long and wide opening is required.

Scalers are described and pictured (Fig. 219), and he warns against corrosive dentifrices, chiefly, however, against vitriol spirits: *Otherwise, however, it is considered the best manner / of maintaining the teeth healthy and clean / to clean them out well in the morning, afternoon, and night after meals, each time with fresh water and the fingers, and at the same time to use a mild tooth powder once every eight or fourteen days*[129]. Hollow teeth should be filled with white wax — Dionis had been translated by him — but this should constantly be renewed. Better yet are finely cut pieces of gold and lead leaf: *Or if a small piece of lead is carved in the shape of the hole, and this is strongly forced into it, then this remains longer and better than the small leaves, and also provides protection against toothaches.* Against pain oil of cloves, which is still useful to us today, is used or acid cauterization or *a fine cautery suitable for this purpose* (Fig. 220), *applied red-hot to the hollowness of the tooth*[130]. He also mentions cauterization of the antitragus because it was described by Nuck, Solingen, and others but as an enlightened man he believed that *such an effect derives from shock and fear, and one pain is displaced by another: similarly toothaches sometimes disappear from people when they see the instruments for tooth extraction*[131]. There are five indications for this procedure: loose primary teeth; congenital teeth if they are a hindrance to nursing; intensely painful teeth, when other means have failed; and teeth which are cosmetically disturbing or fistulous. *If, therefore, a tooth must be pulled out, the Chirurgus should have the patient sit on a low chair or on the ground, if the tooth to be extracted is in the lowermost jaw; if it is in the uppermost jaw, he can have him sit on a high chair or bed*[132]. Thus, we have here no longer the principally low seat as otherwise found with German surgeons, nor exclusively the high one as required by Fauchard[133].

128 Heister (b) p. 558
129 Ibid. p. 560
130 Ibid. p. 561
131 Ibid. p. 537
132 Ibid. p. 563
133 See p. 199

Extraction should never be performed *if there is swelling or inflammation present,* a maxim which even today, in the age of antibiotics, is by no means outdated.

In 1718 in "On Inserting Teeth" there is nothing new reported: *Ivory and sea-horse teeth* serve as materials; . . .*these continue to adhere by themselves, because of their shape;* they remain, therefore, through a clamping effect, or are fastened by silk threads or gold wires. The substitute should be removed and cleaned at night so that it does not quickly decay and become black [134]. In a later work of Heister, the revised third edition from 1755 (according to the preface) of the "Small Surgery," more precise directions are to be found: *The shape, or model, is formed with wax pressed into the hollow, to be similar to the other teeth; and when the thickness and length are obtained in wax, a piece of exactly the same size is sawed from ivory, walrus teeth, or well-bleached ox-bone, which is filed afterwards with a rasp and file, precisely according to the wax impression, in the same size, so that it accurately fills out the gap left by the lost tooth, and it is afterwards made fast to the nearest teeth with silken, silver, or golden threads.* If an entire set of teeth is to be replaced, the teeth must be *differentiated by a fine filed-in groove* [135]. As with Purmann [136] we have here the preparation of a wax model, though, for the first time, an impression is mentioned. On the same page there is a footnote in connection with the description of tooth extraction which refers to settled dentists: *In places where several talented dentists are available, the surgeons are usually glad to put it in their hands.*

In his booklet "Der bey dem Aderlassen und Zahn-ausziehen sicher-geschwindt-glücklich und recht qualificirte Candidatus chirurgiae und Barbiergeselle" (The Journeyman Barber and quite qualified Candidatus chirurgiae who is safe, swift and successful in Bleeding and Tooth Extraction), which was published in 1717, Ludwig Cron, a less prominent court surgeon acting in Thuringia, turned against Dionis' conception (he calls him Dion) that tooth extraction is not worthy work for a surgeon. He maintains that the opposite is the case, pointing out that the well-educated Cornelius a Soling in The Hague had pulled many teeth. After an abundance of case histories, derived in part from his wide knowledge of literature, he comes to the procedural technique [137]. Just as Hemard had done 133 years before, he expressly rejects the loosening of the gingiva before the extraction, which was required since antiquity, as unnecessary torture. Incidentally, the dentists at the markets also refrained from doing this. In principle the patient sits on a cushion on the ground in front of him and wraps his arm of the afflicted side *around the dentist's thigh under the knee* (Fig. 221). The dentist pulls from the right side with his right hand, and from the left with his left. The support surface of the pelican is wrapped in a handkerchief, and the forceps must not be applied to the vitreous parts, but rather to the root, or else the crown will break off. Besides these instruments he recommends the lever, *with which few barbers or surgeons* (are) *familiar.*

The book by the middle German Christoph von Hellwig, which was published in 1732 under the pseudonym Valentin Kräutermann and which contained 220 pages devoted to the eyes and 68 to the teeth, is on a considerably lower level (Fig. 222). In it the junk apothecary and superstitions are revived, and the toothworm and tree frog fat are also to be found. Remedies for toothache include poking with a piece of wood *into which the thunder has hit,* or with *the ossicle from the right hip of a toad, denuded of all flesh,* and also *Transplantation:* a splinter is taken from under the bark of a young tree, and is poked into the painful tooth until bleeding begins. Then the bloody splinter is replaced and a red string is tied around the trunk. *The side of the tree where the cut takes place must face towards evening, and the operator should turn his countenance toward sunrise* [138]. With regard to *Taking Out* of teeth, we find nothing new, and in replacing teeth the dental artist should work with walrus teeth instead of ivory, because the former stays white.

Let us turn from Kräutermann to a shining light of science, Friedrich Hoffmann. This clinician and professor at the university of Halle, who was an extraordinarily fertile man of letters, showed an interest in dentistry far above

134 Ibid. p. 564
135 Heister (d) pp. 236 f.
136 See p. 182
137 Cron pp. 184 f.
138 Kräutermann pp. 243 and 249 f.

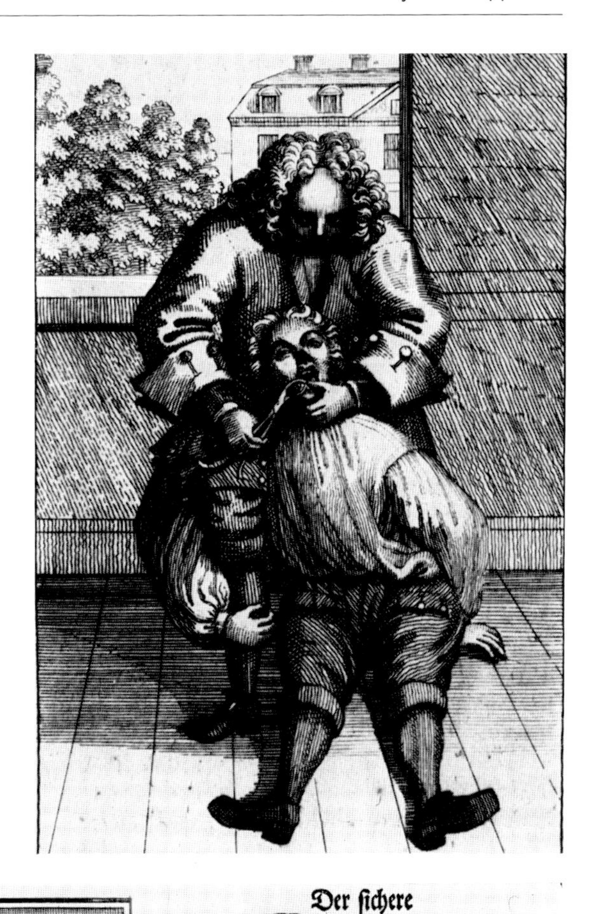

Fig. 221 *Cron: Tooth extraction, 1717*

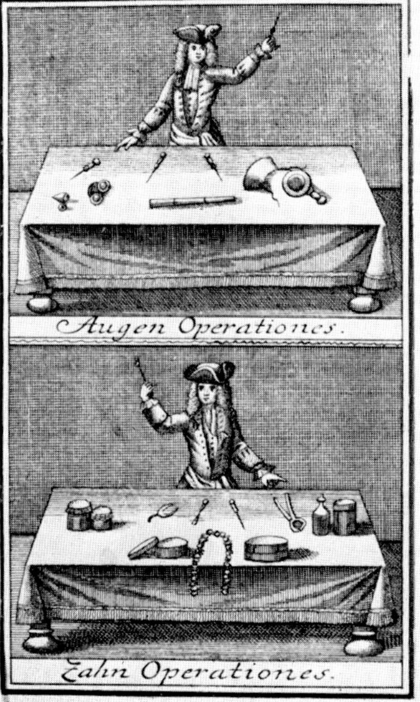

Der sichere
Augen-
und
Zahn-Artzt,
Oder accurate
Beschreibung
Aller und ieden
Augen- und Zahn-Gebrechen,
Nebst
Deutlichen Unterrichte/
Wie solchen bey Zeiten vorzukommen, oder
auch glücklich zu curiren sind.
Aus berühmter Medicorum Schrifften zu-
sammen getragen, und nebst nöthigem Register
ans Licht gestellet
von
VALENT. Kräutermann/ Med. Pr.
Arnstadt/
Verlegts Ernst Ludwig Niedt, 1732.

Fig. 222 *Frontispiece and title page of Kräutermann's "Der sichere Augen- und Zahn-Artzt," 1732*

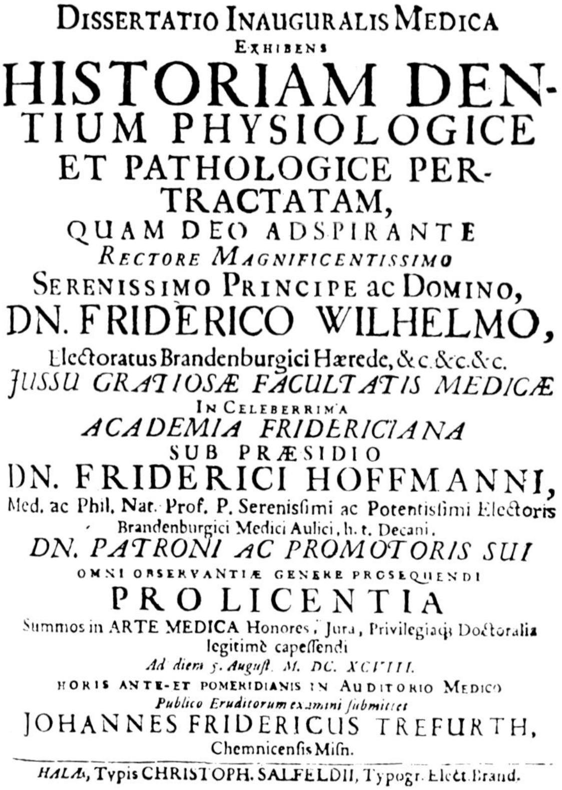

DISSERTATIO INAUGURALIS MEDICA
EXHIBENS
HISTORIAM DENTIUM PHYSIOLOGICE ET PATHOLOGICE PERTRACTATAM,
QUAM DEO ADSPIRANTE
RECTORE MAGNIFICENTISSIMO
SERENISSIMO PRINCIPE ac DOMINO,
DN. FRIDERICO WILHELMO,
Electoratus Brandenburgici Hærede, &c.&c.&c.
JUSSU GRATIOSÆ FACULTATIS MEDICÆ
IN CELEBERRIMA
ACADEMIA FRIDERICIANA
SUB PRÆSIDIO
DN. FRIDERICI HOFFMANNI,
Med. ac Phil. Nat. Prof. P. Serenissimi ac Potentissimi Electoris Brandenburgici Medici Aulici, h. t. Decani.
DN. PATRONI AC PROMOTORIS SUI
OMNI OBSERVANTIÆ GENERE PROSEQUENDI
PRO LICENTIA
Summos in ARTE MEDICA Honores, Jura, Privilegiaque Doctoralia legitimè capessendi
Ad diem 5. August. M. DC. XCVIII.
HORIS ANTE- ET POMERIDIANIS IN AUDITORIO MEDICO
Publico Eruditorum examini submittet
JOHANNES FRIDERICUS TREFURTH,
Chemnicensis Misn.
HALÆ, Typis CHRISTOPH. SALFELDII, Typogr. Elect. Brand.

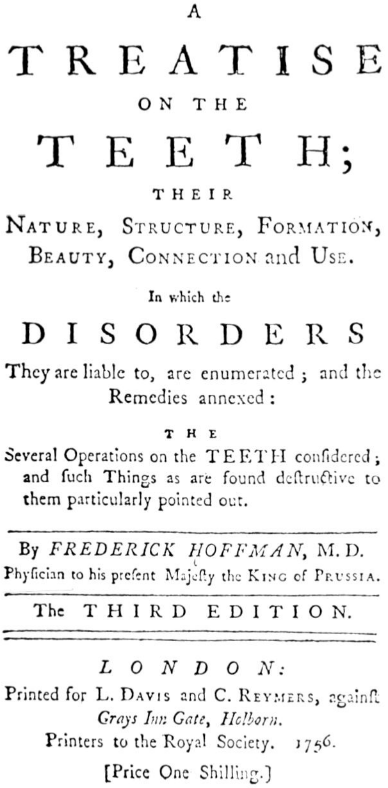

A
TREATISE
ON THE
TEETH;
THEIR
NATURE, STRUCTURE, FORMATION,
BEAUTY, CONNECTION and USE.
In which the
DISORDERS
They are liable to, are enumerated; and the Remedies annexed:
THE
Several Operations on the TEETH considered; and such Things as are found destructive to them particularly pointed out.

By FREDERICK HOFFMAN, M. D.
Physician to his present Majesty the KING of PRUSSIA.

The THIRD EDITION.

LONDON:
Printed for L. DAVIS and C. REYMERS, against Grays Inn Gate, Holborn.
Printers to the Royal Society. 1756.
[Price One Shilling.]

Figs. 223 and 224 *Hoffmann's Dissertation (1698) and its English translation (1756)*

the average. Many pages of his writings, published posthumously in a collected edition in Geneva, are devoted to stomatological problems as are also three dissertations, one of which, the "Historia dentium physiologice et pathologice pertracta" from 1698, came out again under a different title in 1714, and in English translation in London as 3rd edition in 1756 and in Dublin in 1760 [139] (Figs. 223 and 224).

With regard to the anatomy of the teeth, Hoffmann essentially adheres to Eustachi, whom he quotes frequently, but also mentions the structures of enamel and dentin [140] which were observed by Malpighi [141]. In keeping with his iatromechanical system he views toothache as a general disturbance, specifically a rheumatic symptom which is discussed as "Rheumatismus odontalgicus" [142]. Accordingly, the therapy consists mainly of general measures, such as diet, bleeding, purgative baths, and medications such as the anodyne liquor, which is still known today as Hoffmann's drops (1 part ether to 3 parts alcohol). A cure of this kind is minutely described in the XIIth volume of the "Medecina consultatoria": the consulting patient tells how, after his case of gout subsided, an "occurrence" took place in the right side of the maxilla, which we name today as marginal periodontitis. Hoffmann believed that *the Malum was only to be traced to the fact that, because the attacks of gout had disappeared, the bitter arthritic material had fallen upon the membranas and alveolos and of the gum, . . ., that, namely, the gout had turned to a dental disease.* Besides the general measures mentioned, it is recommended that "balsam vitae"

139 Hoffmann (d—h); Wackernagel
140 Hoffmann (e); (f) p. 6; (g) p. 5
141 See p. 171
142 Hoffmann (a) II p. 330; (b) 53—59

and Hoffmann's drops be mixed with rose honey and that the mouth be rubbed with it [143].

There is nothing new in the measures for preventive dentistry. Hoffmann still firmly believed in the toothworm, and decisively antagonized Houllier's denial of its existence [144]: *Therefore, we cannot accept Hollerius who teaches that worms are produced spontaneously from the smoke of henbane seeds . . . Certainly nobody can ever imagine such an origin for a living creature from smoke and flame, unless it is perhaps believed that those worms stem from the mythological family of the Pyraustas* (a kind of moth), *or of the phoenix* [145]. Hoffmann obviously had a fundamental misunderstanding of the Parisian surgeon here.

Hoffmann, the internist, provides no practical measures based on his own personal experience. For sealing cavities he recommends a wax paste similar to Guillemeau's; he also advises, however, probably having read it somewhere and confused it, mixing tin and gold leaf into it beside corals [146]. He suggests to the dental surgeon (Dentarius-Chirurgus) precautionary measures for tooth extraction which are partially reasonable and partially superstitious [147]. He justifiably does not think well of medicamentous tooth loosening; the mild agents seem ineffective to him and the stronger ones he regards with suspicion [148]. All in all this famous man did not advance dentistry by even a single step, and his inclusion of it in his medical system, which gave him fame throughout Europe in his own time, lost all importance as quickly as his system did.

Among Albrecht von Haller's collection of medico-surgical dissertations one is to be found from 1750, by Ludolf Heinrich Runge, a doctoral student at the Rinteln University. He mentions unequivocal cases of maxillary and mandibular cysts, which he quotes from the practice of his father, a surgeon in Bremen [149]. The noise from pressing in on the wall of the cyst, which was later named after Dupuytren, is described here probably for the first time: . . . *and it gave forth a tone, like that of a thin sheet of metal (tenuis Bractea metallica)* and then *returned again to its former position* (page 214). The French translation leaves out this detail in the description of the noise (*se remettait avec bruit à son premier état* [p. 136]). After the opening incision, a viscous fluid flowed *without odor and evaporation.*

The man to whom we owe the first book in German that was equal to the French dental literature was the surgeon Philipp Pfaff, of Berlin who was baptized there on February 27, 1713. Yet his work is still bound up with French medicine in two ways: firstly through his familiarity with Fauchard's work, which was published in Berlin in 1733, and secondly through his father. This man, who had been certified as a surgeon in Berlin since 1710, reports that he was carried off as a child to southern France after the destruction of Heidelberg by French troops, where a major had him trained as a surgeon. From the consultation protocols of the anatomical theatre in Berlin it is proven that he had been a prosector in Montpellier. His son Philipp, after he had completed the curriculum at the Collegium Medico-Chirurgicum, served at first with the Prussian army as company surgeon in keeping with the regulations of the medical edict. Under the young King Frederick II, he applied for a license as surgeon, which he received in 1744 signed by the King's own hand. He practiced at the Fischerbrücke with four helpers in the vicinity of the family home [150].

In 1756 Pfaff's "Abhandlung von den Zähnen des menschlichen Körpers und deren Krankheiten" (Treatise on the Teeth of the Human Body and their Diseases) came out *with the most gracious Royal Prussian Permission.* The book, which comprises 187 pages and engravings, is written in a flowing and uncommonly lively style, and shows its author as an educated man and a practitioner who possibly even mastered the ancient languages. Like Bourdet he used Fauchard's work as a guide, and also presents his own experiences and important new ideas.

Even in the preface he is criticizing the Parisian master, because, although his "French Dentist" ("Frantzösischer Zahn-Artzt" [see Fig. 183] was the title of the German translation from 1733) had brought the author a great deal of fame and

143 Hoffmann (c) XII pp. 243 f.
144 See p. 145
145 Hoffmann (b) p. 678 a, 1—8
146 Ibid. p. 678 a, 21—32
147 Ibid. p. 678 b, 52—679 a, 10; (e) p. 28, 11—29
148 Ibid. p. 679 a, 13—21
149 Dissertatio medico-chirurgica de morbis praecipuis sinuum ossis frontis et maxillae superioris, et quibusdam mandibulae inferioris. In: Hallerus (a) pp. 205—229; (b) pp. 127—148; see pp. 346 f. Jourdain (p. 215) followed in 1778.
150 Witt

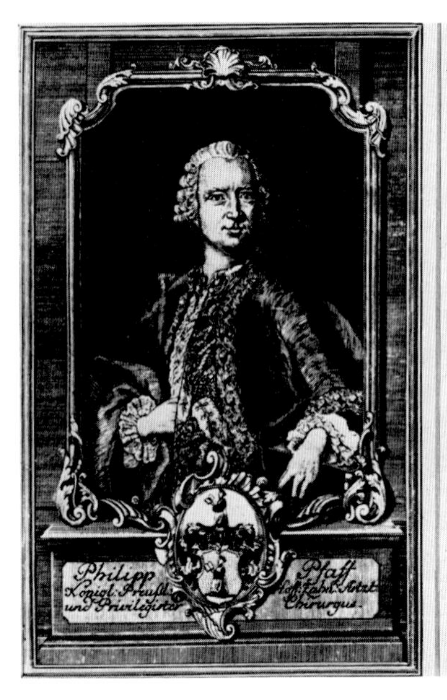

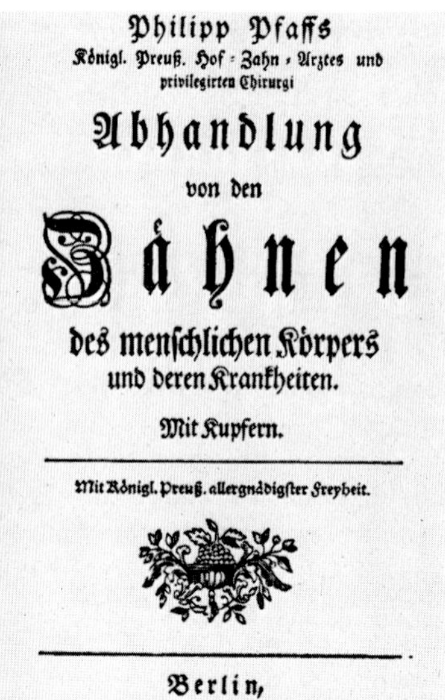
Philipp Pfaffs
Königl. Preuß. Hof-Zahn-Arztes und
privilegirten Chirurgi
Abhandlung
von den
Zähnen
des menschlichen Körpers
und deren Krankheiten.
Mit Kupfern.
Mit Königl. Preuß. allergnädigster Freyheit.
Berlin,
bey Haude und Spener, 1756.

Fig. 225 *Frontispiece and title page of Pfaff's "Abhandlung von den Zähnen," 1756*

praise, it would have been much more useful for the neophyte if the author had avoided an exaggerated lengthiness of scope and provided more order. He himself, as we read later, had taken great pains to achieve brevity always, although he could have written more from his own experiences. Furthermore we learn that Pfaff by the grace of the king had been appointed court dentist a short time before which is not to say, of course, that he had actually treated the great Prussian king. He is portrayed as such and as a privileged surgeon on the portrait engraving. He had himself presented in a proud posture and with rich clothing, as a man who was well aware of his own worth (Fig. 225).

The actual discussions, which are divided into 77 paragraphs, begin with correct explanations of dental anatomy throughout, except that he adopts Vesalius' error in describing the primary teeth as having no roots[151]. The teeth are damaged by venereal disease and venereal cures, by the English disease (rickets) and scurvy as much as by highly spiced foods and external cold influence. Experience also taught him *that confectioners and cake bakers seldom possess good teeth.* Pfaff also gives a theory on caries: cold and heat cause *small fissures* through which contaminants penetrate into the enamel structure and the *porous substance* (dentin), and bring about decay there. One and a half centuries later, the great W. D. Miller named this conception of Pfaff "putrefaction theory." [152]

The smoking of tobacco damages the teeth only accidentally through biting on (clay) pipes, but the smoke irritates the gingiva [153]. Cleansing the teeth to excess is to be avoided. For mouthwashes and dentifrices he refers to the collection of prescriptions in the appendix.

Pfaff writes in great detail about the treatment of pathological conditions of the gingiva and the teeth. A sensible causal therapy is always proposed. For this reason he becomes irritated with those surgeons who see only the abscess and do not worry about the tooth responsible for it.

As to the toothworm he had *despite all possible effort, . . . never encountered* it, but still does not deny its existence with the same certainty as Fauchard did, since he does not *want question the truth and value of learned physician's perceptions* [154].

Tooth extraction, for which Pfaff in contrast to Fauchard prefers the *lower chair* which we also saw in Cron (Fig. 221), is described

[151] Pfaff p. 31
[152] Ibid. pp. 39 f. See p. 401
[153] Ibid. pp. 44 f.
[154] Ibid. pp. 68 f.

with all incidentals and resultant sequelae [155]. If there is pain afterwards, he prepares a ball from poppy juice and places it into the socket.

Cleansing of the teeth must not be performed with acids which are damaging to the enamel, even though quick results can be obtained with them. *An upright dentist, who has the well-being of the patient and his own honor . . . as his noblest aim, must and also will act with greater caution* [156]. He fastens loose teeth with gold wire, after he has freed them from *the tartaric material.*

The devitalization of diseased dental pulp is carried out, as usual, with a cautery (Fig. 226; Figs. I—III), and Pfaff afterwards cleans the cavity and dries it with cotton before he fills it with lead or, *in the case of people of rank,* with gold. First, he recommends that the exposed dental pulp be covered with a piece of gold bent into a concave shape, and that the tooth be filled then, a method which, carried out today under aseptic conditions, is highly up-to-date as direct pulp capping [157].

He prepared artificial teeth mostly from walrus bone, but was familiar with Fauchard's enameled teeth. He used human teeth only seldom, because *most people have a dread of teeth which have been obtained from a corpse* [158]. Pfaff cautions against the transmission of *scurvy and venereal fluids* with the transplantation of teeth from one individual to another. He correctly puts particular stress taking care of the periodontal membrane of the transplanted tooth, the apical hole of which is to be sealed with lead or wax, a very important advice in an evil affair [159].

Pfaff's most important achievement is found in prosthetics: he was the first to describe taking an impression of the jaw, carried out by means of *sealing wax, which had previously been made soft in hot water, so that all elevations on the gingiva can be seen in the wax; thereupon, it is put in cold water until it becomes hard. Now, a dough is made from finely pulverized plaster with water, the mass of wax which has been prepared is previously rubbed with almond oil, and the mixed plaster is poured with a spoon over the wax; it is left to stand until it has become hard, and thus all depressions and elevations can afterward be correctly examined.* In order that the impression not be distorted when it is pulled out, the jaw should be molded in two pieces of wax, which, after being removed individually, are put together outside the mouth [160]. Thus, for the first time a negative is produced from wax, and from it a positive model of the jaw is obtained through plaster casting. If some natural teeth remained, Pfaff had the patient bite into the wax, so that the antagonists could be considered in their correct position of occlusion. With this he gives us the first description of a checkbite, without yet giving one, however, of a primitive articulator, as Bremner believes [161]. The denture itself Pfaff had made by an "artist" [162].

The actual instructional text is followed by a collection of prescriptions, in which an almost medieval variety of dentifrices and mouth washes are enumerated in compositions which are still used. And just as Scribonius Largus recommended a dental powder in the first century after Christ, because the emperor's, Claudius, wife Messalina used it, Pfaff now publicizes a powder, *which was prescribed for our late monarch His Majesty King Frederick William, by his personal regimental surgeon, Holzendorf* [163].

Finally 7 engravings are included on fold-outs, which show Pfaff's overly constructed pelican, cauteries, scalers, dental files, and several pictures of teeth, including of the primary teeth which, according to him, were rootless (Fig. 227; No. VII). In the drawings of the dentures the otherwise so pleasant impression of this talented and creative man is overshadowed lightly, as he copies Fauchard's spring-connected upper and lower dentures without any source acknowledgement (Fig. 227; No. XX). He even admits in the text that he had this picture copied, but regrettably neglects to mention the inventor [164].

In 1764 the author of this first important German manual of dentistry was appointed court councillor. On March 4, 1766 he died from a disease of the chest at the age of 54 in his house, the Black Eagle on the Fischerbrücke [165]. The widowed Madame Councillor Pfaff, however, reported in the *Vossische Zeitung* No. 50 of 1769

155 Ibid. pp. 79 f. See p. 226
156 Ibid. pp. 105 f.
157 Ibid. pp. 123 f.
158 Ibid. p. 132
159 Ibid. pp. 133 f.
160 Ibid. p. 153
161 Bremner p. 221
162 Pfaff p. 148
163 Ibid. p. 180
164 Ibid. p. 152; see Fig. 196
165 Witt pp. 16 f.

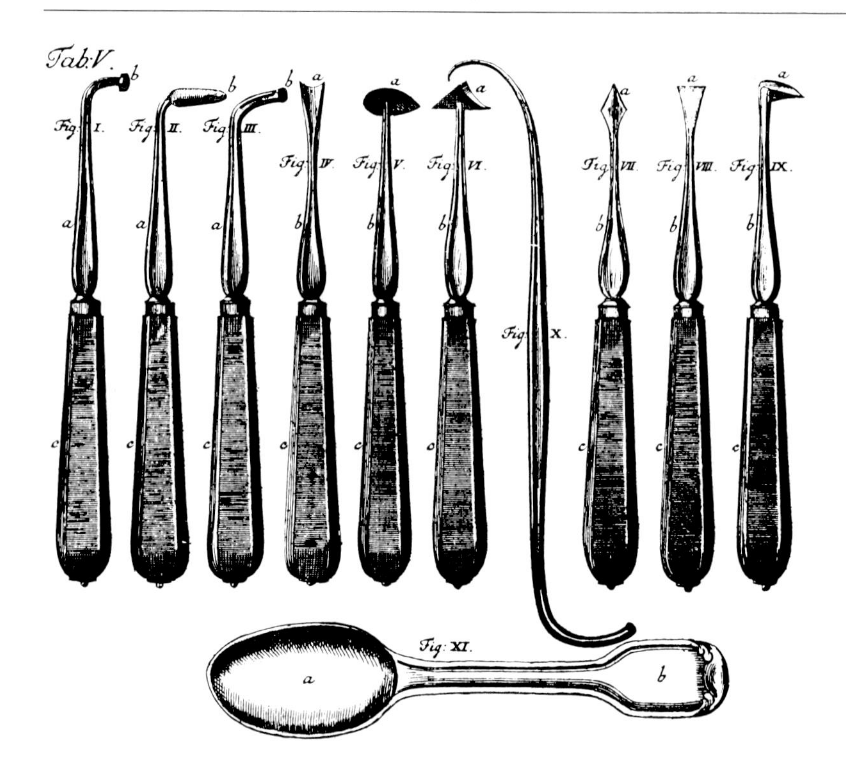

Fig. 226 *Pfaff: Cautery (Figs. I-III), calculus instruments (Figs. IV-VI), probe (Fig. X), caries remover (Figs. VIII-IX), and spoon to retract cheeks during cauterization*

to those who are in need of her help in oral and dental cures, that she has changed her lodgings, and from now on inhabits the Pohlmann House, on the first floor, into the Breite Straße. She will treat the children of all orphanages without fee, if they make their appearance in the afternoons on Mondays and Tuesdays, from 1 o'clock to 2 o'clock.

It is amazing that the most important contribution of Pfaff, namely impression taking, has made its way only hesitatingly, even in German literature. Ten years later the dentist Carl August Gräbner of Hamburg—otherwise quite an enlightened man—described in 1766 in his dental breviary expressly the close fitting of the denture-base on the patient. In his further presentations he kept to Fauchard entirely. It is gratifying that Gräbner recommended the mildest remedies only, such as massage of the gums or chewing on a root of violets soaked in rose-honey, against difficult eruption. His "Zahncalender" (calendar of dentition), in which the parents had to record the dates of the secondary dentition, was something entirely new. The wisdom teeth in females he called "bridal teeth." Regrettably he reported several cases of tooth-transplantation, the case of a singer among them who had rewarded her servant maid with a bridal gown for having donated her tooth[166]. His reticence in behalf of extraction of teeth must be mentioned as something laudable. A sickle-shaped scaler could still be used in our time. As early as 1768, a second edition of this remarkable booklet was printed.

The next significant publication, the "Complete Instructions for Tooth Extraction," appeared in 1782, this time on the side of the physicians and surgeons. This book, comprising 168 pages, was by Johann Jacob Bücking, municipal physician in Wolfenbüttel from 1802 on. Although the author was a prolific writer, he nonetheless provides quite a useful guide to extraction based on practical experience. As academician, he also made profuse reference to older literature, which was amply available to him in the famous Wolfenbüttel Herzog-August Library — its librarian, the great poet of German enlightenment, Gotthold Ephraim Lessing, had just died in 1781.

[166] Gräbner pp. 75 f.

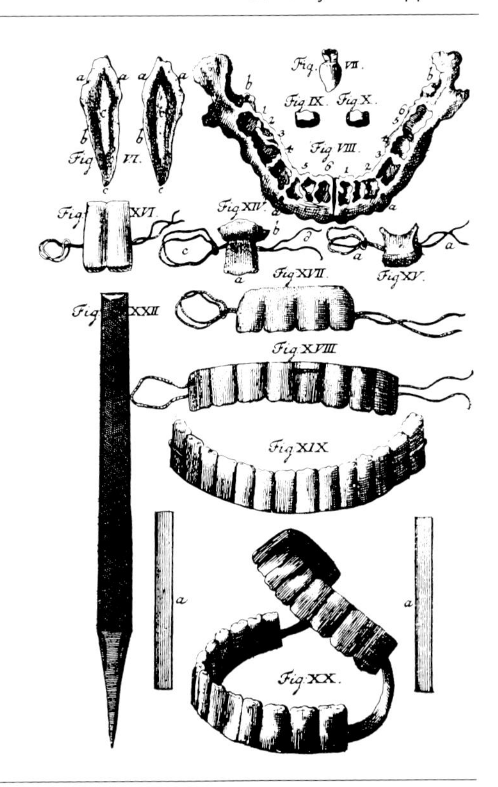

Fig. 227 *Pfaff: Anatomic and prosthetic drawings*

Bücking sang the praises of the forceps together with its variations such as the crow's bill and others as the oldest and most natural instrument, almost as a universal device (Fig. 228), however, he rightly criticized the lever as *one of the quite superfluous instruments*[167] (Fig. 229, Figs. 1 and 2). In discussing the pelican, which he ranked immediately behind the forceps, he — like every other author with any self-esteem — shows his own improved model, with a variable support surface (Fig. 229, Fig. 3). He rejects the "English key" because it pinches the gingiva and easily breaks off the tooth, and he is quite pleased with the pes caprinus because of its simplicity particularly for removing loose roots (Fig. 230). This latter contrasts with Pfaff's too complicated instrument. He requires an exact case anamnesis before an interference in order to exclude the pains caused by venereal diseases or scurvy. He urgently recommends the careful use of a searcher (probe)[168] (Fig. 230; Fig. 15). Like Pfaff and Cron, he placed the patient in front of and below himself on the ground. This seems to have been, in contrast mainly to Fauchard and his adherents, a peculiarity of the German school. He discusses post-extraction hemorrhage in minute detail recommending acid cauterization, packing with punk and lint and compression through biting on cork or wax[169]. As an enlightened man, Bücking had no reservations about extractions on pregnant women. In 1796 we encounter Frederick Hirsch, the court dentist in Weimar (Thuringia) and of many other courts, who had been decorated with the title of Dentist of the University in Göttingen since 1801 and appeared after 1804 under the name of Hirschfeld. His "Praktische Bemerkungen über die Zähne" (Practical Remarks on the Teeth) contained nothing new but still saw a second enlarged edition in 1801. In 1804 it was followed by the even more insignificant "Bemerkungen über die Krankheiten des Zahnfleisches" (Remarks on the Diseases of the Gingiva) which appeared under his new name. As he was well-versed in the literature he quoted Hunter and Bell in the first opus, and saves himself the trouble of describing an artificial

[167] Bücking p. 72
[168] Ibid. pp. 92 f.
[169] Ibid. pp. 97 f. and 128

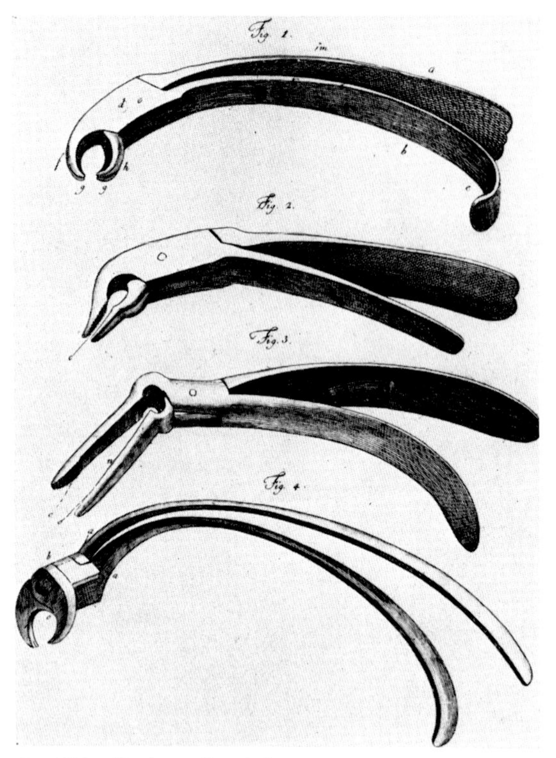

Fig. 228 *Bücking: Tooth forceps, 1782*

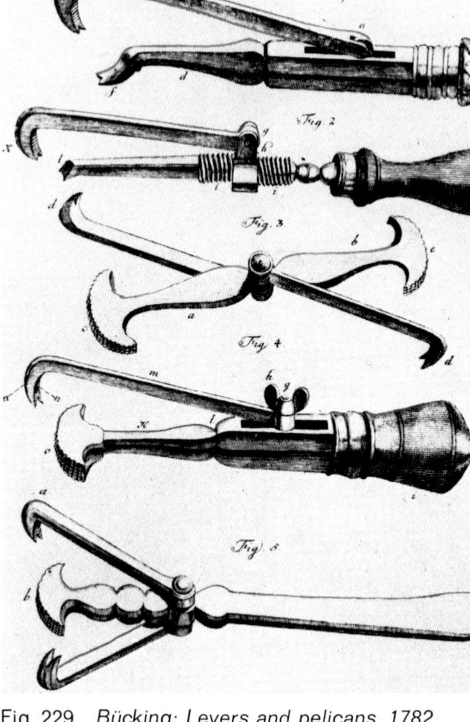

Fig. 229 *Bücking: Levers and pelicans, 1782*

"jaw-bone" by referring to Fauchard. He used tinfoil as a filling material and made the inner space greater than the outside opening for better adherence. Probably because of less salivation in the maxilla he applied there a "stonemass" which consisted of boiled turpentine, unslaked lime, and linseed-oil varnish [170]. In order to avoid postoperative pain the dental pulp was prophylactically destroyed with a cautery. He rejected tooth transplants for the moral reason that he was a practitioner in Germany, and *the exchange of bones between living bodies is the fashion only in England* [171]. Instead he implanted teeth from his stock, derived from young subjects who had died a violent death, directly into the freshly bleeding socket (which naturally heal into place, but their roots are soon absorbed as a result of the devitalized periodontal membrane).

The preface to this book by the anatomist of the university of Jena, Justus Christian Loder, is almost more important to us than its contents. This distinguished scholar expresses his opinion on extraction instruments in detail. He had tested them all on corpses, and could recommend neither the pelican, the lever, nor the key, because they all support themselves on the jaw or on a neighboring tooth and cause *a considerable crushing, quite possibly even fractures of the jaw,* or even loosen the tooth used as a support [172]. It took an anatomist to express these platitudes clearly and unequivocally to the dentists. He agreed with Hirsch that the kinds of curved-shank elevators represented by Bücking in his figures 11 and 12 (Fig. 197) constituted the most suitable instruments. This seems to us today, as Serre had already observed in 1803 [173], somewhat one-sided. In London Loder saw an operation performed with the key by Spence, whom we

[170] Hirsch (a) pp. 58 f. and 131; (b) pp. 54 f. and 180
[171] Ibid (a) p. 102; (b) pp. 100 f.
[172] Ibid. p. XI
[173] Serre pp. 271 f.

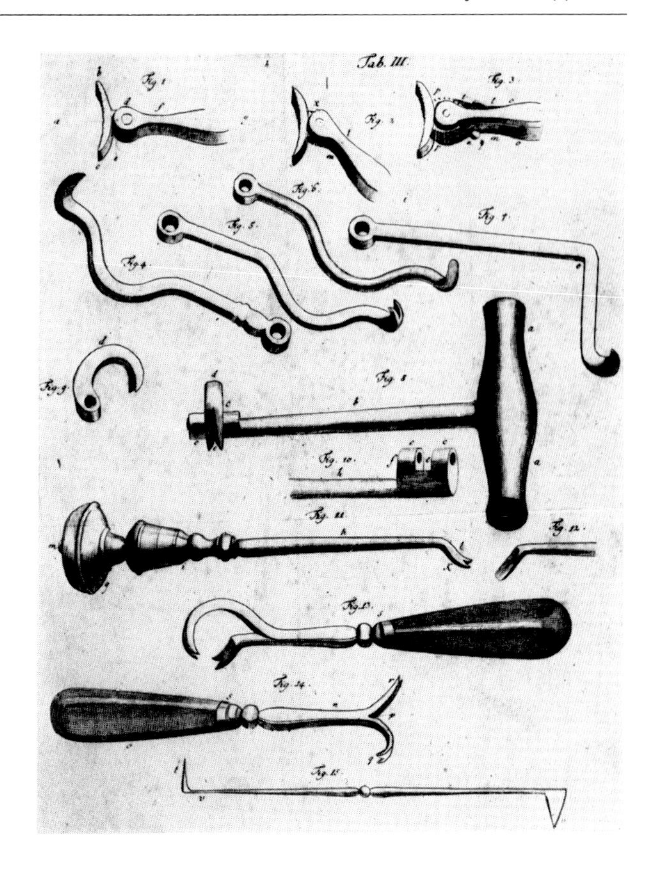

Fig. 230 *Bücking: Keys (Fig. 8) and pes caprinus (Figs. 11 and 12)*

know from Hunter. He calls it the English key, *which carries the name "German key" in England*[174].

The name of the Court Councillor Loder is familiar to us through the anatomical studies which Johann Wolfgang von Goethe, the most distinguished German poet, pursued under him in 1781-1782. In 1784, in the course of comparative investigations of skulls from animals and human fetuses, Goethe recognized on the latter the premaxilla which generally had been disclaimed before (Fig. 231). Enthusiastically he wrote: *I have found neither gold nor silver but still something which gives me unspeakable joy — the human os intermaxillare! I compared human and animal skulls with Loder, caught the scent, and look, there it is . . . because it is like the keystone of man, it is not missing, it is actually there*[175]. Goethe did not know, and it is not prejudicial to him, that the French anatomists Pierre Marie Auguste Broussonet and Felix Vicq d'Azyr had already reported on the premaxilla in humans in 1779 and 1780, respectively[176].

Still another connection of Goethe to stomatology should be mentioned here. We find the following entries in the household book of the 82-year-old poet: on July 7, 1831 *to the man on account of the tooth, 17 silver groschen;* on July 18, *tying of the tooth, 11 silver groschen and 4 pfennigs;* and on July 19, *tying of the other teeth, 11 silver groschen and 4 pfennigs*[177]. This wire splinting of loose teeth cannot, however, have been performed by Hirschfeld, who had become blind later in life and had died already in 1827[178].

Besides other minds of smaller ilk, one of the most important surgeons of the second half of the century expressed his views on dental problems. August Gottlieb Richter, who

174 Hirsch p. XIII
175 Goethe (a) IV 6 No. 1903
176 Bräuning-Oktavio pp. 89 f.
177 Reichenbach
178 Callisen VIII p. 543 f.; XXVIII p. 541

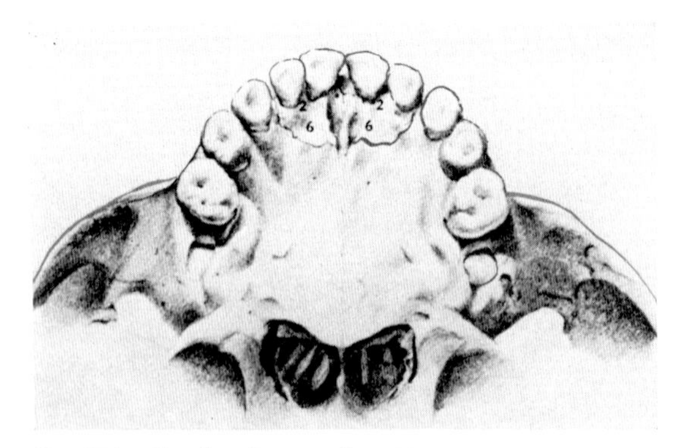

Fig. 231 *Goethe: Premaxilla, 1784*

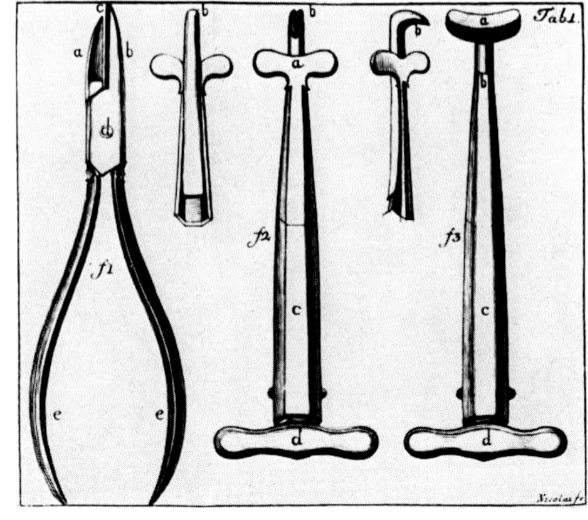

Fig. 232 *Brunner: Instruments for forceful alignment of teeth, 1765*

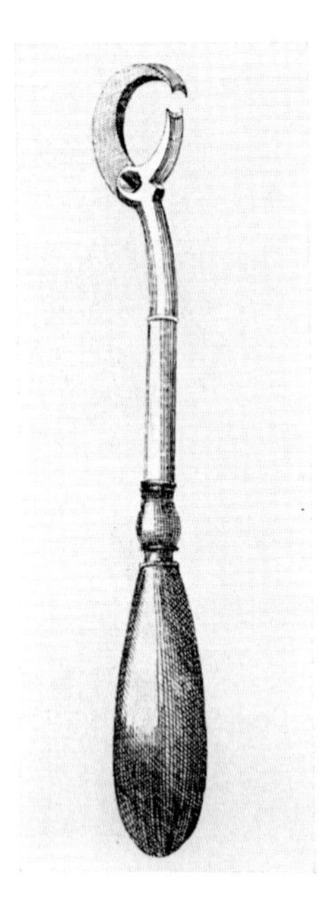

Fig. 231a *Richter: The lever of Görtz, 1798*

was active during his entire life practicing in Göttingen, expressed his opinion on dental problems in 99 pages of the IVth volume of his "Anfangsgründe der Wundarzneykunst" (Rudiments of the Art of Surgery) which appeared in 1798. We cannot expect to find prosthetic insights from the physician in ordinary to His Royal Majesty of Great Britain (Hanover then belonged to the British crown). On this subject reference is made to Fauchard, whom he follows in general, too, and to Jourdain. Richter describes tooth transplants without ethical reservations, but nonetheless he very thoroughly discusses the pros and cons of the possibility of transmitting venereal disease with quotations from Hunter[179]. To alleviate pain he luxates the tooth, which ruptures the neural connection at the apex of the root without, of course, differentiating between pulpal and periodontal causes. *The pulling-out of a tooth* may only be undertaken *if the toothache arises from local causes, if it is not in-*

179 Richter IV p. 139 f.

flamed to a high degree, and if the tooth is conspicuously decayed and useless. The English key, the pelican, and the punch are the instruments used; the first two of these, however, cause crushing of the gingiva, which therefore must be detached before the operation. The goat's foot of Görtz (der Görtzische Geissfuß), not a punch but a kind of lever (Überwurf), is a better device. By means of a hook it *prevents the instrument from slipping* [180] (Fig. 231 a; see Fig. 146).

Richter very pictorially describes how calculus surrounds the tooth below the edge of the gingiva *like a sausage* and penetrates further down until the tooth falls out. Therefore, the *stony material* must be removed and the edge of the gingiva cut off. *An inflammation is thereby stimulated in the detached parts of the gingiva, which effects a new adhesion of same to the tooth* [181]. All things considered this is a thoroughly critical treatise which seems to be based in large part on personal experience.

In contrast we find an amazing passage in the "Commentarii" of 1764 by Gerard van Swieten, a student of the great Boerhaave, and the reformer of Austrian medicine. We read that he did not believe in the existence of roots of deciduous teeth, even though he had studied the theories of Bourdet and Bunon on the absorption of the roots in their books. It becomes even worse when he proceeds: *Nevertheless, observations seem to show that the primary teeth if they do not fall out at the proper time or are not taken out when they are already loose, will put forth roots from their bodies, which, after later becoming firm in the jaws, often remain so for a lifetime.* As early as 1798, the Irishman Robert Blake expressed his astonishment in his dissertation at this error by such an important man [182].

On the other hand van Swieten seems to have been quite open minded toward the practical problems of dentistry. In 1760 he motivated the army surgeons Brunner and Pasch to devote themselves completely to dentistry, which gave rise to each of them writing a book on the subject.

Adam Anton Brunner published an "Einleitung zur nöthigen Wissenschaft eines Zahnarztes" (Introduction to the Science necessary to a Dentist) in Vienna in 1765, the anatomical section of which contains nothing uncommon except a comprehensive bibliography. In the clinical section he adheres wholly to Bourdet, who had advanced beyond Fauchard. Among other things he mentions the smoking of tobacco as a detrimental factor in tooth decay, because *the ignited oil of this plant, dissolved in fine smoke, is pulled into the mouth through puffing . . .* Like Pfaff, he regards *the friction of earthen pipes as even worse* [183]. The treatment *of poorly positioned teeth* is likewise discussed according to Bourdet, except that he constructed two (superfluous) instruments for the forceful straightening (redressement, Fig. 232). Painful dental pulp is, as usual, devitalized with a cautery, after which cotton is placed inside and is filled with gold. This, however, only works for single-root teeth [184]. For extraction he used chiefly the lever but also the punch and the *pelican of M. Bourdet,* for control of bleeding, the particularly effective *oaken sponge* (spunk). He is quite familiar with Hollerius' (Houllier) and Schaeffer's explanations concerning henbane and the toothworm [185]. In the prosthetic section Brunner adheres quite closely to Pfaff with regard to taking impressions, but otherwise owes more to his confidant Bourdet. All in all, this book is not very original which is not surprising considering the author's educational background. The same holds true for the "Abhandlung von der Hervorbrechung der Milchzähne" (Treatise on the Eruption of the Milk [primary] Teeth), which was published in 1771, and which represents an inflation of the corresponding chapter of his first book. The essay ends with the case history of tetanic infants, who recover or die depending on whether the gingiva over the primary tooth has been split or not [186].

The "Abhandlung aus der Wundarzney von den Zähnen . . ." (Treatise on the Surgery of the Teeth . . .) of 1767 by the second army surgeon ordered off to study dentistry, Joseph Georg Pasch, is even more useless. Surely, he published a vitamin remedy for scurvy from van Swieten, consisting of red cabbage, watercress, and horseradish shredded into beer [187]. Then, however, he maintained that extracting

[180] Ibid. IV p. 162 f.
[181] Ibid. IV p. 89
[182] van Swieten IV p. 744; Blake pp. 59 f.
[183] Brunner (a) p. 46
[184] Ibid. p. 115
[185] See pp. 145 and 241 f.
[186] Brunner (b) pp. 131 f.
[187] Pasch p. 62

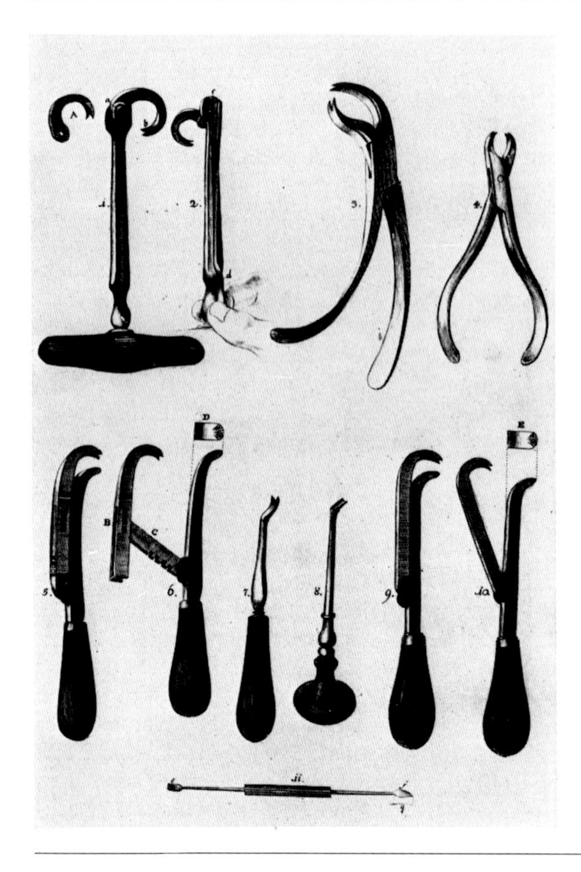

Fig. 233 *Brambilla: Extraction instruments*

teeth from pregnant women caused premature delivery[188]. He devotes several pages to magnetic steel as remedy angainst toothache[189]. (In 1767, that is still before Mesmer's magnetic Viennese cures). He himself did not believe in the magnetic force, but rather presumed that the cold of the iron was able to influence the toothache either beneficially or detrimentally.

Joseph Jacob Plenk, a surgeon in Ofen (then a quarter of Budapest), and later in Vienna, one of the most talented compilers of his time, edited the "Lehre von den Krankheiten der Zähne und des Zahnfleisches" (Instruction Manual on the Diseases of the Teeth and the Gums) in Latin in 1778, in German in 1779, and in Italian in 1786 and in 1790. This work, beginning with Hippocrates and extending to what is probably the last mention of the Arabian frog-fat-therapy for loosening teeth[190], is founded almost exclusively on studies of literature, even though he mixes in an occasional case history of his own, or an experiment which he conducted himself[191]. The most interesting thing about it is the manner in which it is written: the individual disease symptoms are described in concise language and listed under first, second, third, just as in modern manuals. Otherwise, however, it is merely the work of a surgeon who also wrote something about the teeth.

Giovanni Alessandro Brambilla, physician in ordinary to Emperor Joseph II and organizer of the Austrian military health service, also manifests an interest in dentistry. In the Josephinum, the Viennese military medical academy, of which he was the first, but not a particularly important director, there still exists a set of dental instruments made according to his instructions[192]. In his book also, a pompously arranged manual on the knowledge of instruments, he displays these utensils on three plates[193] (Fig. 233).

188 Ibid. p. 96
189 Ibid. p. 98 f.
190 See p. 91
191 See p. 241
192 Driack
193 Brambilla pp 77 f.

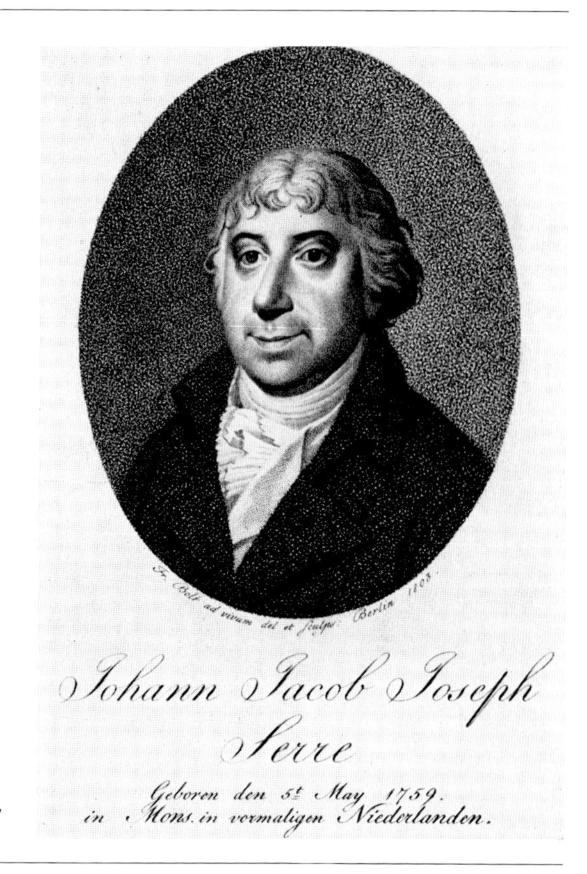
Johann Jacob Joseph
Serre
Geboren den 5t May 1759.
in Mons. in vormaligen Niederlanden.

Fig. 234 *Johann Jacob Joseph Serre: Frontispiece, 1803*

Johann Jacob Joseph Serre, who loved the call of the open air, is by far a more important man in dentistry. He was born in 1759, in the Belgian Mons, and appeared in Vienna in the last quarter of the 18th century, where he passed the surgeons' examination in 1781. In the 19th century, he lived and worked in Berlin until his death in 1830. That he appeared in Frankfurt am Main in 1808 as an itinerant dentist[194] fits into the picture of the tooth-drawer past, which had not yet been overcome (Fig. 234).

His first work, which came out in Vienna in 1788, was the "Geschichte oder Abhandlung der Zahnschmerzen des schönen Geschlechts in ihrer Schwangerschaft" (History or Discussion of Toothache of the Prettier Sex during their Pregnancies) which comprised 131 pages. Serre, like Bunon and Bücking before him, whom he quotes among others, takes a stand against the superstition that the teeth of pregnant women may not even be touched, *because they are always in danger of losing their fruit*[195]. He correctly states that many toothaches have nothing to do with this condition, but rather occur as a result of neglect of the teeth and insufficient oral hygiene. The "Abhandlung über die Flüsse und Entzündungen" (Treatise on the Fluids and Inflammations), which followed in 1791, undertakes, as the title suggests, *a thorough refutation of the prejudice that in the presense of fluids or inflammation the tooth which caused them should not be taken out.* This questionable theory is challenged troughout the entire book with quotations from mostly contemporary authors on the pros and cons. In his own cases he always removes the tooth he views as culpable, without precise indication and without consideration of whether the inflamed condition is acute or chronic. When the osteomyelitis which is to be expected sets in, he even interprets this to his advantage[196]. We come to appreciate Jourdain here, who is

[194] Wiegel p. 22
[195] Serre (a) p. 3
[196] Serre (b) p. 110

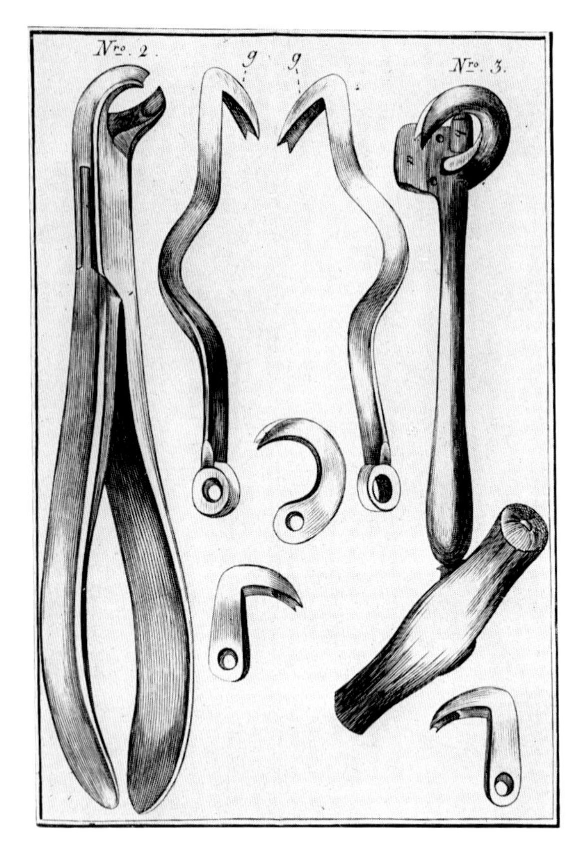

Fig. 235 *Serre: Forceps and key (No. 3)*

attacked by Serre because of the statement (probably taken from Heister) that the *operation itself excites a new degree of inflammation, which joins company with the one already present*[197].

Serre's major work, "Praktische Darstellung aller Operationen der Zahnheilkunst" (Practical Presentation of all the Operations of the Art of Dentistry), appeared in Berlin in 1803 *at the expense of the author,* luxuriously decorated and dedicated to the Czar Alexander of Russia. Quite a detailed history of the profession is put at the beginning, in which he mentions, among others, Hippocrates, Celsus, and Galen, quotes even the Roman Law of the Twelve Tables and Martial's epigrams, and tells of the lead forceps of Erasistratos. He had read "Abulkasis," as well as the French translation of Scultetus; apparently he had a genuine historical interest. Otherwise the book contains all of dentistry with the exception of prosthetics, whereby there is a definite favor shown to instructions for extraction in which he naturally highly recommends the *pyramid-shaped screw* developed by himself for the removal of deeply-seated roots[198].

Beyond what Serre relates of the invention of the *Garengotic key* there is nothing more that we can find out about it: *This instrument is one I have often heard of under the name the key of friar Côme*[199]. *In Germany it is called the English key and in England the German key. What I do not understand is why it is associated with the name of Garengeot in France, since this author does not make even the slightest mention of it; still less one encounters an engraving of it*[200]. *Everywhere the inventor of this key is unknown*[201]. Although Serre improved the key, he always had to *give preference to the*

197 Ibid. p. 110
198 See pp. 326 and 299
199 See footnote p. 191
200 See pp. 210 and 222
201 Serre (c) p. 252

pelican. Nonetheless, the key, which damages the gingiva, having already been mentioned by Bourdet, Bell, Bücking and Loder[202], and others, developed into the most popular extraction-instrument of the 19th century (Fig. 235). The author, however, justifiably praises the "Leklüsischen Hebel" (lever of Lecluse) for removal of the mandibular third molars.

Serre asserted grave scruples in behalf of tooth transplants because of the possibility of transmitting syphilis: *Hunter believes that this disease can only be transmitted by pus. Is it not possible, however, that a drop of impure blood from the alien tooth . . . could infect the entire mass . . .*[203]? The future proved that he, not the great Scot, was right.

For fastening the silk threads in the "Straightening" of teeth he had plates made by a goldsmith from a sulphur or plaster model after a wax impression, and then finished it himself[204]. For drilling the teeth he used a needle-like instrument which was twisted between the thumb and index finger[205].

All in all, Serre's work, comprising 564 pages and 32 copper plates, represents genuine progress. It appears to be based completely and exclusively on personal experience, and for this reason we overlook the author's quite malicious polemics in the preface against his allegedly envious colleagues. In the next year the book underwent a reprinting. In 1856 Joseph Linderer wrote of it that it *with perfect truth was epoch-making at that time, and had been a fundamental help to the practice and the science*[206].

Odontological research

Specialized odontological research first began with Bunon's investigations on the genesis of enamel hypoplasia[207], and Hunter's "Natural History of the Teeth"[208], if we disregard the efforts of the great anatomists of the Rennaissance to explain the development of the teeth. Experimental odontology, even if it was at the most modest level, was pursued by both the professor of anatomy and surgery in Leipzig, Christian Gottlieb Ludwig, in his dissertation "De cortice dentium" (On the Bark of the Teeth), and 25 years later by his colleague in Halle, Johann Christlieb Kemme in his osteological essay "Zweifel und Erinnerungen wider die Lehre der Ärzte von der Ernährung der festen Theile" (Doubts and Memories against the Teachings of Physicians about the Nourishment of the solid Parts). They do not always agree, however: Ludwig believed in the nourishment of the enamel through the humors, while Kemme did not[209]. Both of them tested the behavior of teeth in various acids, whereby Ludwig found that the roots became more decalcified than the crown, while Kemme came to the reverse conclusion[210]. Could it have been that one had removed the periodontal membrane beforehand and the other did not? — Similar experiments were published by Pasch, of Vienna[211], and by the Scots Berdmore and Hunter[212]. Each of the latter pair also studied the behavior of the tooth when heated red hot, and Berdmore even looked into the influence of the toothbrush. Hunter reported on the feeding of young animals with (dyer's-) *madder,* with the result that the dentin turned red while the enamel did not. From this he drew the conclusion that the latter was not vascularized. In 1778 the Austrian Plenk *allowed a healthy tooth to steep in sugar syrup thinned with water for two months, and found the same completely unchanged when it was removed at the end*[213].

In the 18th century authors seldom spoke of the toothworm. The credit, however, for definitively having elucidated mankind about this phantom which came down from the ages, belongs to the evangelical preacher Jacob Christian Schaeffer from Regensburg through his essay, published in 1757, on "Die eingebildeten Würmer in Zähnen nebst den vermeyntlichen Hülfsmitteln wider dieselben" (The imaginary Worms in Teeth and the alleged Remedies against the Same). What Martinez, Houllier, and others had suspected was now proved through a complete series of experiments: the so-called toothworms are nothing other than

[202] See Figs. 203, 215, 230; pp. 210 and 234 f.
[203] Serre (c) p. 336
[204] Ibid. pp. 370 f.
[205] See p. 299
[206] J. Linderer p. 369
[207] See pp. 207 f.
[208] See pp. 219 f.
[209] Ludwig p. X; Kemme pp. 68 f.
[210] Ludwig p. VI; Kemme pp. 84 f.
[211] Pasch p. 4
[212] Berdmore (a) pp. 236 f.; (b) pp. 160 f.; Hunter (b) pp. 34 f.; (c) pp. 38 f.
[213] Plenk (a) p. 70; (b) p. 102

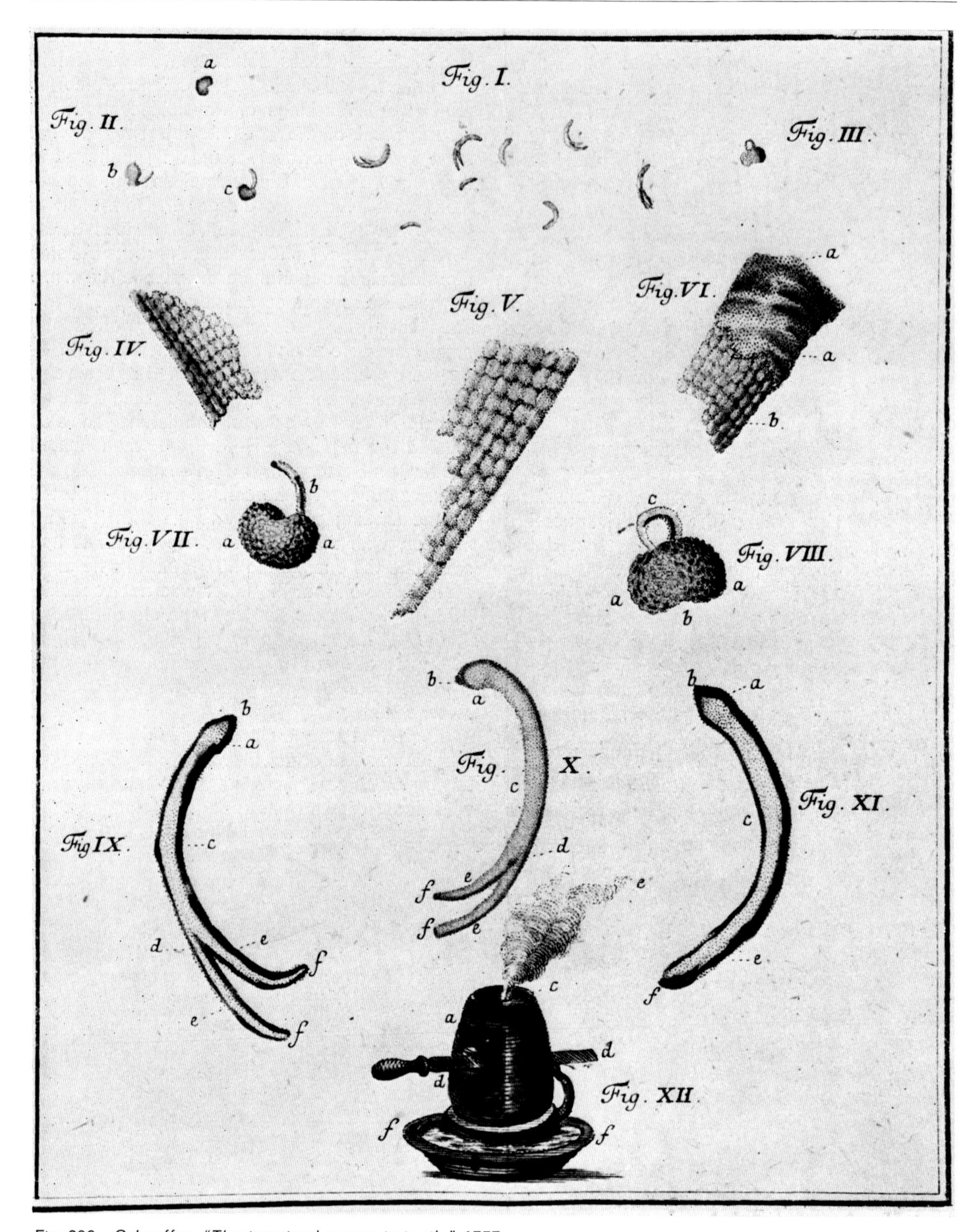

Fig. 236 *Schaeffer: "The imagined worms in teeth," 1757*

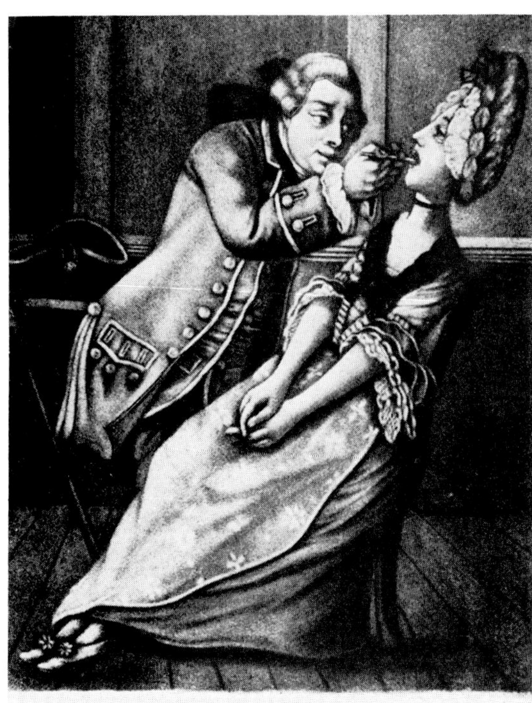
The DENTIST fcaling the LADIES TEETH.
Printed for Carington Bowles, No 69 in St Pauls Church Yard London

Fig. 237 *Anonymous leaflet, second half of the 18th century*

seedlings of the winter cherry, of henbane, the seeds of which, imbedded in wax balls and dropped onto a cautery placed in an earthen vessel (Fig. 236, Fig. XIIdd), leap up with a certain elasticity in the shape of worms and are caught in a water dish (ff) placed below. The patient, however, breathing the slightly narcotic, sialogogic smoke, was brought to believe that the killed worms (Fig. I) were dropping with the saliva into the dish [214].

Social position

The 18th century is not only the time when dentistry became established as an independent profession; the profession was also elevated to a higher plane during this period because it gradually became a resident class, at least in the larger European cities. Therewith the scene shifted from the markets to a room, even if it was at first usually the patient's own one (Fig. 237). As we read on page 209 in Mouton, he counselled an aristocratic lady in her apartment. Pfaff, too, wrote on page 94 of his "Treatise" that *a French merchant here* (a member of the Huguenot community which then led a rather insular life in Berlin) *had me called to him.* In Fauchard's case histories, however, we occasionally read that people came to him and sought him out, both during his stay in the provinces and in Paris. Not till 1834, the Viennese surgeon and dentist Joseph Gall declared unequivocally that *dental operations are better performed in the apartment of the dentist himself, than in that of the sick person, primarily because all the operator's instruments and other aids are available* [215].

The number of resident dentists, who nonetheless still went on journeys now and then, increased only slowly. While there were, according to figure 199, 30 dentists living in Paris, besides to three surgeons who occupied themselves with dentistry, Maury reports that in 1790,

[214] Schaeffer. See pp. 73 and 145
[215] Gall pp. 216 f.

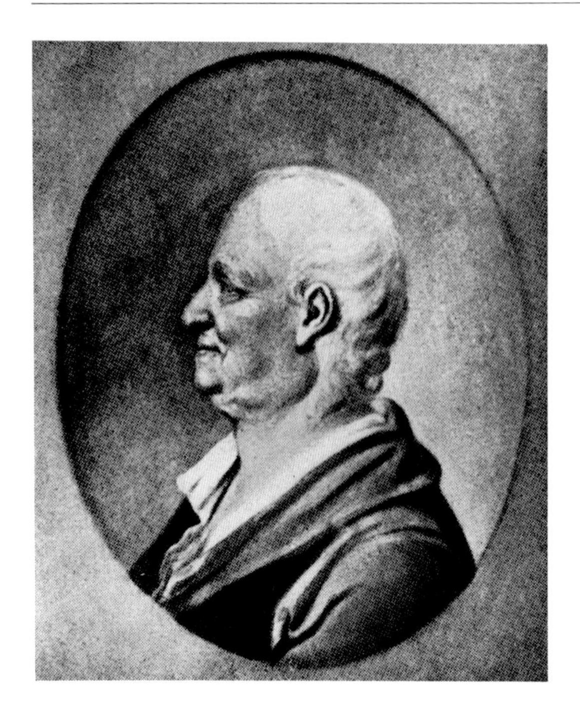

Fig. 238 *Johannes Ehrenreich*

were no more than 5 dentists there, and in all the rest of France, there were perhaps twice as many. In 1800 Dagen counted 34 in Paris according to the "Almanach du Commerce," and in 1828, there were already 140, according to Maury, of whom 100 were registered [216]. The *Vossische Zeitung,* edited in Berlin, reported from Vienna on January 10, 1783 that among 200,000 inhabitants, there were 222 doctores, 75 surgeons, 169 midwives, and 4 dentists [217], and for Berlin itself, a city guide from the year 1786 informs us that *teeth (false ones, including whole and half dentures from walrus and deer teeth)* were made by 2 dentists and one artisan [218].

The Soviet "Great Medical Encyclopedia" states that there were 20 dentists in Russia at the time of the turn from the 18th to the 19th century, all of whom, however, were foreigners, who limited themselves to Petersburg and Moscow. Like all medical men, these had so submit to an examination by the Medical Chancellery, since 1721. Some time around 1790 the first Russians are said to have been educated by them for whose benefit the professional designation "Zubnoj lekar" (Tooth surgeon — probably a reference to the French "Chirurgien dentiste") was initiated in 1818. This became "Dentist" in 1838, and "Zubnoj vrač" (dentist) in 1891. As early as 1829 women officially had the right to practice dentistry [219].

The conditions were similar in North America in the 18th century, while the United States was still in its rough colonial period. Here too, the activity of the predominantly itinerant "Tooth-Drawers" and "Dentists" consisted of pulling teeth. It was essentially carried out by western European immigrants, as well as they could and pursued their bloody calling totally without restraint [220]. Only in the last quarter of the century, as is explained later, a few trained representatives of the profession settled in the large cities. As was the case everywhere pulling teeth was naturally practiced by the surgeons beside their surgical work.

216 Maury p. 438; Dagen p. 328
217 Buchner p. 22
218 Nicolai II pp. 581 f.
219 Bassalyk; Lowarski pp. 11 f.; Muchin. See pp. 412 f.
220 Weinberger has attempted to list the dentists active in the United States in the 18th century by name; see Weinberger II pp. 16 f.

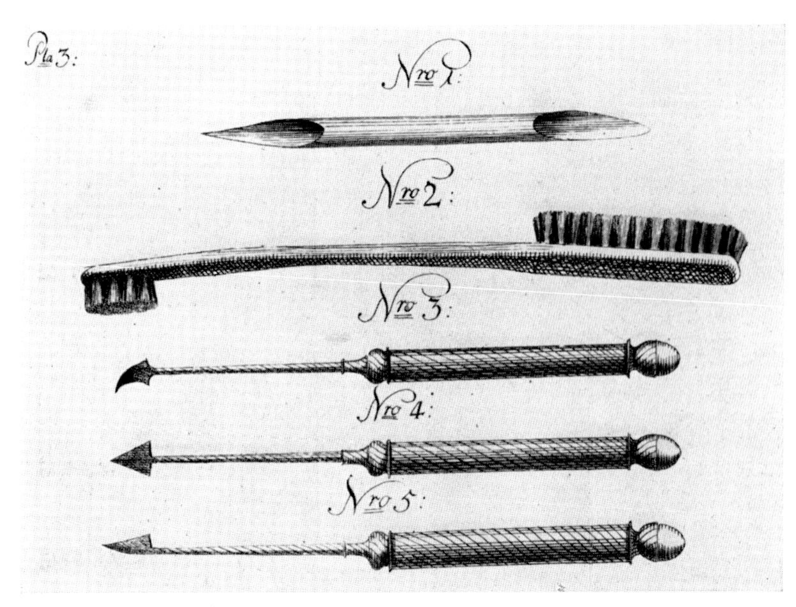

Fig. 239 *Devices for tooth care of J. Girault, court dentist in Braunschweig: toothpick shaped from a quill, toothbrush, and scalers, 1790*

Let us turn back to the situation of the tooth therapists in old Europe: in the free imperial city of Frankfurt am Main, which has been thoroughly investigated in this respect, dental services in the first third of the 18th century still lay entirely in the hands of the surgeons and the itinerant tooth-drawers (Zahnbrecher) who were always present at the fairs. Only in the year 1736 the Hungarian-born (in 1704) Johannes Ehrenreich settled there with the approval of the Council, after a longer period of roving life (Fig. 238). Himself the son and nephew of travelling dentists, he was the only "Mouth and Tooth Operator" there for 28 years. But even such a wealthy and socially accepted man as he was, possessor of an important art and mineral collection, in his 18-page long advertisement essay, "Thoughts on the characteristics of an upright, thoroughly experienced oral and dental surgeon," in which he even mentioned Fauchard, complained about the "baseness" of his class and their low revenue: *Fifty extracted teeth can hardly bring in as much as an amputation often does, or a leg fracture* [221].

Ehrenreich's son, Eberhard Ludwig, went to Stockholm as court dentist in 1747 and was the first important representative of dentistry there. After losing his court position through the change of sovereigns he gave up the profession and founded a porcelain factory, without, as might have been natural, putting the abilities he obtained there to use for his father's profession [222].

In the years from 1736 to 1764, there was only one dentist practicing in Frankfurt; then there were two, and finally, in 1800, six. It is from Frankfurt, however, that we know that this slow increase was not a result of too few applicants but rather of the difficulties which the Councils put in the way of their approval. This was caused, chiefly, by the protests of the surgeons' guild, which was worried about losing its patients [223]. The yearning of the itinerant medical trade to become permanently established was present at the time but it was not yet generally accepted by their environment.

[221] Ehrenreich pp. 6 and 8
[222] Goerke
[223] Wiegel pp. 29 f.

References

Artelt, Walter
Der Zahnarzt im 18. Jahrhundert. Dtsch. med. J. 5 (1954) 269—271

Bassalyk, A.
Zur Geschichte der zahnärztlichen Ausbildung im vorrevolutionären Rußland. "Stomatologija" 1 (1961) 82 f. Transl. Dieter Nüchert in: Zahnärztl. Mitt. 52 (1962) 1199—1201

Baumès, Jean-Baptiste Timothée
Traité de la première dentition et des maladies . . ., qui en dependent. Paris 1806

Bell, Benjamin
A system of surgery. Vol. IV, Edinburgh 1786

Berdmore, Thomas
a) A treatise on the disorder and deformities of the teeth and the gums. London 1768
b) Abhandlung von den Krankheiten der Zähne und des Zahnfleisches . . . Altenburg 1771

Besombes, André, Georges Dagen
Pierre Fauchard et ses contemporains. Paris 1961

Blake, Robert
An essay on the structure and formation of the teeth in man and various animals. (Med. Diss. Edinburgh 1798) Dublin 1801

Böhmecke, Mathilde
Lécluse. Med. Diss. Berlin 1931

Botot
Sur la suppuration des gencives. Medecine, Chirurgie, Pharmacie, etc. 32 (1770) 356—372

Bourdet, (Etienne)
a) Soins faciles pour la propreté de la bouche, . . . Paris 1760/1771
b) Leichte Mittel, den Mund rein zu halten . . . Leipzig 1762
c) Recherches et observations sur toutes des parties de l'art du dentiste. 2 vols., Paris 1786

Bräuning- Oktavio, Hermann
Vom Zwischenkieferknochen zur Idee des Typus. Nova Acta Leopoldina 18 (1956) Nr. 126

Brambilla, Ioan. Alexander
Instrumentarium chirurgicum viennese. Wien (1781)

Bremner, M. D. K.
The story of dentistry. 3rd ed., Brooklyn, London 1964

Brethauer, Karl
Der Chirurg Eisenbart im Urteil eines Zeitgenossen. Materia Med. Nordmark 18 (1966) 762—773

Brunner, Adam Anton
a) Einleitung zur nöthigen Wissenschaft eines Zahnarztes. Wien 1766
b) Abhandlung von der Hervorhebung der Milchzähne. Wien 1771

Buchner, Eberhard
Ärzte und Kurpfuscher. München 1922

Bücking, J(ohann) J(akob) H(einrich)
Vollständige Anweisung zum Zahnausziehen für angehende Wundärzte. Stendal 1782

Bunon, (Robert)
a) Essay sur les maladies des dents . . . Paris 1743
b) Expériences et demonstrations faites à l'Hôpital de la Salpêtrière . . . Paris 1746

Callisen, Adolph Carl Petere
Medicinisches Schriftsteller-Lexicon . . . Bd. VIII, Copenhagen 1831; Bd. XXVIII, Copenhagen 1840

Campani, Antonio
Odontologia, ossia trattado sopra i denti. Firenze 1786

Campbell, J. Menzies
Dentistry then and now. Glasgow 1963

Cohen, R. A.
Notes on the identification, description and dating of ivory dentures. Brit. Dent. J. 113 (1962) 259—263

Courtois, Honoré-Gaillard
Le dentiste observateur. Paris 1775

Cron, Ludwig
Der bey dem Aderlassen und Zahn-aus-ziehen . . . qualificirte Candidatus chirurgiae oder Barbiergeselle . . . Leipzig 1717

Dagen, Georges
Documents pour servir à l'histoire de l'art dentaire en France. Paris (1926)

Driak, Fritz
Anteil der Wiener Schule an der Zahnheilkunde des XVIII. und XIX. Jahrhunderts. Wien. klin. Wschr. 49 (1936) 951—964

Duval, (Jacques René)
Notice historique sur la vie et les ouvrages de M. Jourdain. Paris 1816

Ehrenreich, Johannes
Gedancken von den Eigenschafften eines rechtschaffenen gründlich erfahrnen Mund und Zahn-Artztes. Franckfurt am Mayn (1755?)

Fauchard, Pierre
a) Le chirurgien dentiste, ou traité des dents. 2nd ed., 2 Tomes, Paris 1746
b) Frantzösischer Zahn-Artzt, oder Tractat von den Zähnen. 2 Teile, Berlin 1733
c) The surgeon Dentist or Treatise on the Teeth. Transl. from the 2nd ed., 1746, by Lilian Lindsay, London 1946

Gall, Joseph
Populäre Anleitung über die wichtigsten Gegenstände der Zahnheilkunde . . . Wien 1834

Geraudly, (Claude)
L'art de conserver les dents. Paris 1737

Girault, J.
La bonne mère. Bronsvic 1790

Goerke, Heinz
Johann Eberhard Ludwig Ehrenreich. Sudhoffs Arch. Gesch. Med. Naturw. 40 (1956) 29—40

Goethe, Johann Wolfgang von
a) Goethe's Werke (Sophien-edition). Part IV, vol. VI, Nr. 1903, Weimar 1890
b) Abhandlung vom Zwischenkieferknochen. Reprint ed. by Hermann Bräuning-Oktavio, München 1968

Gräbner, C(arl) A(ugust)
Gedanken über das Hervorkommen und Wechseln der Zähne bey Kindern; . . . Hamburg 1766. Reprint Ed. A. Geus, Marburg 1978

Guerini, Vincenzo
Italian writers on dental science and their works. Dent. Cosmos 46 (1904) 1010—1017

Hallerus, Albertus
a) Disputationes chirurgicae selectae. Tomus I, Venetiis 1755
b) Collection de Thèses medico-chirurgicales. Tome I, Paris 1757

Heister, Lorenz
a) Dissertatio anatomico-physiologica de masticatione. Noricorum 1711
b) Chirurgie, in welcher alles, was zur Wund-Artzney gehöret . . . 2. Aufl., Nürnberg 1724
c) Institutiones chirurgicae, 2 vols., Amstaeldami 1750
d) Kleine Chirurgie oder Handbuch der Wundtartzney, 3rd ed., Nürnberg 1767

Hirsch(feld), Friedrich
a) Practische Bemerkungen über die Zähne und einige Krankheiten derselben. Jena 1796
b) Idem, 2nd ed. Jena 1801
c) Bemerkungen über die Krankheiten des Zahnfleisches . . . Erfurt 1804

Hoffmann, Friedrich
a) Medicina rationalis systematica (1718—1739), in: Opera omnia physico-medica, vols. I—III, Genevae 1748
b) Disputatio medico-practica de remediis ant-odontalgicis, in: Opera omnia, Suppl. II, pars I, Genevae 1753
c) Medicina consultatoria, . . . Vol. XII, Halle 1721—1739
d) Disputatio inauguralis medico-practica de remediis ant-odontalgicis. Resp.: Johannes Süsse (Halae) 1700

e) Dissertatio inauguralis medica exhibens historiam dentium physiologice et pathologice pertracta, . . . Resp.: Joh. Fredericus Trefurth. Halae 1698

f) Dissertatio solemnis de dentibus, eorum morbis et cura, . . . Resp.: J. F. Trefurth. Halae 1714

g) A treatise on the teeth; . . . 3 rd ed., London 1756

h) Dissertatio chirurgica de fistula maxillari. (primum ed. 1735) in: Opera omnia, Suppl. II, pars II, Genevae 1753

Hoffmann-Axthelm, Walter
Robert Bunon (1702—1748), der erste Krankenhauszahnarzt. Zahnärztl. Mitt. 57 (1967) 1110—1112

Hunter, John
a) The natural history of the teeth . . . 1st ed. London 1771; 2nd ed. London 1778
b) A practical treatise on the diseases of the teeth. London 1778
c) Natürliche Geschichte der Zähne und Beschreibung ihrer Krankheiten in zween Theilen. Leipzig 1780

Hurlock, Joseph
A practical treatise upon dentition . . . London 1742

Jourdain, (Anselme)
a) Traité des maladies et des opérations . . . de la bouche . . . 2 Tomes, Paris 1778
b) Abhandlungen über die chirurgischen Krankheiten des Mundes . . . 2 vols., Nürnberg 1784

Jöcher, Christian Gottlieb
Fortsetzung und Ergänzungen zu Jöchers allgemeinem Gelehrten-Lexikon, . . . Vol. IV, Bremen 1813

Kemme, Johann Christlieb
Zweifel und Erinnerungen wider die Lehre der Aerzte von der Ernährung der festen Teile. Halle 1778

Kowarski, M. O.
Die Zahnheilkunde in Rußland im 18. und 19. Jahrhundert. Greifswald 1933

Kräutermann, Valentin
Der sichere Augen- und Zahn-Artzt, . . . Arnstadt 1732

Lecluse, (Louis)
Nouveaux éléments d'odontologie. Paris 1754

Linderer, J(oseph)
Die Zahnheilkunde nach ihrem neuesten Standpunkt. Erlangen 1851

Lindsay, Lilian
Thomas Berdmore. Brit. Dent. J. 49 (1928) 225—238

Ludwig, Christianus Gottlieb
De cortice dentium. Lipsiae 1753

Magitot, Emile
Etude sur le développement et la structure des dents humaines. These Mèd. Paris 1857

Matheson, Leonard, J. Lewin Payne
The history of dentistry in Great Britain. J. Am. Dental Ass. 15 (1928) 441—461

Maury, F.
Traité complet de l'art du dentiste. Nouv. Ed., Paris 1833

Medicinal-Edict, Königl. Preuß. u. Churfürstl. Brandenburgisches, und Verordnung . . . Berlin 1725

Medizinisch-chirurgische Zeitung. Bd. 4 (1804) 352, Salzburg

Meusel, Johann Georg
Lexikon der vom Jahre 1750 bis 1800 verstorbenen teutschen Schriftsteller. Vol. VIII, Leipzig 1808

Mouton, (Claude)
Essay d'odontotechnie . . . Paris 1746

Muchin, M.
"Stomatologija". In: Bol'šaja medicinskaja enciklopedija, 2nd ed., vol. XXXI, Moskva 1963. coll. 544—561

Mylius, Christian Otto
Corpus constitutionum marchicarum . . . Vol. V, part 4, Halle 1740

(Nicolai, Friedrich)
Beschreibung der Königlichen Residenzstädte Berlin und Potsdam . . . 3 vols., 3rd ed., Berlin 1786

Pasch, Joseph Georg
Abhandlung aus der Wundarzney von den Zähnen, . . . Wien 1767

Petit, (Jean Louis)
a) Traité des maladies des os. Paris 1767
b) Abhandlung von denen Kranckheiten derer Knochen . . . Berlin 1725

Pfaff, Philipp
Abhandlung von den Zähnen des menschlichen Körpers und deren Krankheiten. Berlin 1756. Reprint ed. Walter Hoffmann-Axthelm, Hildesheim 1966

Plenk, Joseph Jacob
a) Doctrina de morbis dentium ac gingivarium. Viennae 1778
b) Lehre von den Krankheiten der Zähne und des Zahnfleisches. Wien 1779
c) De morbi de denti e delle gengie. Venezia 1786

Proskauer, Curt, Fritz H(einz) Witt
Bildgeschichte der Zahnheilkunde. Köln 1962

Rau, Iohannes Iacobus
De ortu et regeneratione dentium. Med. Diss. Lugduni batavorum 1694

Reichenbach, Erwin
Goethe und die Stomatologie. Dtsch. Stomat. 11 (1961) 556—568

Richter, August Gottlieb
Anfangsgründe der Wundarzneykunst. Vol. IV, Wien 1798

Ruspini, Barth(olomeo)
A treatise on the teeth . . . 2nd ed., London 1768

Ruyschius, Fredericus
Observationum anatomico-chirurgicarum centuria. Amstelodami 1691

Schäffer, Jacob Christian
Die eingebildeten Würmer in Zähnen nebst dem vermeintlichen Hülfsmittel wider dieselben. Regensburg 1757

Serre, Johann Jacob Joseph
a) Geschichte oder Abhandlung der Zahnschmerzen des schönen Geschlechts in ihrer Schwangerschaft. Wien 1788
b) Abhandlung über die Flüsse und Entzündungen, von denen die Geschwulsten oder Zahnfleischgeschwüre herrühren . . . Wien, Leipzig 1791
c) Praktische Darstellung aller Operationen der Zahnheilkunst. Berlin 1803

Smitt, Kurt Willem:
Der Zahnarzt Bartholomeo Ruspini und sein Werk. Med. Diss. Leipzig 1924

van Swieten, Gerardus L. B.
Commentaria in Hermanni Boerhaave Aphorismos. Lugdunum Batavorum 1764

Tolver, A.
A treatise on the teeth. London 1752

Wackernagel, Imme
Friedrich Hoffmann (1660—1742) und seine Beziehungen zur Zahn-, Mund- und Kieferheilkunde. Med. Diss. Berlin (FU) 1969

Weinberger, Bernhard Wolf
An introduction to the history of dentistry. Vol. I and II, St. Louis 1948

Wiegel, Paul
Zahnärzte und Zahnbehandlung im alten Frankfurt am Main bis zum Jahre 1810. München 1957

Winslow, Jacobus Benignus
An anatomical exposition of the structure of the human body. Vol. I. London 1733

Witt, Dirk
Beiträge zum Leben und Werk von Philipp Pfaff. Med. Diss. Berlin (FU) 1969

Part 2

Dentistry in the Industrial Age

Introduction

After dentistry had established itself largely on its own base in the 18th century, there followed in the 19th century an increasing professional consolidation, but especially an expansion of the therapeutic methods and the means for treatment, corresponding to the technology being developed in dentistry's environment. This entry into the general economic system of the industrial age had already begun in England in the 17th century, if with some hesitation. Technical advance was signalled by the change from single piecework in small workshops to factory manufacture. In the late 18th and in the 19th centuries, the sudden introduction of machine technology brought along its own problems. This change took place according to the state of development of the various individual nations and their own requirements, over significant intervals of time and insolubly coupled with the political situations existing locally.

These political circumstances were determined at the turn of the century in Europe by the French Revolution and the Napoleonic wars, from which only the British island kingdom came out strengthened. In the second half of the century also, almost all of the nations met on the battlefield, e. g., in the Crimean wars, the Italian and the German wars of unification, and the Russo-Turkish conflict. The national fronts, in consequence, became more rigid, a condition which, increased by the economic and colonial contrasts, led to the far more serious tumults of war of the 20th century.

Liberal trends, which arose in the central European middle classes after Napoleon's abdication initially in industrially advanced England and in France changed by its revolution, failed through the restorative measures of monarchial governments which withstood the revolutionary waves of 1848, if not entirely without damage. Social tensions, developed by increasing population shifts from agrarian to industrial societies, became stronger. Toughtlessly developing wholesale industry was gradually confronted by a slowly organizing workers' movement.

Continuously and with increasing acceleration, industrialization developed in the United States of America, the process being interrupted only by the bloody war between the southern and the northern states, with the result being the emancipation of slaves. The developing feelings of political and economic freedom and also America's technical development was not without effect on the nations of Europe. Dentists such as Harris, Kingsley, Morrison, Black, Bonwill and Angle had in this sense a world-wide stimulating effect on practical dentistry.

When the phase of natural philosophy, based largely on speculation, had been overcome in medicine an unprecedented advance began in the fourth decade of the 19th century. The resulting progress was based on purely scientific research in natural history, in which dentistry participated. In addition to the development of the very important mechanical and technical components of the subject, taking place chiefly in the New World, fundamental research as intensive as it was successful was stimulated in Europe. The stimulus was provided directly or indirectly by the work of outstanding scientists such as Johannes Müller, Owen, Purkinje, Retzius, Virchow, Broca, Pasteur and Koch, and by important dentists such as Tomes, Linderer, Heider, Magitot, Witzel, Miller and Preiswerk.

The fusion of knowledge in Europe and America led in practical dentistry, as in general medicine, to the initiation of specialties. The benefits from this development were restricted, however, in this century to the wealthy, while the poor continued as they had done before to take their toothaches to the tooth-drawer, the barber, and — in the second half of the century — to a growing number of unlicensed dental therapists. In Europe these conditions were eliminated only in the 20th century largely through the installation of social health insurance systems. The coalescence to an academically trained profession of the two groups of persons treating dental diseases is not yet entirely completed in all the nations.

These developmental tendencies of the 19th and of the beginning of the 20th centuries will be

described on the following pages. In contrast to the arrangement used up to this point, the developing branches of dentistry will be described separately in their growth. The section will close with a look at research in selected fields of odontology and with a review of dental education in some of the leading nations. Broad-based academical training of new dentists, beginning in the United States in the third and in Europe in the last quarter of the 19th century, has been gradually and systematically controlled by governments of progressive nations.

Chapter 11

Prosthetics

The desire to close disfiguring gaps between the teeth might well be almost as old as humanity itself. The first woman ever to dress and adorne herself probably tried to replace a tooth lost by external forces, by caries or periodontal atrophy with a bit of wax, a skein of flax, or even with a suitably shaped piece of bone. As these efforts always involved perishable materials, no trace of these attempts have remained for study.

As we have read, the oldest relics found so far are the two gold wire ties from Egypt from the middle of the third millenium before Christ. A similar technique is encountered 2,000 years later in Syria for the fastening of two crowns of natural teeth as replacements for incisors[1]. This came to be included in Hippocrates' writings in the recommendation of tying traumatically loosened teeth[2], and thus became a component part of the Greek and Roman, and later the Byzantine and Islamic literatures. In the writings of the high Middle Ages, for example, in Guy de Chauliac, we find that this binding technique and its application for the fastening of a primitive dental prosthesis carved from bone had been taken from the Arabs[3]. Information on the far more advanced Etruscan and Roman gold band techniques[4], on the other hand, was lost in the chaotic period of tribal migrations.

Early pictures of dental prostheses are delivered to us by Abulcasim and the father of modern surgery, Ambroise Paré (see Figs. 81 and 121). Their development was advanced by the reports by the surgeon in Breslau Purmann and by the professors Nuck and Heister[5] as well as by the efforts of anonymous talented craftsmen. Their insights achieved through quiet activity, were compiled in 1728 by the great Parisian dentist Pierre Fauchard who combined traditional knowledge of literally active surgeons with his own experience in his fundamental book[6]. In 1746 Mouton in Paris described the first gold crown; Philipp Pfaff in Berlin was the first with a wax impression from the jaw and a plaster casting from it for prosthetic purposes in 1756, and Bourdet in Paris was the first to try a gold base[7]. The materials used for the teeth, in addition now to bones, ivory, and tusks from hippopotamus and walruses, were human teeth obtained from corpses, which, however, like every other organic substance in the oral cavity, fell prey all too quickly to caries (Fig. 240). Only toward the end of the 18th century attempts began to use a durable material which had been manufactured in Europe since the beginning of the century for dental prosthetics.

[1] See pp. 25 f. and 34
[2] See p. 64
[3] See p. 99
[4] See pp. 68 f.
[5] See pp. 182 f., 185 and 226
[6] See pp. 202 f.
[7] See pp. 209, 231, 213 f.

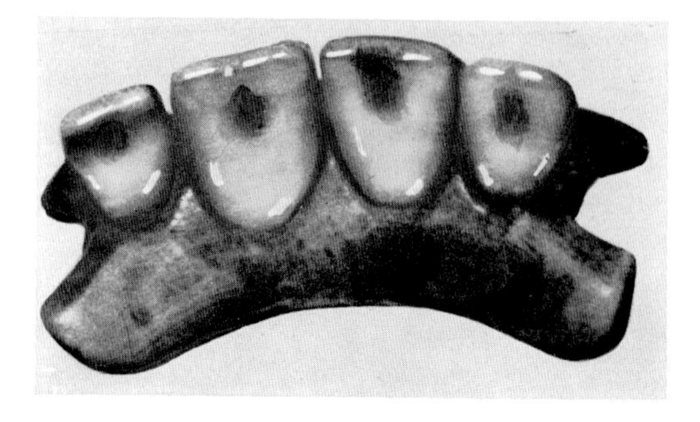

Fig. 240 *Incisor replacement, made of carved ivory base to which are fastened human teeth mounted on wooden connecting posts, 18th century (Forschungsinstitut für Geschichte der Zahnheilkunde, Cologne)*

Plate Prostheses and their Materials

Even before the French Revolution began with the storming of the Bastille in 1789, bringing with it a sudden end to the cultivated court dentistry of the Ancien régime, the bases for the fabrication of porcelain teeth had been worked out through great effort in Paris. In the course of the following century these were to push from the scene the grisly corpses teeth obtained in hospitals, from the executioner, from cemeteries, and, chiefly, from battlefields. Not until modern times artificial teeth assumed an importance equal to these. Here previous inadequate experiments come to mind, such as Guillemeau's artificial teeth produced from a mineral paste, and those of Fauchard, painted in enamel on a metal capsule [8].

The interesting history of this invention has been passed on to us by the Parisian dentist Joseph Audibran in a book published in 1821 which is not, however, to be regarded in any way as an objective source. According to this report an apothecary in the Parisian suburb of St. Germain, named Alexis Duchâteau, who was dissatisfied with the decomposing and smelly bone prostheses, had a porcelain denture fired by the Guerhard porcelain factory in Sèvres near Paris in 1774. The results were so totally successful that he communicated his findings to the Surgical Academy in 1776 [9]. The attempt to make use of the invention for other patients too, however, failed because of the apothecary's insufficient special training, and the porcelain denture fell into oblivion.

It was not forgotten, however, by the Parisian dentist Nicolas Dubois de Chémant (Fig. 241). He succeeded in eliciting from Duchâteau the prescriptions for it, and a "Dissertation sur les avantages des nouvelles dents et rateliers artificiels" (London edition: "A Dissertation on Artificial Teeth") came out from his pen in 1788 in Paris and London. Here he characterizes the dentures as *incorruptibles et sans odeur (imperishable and odorless): . . . I have found incorruptible substances among the minerals, . . . I have finally succeeded after many experiments in compounding a mineral paste capable of being shaped (modelled, ductile), which is suitable for taking the correct and exact impression from gingiva and from parts of the teeth, without it being necessary to extract these*[10] (Fig. 242). With this the descriptive

[8] See pp. 151 and 206
[9] Verchere was unable to find any indication thereof in the files of the Academy in 1974
[10] Dubois de Chémant pp. 5 f.

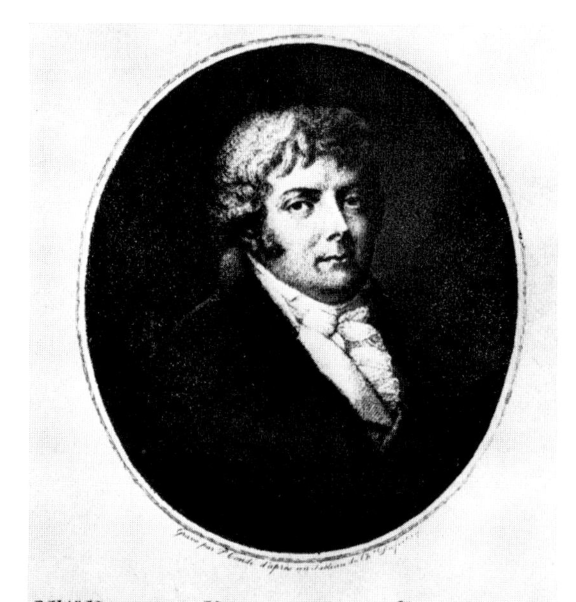

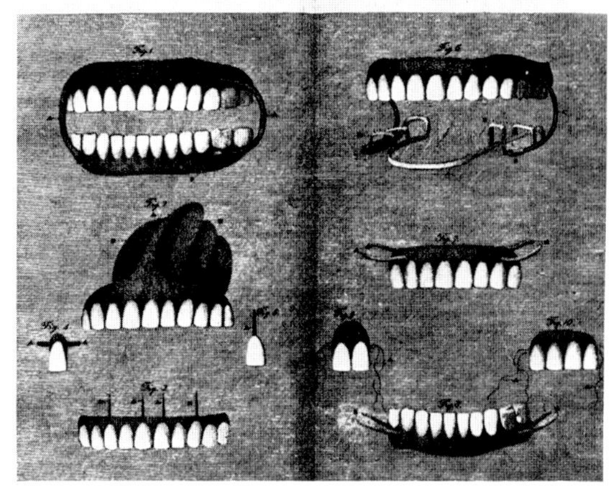

Fig. 242 *Dubois de Chémant: Porcelain dentures and an obturator in the English flyer "A Dissertation on artificial Teeth," 1797*

Fig. 241 *Nicolas Dubois de Chémant*

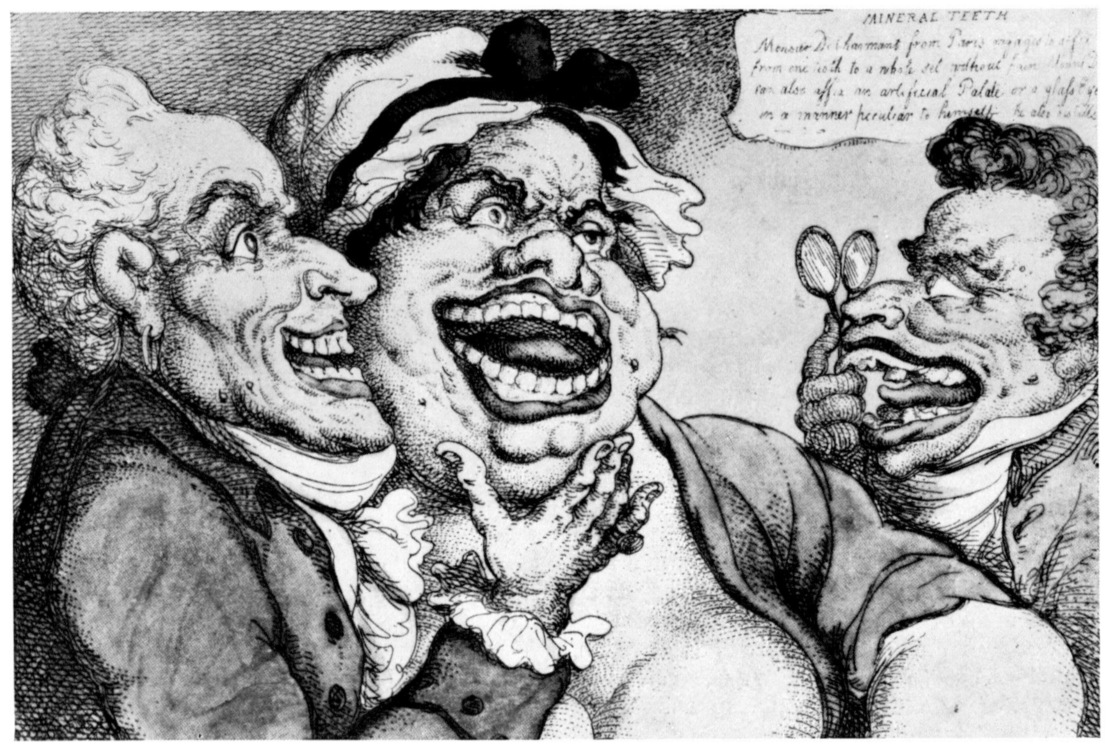

Fig. 243 *Caricature of Dubois' porcelain dentures, copper etching by Thomas Rowlandson, about 1790*

word *incorruptibles* became the term for the porcelain denture.

Nonetheless, we must give this plagiarizer credit for having understood how to increase his ill-gotten gains, because his porcelain dentures, which were shaped according to models [11], seem to have stood the test of use. Herewith they not only brought him the desired financial rewards, but also honors from the Royal Medical Society and the Faculty, both of which were expressly mentioned in his book. The approval of the Association was certified in 1788 by the permanent secretary, the anatomist Vicq d'Azyr, whom we have already encountered as one of the first to describe the premaxilla bone [12]. On the basis of these certificates Dubois de Chémant obtained a patent in 1791 which assured him a monopoly on manufacture for 15 years[13]. Later he sold his methods of fabrication under a promise of secrecy to some Parisian colleagues, including Jean Baptiste Gariot and others. In his book of 1805 Gariot strongly condemned the secrecy surrounding a technique which could have been useful everywhere, but he still had to submit to it [14]. On the other hand Louis Laforgue in 1802 had rejected porcelain dentures from the outset because of their fragility and because in use they sounded like cracked bells[15].

The issuance of the patent induced the apothecary Duchâteau to return to his idea, but his claims were rejected because the patent was irrevocable. Dubois de Chémant, however, betook himself to London in 1793, *in order to escape the dangers* (of revolution) *which then existed in France* (Audibran, 1821), and *because he was weary of struggling with his colleagues* (Désirabode, 1843). There, too, as early as 1791, a royal patent for 12 years was awarded to him. In 1806 Joseph Fox in London praised the artificial teeth *made of a porcelain composition, which has been introduced by M. de Chamant* [16]. His products attained such a

11 Ibid. p. 13
12 Ibid. p. 10. See p. 235
13 Dagen p. 188
14 Gariot pp. 296 f.
15 Laforgue (a) pp. 361 f.; (b) p. 310
16 Audibran p. 42; Désirabode p. 576; Cohen (b); Fox pp. 127 f

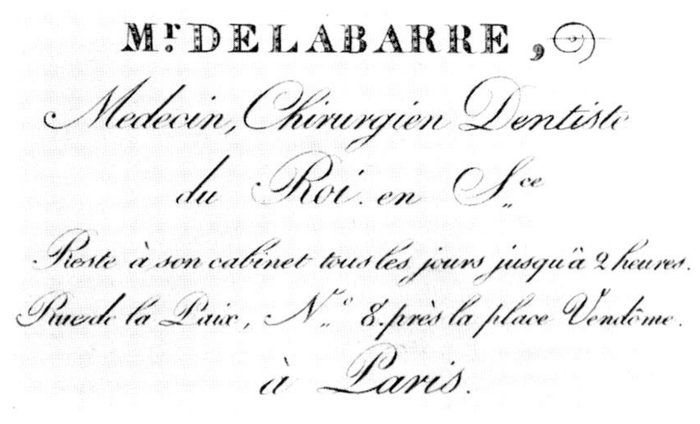

Mr DELABARRE,
Médecin, Chirurgien Dentiste
du Roi. en Sce
Reste à son cabinet tous les jours jusqu'à 2 heures.
Rue de la Paix, No. 8. près la place Vendôme.
à Paris.

Fig. 244 *Business card of Ch. F. Delabarre, glued into his "Odontologie" Paris, 1815*

degree of popularity there that the famous English caricaturist Thomas Rowlandson devoted a colored copper etching to them; in it, under the title of "Mineral Teeth," we find a commendation of "Monsieur De Charmant from Paris" (Fig. 243).

This representation of the invention of the porcelain denture, which was based on Audibran, contrasted somewhat with the report by the man to whom we owe thanks for the first scientifically written textbook of prosthetics: the physician and court dentist Christophe François Delabarre (Fig. 244). In his two-volume "Traité de la partie mécanique de l'art du chirurgien-dentiste" (Treatise on the mechanical portion of the art of dentistry), which was published in Paris in 1820, we learn that several respected dentists, who were worried about their clientele because of Dubois de Chémant's successes, had jointly brought an action against him. In it they attributed the credit to an apothecary named Duchâteau; the suit was lost, however, because of insufficient evidence. They also demolished Dubois' furnace in the factory at Sèvres, but its director, Jean Darcet, provided him with a new one. He was also the man who had introduced Dubois into this famous porcelain manufactory, where the craftsmen had given him the idea of taking oral impressions (moules de la bouche) and casting them in plaster of Paris. This was the same method which Pfaff had recommended thirty years before [17]. In those centuries when Latin still prevailed as the universal language of scholars international communication was better as we can see.

Another opponent of Dubois de Chémant, the court dentist to Louis XVI (and later also to Napoleon, Louis XVIII, and Charles X), Jean-Joseph Dubois-Foucou, also had become acquainted with the new material as the assessor of the Surgical Academy. On the base of his familiarity with the composition of the porcelain paste, which was not exactly honestly come by, Dubois-Foucou, who had bitterly opposed the mineral teeth 15 years before [18], continued the work in Paris on the day after the patent expired [19]. He modified firing temperatures and mixtures and fabricated dentures with teeth in three different shades through the addition of metal oxides, blue-white, gray-white, and yellow-white [20]. He deserves credit, however, for being the first to reveal the compositions of these ceramic mixtures in 1808. The identity of the genuine inventor of the porcelain denture can hardly be established toady. Since later authors, however, such as Maury, Lefoulon, and Désirabode, believed that the apothecary Duchâteau was the first, the pithy summary by a contemporary might be close to the mark: the thief (Dubois-Foucou) had robbed the thief (Dubois de Chémant). There is no dispute, on the other hand, that Dubois de Chémant's efforts had kept the idea of the "incorruptibles" from falling into oblivion.

The decisive progress made in the beginning of the 19th century by Giuseppangelo Fonzi (Fig. 245), who was working in Paris, was met, in contrast, with unqualified general acclaim. This man, who was born in Teramo in central Italy, had a life of adventure behind him. At the age of 16 he went to Naples to attend the university. Instead he joined the Spanish mer-

17 Ch. F. Delabarre pp. 86 f.
18 Dubois de Chémant p. 15; Désirabode pp. 576 f.
19 A. Delabarre p. 31
20 Audibran p. 45

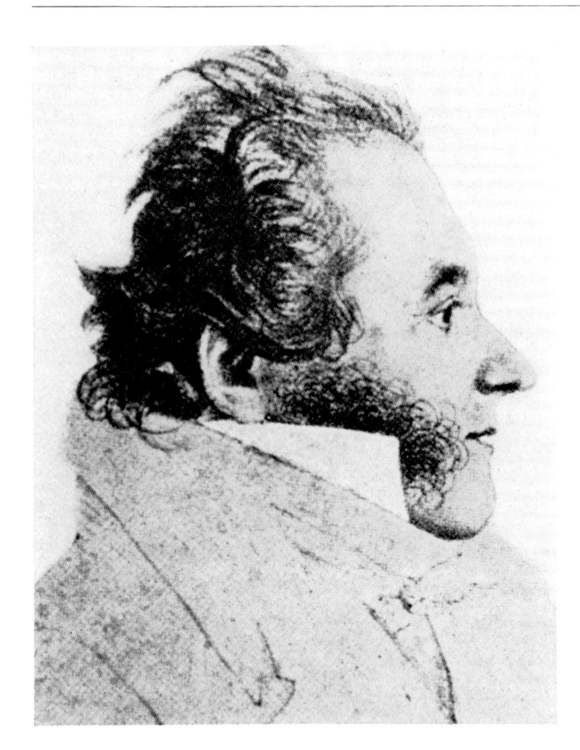

Fig. 245 *Giuseppangelo Fonzi*

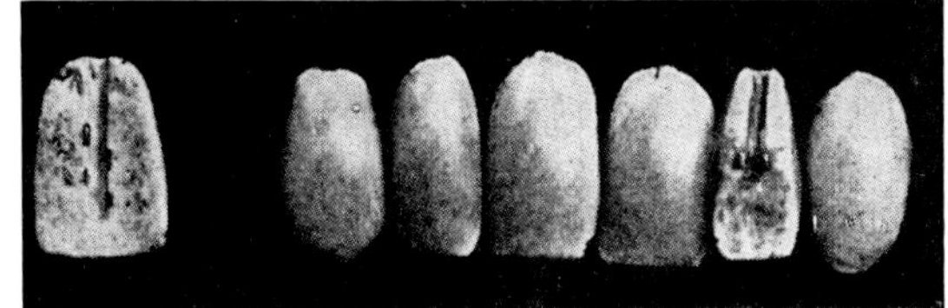

Fig. 246 *Dents terro-métalliques*

chant marine and spent a long time at sea. When one day he became displeased with the strict discipline he left the ship in Spain, and found himself completely destitute in a foreign country. In the marketplace he observed a tooth-drawer, memorized the man's techniques, fitted himself out with a few instruments and embarked on the new profession, in which he was rapidly successful. Soon he found his knowledge insufficient, and read the book by Martinez[21] followed by those of the French authors. Then, in 1795, he moved to Paris, where the situation was beginning to be consolidated under the government of the Directorate. He soon had a brilliant practice there and was summoned to the courts of Munich, St. Petersburg and Madrid in the twenties. He returned to Spain where the king had granted him a pension as an impoverished old man. Still longing for his Italian homeland, however, he died on the way there, in Barcelona, at the age of 72[22].

While previously the entire mineral denture, both base and teeth, had been fired as a single piece, Fonzi in 1808 published a method for the manufacture of individual teeth with platinum hooks fired into them (in French, "crampons"). Whith the invention of these "Dents terro-metalliques" (Fig. 246), or "Calliodontes" (from "dents de caillon," or "flint teeth," as they were called by his countryman, the Parisian dentist François-Dominique Ricci) which could be soldered to a metal bar, the determining step towards modern dental prosthetics had been taken.

Soon, the colors too were significantly improved which gave the porcelain the *very necessary semi-transparency* as it was described by Linderer[23]. J. C. F. Maury, a dentist at numerous Parisian hospitals and at the Royal Polytechnical College, boasted in 1820 of being the first to have publicized this method. According to him the teeth, already in two correspondingly colored layers, were molded in a single matrix to a porcelain anchor and covered with a varnish coating, dried, fitted with platinum pins and then fired[24].

Nonetheless human and animal materials continued to be used until into the second half of the 19th century. In 1820, a melancholy Dela-

[21] See pp. 151 f.
[22] Guerini
[23] J. Linderer p. 402
[24] Maury (a) pp. 289 f.; (b) p. 228

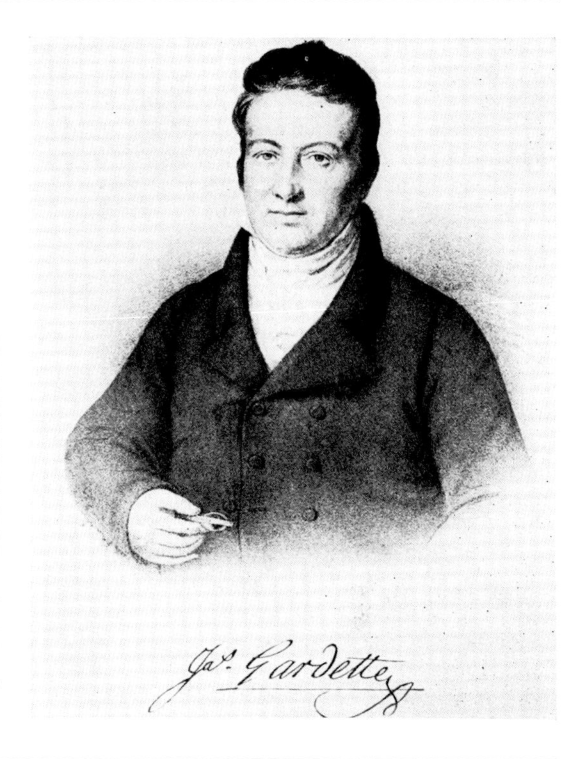

Fig. 248 *Jaques (James) Gardette*

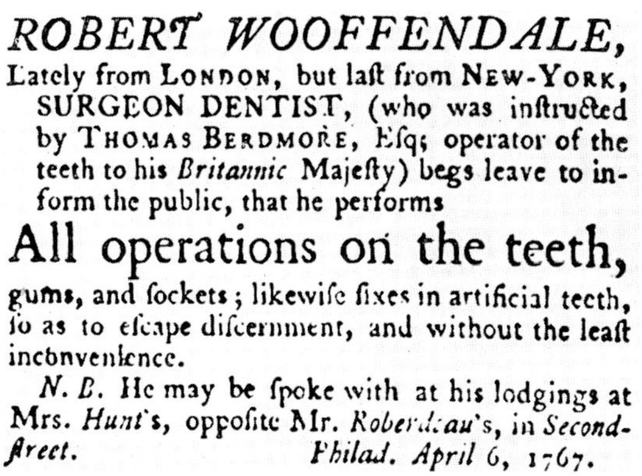

ROBERT WOOFFENDALE,
Lately from LONDON, but laſt from NEW-YORK, SURGEON DENTIST, (who was inſtructed by THOMAS BERDMORE, Eſq; operator of the teeth to his *Britannic* Majeſty) begs leave to inform the public, that he performs

All operations on the teeth,

gums, and ſockets; likewiſe fixes in artificial teeth, ſo as to eſcape diſcernment, and without the leaſt inconvenience.

N. B. He may be ſpoke with at his lodgings at Mrs. *Hunt's*, oppoſite Mr. *Roberdeau's*, in *Second-ſtreet*. *Philad. April 6, 1767.*

Fig. 247 *Advertisement of Robert Wooffendale (from Weinberger)*

barre reflected on the times, *when wars yielded their harvests, and the most beautiful teeth were to be had, healthy and suitable for the replacement of those lost by so many persons.* During times of peace, however, men were forced to fall back on the anatomical theater or on supernumerary teeth, and these were as ill-suited as those from graves and cemeteries [25].

The pioneer of a prominent family of dentists also, Levi Spear Parmly, who later practised in New York, mentioned in his textbook in 1819 that he had *in his possession thousands of teeth, extracted from bodies of all ages, that have fallen in battle.* Even in the Crimean war, from 1853 to 1856, thousands of dead men's teeth were harvested by the "hyenas of the battlefield".[26] Not until industry adopted the mineral tooth and developed products which were acceptable with regard to statics and color, was the new material generally accepted by practitioners of dentistry.

This production first began in the United States of North America, the country, to which the development of dentistry had moved in the beginning of the 19th century. The New World had now transcended its pioneer period and had begun an unparalleled period of technological progress. The young American dentists were not burdened by the traditions and theories under which Europe had labored for centuries, nor were they limited by guild restrictions or other constraints. Equipped with their practical common sense and the right to pursue their profession freely, they followed their predecessors, France and Germany in specialized surgery and plate prosthetics, and England in investigations of the anatomy and physiology of the dental system by pioneer work chiefly in the area of dental preservation and metal technology.

In the 18th century, on the other hand, it had mostly been immigrants from France and England who had represented the profession in this young country. The first prominent dentist was a student of the court dentist Thomas Berdmore, the Englishman Robert Wooffendale, who landed in New York in 1766. He was disappointed by his financial success, however, and re-embarked for England again after two years. He left behind a few newspaper advertisements and ivory prostheses, which now

[25] Ch. F. Delabarre pp. 82 f.
[26] Parmly p. 84; Paulson

seem somewhat primitive in contrast to the contemporary French "pièces" (Fig. 247). In Liverpool he compiled the popularly written "Practical Observations on the Human Teeth," which was published in London in 1783. There he gained an exclusive practice after the death of his teacher, Berdmore. In 1795 he went again to New York, where he practiced for another two years. Afterwards he withdrew to a farm until the end of his days, apparently not only an artist in his profession but also an artist at living.

Of incomparably greater importance for prosthetics, and not only in North America, was the former naval physician Jacques (James) Gardette (Fig. 248), who immigrated in 1778. After numerous changes of location this man, who like Bourdet came from Agen in southern France, finally settled permanently in Philadelphia in 1784. His son Emil reports that he had constructed the first self-adhering upper prosthesis, even though it was by accident. He had put a complete denture made from the enamel of hippopotamus teeth ("enameled Hipps") into the maxilla of a female patient, with her approval, however, without the normal support by springs on the mandible. She had wanted to accustom herself to the unfinished piece by keeping it in her mouth, and this was granted. Not until months later did Gardette see his patient again; to his complete amazement, with the prosthesis in place *she had been conversing with her usual facility.* She was delighted to continue to do without the springs which then were to have been inserted. *The principle,* so reports the son, *upon which the artificial piece thus adhered to the gum, at once suggested itself to his mind, and suction, or athmospheric pressure, was henceforth depended upon in numerous cases of the same kind* [27]. In any case, a suction effect from a carved bone prosthesis seems rather improbable to us now; on the other hand, these pieces were then very carefully adapted with a drill and an engraving blade to the model, and furthermore the patients were not exacting.

In writing further about his father, who also had provided George Washington with a dental prosthesis, Gardette's son claims for him the invention of the gold clasp, and also a method of making natural teeth firm with gold pins on a gold plate. We find the first one of these already anticipated in Mouton's "Dent à coulisse" and read of the second in Bourdet. In a medical journal of 1827 Gardette himself spoke out in unequivocal opposition to dental prostheses with transplantation of living teeth, not for ethical reasons but because he had never seen lasting success with them. In 1829, after a half century in the New World, he shook its dust from his boots and returned, shortly before his death, to his native France. He settled in Bordeaux, somewhat disappointed with his old homeland. There, *he was attacked by his old enemy, the gout, and died in August 1831* [28].

In 1788 Richard Cortland Skinner, a student of Ruspini's, immigrated from his native London first to Philadelphia and then to New York, where he practiced from 1791 until his death in 1834. In 1801, he published the first American book for the profession: a small popular dental book of the type customary in Europe, which fundamentally served purposes of advertisement [29].

The dental dynasty of the Greenwoods, in contrast, was long-established. The older, Isaac, was a turner in Boston, who also produced dentures, and gradually devoted himself completely to dentistry. Four sons followed his example, among whom John Greenwood was outstanding (Fig. 249). He was an efficient and creative practitioner in New York of whom it is known that he studied Hunter's works thoroughly. Weinberger [30] believes the first gold plate in America was prepared in 1798, not by Gardette but by Greenwood for George Washington, who had him as his last "Surgeon-dentist" from 1789 on [31] (Fig. 250). Other dental operators worthy of mention were John Baker, an excellent advertiser who had also treated the father of his country and his pupil, Paul Revere.

The firing of porcelain teeth crossed the ocean to North America in 1817 through Antoine (Anthony) Plantou, a dentist who immigrated from Paris. The procedure was then adopted by the universal genius Charles Willson Peale, but was first produced in large quantities by a jeweler in Philadelphia, named Samuel Wesley Stockton, starting in 1825. This man was soon manufacturing a half million teeth per year and was forced

27 Gardette p. 380, footnote
28 Ibid. p. 383; Weinberger pp. 147 f.
29 Skinner, Geshwind
30 Weinberger p. 142
31 Bremner pp. 129 f.; Weinberger pp. 306 f.

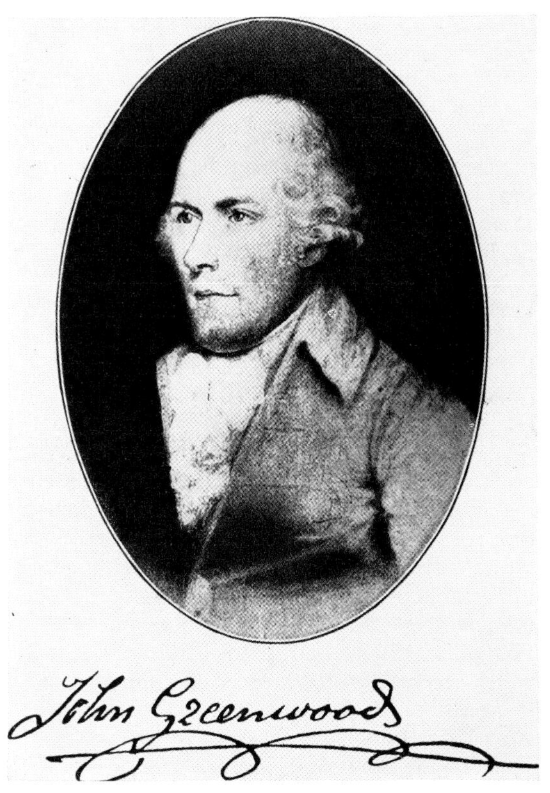

Fig. 249 *John Greenwood, 1805*

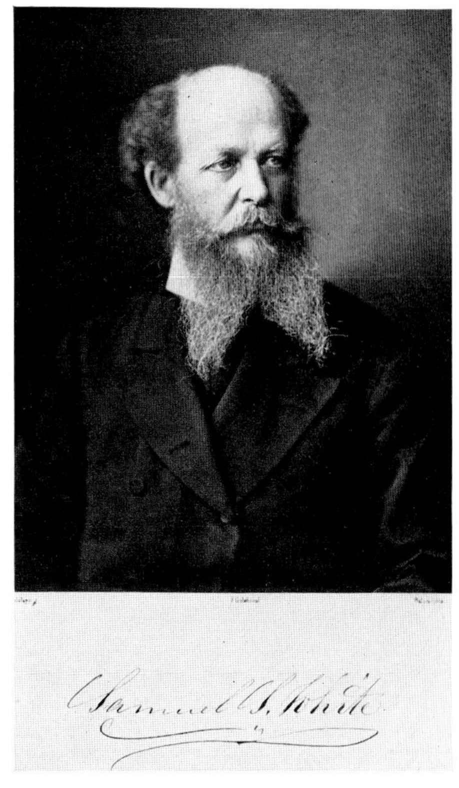

Fig. 251 *Samuel Stockton White*

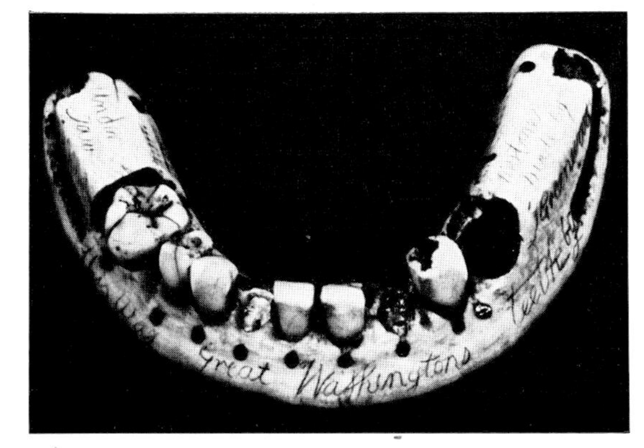

Fig. 250 *John Greenwood: George Washington's denture, carved from hippopotamus bone and fitted with 8 human teeth, 1789 (Academy of Medicine, New York)*

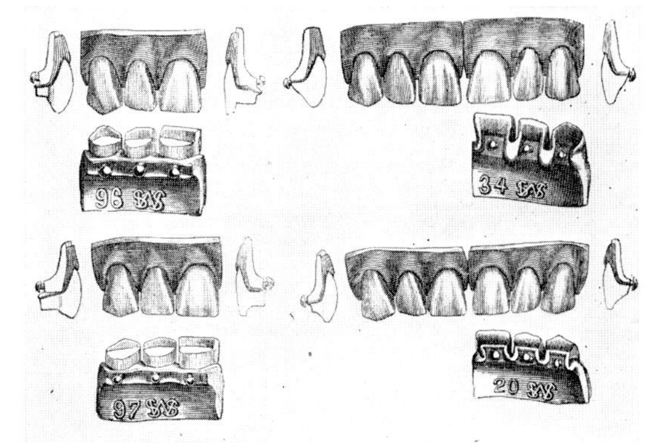

Fig. 252 *"Continuous Gums"*

to take two nephews into the business for assistance. A story is told about one of them to the effect that after seven years of apprenticeship at six dollars per week he had asked for a raise of one dollar. The uncle said, *That is enough, Sam,* whereupon the nephew, who had just come of age, quit the business, established himself as a dentist in 1843, and started fabricating his own improved teeth independently in 1844. He was Samuel Stockton White Fig. 251), and was the founder of the S. S. White Company, which is still flourishing today, and whose products soon spread throughout the entire world [32].

White also exerted a great and beneficial influence on the advancement of the dental profession. In 1847 he founded the journal, *Dental News Letter,* which gave rise in 1859 to the professional periodical, *Dental Cosmos,* which was for a long time the leading journal in the United States and elsewhere too. More than a half century after White's death (1879), his heirs, that is the S. S. White Company, decided they did not wish to suffer losses from the journal, which was gradually declining in reputation. Therefore the *Dental Cosmos* was transferred to the American Dental Association which combined it in 1936 with its own professional periodical founded in 1913, and had been published since 1922 as the *Journal of the American Dental Association.* For two years it bore both names but then the title, *Dental Cosmos,* which had already become a historical concept, unfortunately sank under the waters of oblivion.

The "Continuous gums" constituted a variation of the porcelain teeth which continued to be used into our own century. They were patented in 1851 by John Allen, a dentist in Cincinnati. The patent quickly brought him the opposition of another dentist in residence there, William M. Hunter. The apparatus involved rows of teeth, consisting, for example, of two incisors and a canine which were united by a common gingiva (Fig. 252). Delabarre had already publicized a first step to these block-teeth in 1820. To produce his "placage minéral", he applied a reddish colored mineral mass to the model, let it dry, and then made indentations in it, wherein he cemented the corresponding teeth, the very thin, cramp-less "Calliodontes." Then he fired the entire piece, whereby the teeth were inseparably fused together with the gingival base [33].

Claudius Ash (Fig. 253), who industrialized the dental kilns, operated in London by other French immigrants after Dubois de Chémant, was, like Stockton, initially a goldsmith. He became the founder of the British international firm of Ash, Sons, and Co., which produced the first truly high-quality teeth, starting in 1837. Around 1840 they introduced the tube tooth, a type with a central canal, which could be firmly riveted to the metal base with a post (Fig. 254).

Paris, the birthplace of the mineral tooth, now fell behind. Here a few dentists only such as Louis Alexandre Billard were engaged in production for the use of their colleagues [34], until these products yielded to the higher-quality offerings from the S. S. White and Ash firms. These were able to establish a monopoly in the world market which lasted for the rest of the 19th century. Not until 1893 Friedrich August Wienand, a dentist in Pforzheim, founded the first continental dental manufactory able to offer competitive products.

Thoughts about the forms of artificial teeth, which were offered by each manufacturer in an immense number of varieties, came very late. It was not until 1911 that the American dentist James Leon Williams (see Fig. 192), then working in London, put this confuse abundance in order. After a long period of anatomical research he established three typical basic shapes, a classification which was accepted rapidly in all the world.

The anchoring of partial dentures with clasps, which we see in the simplest possible form in Dubois de Chémant's brochure of advertisement, became better. Delabarre already had constructed a kind of supported prosthesis in 1820, and the *saddle-shaped spring* by the London dentist J. P. de la Fons (1826), which exerted its force partially in the open position and partially in the closed and extended within the row of teeth over the points of contact, is similar in all respects to the later Jackson clasp (Figs. 255 and 256; see Fig. 469). Besides upper prostheses were generally attached with the help of dowels which, suitably fastened to the plate, were inserted into the prepared canals of the roots. These were preserved and filed flat [35] (Fig. 257). The fact that

[32] S. S. White; Bremner p. 110; Geist-Jacobi p. 221
[33] Ch. F. Delabarre pp. 235 f.
[34] Désirabode pp. 583 f.
[35] See p. 204

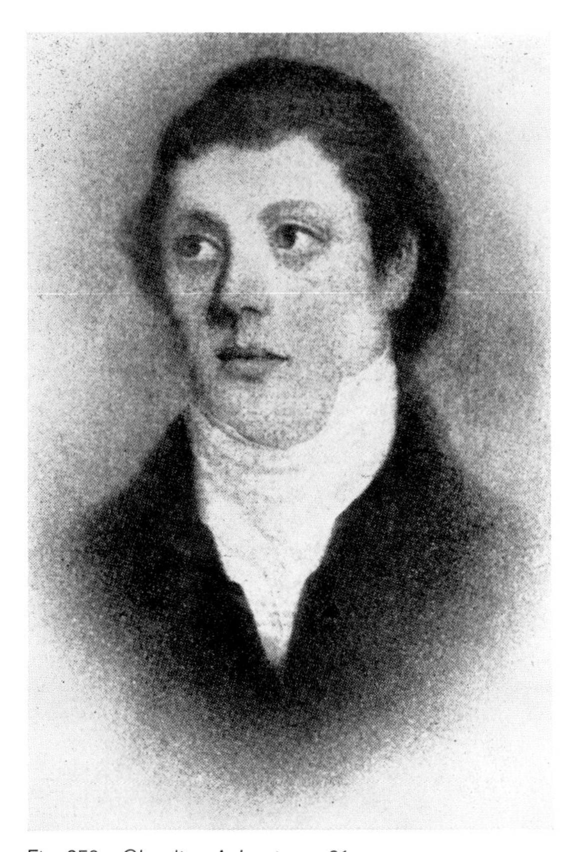

Fig. 253 *Claudius Ash, at age 21*

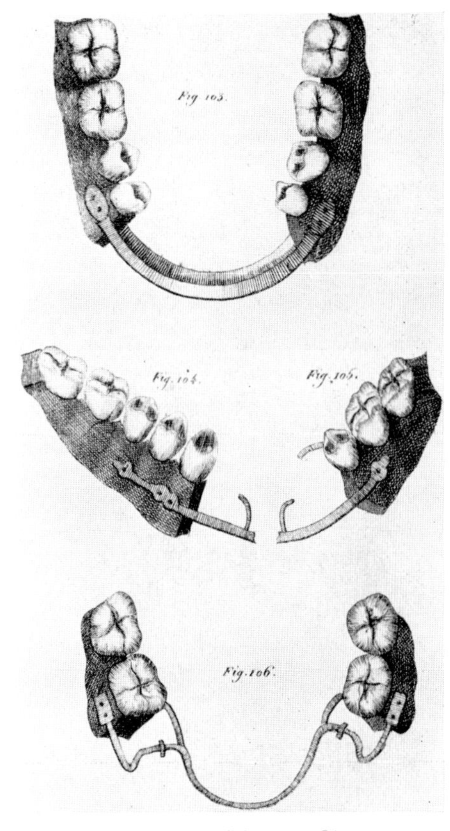

Fig. 255 *Ch. F. Delabarre: Clasp retentions, 1820*

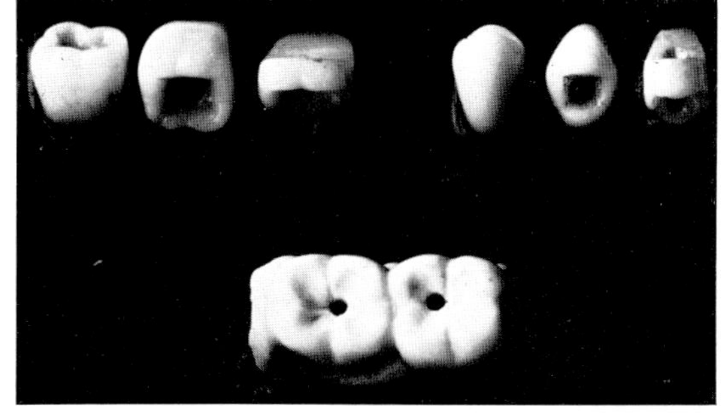

Fig. 254 *Tube teeth of the Ash Co., approximately 1840*

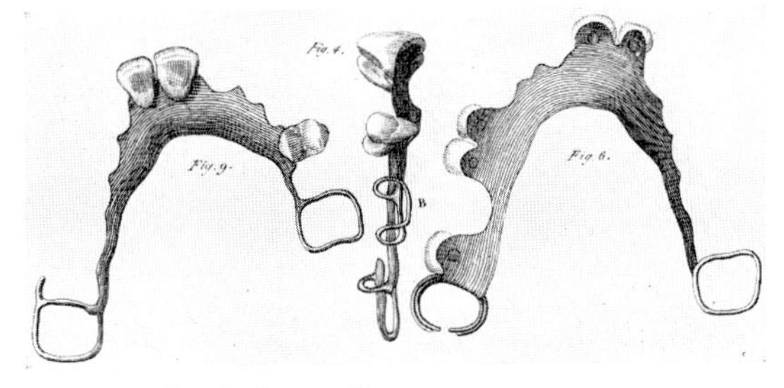

Fig. 256 *De la Fons: Clasp retentions, 1827*

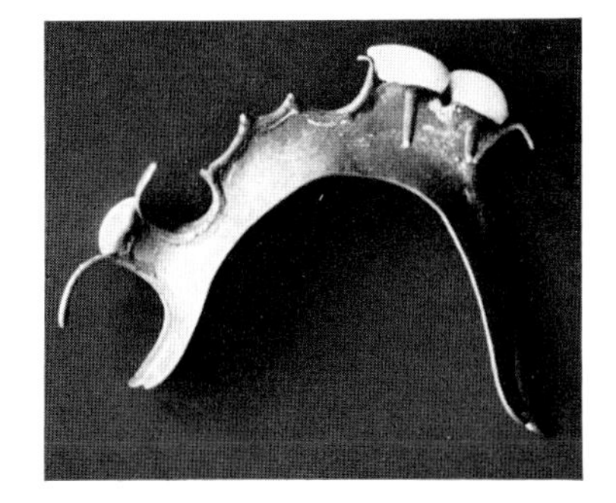

Fig. 257 *Metal prosthesis with human teeth and posts for retention in the tooth root, 1st half of the 19th century (Forschungsinstitut für Geschichte der Zahnheilkunde, Cologne)*

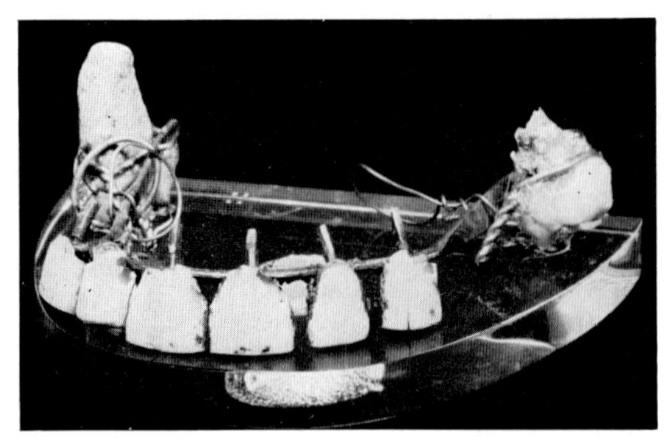

Fig. 258 *Gold bar denture with post retention of a woman who died in 1791 at age 32 years; found in 1964 in the Church of St. Anna, Augsburg (Forschungsinstitut für Geschichte der Zahnheilkunde, Cologne)*

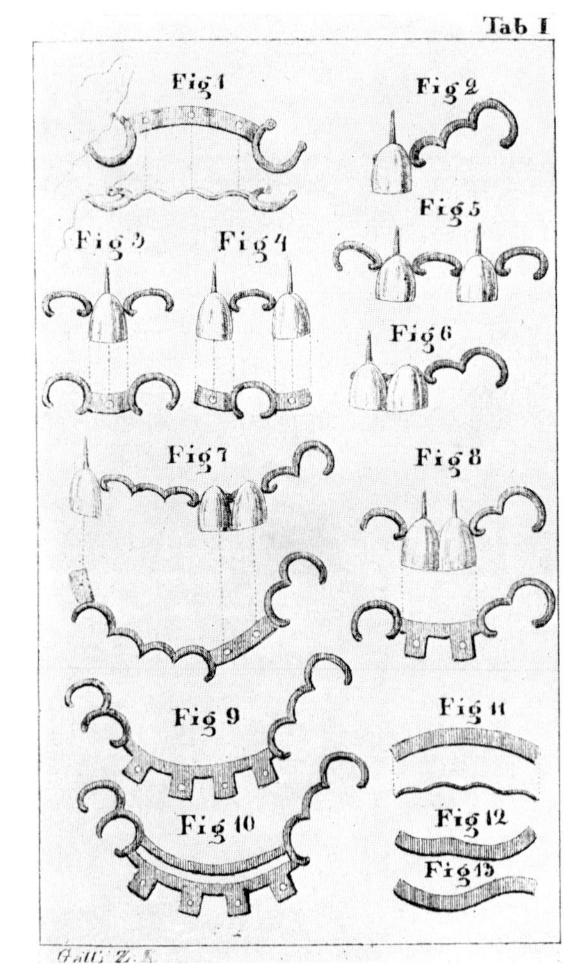

Fig. 259 *Gall: Clasp retentions, 1834*

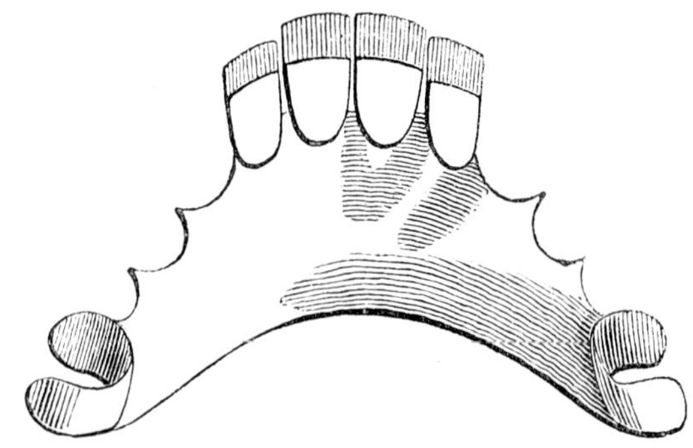

Fig. 260 *Robinson: Clasp retentions, 1846*

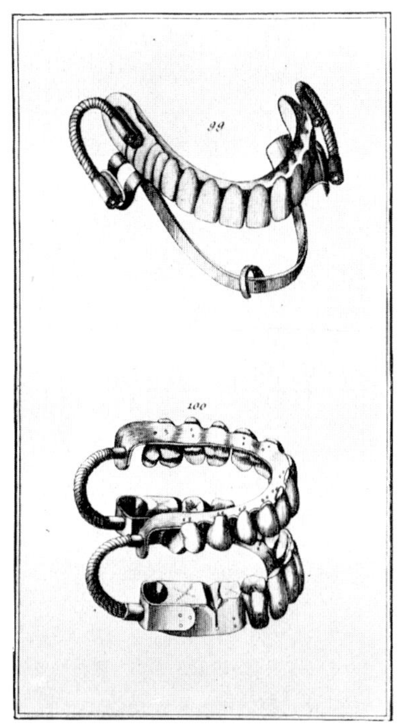

Fig. 261 *Laforgue: Denture with gold spiral springs, 1802*

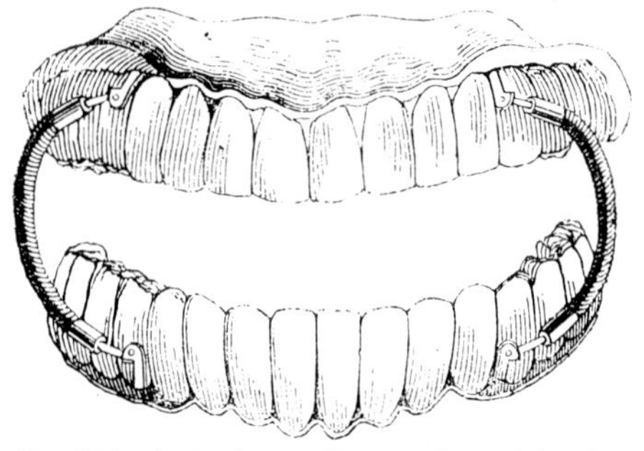

Fig. 262 *Lefoulon: Stamped gold denture with springs, 1841*

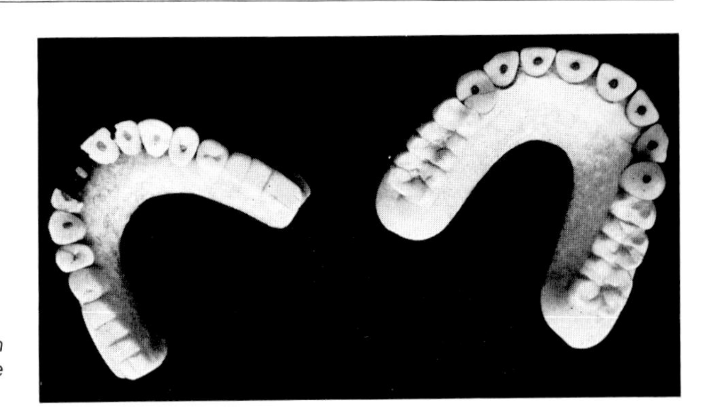

Fig. 263 *Carved bone denture with porcelain anterior teeth (Forschungsinstitut für Geschichte der Zahnheilkunde, Cologne)*

this technique reaches back as far as the 18th century is shown by the gold prosthesis of a 32-year-old woman interred in the St. Anne's Church in Augsburg in 1791: posts which carry crowns of human teeth on one side and are implanted on the other in the root canals of the front teeth are soldered to a gold bar which is wired to a molar on each side (Fig. 258).
Variations of the clasp technique are shown by a lithograph in a "Popular Introduction" by Joseph Gall in Vienna from 1834. Gall, who had been trained under Carabelli in 1821 to 1824, was now "Master of dentistry and midwifery, then veterinarian, practical surgeon and practicing dentist" (Fig. 259). In comparison to these ornamental denominations we feel much more confident with the clasps from James Robinson in London which lie flat against the tooth [36] (Fig. 260; see Fig. 386). He is the man British dentistry has to thank for the first precise instructions in the field of prosthetics, and also for the composition and firing of the "mineral teeth" from his textbook, which came out in 1846 [37]. One year before this the professional journal which Robinson had founded in 1844, *The Forceps*, had disappeared, following the 1843 *British Quarterly of Dental Surgery* which had also been edited by him, and which was just as short-lived.
Upon Bourdet's recommendation (1757), Fauchard's flat steel springs for the fixation of complete upper prostheses which were subject to rust were finally replaced in most cases by spiral springs of gold or platinum (Fig. 261). In 1805, Gariot found the whale-bone springs also to be completely impractical [38]. In this field Delabarre was mainly successful in the invention of increasingly complicated spring devices. The first application of spiral springs which also allow lateral deviations is believed to be discernible as early as 1788, in the illustrations of Dubois de Chémant [39] (see Fig. 242).
The gold and platinum plates were stamped in a die, consisting usually of a matrix cast from copper and a counter-die of softer lead (Fig. 262). In 1836, Eduard Blume, the court dentist practicing in Berlin, described the manufacture of bone dentures then customary. The piece was initially roughly formed with a rasp, and then *an ink was prepared from lamp-black and oil, and the model was painted with it; the piece was then held against it, whereby the plate also was inked.* These sites were then removed with a graving tool [40]. In 1845, John Tomes [41] in London patented a machine for the manufacture of dentures, which he called the "Dentifactor." This was an apparatus equipped with a drill which transmitted the shape of the model to the bone material through a touch arrangement [42]. Robinson characterized the apparatus as an *ingenious machine*, but criticized it for its inability to transmit any *undercutting* areas [43].
Still, even well into the 19th century, dental prostheses were the privilege of very well-to-do circles. We read in Callman Jacob Linderer, the Berlin dentist [44], that in his capacity as court dentist in Bad Pyrmont around the turn of the century he had very frequently replaced

36 C. J. Linderer p. 25
37 Robinson pp. 259 f.
38 Gariot pp. 320 f.
39 Cohen (a)
40 E. Blume p. 176
41 See pp. 391 f.
42 Cope pp. 25 f.
43 Robinson pp. 237 f.
44 See p. 273

entire sets of teeth for persons of the highest rank, *which was at that time a rarity, since the middle classes knew of this operation almost solely from hearsay, and if anyone ever had a few teeth inserted, he could not afford to let it come to anyone else's knowledge unless he wanted to become the talk of the town* [45]. In 1830, the same man announced in the *Vossische Zeitung, that again* (there has been) *a complete set of teeth prepared for a patient, through the mechanism of which the upper denture cannot deviate either forwards or to the side; . . . this denture will be shown only for the next eight days to those who wish to have teeth put in, because then it will have to be delivered.*

With the production of industrially manufactured mineral teeth only one initial obstacle in the path of affordable dental prostheses was eliminated, for a simplified production of the base was still lacking (Fig. 263). The dentures prepared from bone demanded complicated lathe work, and quickly fell prey to caries. Likewise, the stamped gold and platinum plates were very expensive. Experiments with tortoise-shell—Harrington in Portsmouth had constructed a special press for this in 1849—and horn were not satisfactory. In 1820, Edward Hudson [46] in Philadelphia was the first to cast the base of a prosthesis from tin; because of its weight, however, it was suitable only for lower dentures. For precisely this reason it is still used today occasionally when condition of the jaw is unfavorable. Therefore, as before, the enamel from hippopotamus tusks remained the preferred material for bases. According to an estimate from 1861 *no fewer than 1,100 of these gigantic creatures must be slaughtered each year in order to supply our markets* [47].

In 1848, Antoine Delabarre, the son of the often quoted Parisian dentist, recommended guttapercha, which is still used today as a temporary filling material, for the bases of prostheses. He used this resin material for the first time to fill in the underside of a hippopotamus prosthesis which did not fit. Later he set a gold framework, to which the teeth were firmly soldered into a wax model, formed a mold and counter-mold from plaster-of-Paris, and replaced the wax with heated guttapercha. He compressed the entire piece for hours in an iron press. He also used the new material for lining metal prostheses [48]. This procedure also was unable to become established, because the quite unstable guttapercha required complicated but statically necessary metal support.

As Geist-Jacobi assumes, William Rogers, the American working in Paris, used the same material for his mysterious "Osanores" [49], which he enthusiastically publicized in the conclusions of two books in 1845, one directed to the professional world and another *to all classes and professions* [50]. After studying both texts, the reader knows just as much as he did before; he only learns that the "râteliers osanores" adhere to the gingiva without springs, clasp or ligatures, and that they are unbreakable.

Not until the second half of the century was the way prepared for the much-sought progress with the introduction of vulcanized hard rubber as a prosthetic material. In 1851, after numerous previous experiments by others and after a great deal of his own effort, the American Charles Goodyear succeeded in hardening the resin of the rubber tree, which had been used before only for erasers, through treatment with sulfur and heat.

Thomas W. Evans, an American dentist who emigrated to Paris in 1848 was probably one of the first to use the new prosthetic material (Fig. 264). As he was discussing this problem with Goodyear in Paris in 1851, he answered—according to Evans [51]—as follows: *"Here again is a new application which I never thouht of." I urged him to make him a set of teeth with caoutchouc on the base, and did make him not only one, but several pieces for his mouth.* Exactly the same thing occurred during a visit in 1855 by Charles Goodyear, Jr., who had taken a patent out on it in America and Britain; the first of these, however, soon expired [52]. In 1864 new improvements by John A. Cummings made possible a resurrection; the Goodyear Dental Vulcanite Company was founded, the licences were distributed, and the fees were mercilessly exacted in the United States (Fig. 265). Only after a few lawsuits were

[45] C. J. Linderer p. VIII
[46] French p. 356. See Fig. 360
[47] Rock
[48] A. Delabarre p. 29
[49] The name may be derived from the Latin os, ossis (bone), an (Greek, negation) and the Latin os, oris (mouth), i. e., a material for the mouth, not consisting of bone
[50] Rogers (a) pp. 441 f.; (b) pp. 283 f.; Geist-Jacobi p. 223
[51] Evans (a). Evans played a small historical role in 1871 when he saved the Empress Eugénie, wife of Napoleon III, from the revolutionaries of the Parisian Commune and aided her escape to England (Evans b). The carriage used for the purpose is exhibited in the Thomas W. Evans Dental Institute in Philadelphia
[52] Heider

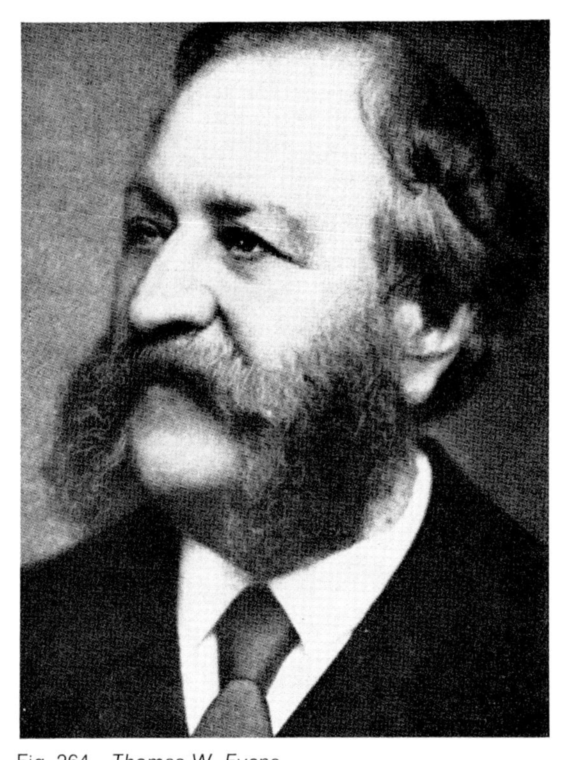

Fig. 264 *Thomas W. Evans*

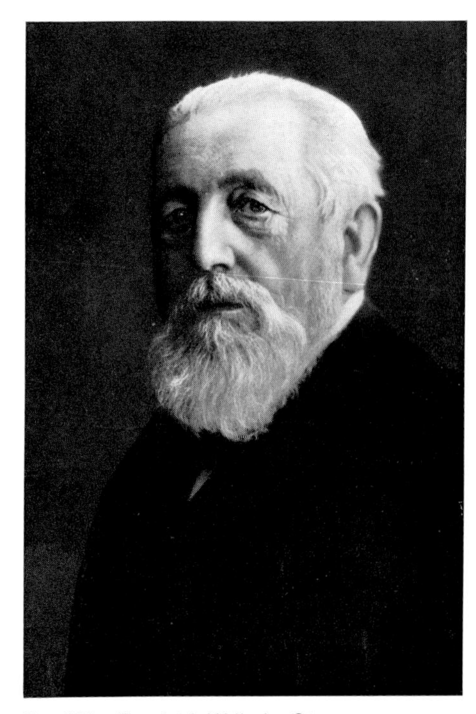

Fig. 266 *Friedrich Wilhelm Süersen*

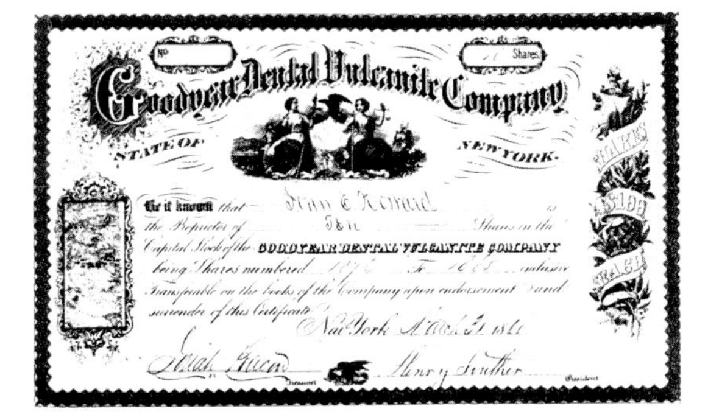

Goodyear Dental Vulcanite Company

State of New York.

Be it known that ... is the Proprietor of ... Shares in the Capital Stock of the GOODYEAR DENTAL VULCANITE COMPANY being Shares numbered ... To ... inclusive Transferable on the books of the Company upon endorsement and surrender of this Certificate.

New York

Treasurer

President

Fig. 265 *License issued by the Goodyear Co. for the manufacture of vulcanized dentures, with signature of Josiah Bacon*

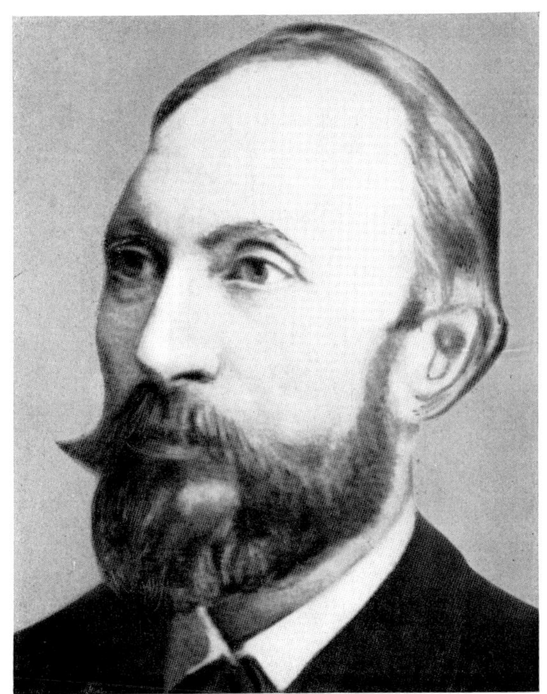

Fig. 267 *Carl Sauer*

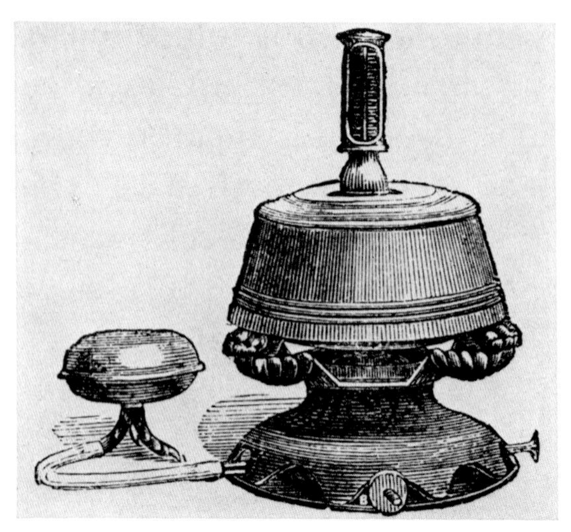

Fig. 268 *Vulcanizer, approximately 1870*

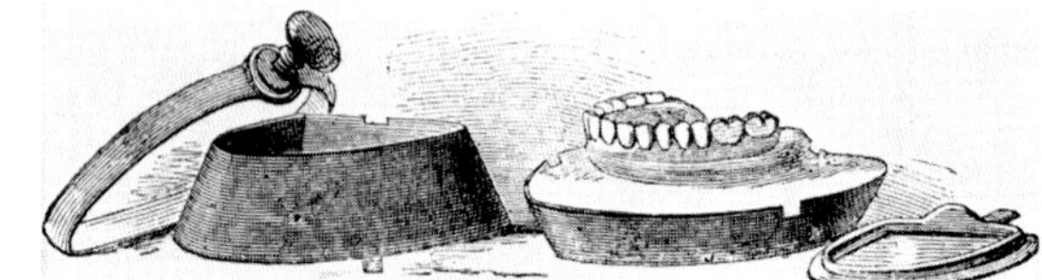

Fig. 269 *Flasks, approximately 1870*

won, and after the particularly hard-boiled director of the organization, Josiah Bacon, had been shot to death in 1879 in a San Francisco hotel by a despairing dentist, dealings with the licences became less harsh. Then, starting in 1881, American dentists were allowed to use hard rubber unmolested and without cost.

The New York dentist Clark Samuel Putnam, who had moved to Paris, unabashedly claimed the "Vulcanite system" as his own[53]. In 1858 he obtained patents in Europe for his vulcanizer which he sold in Germany also. In Berlin, this was acquired by Friedrich Wilhelm Süersen (Fig. 266) who was the royal, and later the imperial, court dentist. His technician, Carl Sauer, developed the method which was then still unknown there through great efforts, and Süersen then made it public[54]. Sauer, however, after completing his studies, in 1884 became the first German professor of dental prosthetics at the newly founded Berlin University Institute[55] (Fig. 267). Putnam was probably astonished when he tried to sell his licence to Christian Friedrich Wehner, a dentist in Frankfurt, because the man had already secured some raw rubber and treated it with sulfur and red mercury sulfide with the aid of a chemist. He had samples obtained from it, vulcanized in the locomotive boiler of the Frankfurt-Taunus Railroad on a trip to Kassel. Later he constructed a gigantic vulcanizer which produced dentures allegedly far superior to Putnam's in quality of color[56].

In 1856, i. e., soon after the introduction of hard rubber, Alfred A. Blandy in London, a son-in-law of Harris, recommended an easily melting metal as a base material. His "cheoplastic metal" was a compound of silver and bismuth with traces of antimony. Even though this material also fell into disuse soon, the author's recommendation of embedding a wax model of the plate in plaster-of-Paris was put to use in the vulcanization of hard rubber dentures[57]. Celluloid, which was introduced in the sixties, also did not last because of its insufficient durability in the mouth. Similarly aluminum, from which prostheses had been cast in Paris by Berthé and in 1866 by James B. Bean in Baltimore, also fell by the wayside.

After vulcanized hard rubber was generally established, the development became somewhat smoother. The technical means of production were improved: the vulcanizers were built smaller in accordance with the principle of the Papin vessel, and convenient flasks corresponding to this were produced (Fig. 268 and 269). The clasps which had been soldered before were then adapted to the method of vulcanization through according retentions (Fig. 270). Above all effort was devoted to manufacturing dentures which adhered to the palate, whereby Gardette generally was given credit for being the first one

53 Putnam pp. 68 f.
54 Süersen (a)
55 See p. 410
56 Paulson
57 Harris (c) pp. 759 f.

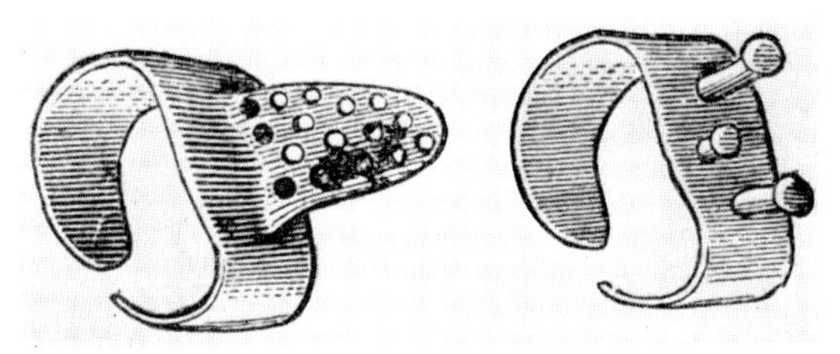

Fig. 270 *Clasps for vulcanized denture bases (from Harris and Austen, 1874)*

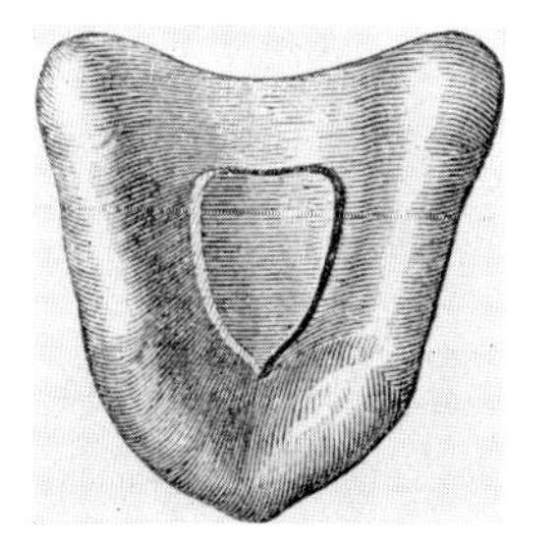

Fig. 271 *Harris: Suction chamber, 1835*

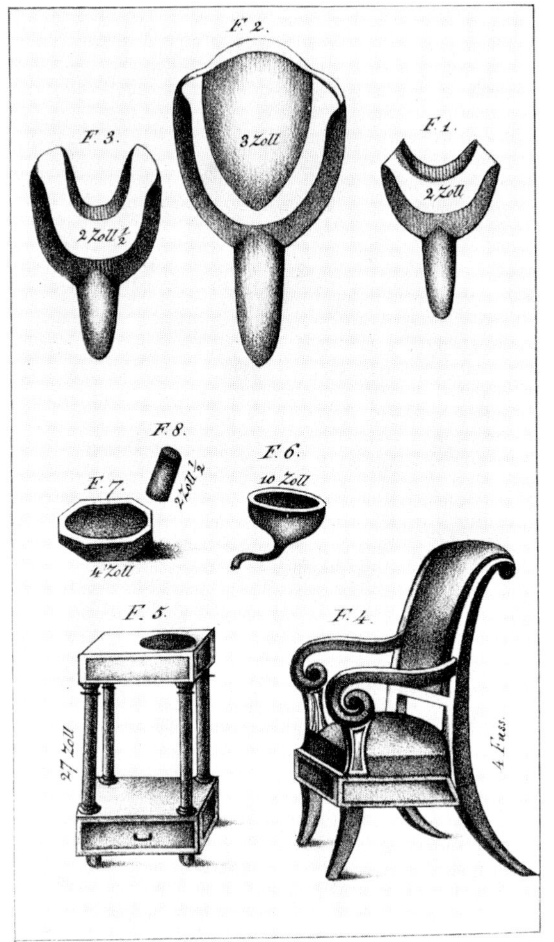

Fig. 272 *Maury: Impression tray; also treatment chair and table with cuspidor, 1830*

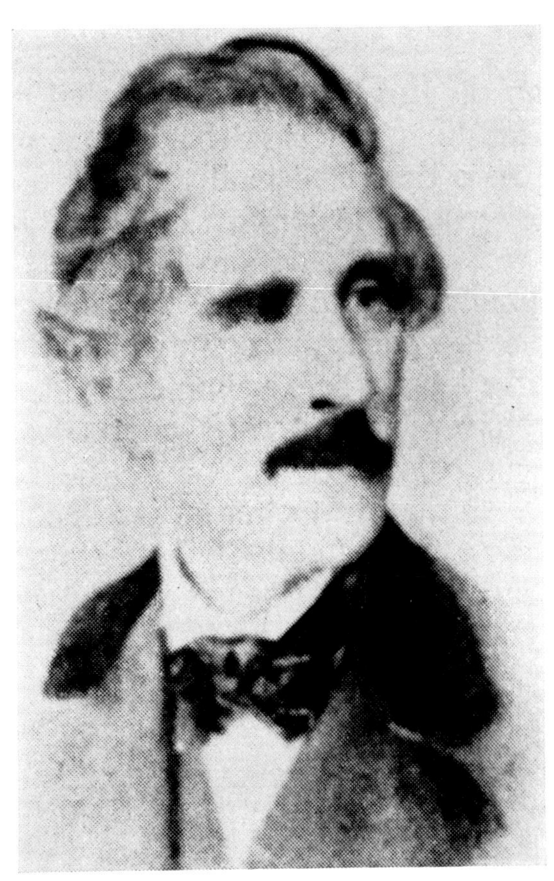

Fig. 273 *Charles Stent*

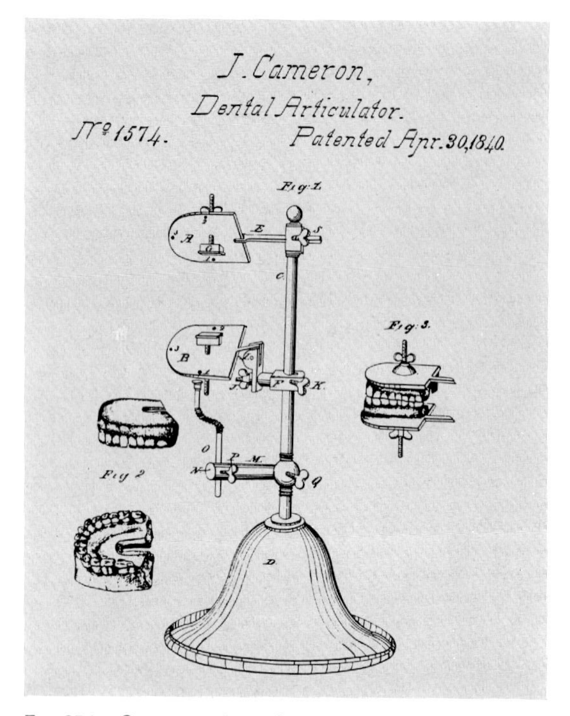

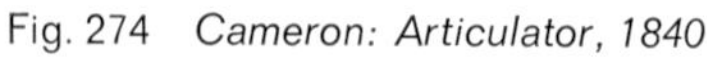
Fig. 274 *Cameron: Articulator, 1840*

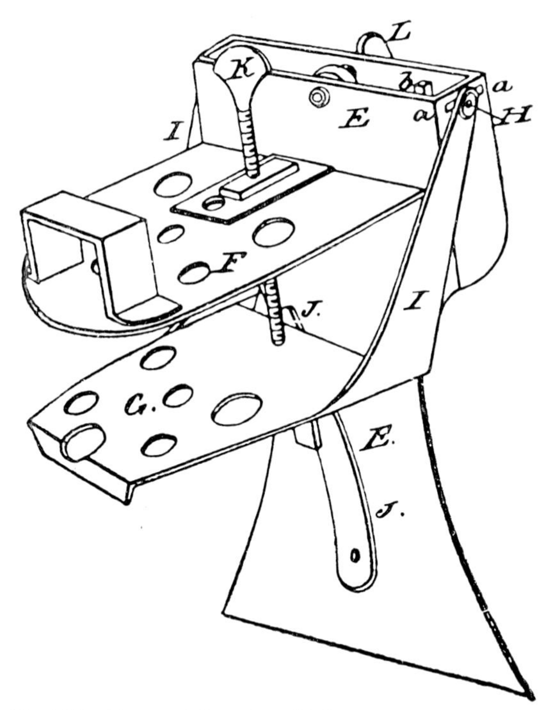

Fig. 275 *Evans: Articulator, 1840*

to succeed. Chapin A. Harris claimed to have introduced the suction chamber in 1835 [58] (Fig. 271), but this is not mentioned in the first edition of his work of 1839. Herein he indicates that he had initially made use of atmospheric pressure, independent of his predecessors, with gold dentures [59]. In 1848 Levi Gilbert, New Haven, claimed that he was its inventor [60].

A prerequisite necessary for this development was the fact that improvements in the techniques of making impressions had been made in the meantime. The first step forward was the introduction of the impression tray, which the elder Delabarre had recommended in 1820. According to him softened wax is to be placed *in a small track, or semi-elliptical cast of white metal or silver, on the front side of which a haft or handle is mounted. The walls of this instrument provide resistance and keep the pressure of the cheeks away from the wax.* After the cast has been pressed on firmly, it is carefully pulled off in the direction of the teeth and immersed in cold water. Then the excess is removed with a spring blade, and it is replaced briefly once more [61] (Fig. 272). As a whole, it is a procedure with which we cannot find fault, even today. In this respect Delabarre unjustly celebrated the business-like Dubois de Chémant as the inventor of the impression method; we know that it had already been developed by Philipp Pfaff in 1756.

In 1857 the London dentist Charles Stent (Fig. 273) tested a combination of different kinds of waxes hardened at oral temperatures, which is still used today under the name of Stents composition [62]. In 1860 a professor at Ohio College, Joseph Richardson, recommended in his textbook on "Mechanical Dentistry" *the Gutta Percha . . . rarely used except in obtaining impressions for partial pieces* [63], because of its elasticity. The plaster-of-Paris impression seems to have been developed in the forties by various authors in the USA (Levi Gilbert, and W. H. Dwinelle). In 1843 Désirabode in Paris did not know of it yet,

58 Harris (c) pp. 628 f. See p. 258
59 Ibid. (a) pp. 327 f.
60 J. D. White
61 Ch. F. Delabarre pp. 159 f.
62 Ward (a)
63 Richardson pp. 132 f.

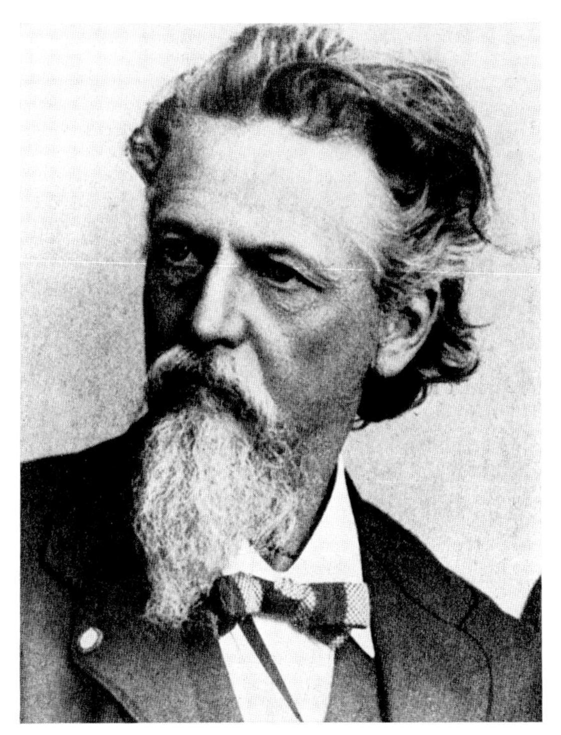

Fig. 276 *William Gibson Arlington Bonwill*

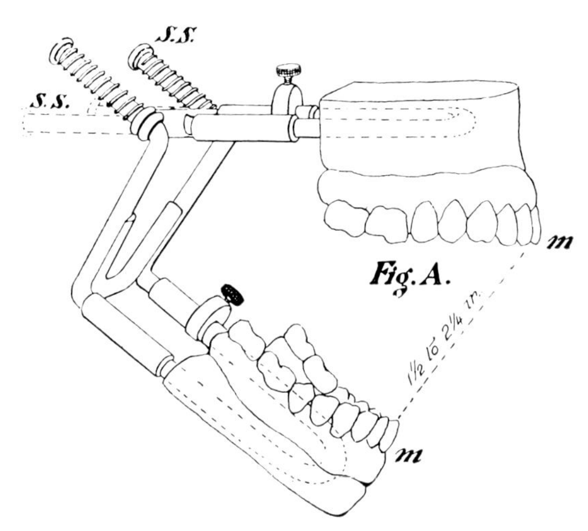

Fig. 277 *Bonwill articulator*

and in 1853 it was presented as an innovation by Harris at the sixth annual convention of the American Society of Dental Surgeons, which was founded in 1840 [64]. In 1864 Johann Joseph Schrott, a dentist from Mühlhausen in Alsace, lectured on the functional impression at the meeting of the Central Verein Deutscher Zahnärzte in Munich. After taking wax impressions, he stamped individual upper and lower impression trays, fastened them together with springs as was customary with complete dentures and impregnated them with heated gutta-percha. With this he at first took an impression from the model and then inserted the apparatus, whereupon the patient was to perform normal functional oral movements for ten minutes. Schrott thus defined the principle of the functional impression exactly as we know it today. As we read in the report of the meeting *the collegium concludes unanimously that a prize of forty Thaler is to be awarded to our colleague Schrott* [65].

Philipp Pfaff, who had first described preparation of impressions, was probably also the first in 1756 to direct his attention to the problem of articulation, more properly at first, to occlusion: *The patient, for whom I measure the dimensions in this fashion, must close his mouth during the process,* that is, he must bite into the wax of the impression [66]. Gariot proceeded similarly in 1805, but he too describes a simple plaster articulator [67].

In April of 1840 James Cameron, a dentist in Philadelphia, patented *a new and improved instrument for adjusting artificial teeth* with which the models were fastened in place on a support (Fig. 274). This, too, allowed opening and closing movements only. In contrast Daniel T. Evans' articulator which was patented in August of the same year represented a step forward, because this apparatus, which was *so constructed as to imitate the motion of the lower jaw,* also provided for lateral and forward movements. This way it was already oriented in three dimensions [68] (Fig. 275). It was manufactured by

[64] J. D. White; Harris pp. 637 f.
[65] Schrott (a and b)
[66] See p. 231
[67] Gariot pp. 306 f.
[68] Quotations from the patents; cf. Hall (a and b)

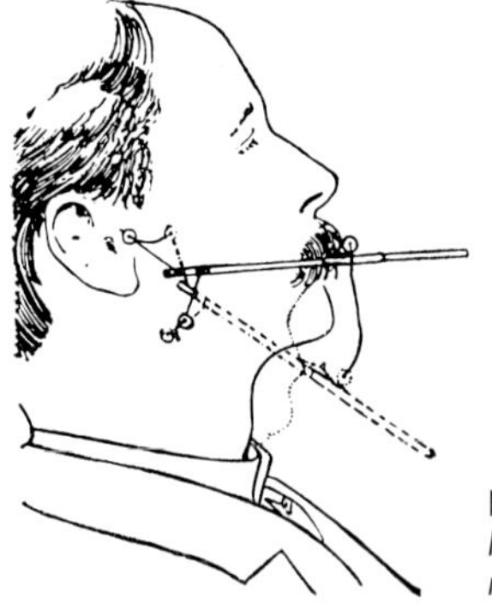

Fig. 278 *Luce: Paths of movement in mouth*

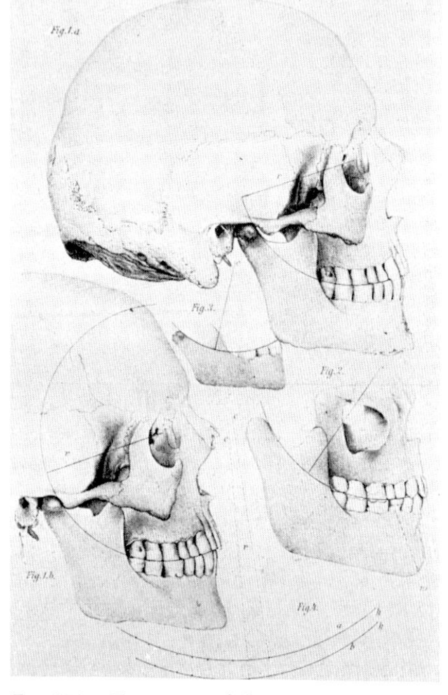

Fig. 279 *The curve of Spee, 1890*

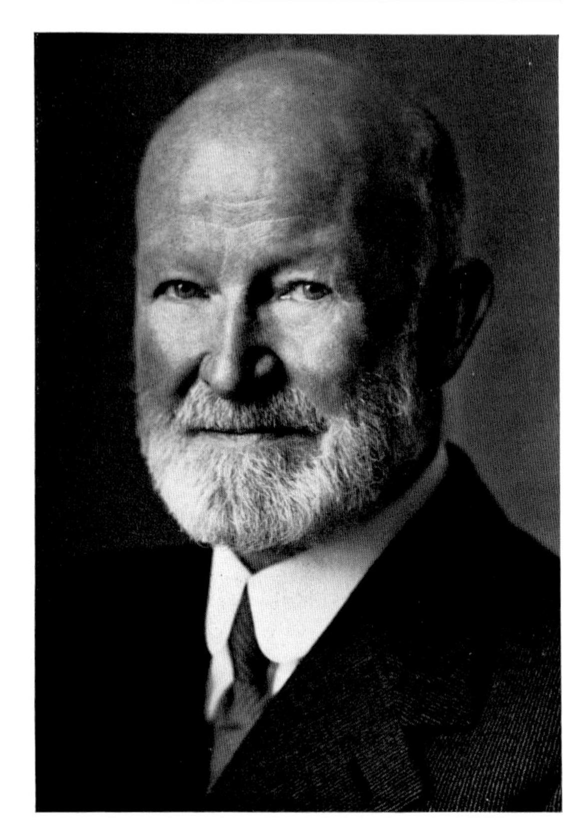

Fig. 280 *Alfred Gysi*

Horatio G. Kern in Philadelphia, one of the first producers of dental materials.

The first truly useful articulator, *founded on geometrical, mathematical, and mechanical laws,* was presented in 1864 at the meeting of the Delaware Dental Society by William Arlington Gibson Bonwill also from Philadelphia[69] (Figs. 276 and 277). It was based on a balanced three-point contact occlusion and set the standard for all successive types even though the condyle path was still vertical and not in a slanted curve. Bonwill provided it with the triangle named after him: he had demonstrated on several thousands of skulls that an equilateral triangle exists (at least in Europeans) between the middle of the condyles of the temporomandibular joints and the contact point of the mandibular central incisors' edges. Thus, at least one fixed point was given for the set up of complete dentures in the laboratory. It is worthy of mention that Bonwill did not patent his invention, but rather presented it as a gift to the entire dental profession. Others, however, were slow to recognize the

[69] Bonwill

importance of the new device; because of this, his manuscripts were rejected twice (in 1864 and 1888) by the editors of the *Dental Cosmos* and the first publication on this subject from his pen is not found until 1899 [70].

The British dentist Francis Hancock Balkwill, who practiced in Plymouth, had already made research on the fundamentals of articulation more than twenty years before, and publicized his findings in 1866 at a meeting of the Odontological Society of Great Britain in London. He did this, however, without evaluating them from a practical standpoint or constructing a corresponding articulator. Even then Balkwill described the condyle as a hinge, and he was also familiar with the various directions of the joint movements, the significance of the conical shape of the molar cusps, of the canines as guiding elements, and that of the fissures as *channels of clearance* for food remnants. Even an intimation of knowledge of the curve of occlusion, and a great deal of other things is to be found [71]. In 1912 Gysi in Zurich paid his respects to the contributions of this unjustly forgotten pioneer of the problem of articulation: in his papers presented at the Odontological Society's meetings and buried in its publications, there was *to be found everything already there, which had to be arduously and gradually rediscovered by articulation researchers over the course of these last 46 years* [72].

The anatomists, too, devoted their attention to this field. In 1889 Charles Elmer Luce in Boston investigated the physiology of the temporomandibular joint with the help of photography. By means of a structure mounted on the mandibular incisors, he fastened shiny silver pearls to the angle of the jaw and to the condyle as well as in front of the incisors; then he captured the curves formed during the movement of opening on a photographic plate [73] (Fig. 278).

In 1890 the discovery of the curve of occlusion or compensation, which is named after its inventor, the anatomist Ferdinand Count of Spee of Kiel, became a particularly important aid for the set-up of artifical teeth in articulators (Fig. 279) [74]. This idea was modified and later transferred to prosthetic practice by the Danish dentist, Carl Christensen, in 1901 [75]. In 1908 Sir Norman Godfrey Bennett, an oral surgeon in London, spoke before the Royal Society of Medicine on experiments he had performed on himself with small glowing lamps attached to the mandible. With these, he had ascertained the lateral movement of the condyle during mastication and its angle which are named after him [76].

Among the men who occupied themselves with the problem of articulation, Alfred Gysi of Zurich (Fig. 280) is outstanding. Starting in 1894 he spent half a century on the subject, and was as successful as he was indefatigable. Progress in this area was made in the twenties of our century by the Berlin prosthodontist Hermann Schröder, who saw in the creation of a satisfactory articulator more a functional problem than a purely mechanical one [77].

Crown and Bridge Prostheses

For a long time still natural teeth were preferred in the preparation of dowel crowns (Fig. 281). While Maury (1830) was still filing them to size in the mouth, Lefoulon (1841) was taking a wax impression from the stump of the root with an inserted post and adapting the tooth to a plaster cast from it.

Before the introduction of cement in the sixties, the main problem was the fastening of the post in the enlarged root canal which was made of gold, platinum, or hardwood such as hickory or box-tree. In addition to the old method, such as wrapping it with hemp, cotton, or silk. Maury recommended enveloping the post with the outer layer of birchbark [78].

Malagou Antoine Désirabode, who was the surgeon-dentist to the king, was the first to entitle a chapter in his textbook "Prothèse." This comprehensive work of 1843, "Nouveaux éléments complets de la science et de l'art du dentiste" (New Complete Elements of the Science and Art of the Dentist), summarized all the customary methods. Fauchard's cemented post (which was misleading, as he had only glued the post to the crown), Bourdet's screw-in post, Maggiolo's, a dentist in Nancy, spring-lock post (tenon à cliquet, Fig. 249, No. 142), that of Ricci which was

70 Schwarze
71 Balkwill
72 Gysi (b)
73 Luce
74 Spee
75 Christensen
76 N. G. Bennett
77 Gysi; Schröder
78 Maury (a) pp. 243 f.

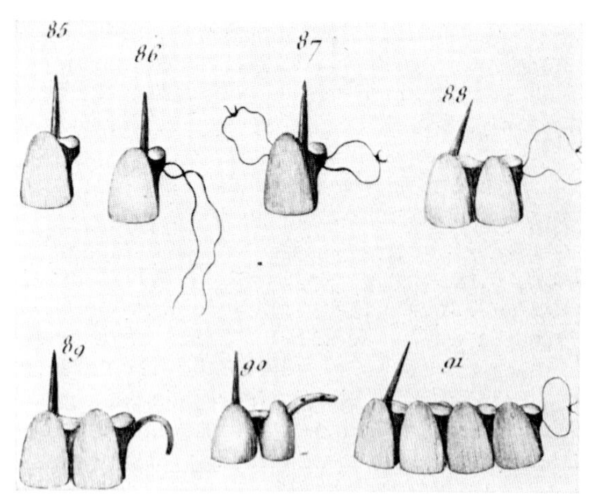

Fig. 281 *Laforgue: Pivot teeth and pivot bridges, 1802*

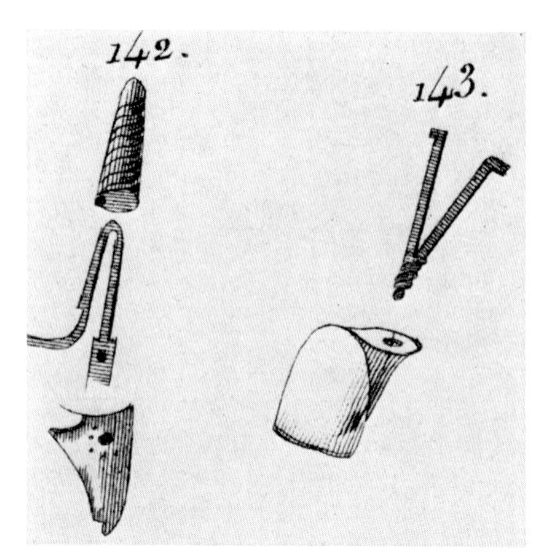

Fig. 282 *"Tenon à cliquet" and "tenon des antennes" (from Delabarre, 1820)*

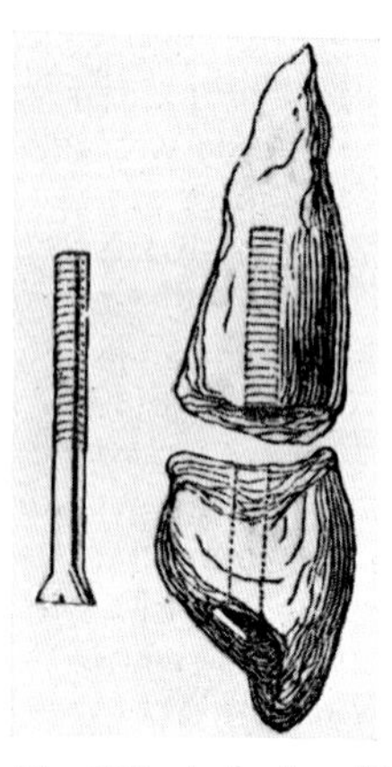

Fig. 283 *Lefoulon: The screw-in post, 1841*

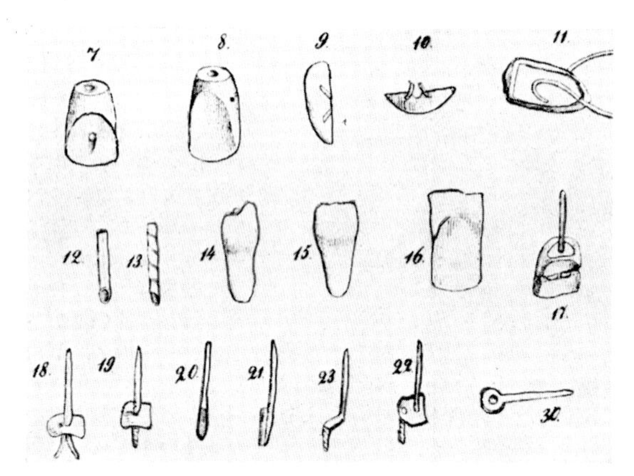

Fig. 284 *Joseph Linderer: Root posts with gold plate, 1848*

fastened with (swelling) cork, the "tenon des antennes" (Fig. 282, No. 143), and finally the perforated post (tenon perforé) which could serve as a drainage tube for secretions from the root canal. At that time there were not yet any root fillings in Europe; the procedure was limited to partial removal of the dental pulp tissue, so that chronic inflammation was unavoidable. Lefoulon's recommendation was even more involved: that a gold cylinder with threads on the inside be inserted in the root canal, in which he fastened the crown with a corresponding screw-in post (Fig. 283). Désirabode thought little of this complicated method of attachment; he preferred the simple pin (pivot simple) and regarded Lefoulon's idea as purely theoretical, and likewise rejected the suggestion[79] that the post be inserted with metal with a low melting point[80].

Callman Jacob Linderer, a dentist in Berlin, in 1834 was probably the first to protect the root with a precisely adapted *small gold plate, onto which the tooth is placed*[81]. His son Joseph also covered the root of the dowel crown with a small gold plate (Fig. 284), accord-

[79] See p. 287
[80] Desirabode pp. 672 f.; Lefoulon p. 371
[81] C. J. Linderer pp. 11 f.

ing to his "Handbook" of 1848. But this method is not mentioned again in his work of 1851 [82].

The credit for the first scientific handbook of German dentistry goes to both Linderers, father and son, whom we will meet frequently again. The father, a practitioner far above the average, was still a child of the 18th century with perceptible traces of the tooth-drawer past. Born in Elgershausen near Kassel in 1771 he was certified in 1804 by the Königlich Preussische Obercollegium in Berlin for practice in Halberstadt and the provinces there after ten years of activity in Hildesheim. Between 1805 and 1808 he appended the name "Linderer" (soother, in German), which was full of connotations for a dentist, to his previous name of Calmann Jacob, and changed his first name to Callman. In 1810 he appeared in Göttingen, and in 1812 was appointed dentist of the University by the general director of public instruction in Kassel, residence of Jérôme, king of Westphalia and brother to Napoleon, but during the season he practiced (since 1802) in Bad Pyrmont as the Waldeck ducal court dentist. After Bonaparte's down-fall he was forced to reapply for his title in December of 1813 with the then new government in Hannover. In the assessment by the university his demonstrated talent is recognized, but the opinion is in a negative one, *especially because of his populous family of Jewish heritage, who could become very annoying to the university if the father should die at a young age.* He had also demanded disproportionately high fees at different times. Furthermore, members of the faculty complained in their expressed opinions that he had operated a horse and wagon rental service on the side and feared difficulties with the other (itinerant) university dentist, Friedrich Hirschfeld [83]. Therefore his request was denied, but he obtained a concession as a dentist contingent on paying an honorarium tax, with an interdiction on selling drugs. He seems to have broken both conditions despite repeated warnings frequently, and complaints were also submitted against him for deception and fraud, so that the concession was withdrawn at the request of the police.

This occured on the 28th of March, 1818. On the 18th of April Linderer had already announced his presence in Erfurt, where he had previously practiced as itinerant and where, with foresight, he had previously obtained the status of a Prussian citizen in 1816. He arrived there *in the uniform of the militia, and requested* (with the following signature) *that he might fulfill his duty as a citizen there* [84]:

Callman Jacob Linderer

He practiced there until 1826 and then moved to Berlin, where he lived until his death on February 23, 1840, and where his books were published: the "Lehre von den gesammten Zahnoperationen" (Instruction for all Dental Operations), in 1834, and his collaborative work with his son, the "Handbuch der Zahnheilkunde" (Handbook of Dentistry) in 1837. Both of these books were substantial works and earned him the Prussian and the Austrian medals for Art and Science.

Linderer's son Joseph was born on February 26, 1809 in Göttingen and trained in Berlin. There, in addition to his practical activity under the great physiologist Johannes Müller, he received instructions in microscopic work, which he put to use in odontological investigations [85]. He published his important research findings in his father's handbook, in the second edition of 1842 and in the second volume of 1848. Although these researches were not acknowledged by his German colleagues, they earned him an honorary doctorate from the Philadelphia Dental College. After he had written still another book in 1851 on "Die Zahnheilkunde nach ihrem neuesten Standpunkte" (Dentistry According to the Most Recent Points of View), he retired a resigned but well-to-do man and died on July 20, 1878 in Berlin [86].

We have reserved a great deal of space for the life of this family, because it is representative of the transition of dentistry from itinerant tooth-drawers to scientifically educated dentists such as the Ehrenreichs in Frankfurt or the Greenwoods in the USA.

Leonard Koecker's (Fig. 285) life at the same time is an even more colorful example. This man, who was born as the son of a cleric in 1785 in Bremen, and who was later an honorary doctor of several universities, began as an almost completely self-taught man. As an appren-

[82] J. Linderer (a) p. 361
[83] Fenner pp. 9 f. and 88 f. See p. 233
[84] Romeick pp. 38 f. See pp. 263 f.
[85] See pp. 390 f.
[86] Baume

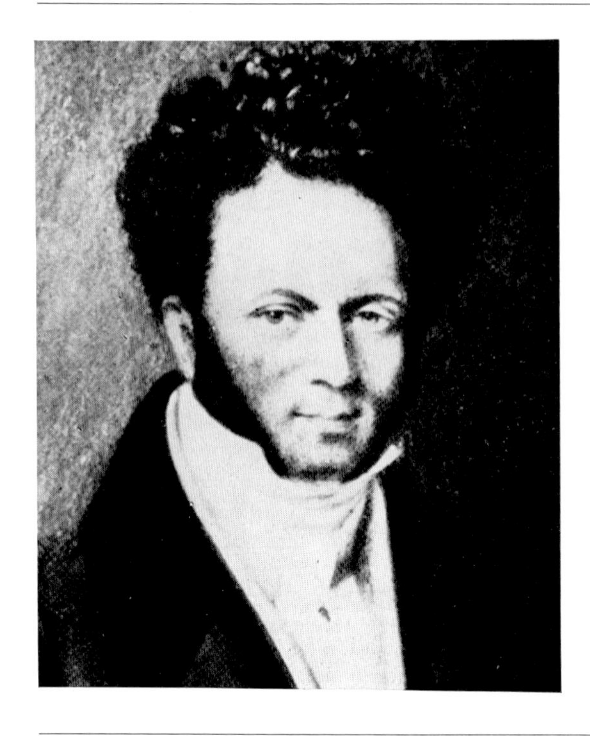

Fig. 285 *Leonard Koecker*

tice to a merchant in his native city he became friends with an itinerant tooth-breaker and learned a few procedures from him. Then, in 1807, he went to Baltimore as a trade agent. As he was not successful in this business, he settled there as a dentist and soon developed a lucrative practice on the basis of his adeptness and his courteous manners. In 1812 we find him for a short time in Lancaster, Pennsylvania, and in the same year in Philadelphia. After an intestinal disease he went from there to Europe to regain his health and remained in London, where he continued to be just as successful and where he published his textbook in 1826, "Principles of dental surgery ..." It was published in German in Weimar in 1828 and once again in the original text in Baltimore in 1842. Koecker remained comfortably well off until his death which came as a result of burns on August 8, 1850.

As an early advocate of the theory of odontogenic focal infections Koecker rejected the dowel crown, which was still actually mounted on untreated roots in 1826. He insisted that before the insertion of any dental prosthesis a sanitation of the oral cavity be undertaken through the extraction of all roots because they could give rise not only to local symptoms, but also to secondary infections affecting the entire body [87].

Koecker had adopted this hypothesis from a physician and philanthropist, also working in Philadelphia, Benjamin Rush, who was probably the first ever to raise the possibility of such connections in a casuistry [88]. Independent of these efforts and motivated by a lecture of W. D. Miller ("The Human Mouth as a Focus of Infection"), Sir William Hunter in London began to develop and promulgate his theory of "Oral Sepsis" [89] in 1890.

In a later specialized essay dating from 1835, "An Essay on Artificial Teeth", Koecker had described, however, the preparation of "pivoted teeth": they should be constructed in such a fashion that the patient himself could remove them in case of an infection. He was also to clean the root canal himself every fortnight and then replace the dowel crown again with fresh cotton [90].

In the second half of the century new ways of attaching the dowel crown began to be suggested. In 1850 Gustav Blume, a dentist

[87] Koecker (a) pp. 256 f.
[88] Ibid. pp. 117 f.
[89] Hunter; Miller
[90] Koecker (b) pp. 151 f.

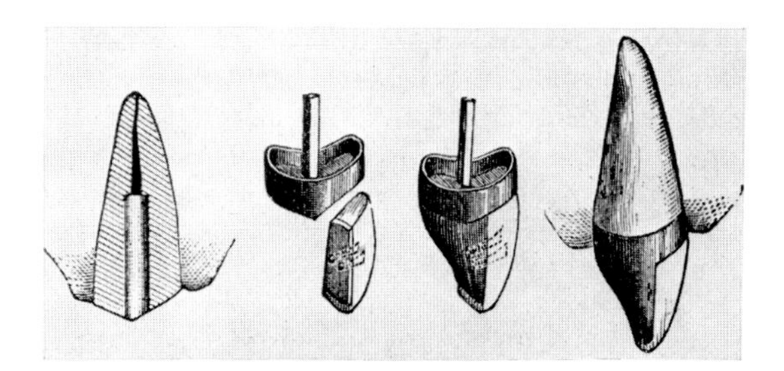

Fig. 286 *Richmond crowns, 1880*

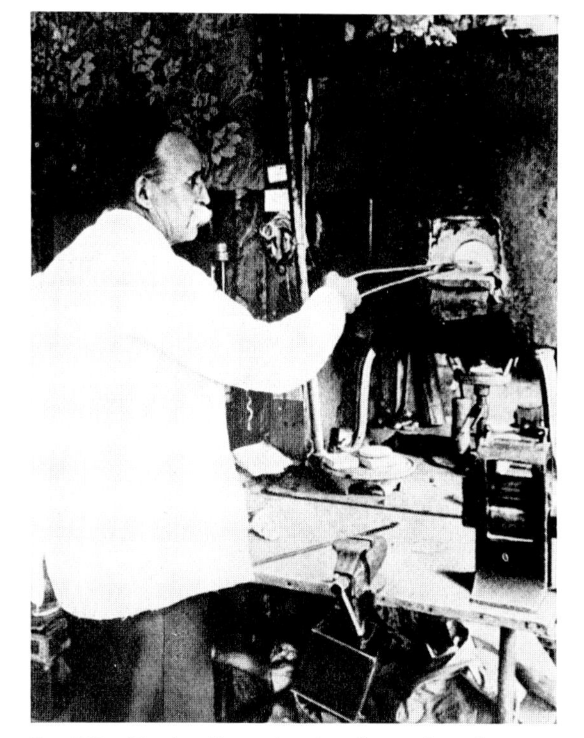

Fig. 287 *Charles Henry Land in front of his furnace*

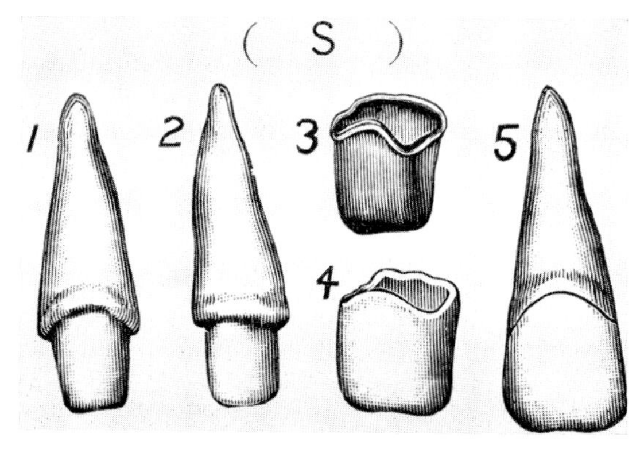

Fig. 288 *Land: Porcelain jacket crowns, 1903*

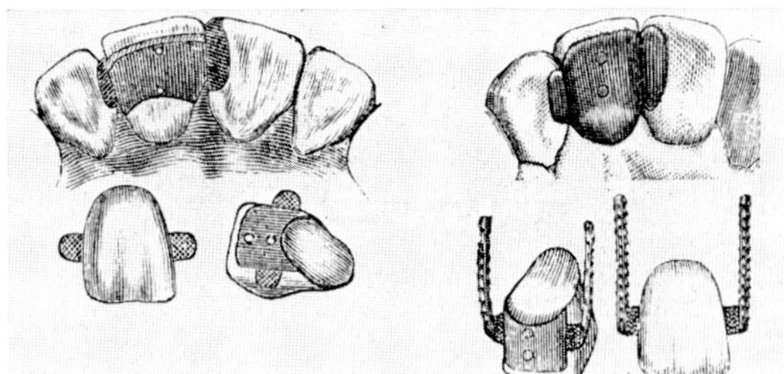

Fig. 289 *Bing: Inlay bridge, 1869*

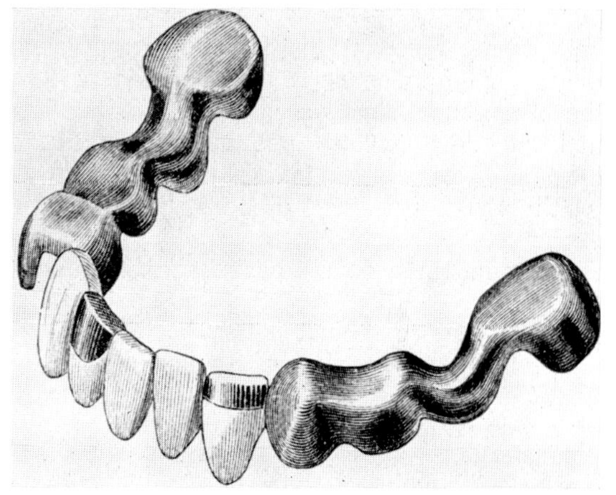

Fig. 290 *Dexter: Removable partial denture, 1883*

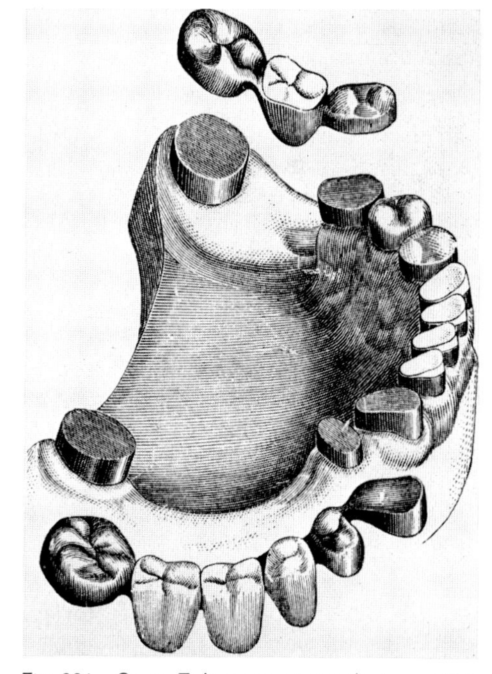

Fig. 291 *Starr: Telescope crown denture, 1886*

in Solothurn, Switzerland, fastened a notched gold post with gold foil in a root canal cleansed of all dental pulp tissue and enlarged with a five-sided reamer[91]. In Cincinnati Jonathan Taft recommended guttapercha for the same purpose in 1859: *The canal in the root above the pivot should be filled with gold*[92]. The same subject brought a lively discussion to the first annual meetings of the Central-Verein deutscher Zahnärzte, which was founded in 1859. As usual there was wavering between gold and wooden posts[93].

This problem was finally resolved temporarily only after the invention of cements, and in 1880 the American Cassius M. Richmond had the dowel crown patented which bears his name. This modified form of the dowel crown, which is still used today, consists of a root stump coping connected to a gold post, upon which is mounted a gold base bearing the porcelain veneer[94] (Fig. 286). These facings were ordinary denture teeth but with platinum pins. Later, in 1904, Thomas Steele of New Jersey produced replaceable veneers attached by a vertical mortise in their backs to a corresponding tenon of the gold backing.

The full porcelain crown was devised by Marshall L. Logan, a dentist in Tyrone, Pennsylvania. Patented in 1884 it achieved rapid and long-lasting popularity. This Logan crown, which had a fired cylindrical post could, indeed, be put in place easily and quickly, but it was not able to provide protection to the root stump in any way[95].

The gold crown, which had already been mentioned by Mouton in 1746 and had been employed in 1829 as a bite-block by Thomas Bell[96] was rediscovered in 1873 by the Californian dentist B. B. Beers, who immediately had it patented. *The suitable basis for cement for fixing is the German os-artificial*[97]. According to another interpretation, the first crown had been manufactured already in 1869 by a dentist in St. Louis, William Newton Morrison, the elder brother of the man who has invented the pedal drilling engine.

The first mention of the half crown is found in 1888 in the discussion of a lecture by A. G. Bennett in the report of a meeting of the Odontological Society of Pennsylvania. This Philadelphia dentist demonstrated the model of a *new attachment or anchorage for bridgework. It consists of a vertical half-cap, which incloses the inner part of molars and bicuspids, and is retained in grooves on the approximal surfaces and between the cusps*[98]. This important device was modified and improved in 1896 by Charles L. Alexander[99], and in 1900 by John P. Carmichael and others[100].

The esthetic climax of the crown technique was attained by Charles Henry Land, a dentist in Detroit (Fig. 287), with the introduction of an individual *enameled Cap or Jacket Crown* fired of porcelain. He had already patented the principle of shaping gold or platinum foil to produce a matrix for fillings of gold, porcelain, glass, or hard rubber in 1887-1888. He published it in 1903 as a method to be used for complete crowning[101] (Fig. 288). His jacket crown differed fundamentally from the conventional ones in resting on a prepared shoulder placed under the edge of the gingiva. It is odd that this type of crown, which is cosmetically so satisfactory, was not generally appreciated until the nineteen-twenties.

The development of the crown prosthesis followed closely after that of bridges. The first bridgework which advanced beyond Fauchard's dowel crown bridge was produced in 1869 by an American dentist in Paris, B. J. Bing, who anchored an anterior tooth veneer by pin inlays on each of the adjacent teeth[102] (Fig. 289). Constructions of removable bridges followed in 1883 and 1886 by James E. Dexter in New York (Fig. 290) and R. Walter Starr (Fig. 291). The latter was a telescoping crown bridge placed on abutments protected by cylindrical copings[103]. James Leon Williams (Fig. 292), a dentist and writer in New Haven and from 1887 to 1912 in London, used the Richmond crown to bear laterally hung replacement teeth, and then, in 1885, as a true bridge abutment[104] (Fig. 292 a). In 1899 Charles Wesley Stainton in Buffalo devised the *open posterior bridge,* a hygienically irreproachable device which represents a true

[91] G. Blume
[92] Taft p. 227
[93] Heider; Mühlreiter; Tomes pp. 624 f.
[94] Talbot (b)
[95] Prothero. I thank Dr. Donald Washburn, Chicago, for a copy of the patent
[96] See pp. 209, 370, and Fig. 311
[97] Talbot (a). See p. 294
[98] A. G. Bennett
[99] Alexander
[100] Carmichael; Evans pp. 311 f. and footnote
[101] Land
[102] H. D. Bennett
[103] Dexter; Starr
[104] Williams (a); (b)

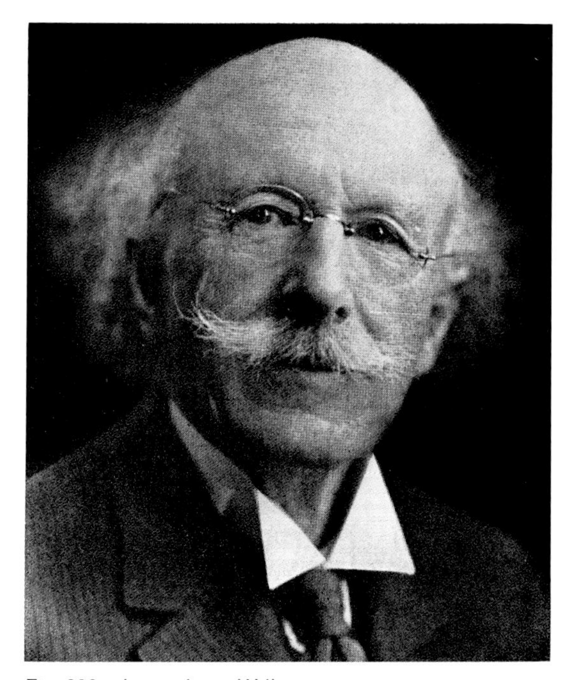

Fig. 292 *James Leon Williams*

Fig. 292 a *Williams: Richmond crown bridge, 1884*

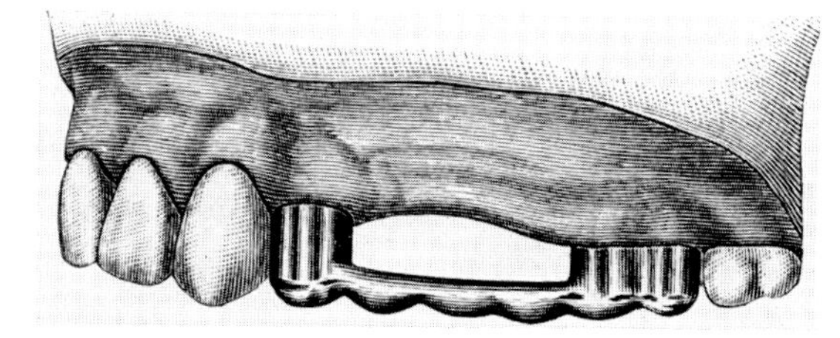

Fig. 293 *Stainton: "Open posterior bridge," 1899*

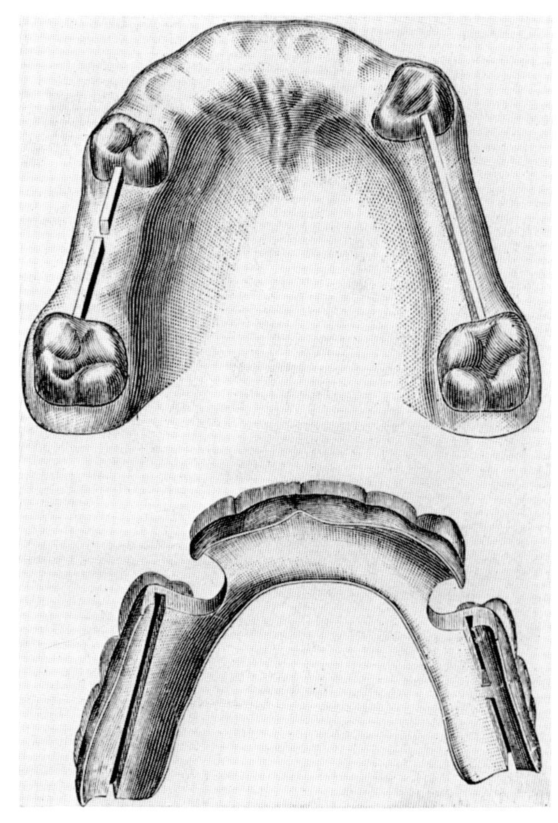

Fig. 294 *Parr: Bar denture, 1890*

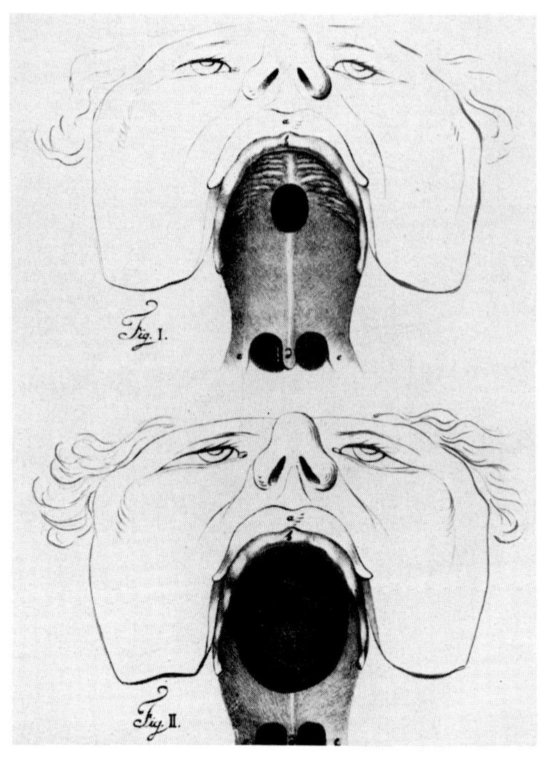

Fig. 295 *Ballif: Enlargement of a palatal perforation over a 16-year period as the result of the use of a sponge obturator*

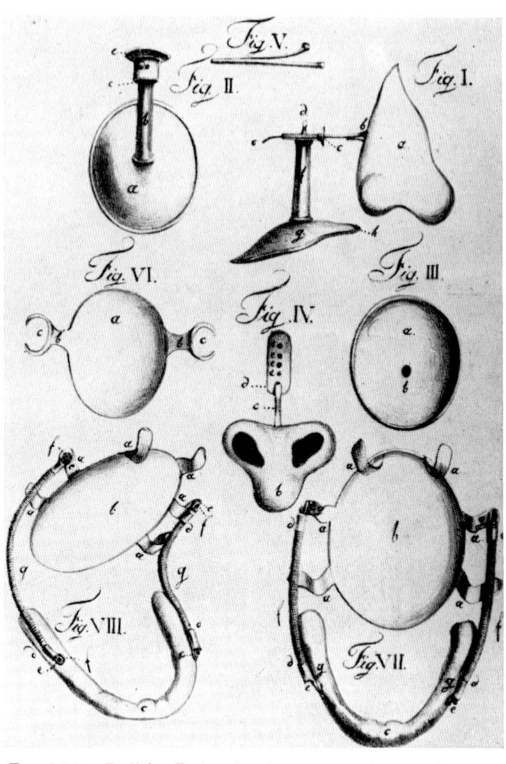

Fig. 296 *Ballif: Palatal closure and nasal prosthesis 1826*

advance, because it permitted cleansing of the gingival surfaces [105] (Fig. 293). In 1890 we are led back again to the removable dental prosthesis introduced by the New York dentist Henry A. Parr which was fastened to crowns and supporting bars [106] (Fig. 294), a real precursor of the supported denture base of our days.

Decisive improvements were made in the preparation of crowns and bridges through metal casting techniques which were introduced in the beginning of the 20th century. This technology is connected with the names of Arthur Ollendorf (1904), a German, and William H. Taggart (1907), an American [107].

Obturators

The development of palatal obturators had stagnated for a long time after Renner, Amatus Lusitanus, and Paré [108] who had almost simultaneously constructed the first ones with the sudden outbreak of central perforations, the sequelae of syphilis brought into Europe by the discoverers of America [109]. Fauchard and Bourdet had improved these devices in the 18th century [110], but no significant progress was made until the 19th century when they began to show a functional shape.

The court dentist to the Prussian king, Pierre Ballif (Baillif), who came from Lausanne and worked in Berlin, used two spiral springs which were supported on the mandible to fasten his obturator, fashioned similarly to Fauchard's "dentier," in 1826. He demonstrated with illustrations of a case how the sponge obturator (see Fig. 122), which was still dominant in spite of all recommended improvements, had widened a coin-sized perforation. Through its swelling

105 Stainton
106 Parr
107 See pp. 295 f.
108 See pp. 167 f. and 148 f.
109 See p. 143 f.
110 See pp. 206 f. and 214

effect alone it included the entire palatine vault within a period of 16 years (Fig. 295). In the case of a syphilitic patient he had combined the obturation of a palatal perforation of this excessive size with a nose prosthesis of his own conception [111] (Fig. 296).

In 1820 Ch. F. Delabarre in Paris established a clear differentiation between the obturation of a central perforation and of a congenital or acquired complete cleft palate in his excellent textbook on prosthetics [112]. With the central type he followed Bourdet in fundamentally simplifying the prosthesis by omitting all nasally placed mechanisms—which are always traumatic to the tissue—and fastening it to the teeth with gold clasps (Bourdet still used gold threads. See Fig. 205).

Delabarre was the first to dare the replacement of the soft palate. The case he described concerned a syphilitic patient whose entire palate, both soft and hard, had been destroyed by perforation, and who had no teeth in his maxilla. The platinum plate which was prepared and provided with mineral teeth was attached to the mandibular teeth by springs and a framework. The separation between the mouth and nose was perfect for eating, but the patient had a nasal speech. Then an artificial velum palatinum made from *gomme élastique* was fastened to the posterior edge of the plate by means of a mechanism which opened the passage only during the act of swallowing; this was effected by a lever on the palatal plate, activated by tongue pressure which occurred during swallowing (Fig. 297).

In the appendix to his book on the straightening of the teeth (redressement des dents) [113], J. M. Alexis Schange recommended in 1842 that Delabarre's obturator, which he praised highly, be provided with his own solid retainers developed for orthodontic purposes. He also constructed artificial soft palates: metal plates movable on a hinge (Fig. 298) which were pressed against the remaining portions of the soft palate by a spring (palatally mounted in No. 15 and nasally in No. 16) so that the plates followed their movements [114].

In 1824, James Snell in London fastened *a spring of highly elastic gold, . . . of which was attached another small silver plate of a long oval form, which exactly covered the fissure of the soft palate* to the silver obturation plate. The little plate, covered on the back with chamois, took part in all swallowing movements [115]. The American Charles Woodward Stearns, who was himself a sufferer from a cleft palate, also constructed a simplified velum. Above everyone, however, Norman W. Kingsley of New York deserves credit here: in 1859 he made use of the functioning of the muscles for sealing the pharynx [116]. Kingsley's soft palate was made from elastic hard rubber, therefore being quite sensitive to deterioration [117], and was attached to the hard rubber plate with a gold peg. It was in contact with the residual portions of the soft palate in such a fashion that it followed their movements without springs, and therewith completely served its function [118] (Fig. 299).

The investigations by the surgeon in Frankfurt Gustav Passavant on the physiology of the closure of the pharynx furnished important, perhaps decisive, progress. In 1863 he demonstrated that the closing of the nasal cavity was not achieved through lifting of the soft portions of the palate alone, but rather also through the simultaneous formation of a transverse cushion on the posterior wall of the pharynx, which extended towards the velum [119] (Fig. 300).

In 1867 Süersen, the Berlin court dentist, took this phenomenon into account when he let soft guttapercha be formed by the function of the musculature of the palate and of Passavant's cushion of the pharynx into the obturating lump. This product of the muscle movements which was firmly connected with the palatal plate, was then vulcanized in hard rubber (Fig. 301). As he himself emphasized, he had derived this idea from a recollection of Schrott's impression procedure [120]. In Kingsley's assessment of Süersen's construction it is pleasant to observe the objectivity with which he undertakes the *consideration of the most scientific obturator which has ever been applied to natural deformities* [121].

This principle was modified in 1881 by the "dental artist" Otto Schiltsky in Berlin: in order

111 Ballif; Hoffmann-Axthelm
112 Ch. F. Delabarre pp. 291 f.
113 See p. 366
114 Schange pp. 145 f.
115 Snell pp. 61 f.
116 Kingsley pp. 261 f. See p. 269 and Fig. 462
117 Brugger p. 16
118 Kingsley (a) pp. 278 f.; (b) pp. 199 f.
119 Passavant
120 Süersen (b); see Fig. 266
121 Kingsley p. 230

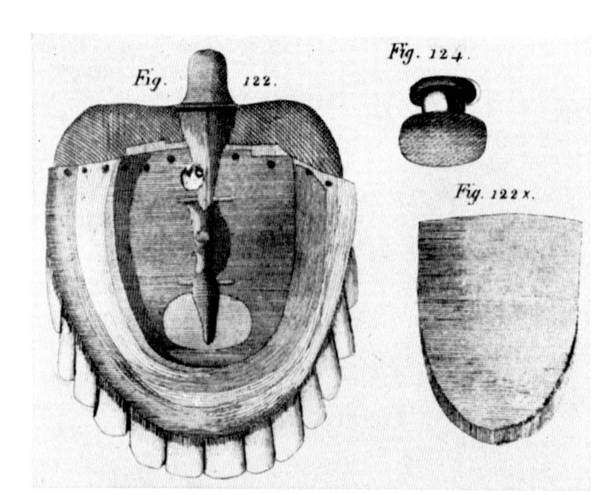

Fig. 297 *Delabarre: Obturator with mechanical soft palate, 1820*

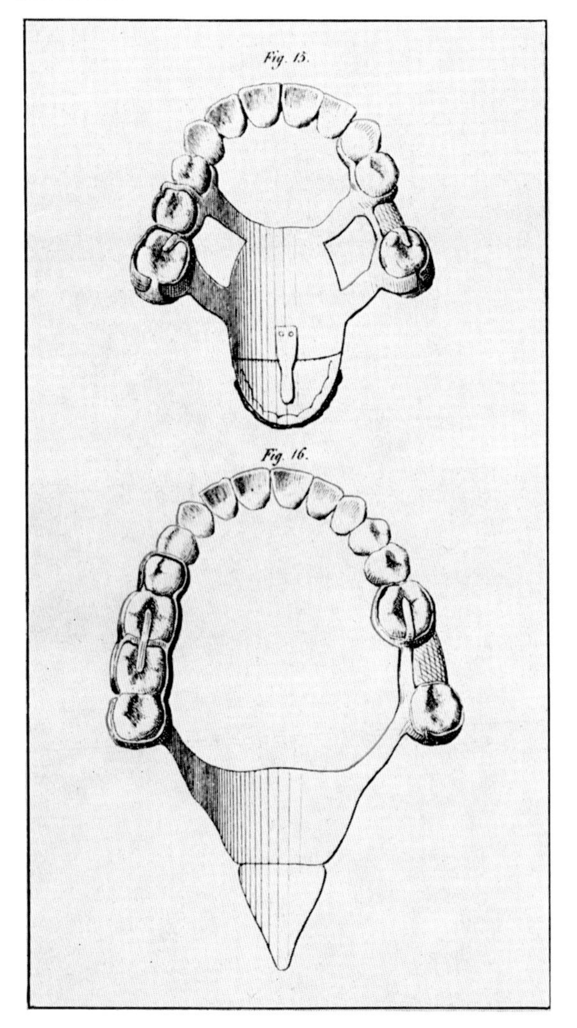

Fig. 298 *Schange: Obturator with mechanical soft palate, 1842*

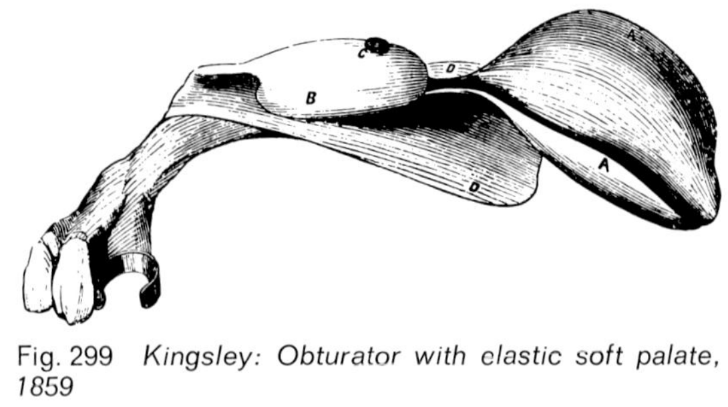

Fig. 299 *Kingsley: Obturator with elastic soft palate, 1859*

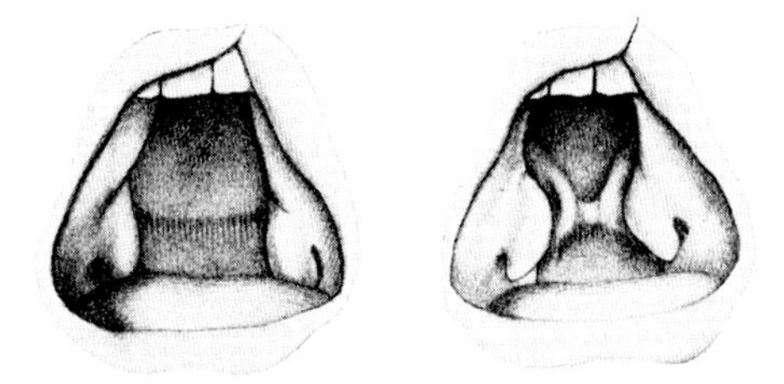

Fig. 300 *Passavant's cushion, 1863*

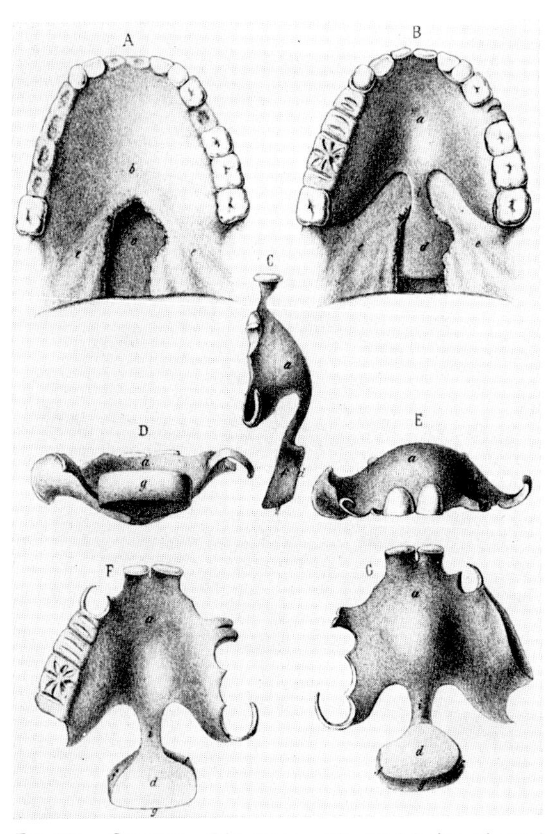

Fig. 301 *Süersen: Obturator with rigid bulge shaped through function, 1867*

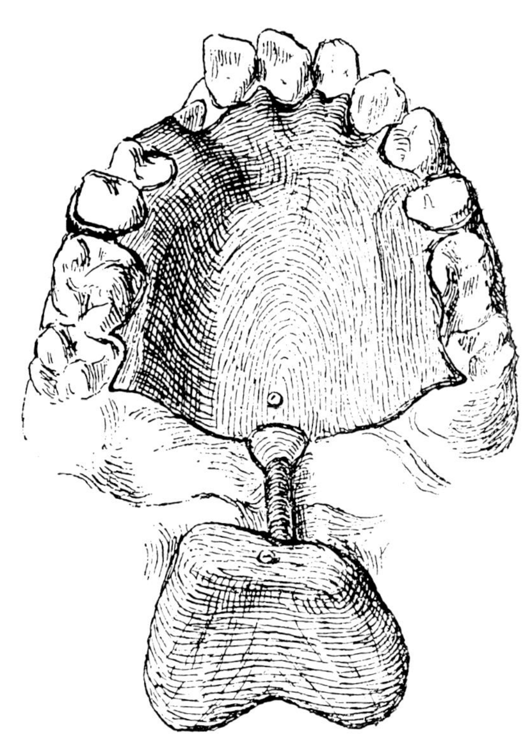

Fig. 302 *Schiltsky: Obturator with pedicled bulge, 1881*

to decrease weight, he formed a hollow lump from *vulcanized soft rubber,* and fastened it to a movable strut [122]. This type, equipped nowadays with a fixed strut, is used chiefly when there is incomplete postoperative closure of the soft palate (Fig. 302). The rigid obturator was developed further in 1896 by Ludwig Warnekros, a professor of prosthetics at the Berlin University. He used the Süersen lump but formed it significantly narrower [123], and therewith gave it the form it still maintains today (Fig. 303). In contrast to this, the obturators described in 1889 by Claude Martin, an important dentist in Lyon, did not present any special advances. He surely departed from the mobile velum palatinum, but his devices still seem exceptionally large—apparently Passavant's investigations had not come to his attention [124] (Fig. 304).

The MEAT-obturator is based on a very different principle. He achieves its speech improving action by closing the nasopharyngeal opening (MEATus nasopharyngeus). In 1928 this apparatus was developed by an assistant at the maxillofacial clinic of Vienna, Albert Schalit, based on the investigations of the Viennese logopedist Emil Fröschels, later in New York. It is composed of a palatal plate with a lump vertically and stiffly attached to it which closes the nasal passages from behind. This closure is made of black guttapercha, formed while functioning then completed in caoutchouc, toady in resin (Fig. 305). A funnel-shaped opening is drilled in this lump until it is large enough

[122] Grunert; Schiltsky pp. 31 f.
[123] Warnekros
[124] Martin pp. 387 f. See pp. 355 f.

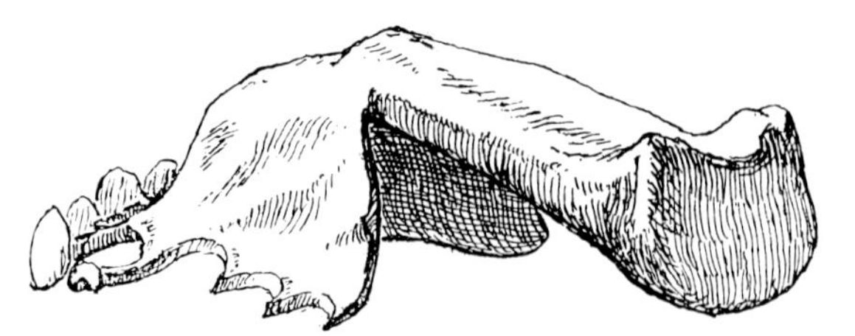

Fig. 303 *Warnekros: Functional obturator, 1896*

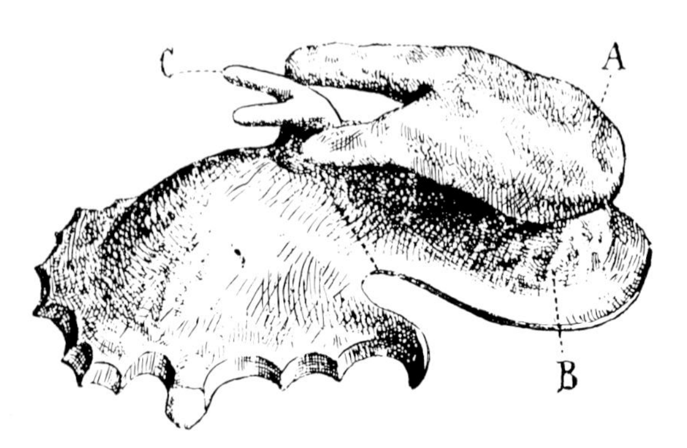

Fig. 304 *Martin: Obturator, 1889*

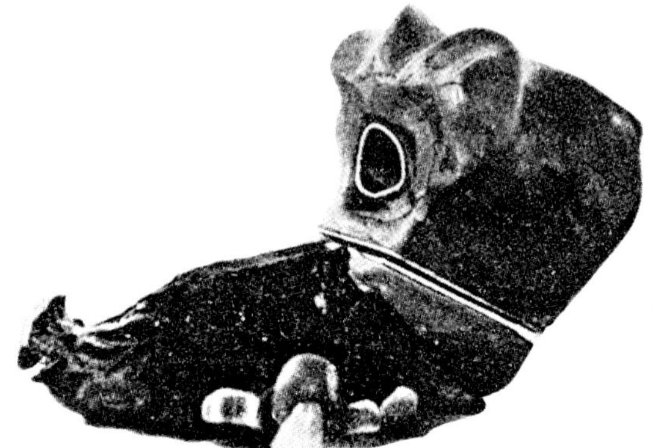

Fig. 305 *Fröschels and Schalit: The Meat obturator, 1928*

for nasal respiration and normal sound of speech [125].

The great progress in the 20th century in the surgical treatment of congenital and acquired palatal defects significantly diminish the importance of obturators, the development of which had claimed the attention of surgeons and dentists for more than five hundred years. Nonetheless, they are still indispensable for the closure of fresh defects after maxillary resection.

Dental Technique and New Materials

In the 19th century the technological manufacture of dental prostheses and palatal obturators was in part in the hands of dentists and in part in the hands of craftsmen. In 1805 Gariot took impressions only leaving everything else to an adept craftsman (ouvrier): *It is better if he* (the dentist) *leaves himself a few free moments from his practice, to be used for the scientific part of his profession, than to make all the pieces himself, like a workman* [126]. The Parisian advertising genius Georges Fattet, a sort of "Great Thomas" of the 19th century, showed himself dressed in a silk morning coat in an advertising brochure around 1850, supervising the craftsmen in his "Laboratoire" (Fig. 306). Serious dentists, on the other hand, such as Laforgue (1803), Lefoulon (1841), and Désirabode (1843), supported the view that the surgeon-dentist should prepare his own technical devices. Joseph Linderer gave this precise definition in 1851: *As mechanical dentistry (Prothèse dentaire, Technik der Zahnheilkunde) is to be understood the art of fabricating artificial teeth, both individual ones and whole dentures, and furthermore the fabrication of artificial palates, artificial noses, and the machines for straightening the teeth.* He classified gold working into two categories: those things which are not a dentist's concern, such as alloying, melting, fabrication of plates and wire and goldplating; and in everything else, which a dentist should perform personally [127]. Not until the sec-

[125] Fröschels; Schalit
[126] Gariot p. 299
[127] J. Linderer (b) p. 235

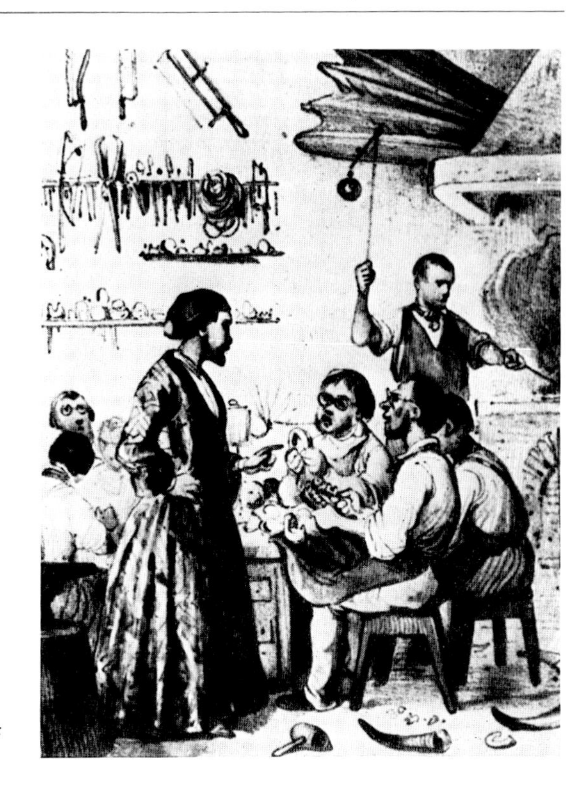

Fig. 306 *The dentist Georges Fattet in his laboratory; lithograph by Edouard Pingret, 1850*

ond half of this century the increasingly complicated production methods and apparatuses, necessary for them, moved the manufacture of dental prostheses more and more into the laboratory of the dental technician.
All the principles of construction in the field of dental prosthetics had been determined by the turn of the 20th century. Corresponding to advances in technology overall significant developments grew from the use of new materials and the inferences drawn from them.
The first stainless steel, an alloy of steel and chromium, was discovered by the French mineralogist Pierre Berthier as early as 1821. It was not until 1919, however, that the dentist Friedrich Hauptmeyer, head of the Krupp dental clinic in Essen, demonstrated the first prosthesis from a stainless nickel-chrome-steel alloy, the so-called V 2-A steel, which had been developed by Benno Strauss, the director of the Chemico-Physical Experimental Institute of the Krupp company[128]. In 1911 Gustav Tammann, a chemist in Göttingen, had developed a forgeable and corrosion resistant alloy of chromium, cobalt and nickel for the same firm, only nowadays used for wires, clasps and bands.
From among the myriad synthetic products which had been recommended since the end of the 19th century as substitutes for vulcanized rubber, such as, for example, celluloid, glyptal and vinyl resins, only the methacrylic esters were able to establish themselves; initially, these were only processed thermoplastically. They were developed in the 1920s by the German chemist Walter Bauer, of the Röhm and Haas Company in Darmstadt, and patented generally in 1928, and specifically as a dental technical material in 1930. The first methacrylate dental preparation in England appeared in 1935 as "Kallodent," in Austria, it was called "Gingivist," and in Germany, "Heliodon." Then, in 1936, the Kulzer company in Frankfurt am Main brought out its own patented thermoplastic "Paladon," which could be polymerized easily in offices by the mixture of liquid monomers and powdered polymers, and soon dominated the European market. The first Amer-

[128] Hauptmeyer

ican polymer preparation of this kind was "Vernonite," which was introduced in 1937 as a collaborative development of the Vernon Benshoff Company in Pittsburg and the American Roehm & Haas Company in Philadelphia. Since then methacrylate products have undergone a tremendous development, particularly after the introduction of cold-curing resins [129].

In a "Short Introduction" of 1924, the Viennese physician Alphons Poller publicized the first usable impression material which remained elastic even after setting. He produced it in somewhat different compositions for molding of body parts (Negocoll), and of dentitions (Dentocoll). The patent for this preparation, which was based on agar-agar, was acquired by dental firms which successfully developed it further after the inventor's death in 1931 [130]. When the types of algae used for the manufacture of agar-agar from the Japanese coast were no longer available in unlimited supply in the United States during the second World War, work was begun there with alginates derived from the native brown algae. Chemical processing of this organic product yielded new impression materials capable of extreme alteration. Besides elastic impression materials were developed from synthetic rubber by S. L. Pearson at the University of Liverpool in 1955 [131], and from resin bases, so that now a wide variety of preparations is available which can be variously employed, depending on the indications at the time. These allow impressions of the highest possible precision.

Today man can expect to live decades longer than in the past, and dental prosthetics is well prepared for this. As a result of development over the course of the millenia, it is now capable of providing older persons with the means of mastication which, in this respect at least, practically eliminate the burden of age, both functionally and cosmetically.

[129] Worner/Guerin; Bauer
[130] Poller (a and b)
[131] Pearson

References

Alexander, C(harles) L(ee)
Casting fillings and abutments for bridges. Dent. Cosmos 38 (1896) 850—854

Ash, Claudius, Sons & Co
A century of dental art. London 1921

Audibran, Joseph
Traité historique et pratique sur les dents artificielles incorruptibles . . . Paris 1821

Balkwill, (Francis Hancock)
a) The best form and arrangement of artificial teeth for mastication. Trans. Odont. Soc. G. B. 5 (1866) 133—158
b) The work of Francis Hancock Balkwill. Dent. Record 42 (1922) 549—553

Ballif, Pierre
Description d'un nez artificiel et de plusieurs obturateurs. Berlin 1826

Bauer, Walter
Die Methacrylära in der Zahnheilkunde. Dtsch. zahnärztl. Zschr. 4 (1949) 1165—1173

Baume, Robert
Nekrolog auf Joseph Linderer. Dtsch. Vjschr. Zahnheilk. 19 (1879) 105—107

Bennett, A. G.
a) Odontological Society of Pennsylvania. Dent. Cosmos 30 (1888) 355
b) The vertical half-cap or bridge-work anchorage. Dent. Cosmos 46 (1904) 367—369

Bennett, H. D.
Partial sets of teeth without plate, clasp, or pivot. Dent. Cosmos 11 (1869) 509—510

Bennett, Norman G(odfrey)
A contribution to the study of the movements of the mandible. Proc. Roy. Soc. Med. London, vol. I, part 3, Odont. Section, pp. 79—98

Blume, E(duard)
Der praktische Zahnarzt . . . Berlin 1836

Blume, G(ustav)
Über das Einsetzen der Stiftzähne. Der Zahnarzt, Berlin 5 (1850) 129—146

Bonwill, W. G. A.
Scientific articulation of the human teeth as founded on geometrical, mathematical and mechanical laws. Dent. Items Int. 21 (1899) 617—636; 873—880

Bremner, M. K. D.
The story of dentistry. Rev. 3rd ed., Brooklyn, London 1964

Brown, Laurence Parmly
The antiquities of dental prosthesis. Dent. Cosmos 76 (1935) 1155—1165

Brugger, Heinrich
Die Behandlung der Gaumenspalten . . . Leipzig 1895

Carmichael, J(ohn) P.
Proceedings of societies. Dent. Rev. 14 (1900) 141—142

Christensen, Carl
A rational articulator. Ash's Quart. Circ. (1901) 401—420

Cohen, R. A.
a) Notes on the identification, description and dating of ivory dentures. Brit. Dent. J. 113 (1962) 259—263
b) Messrs Wedgwood and porcelain dentures correspondence 1800—1815. Brit. Dent. J. 139 (1975) 27—31; 69—71

Cope, Zachary
Sir John Tomes. London 1961

Dagen, Georges
Documents pour servir à l'histoire de l'art dentaire en France . . . Paris (1926)

Delabarre, A(ntoine)
Über die Guttapercha und ihre Verwendung zu künstlichen Zähnen . . . Transl. C. W. L. Schmedicke, Berlin 1852

Delabarre, C(hristophe) F(rançois)
Traité de la partie mécanique de l'art du chirurgien-dentiste. Paris 1820

Désirabode, (Malagou) A(ntoine)
Nouveaux éléments complets de la science et de l'art du dentiste. 2 vols. Paris 1843

Dexter, James E.
The cap plate: A new appliance in mechanical dentistry. Dent. Cosmos 25 (1883) 344—350

Dubois de Chémant, Nicolas
Dissertation sur les avantages des nouvelles dents et rateliers artificielles, . . . Londres, Paris

Evans, George
A practical treatise on artificial crown-, bridge-, and porcellainwork. 9th ed. London 1923

Evans, Thomas W.
a) The discovery of vulcanized caoutchouc and the priority of its application to dental purposes. Paris 1867
b) Mémoires du Dr. Th. W. Evans. Trad. E. Philippi, Paris 1910
c) Obituary Dr. Thomas W. Evans. Dent. Cosmos 40 (1898) 71—76

Fenner, Jörg
Die Zahnärzte an der Universität Göttingen im 19. Jahrhundert . . . Med. Diss. Göttingen 1971

Fons, J. P. de la
A description of the new patent instrument for extracting teeth; also of a patent method of fixing. London 1826

Fox, Joseph
The history and treatment of the diseases of the teeth, . . . London 1806

French, (A. J.)
Bericht über die Fortschritte der dentistischen Mechanik, . . . Der Zahnarzt, Berlin 10 (1855) 353—364

Fröschels, Emil
Sprachärztl. Gedanken die Herstellung eines neuen Obturators . . . betreffend (Meat-Obturator). Österr. Zschr. Stomat. 26 (1928) 882—888

Gall, Joseph
Populäre Anleitung über die wichtigsten Gegenstände der Zahnheilkunde . . . Wien 1834

Gardette, Emi!e B.
Biogr. Notice on the late James Gardette, . . . Amer. J. Dent. Sci. 2/1 (1851) 374—382

Gariot, J(ean) B(aptiste)
Traité des maladies de la bouche. Paris 1805

Geist-Jacobi, G(eorge) P(ierce)
Geschichte der Zahnheilkunde . . . Tübingen 1896

Geschwind, Max
Historical Introduction, in Reprint Skinner, New York 1967

Grunert, Otto
Anleitung zur Anfertigung weicher Obturatoren nach Schiltsky. Dtsch. Mschr. Zahnheilk. 21 (1881) 141—147

Guerini, Vincenzo
Life and works of Guiseppangelo Fonzi. Philadelphia, New York 1925

Gysi, Alfred
a) Beitrag zum Artikulationsproblem. Berlin 1908
b) Neuere Gesichtspunkte im Artikulationsproblem. Schweiz. Vjschr. Zahnheilk. 22 (1912) 118—151

Hall, Rupert H.
a) An analysis of the work and ideas of investigators and authors of relations and movements of the mandible. J. Amer. Dent. Ass. 16 (1929) 1642—1693
b) An analysis of the development of the articulator. J. Amer. Dent. Ass. 17 (1930) 3—51

Harris, Chapin A(aron)
a) The dental art, a practical treatise on dental surgery. Baltimore 1839
b) The principles and practice of dental surgery. 5th ed. Philadelphia 1853
c) Ibid., 9th ed., rev. and ed. by Philip H. Austen Philadelphia 1871

Hauptmeyer, Friedrich
Über die Verwendung von nicht rostendem Stahl in der Zahnheilkunde. Dtsch. Mschr. Zahnheilk. 38 (1920) 1—7

Heider, (Moriz)
Quelques détails sur l'introduction du Caoutchouc vulcanisé dans la chirurgie dentaire par Thomas W. Evans. Paris 1856. Dtsch. Vjschr. Zahnheilk. 6 (1866) 108—110

Hepburn, Christian
Die Geschichte der Hersteller und Verkäufer zahnärztlicher Bedarfsartikel bis um 1900. Köln 1965

Hesse, (Friedrich)
Nachruf an Carl Sauer. Dtsch. Mschr. Zahnheilk. 10 (1892) 175—181

Hoffmann-Axthelm, Walter
Die Brücke des königl. preuß. Hofraths und Leibzahnarztes Pierre B. Ballif (Baillif). Zahnärztl. Mitt. 58 (1968) 1259—1265

How, W. Storer
Some phases of crown and bridge work. Dent. Cosmos 48 (1906) 290—302

Hunter, William
The relations of dental diseases to general diseases. Trans. Odont. Soc. G. B., N. S. 31 (1899) 92—115

Kingsley, Norman W(illiam)
A treatise on oral deformities . . . New York 1880

Koecker, Leonard
a) Principles of dental surgery, . . . London 1826
b) An essay on artificial teeth, . . . London 1835

Laforgue, Louis
a) L'art du dentiste. Paris 1802
b) Die Zahnarzneikunst. Transl. C. F. Angermann, Leipzig 1803/1806

Land, Charles H(enry)
Porcelain dental art. Dent. Cosmos 45 (1903) 437—444, 615—620

Lefoulon, J(oachim)
Nouveau traité . . . de l'art du dentiste. Paris 1841

Linderer, C(allman) J(acob)
Lehre von den gesammten Zahnoperationen . . . Berlin 1834

Linderer, Joseph
a) Handbuch der Zahnheilkunde. Vol. II, Berlin 1848
b) Die Zahnheilkunde nach ihrem neuesten Standpunkte. Erlangen 1851

Luce, Charles E(lmer)
The movements of the lower jaw. Boston Med. Surg. 121 (1889) 8—11

Martin, Claude
Prothèse immédiate appliquée à la résection des maxillaires. Rhinoplastie sur apparail prothétique permanent. Restauration de la face: lèvres, nez, langue, voute et voile du palais. Paris 1889

Matheson, Leonard; Lewin J. Payne
The history of dentistry in Great Britain. J. Amer. Dent. Ass. 15 (1928) 441—461

Maury, F.
a) Vollständiges Handbuch der Zahnarzneikunde. Weimar 1830
b) Traité complet de l'art du dentiste. Nouvelle éd., Paris 1833

Miller, W. D.
The human mouth as a focus of infection. Dent. Cosmos 33 (1891) 689—713; 789—804; 913—919

Mühlreiter, Eduard
Physikalische Studie über das Festhalten der Stiftzähne. Dtsch. Vjschr. Zahnheilk. 7 (1867) 88—102

Parmly, L(evi) S(pear)
A practical guide to the management of the teeth, . . . Philadelphia 1819

Parr, H. A.
Proceedings of dental societies. Dent. Cosmos 32 (1890) 439—440

Passavant, Gustav
Über die Verschließung des Schlundes beim Sprechen. (Virchows) Arch. path. Anat., Berlin 46 (1869) 1—31

Paterson, Alexander H(orn)
Seeing prosthesis through the eyes of the "Dental Cosmos". Dent. Cosmos 76 (1934) 67—88

Paulson, G(erhardt)
Erinnerungen eines alten Zahnarztes. Dtsch. Mschr. Zahnheilk. 26 (1908) 369—392

Pearson, S. L.
A new elastic impression material: a preliminary report. Brit. Dent. J. 99 (1955) 72—76

Pfaff, Philipp
Abhandlung von den Zähnen . . . Berlin 1756

Poller, Alphons
a) Kurze Anleitung zum Abformen am lebenden und toten Menschen, sowie an leblosen Gegenständen. Apotela, Wien (1924)
b) Das Pollersche Verfahren zum Abformen . . . Berlin, Wien 1931

Prothero, J. H.
Prosthetic dentistry. 4th ed. Chicago 1928

Putnam, C(lark) S(amuel)
Zahnarzneikunde wie sie sein sollte. Leipzig 1861

Richardson, Joseph
A practical treatise on mechanical dentistry. Philadelphia 1860

Robinson, James
The surgical, mechanical, and medical treatment of the teeth. London 1846

Rock, Thomas D.
Über die Hippopotamus-Zähne oder Hauer. Der Zahnarzt, Berlin 16 (1861) 238—246

Rogers, William
a) L'encyclopédie du dentiste . . . 2nd ed., Paris 1845
b) Manuel d'hygiène dentaire . . . Paris 1845

Romeick, Dietrich
Die Erfurter Zahnärzte von 1587 bis 1967. Erfurt 1968

Schalit, Albert
Über einen neuen Obturator (Meat-Obturator). Österr. Zschr. Stomat. 26 (1928) 888—898

Schange, J. M. A(lexis)
Précis sur le redressement des dents, . . . réflexions sur les obturateurs du palais. 3rd ed , Paris 1842

Schiltsky, Otto
Über neue weiche Obturatoren . . . Berlin 1881

Schröder, Hermann
Über die Aufgaben der zahnärztl. Prothetik und die Versuche zu ihrer Lösung. Berlin 1929

Schrott, (Johann Joseph)
a) Bericht VI. Jahresvers. Central-Verein dtsch. Zahnärzte. Dtsch. Vjschr. Zahnheilk. 4 (1864) 267—270
b) System den genauesten Abdruck und die sicherste Artikulation zu erhalten. Dtsch. Vjschr. Zahnheilk. 4 (1864) 296—304

Schwarze, Paul
Über die Bonwill'sche Articulationsmethode. Dtsch. Mschr. Zahnheilk. 7 (1889) 1—12

Skinner, R(ichard) C(ortland)
A treatise of human teeth . . . New York 1801 (Reprint 1967)

Snell, James
Observations on the history, use, and construction of obturateurs, or artificial palates. (London 1824) 2nd ed. London 1828

Snow, G. B.
Present status of articular question. Dentist's Mag. 2 (1906—1907) 635—647

Spee, Ferdinand Graf
Die Verschiebungsbahn des Unterkiefers am Schädel. Arch. Anat. Physiol. 16 (1890) 285—294. English transl. J. Amer. Dent. Ass. 100 (1980) 670—675

Stainton, C(harles) W(esley)
Open posterior bridges. Dent. Cosmos 41 (1899) 278—282

Starr, R. Walter
Removable bridge-work, — porcelain cap crowns. Dent. Cosmos 28 (1886) 17—19

Süersen, W(ilhelm)
a) Über die Anwendung des vulkanisirten Kautschuks . . . und die Anfertigung der sog. Luftdruckgebisse. Der Zahnarzt, Berlin 18 (1863) 33—46
b) Über die Herstellung einer guten Aussprache durch ein neues System . . . Dtsch. Mschr. Zahnheilk. 7 (1867) 268—287

Taft, J(onathan)
A practical treatise on operative dentistry. Philadelphia 1859

Talbot, E. S.
a) Gold crowns. Dent. Cosmos 22 (1880) 463—466
b) Proceedings of the first district dental society, State of New York. Dent. Cosmos 26 (1884) 411—413

Tomes, John
A system of dental surgery. Philadelphia 1859

Verchere, Louis
Le pharmacien Alexis Duchateau, inventeur des dents de porcelaine. Rev. d'odonto-stomat., Paris 3 (1974) 423—426

Ward, G.
a) Impression materials and impression taking. Brit. Dent. J. 110 (1961) 118—119
b) Mr. Goodyear's preparation of caoutchouc. Brit. Dent. J. 114 (1963) 449—451

Warnekros, Ludwig
Demonstration über Obturatoren und ihre Anwendung bei angeborener Gaumenspalte. Verh. Dtsch. odont. Ges. 7 (1896) 145—152

Weber, I. H. C.
Verschiedenes. Dtsch. Vjschr. Zahnheilk. 7 (1867) 257—265

White, John DeHaven
Practical hints. Dent. Cosmos 3 (1862) 177—179, 289—290

White, Samuel Stockton
Obituary. Dent. Cosmos 22 (1880) 57—63

Weinberger, Bernhard Wolf
An introduction to the history of dentistry in America. Vol. II, St. Louis 1948

William, J(ames) L(eon)
A consideration of the merits and claims of the artificial crown- and bridge-work. Dent. Cosmos 25 (1883) 622—631, 26 (1884) 1—8, 27 (1885) 705—716

Wooffendale, Robert
Practical observations on the human teeth. London 1783

Worner, H. K.; B. D. Guerin
Acrylic resins in dentistry. Austral. J. Dent. 46 (1942) 202—211

Chapter 12

Conservative Dentistry

Restorations and Restorative Materials

The demand for systematic conservation of teeth is largely an idea of the 19th century. Whatever had transpired before as regards this subject was generally related only to the removal of tartar and of sharp edges on the teeth, as also the unmethodical filling of cavities with a variety of materials to which occasionally, especially in Islamic medicine, analgesic drugs had been added.

The first recommendation of gold foil as a filling material of which we know was made in the 15th century by Giovanni d'Arcoli. In the following century Giovanni da Vigo proposed previous removal of the "corrosio" with drills, files and scrapers. Pierre Fauchard removed caries with strong probes and plugged the dried cavities with lead or tin[1].

The Parisian authors of the first half of the 19th century dealt with the subject, known today as restorative dentistry, in three brief chapters of their textbooks stereotypically as filing, cauterization, and "filling" of the teeth. Their term for filling, "plomber," is derived from the Latin "plumbum" (lead), because this material in general was used to restore the cavities. Louis Laforgue also preferred it (Fig. 307), using gold foil only in visible places. Jean-Baptiste Gariot in 1805 filled only those teeth which were painless. These he carefully cleaned of caries and dried the cavity with cotton. Then he filled them with foils of lead, silver or gold, as obtained especially for this purpose at the gold-beater's[2].

Filing was largely limited to the anterior teeth and consisted of removal of the carious matter and, preventively, in reduction of the adjacent surfaces of neighboring teeth, a process through which food particles were prevented from adhering. The shoulder at the neck of the tooth was left to forestall closure of the interdental space (Fig. 308). Joseph Fox of London determined in 1806 that a filling ("stopping") at the sides and between the teeth tended to fall out by the pressure exerted by food, and that, therefore, frequent replacement was requested[3].

In these cases, filing between the upper incisors was indicated, prophylactically as well as in the presence of caries. As early as 1815 Christophe François Delabarre objected to this procedure, which he blamed justifiably that the good was being taken away with the bad. He used a burin to remove only the caries and spared the enamel layer as much as possible[4].

Invention of the probe in its present form is claimed by C. F. Maury, who also described a dental mouth mirror (miroir du dentiste, Fig. 309). In his "Traité complet de l'art du dentiste" (Complete Treatise on the Art of Dentistry), published several times since 1820 in its original language and translated into German (1830), English (1843), Italian, and Dutch, lead is rejected because of its blackening, in favor of tinfoil, even better is gold or platinum foil, especially for the anterior teeth. Joachim Lefoulon, in 1841, removed caries with spoon-shaped excavators and shaped the cavities as reverse funnels with hand drills. He dried them with alcohol and cotton, inserted metal foils in the shape of small cylinders or pellets with the probe, and packed them with pluggers (Fig. 310).

In 1826 Leonhard Koecker of London recognized only gold foil as filling material; most important for him, however, was the complete removal of the caries before filling lest the disease expand more quickly[5]. In lengthy explanations[6], he rejected a low-melting alloy which had been composed independently by Isaac Newton and, approximately a century later, by the Parisian chemist and mint-warden Jean Pierre Joseph Darcet[7] from bismuth, lead and tin (8 : 5 : 3).

Probably as the first, Joseph Fox in 1806 proposed the use of this material as a filling[8]. In 1818, the Parisian dentist Louis Nicolas

1 See pp. 133, 134, and 200
2 Laforgue (a) pp. 167 f.; (b) pp. 148 f.; Gariot pp. 266 f.
3 Fox p. 138
4 Delabarre pp. 59 f.
5 Koecker pp. 383 f.
6 Ibid. p. 395
7 Son of the sponsor of Dubois de Chémant. See p. 255
8 Fox p. 139

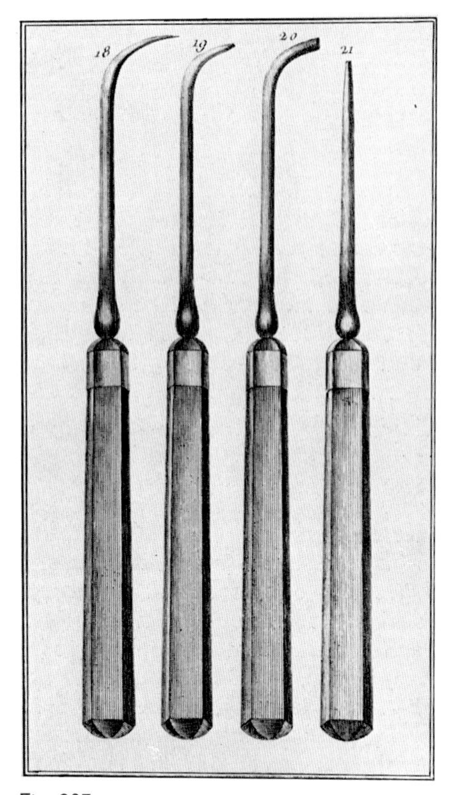

Fig. 307

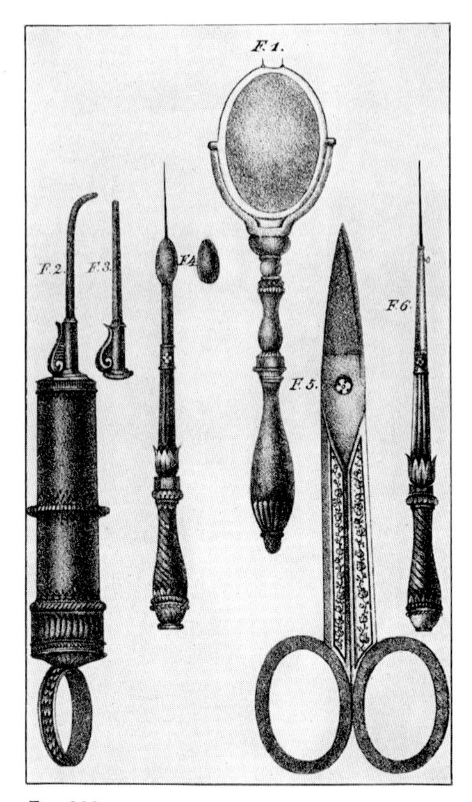

Fig. 309

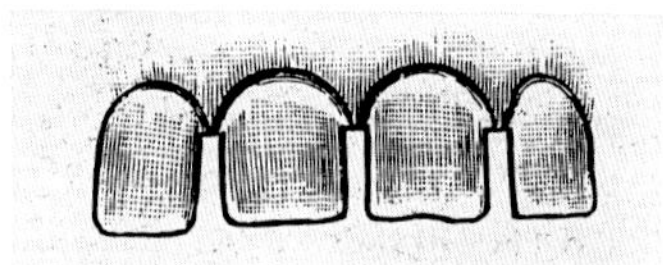

Fig. 308

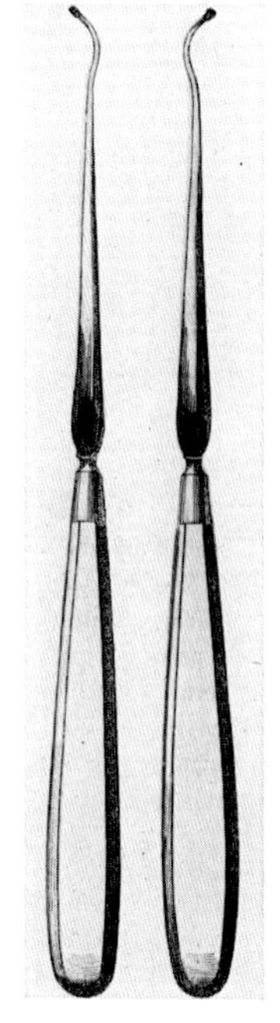

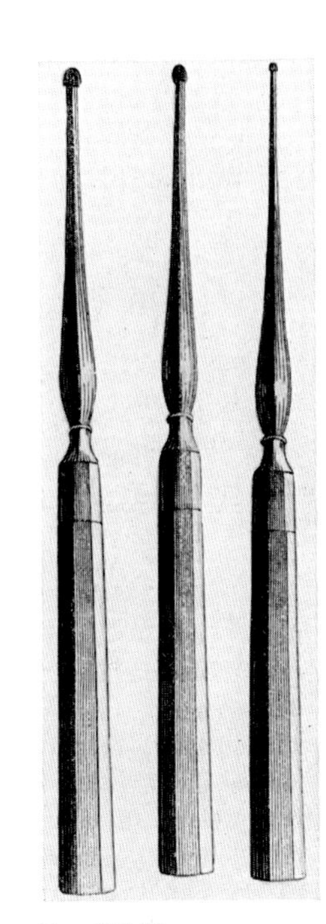

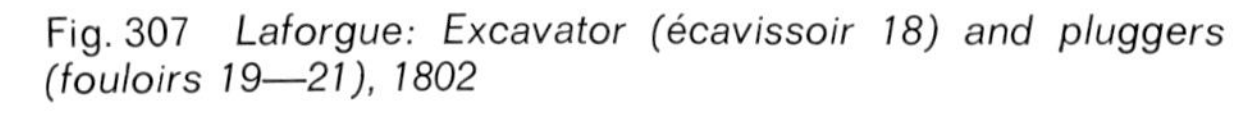

Fig. 307 *Laforgue: Excavator (écavissoir 18) and pluggers (fouloirs 19—21), 1802*

Fig. 308 *Filing to remove a flat carious lesion and as a preventive measure (from Willoughby D. Miller)*

Fig. 309 *Maury: Mouth mirror, water syringe, probes, etc., 1822*

Fig. 310 a) and b) *Lefoulon: Spoon-shaped excavators and hand drills, 1841*

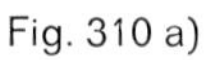

Fig. 310 a)

Fig. 310 b)

Regnart suggested in his "Mémoire sur un nouveau moyen d'obturation des dents" (Note on a new Means for Obturating the Teeth) that the alloy be placed in the cavity in small pieces, and that it should be melded there through the use of a heated plugger. By addition (of one-tenth) of mercury to the mass of the alloy he was able to reduce the melting point significantly. Regnart, a physician who devoted himself entirely to dentistry, became the first president of the Société de Chirurgie Dentaire de Paris, founded in 1845[9].

Perhaps stimulated by Regnart's publication, Auguste Onésime Taveau between 1826[10] and 1835[11] introduced amalgam in Paris which we have encountered as a filling material in the 16th century in China and approximately simultaneously as a prescription of Ulm's municipal physician Stockerus[12]. Taveau prepared it from pulverized silver and mercury and called it "pâte d'argent" (silver paste).

This significant suggestion was not greeted with excessive zeal. Lefoulon, who mentioned it once in 1841 and who used the designation "amalgame" probably as the first after Stocker, rejected it because of the black discoloration, the tendency to shrink with volatilization of the mercury, and its porosity[13]. He and Désirabode also voiced serious qualms because of the mercury content, a hesitation entirely understandable because in those times they probably saw severe stomatitis nearly every day, in consequence of treatment of syphilis with ointment of mercury[14]. In 1851 the younger Linderer revised the doubts expressed three years before in the second volume of his handbook and wrote: *The amalgam filling is an excellent means for conservation of the teeth.* He provides exact methods for preparation, also for the copper amalgam used for several years in Paris. He turns decisively against the amalgam-rejecting position of Chapin A. Harris of Baltimore, whose countryman Thomas W. Evans, working in Paris, added cadmium to the tin-silver mixture (1 : 3 : 1) in 1848. This amalgam surely expanded less but was not satisfactory on the whole because it crumbled in time[15].

As early as 1819 Charles Bell, a chemist, is said to have produced a kind of silver amalgam which was distributed as "Bell's Cement," later as "Mineral succedaneum" (replacement mineral). However, it is not mentioned in "The Anatomy, Physiology and Diseases of the Teeth" published in 1829 by Thomas Bell, who was Fox's successor as lecturer in dentistry at the London Guy's Hospital (Fig. 311). This dental surgeon, zoologist and president of Linnaean Society knew only Newton's metal by hearsay and, like Koecker, rejected it[16]. Broader acceptance was gained only in 1830 with the introduction of an amalgam made of filings of French silver coins by the family of the London dentist Crawcour, poor representatives of their profession, who sought to add greater esteem to the "mineral succedaneum" by appending the prefix "Royal." When they used the material themselves they did not make the effort to remove the caries beforehand. They rather filled the teeth *in about two minutes without the slightest pain, inconvenience or pressure,* as Campbell tells us from newspaper advertisements and conversations with the descendants of the Crawcours[17]. After they had grazed all over England and Paris, too, in such manner, two of the brothers went to New York in 1833, where they distributed their "Royal Mineral Succedaneum" widely and made a fortune in a short time. With these methods they paved the way for the "amalgam war" that split American dentistry into two camps well into the second half of the century, and that was carried out with such passion that it resembled that of European religious conflicts.

The prominence in dentistry in the United States, led by Eleazar Parmly (Fig. 312) and Isaac John Greenwood of the third generation of this dental family, and later by Chapin Aaron Harris and Jonathan Taft, supported gold fillings with fanaticism and banned completely all those who would prefer the less complicated and less expensive amalgam. The American Society of Dental Surgeons, founded in 1840 by Horace Hayden, caused its members in 1843 to sign an agreement that they would never, under any circumstances, use amalgam—on the penalty of expulsion[18]. In London, too, in 1846 James Ro-

[9] Dagen p. 295
[10] Ibid. p. 360
[11] de Maar
[12] See pp. 43 and 156 f.
[13] Lefoulon pp. 264 f.
[14] Désirabode pp. 408 f.
[15] J. Linderer (a) p. 409; (b) p. 331
[16] Bell pp. 144 f.
[17] Campbell pp. 265 f.
[18] See p. 408

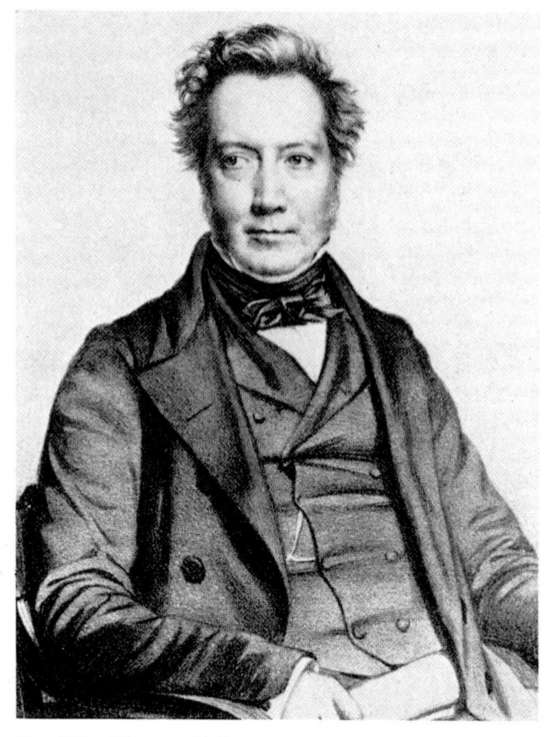

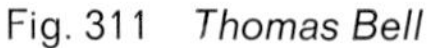

Fig. 311 *Thomas Bell*

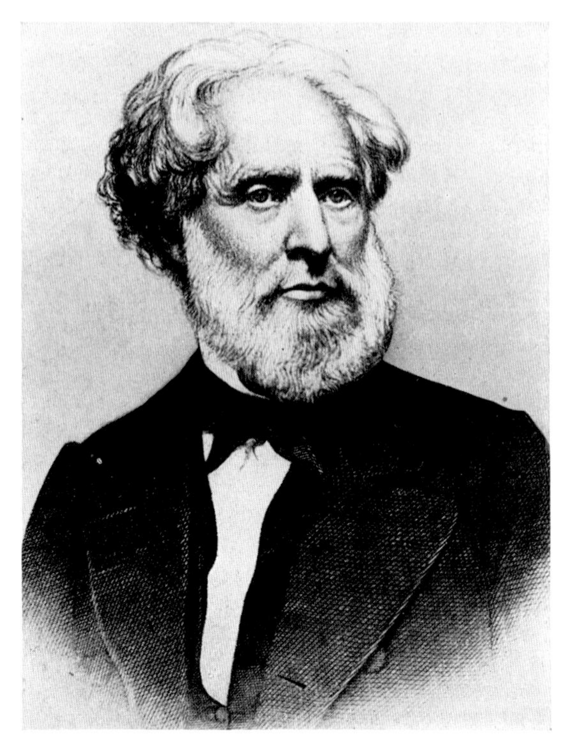

Fig. 312 *Eleazar Parmly*

binson took the side of gold fillings completely, recommending that an asbestos layer be used to protect the pulp from severe temperature changes in large defects[19].

The technique of fillings with gold or amalgam was improved significantly after mid-century. In 1857, Robert Arthur, one of the first students of the "Baltimore College of Dental Surgery" and later dentist in Washington, Philadelphia, and from 1857 on in Baltimore, published his system of filling teeth with an "adhesive" gold. This rested on the fact that annealed pellets of gold foil could be welded without heat by pressure[20]. This pressure was exerted at first by hand with specially designed instruments. From 1861, hammer blows were used on the recommendation of William Henry Atkinson of New York[21].

Following the introduction of the foot-powered drill, mechanical hammers also were used[22]. In any case it was a tedious, difficult task, and also embarrassing for the patient. But the technique made possible restoration of the anatomical shape of the tooth and the re-establishment of contact points. As the procedure was possible only in perfect dryness, air blowers and saliva ejectors with rubber balls were constructed. Increased usefulness was established in 1864 when Sanford Christie Barnum, a New York dentist, invented the rubber dam and had publish his concept in the *Dental Cosmos* in 1866, thereby making a gift of this idea to the dentists, an action then quite unusual. *Unfortunately, he shared the fate of so many benefactors of mankind for he died without means, even needy*[23]. The technique, then as now, consists of placing a highly elastic punched rubber sheet over the tooth to be treated and its neighbors, thus isolating it as if outside the oral cavity (Fig. 313).

The leading position of North Americans in the field of condensed gold foil fillings continued up to the turn of the century. Europe's dentists flocked to the New World to learn the technique

19 Robinson pp. 112 f.
20 Arthur (a) pp. 25 f.
21 Miller (c) p. 125
22 See p. 306
23 Latimer; Christen; Miller (c) p. 80; Francis

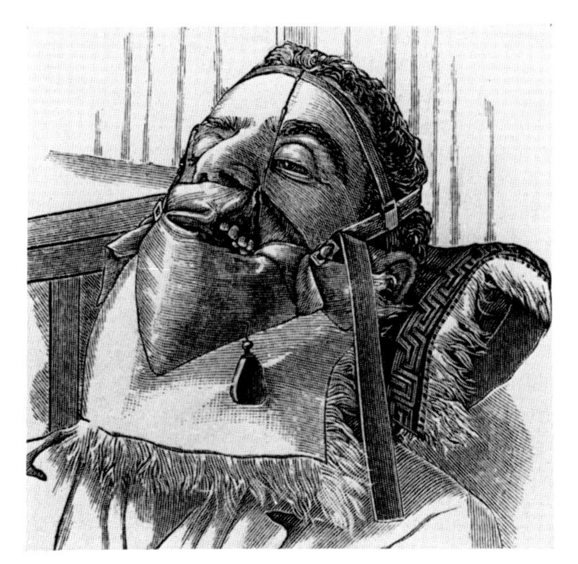

Fig. 313 *Placement of a rubber dam*

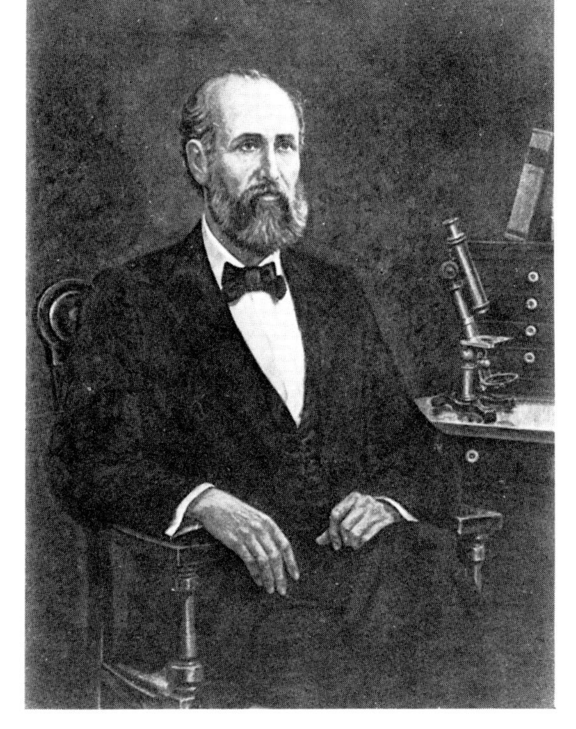

Fig. 314 *Greene Vardiman Black, age 35, painted by Floyd Ostendorf, 1870 (Illinois State Dental Society)*

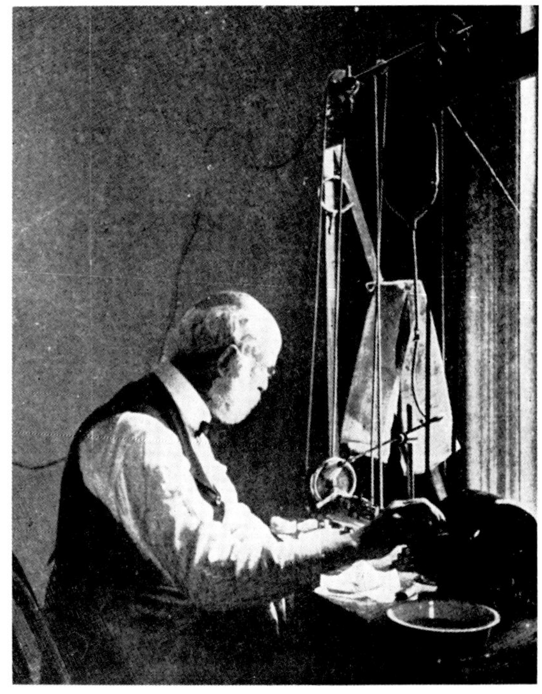

Fig. 315 *"Dr. Black at Work in His Laboratory" (from Thorpe)*

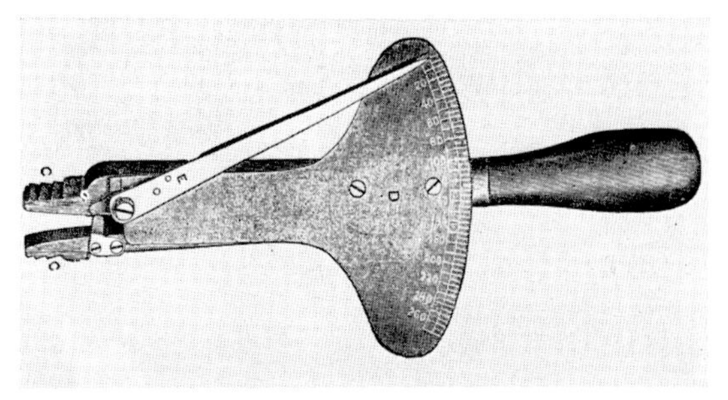

Fig. 316 *Black: Gnathodynamometer*

in its home—and many American dentists came to Europe, too, to settle and practice in its metropolitan centers[24].

But amalgam made progress also. In 1855, the Cincinnati dentist William M. Hunter and, inspired by Hunter, Philadelphia's Elisha Townsend published a formula consisting of a combination of 4 parts silver and 5 parts tin, a ratio approaching that of today's material[25]. Shortly before his death in 1859, Townsend, it may be noted, went over to the side of the amalgam opponents, an event that John DeHaven White, a Philadelphia dentist and first editor of *Dental Cosmos,* founded in 1859 and for more than 75 years the leading professional journal, triumphantly reported even as late as 1878[26]. In 1859, Taft wrote in his textbook that amalgam should be regarded by no means as a durable material, and in 1873, a Dr. Payne proclaimed in the *Chicago Medical Journal* that *neither Asiatic cholera, nor smallpox, nor any malarious disease, is doing half the mischief in the world that is done by this poisoning*[27]. Then, however, in the 1870s, strong opposition began to form under the leadership of the skilled orator and writer Joseph Foster Flagg, a grandson of one of the first important dentists born in the nation (1763), Josiah Flagg. The opposition was characterized, with some degree of propriety, as being one-sided and as taking an anti-social and uncollegial attitude. But only when Chicago's prominent teacher of dentistry, Black, stood up for the new material and improved it significantly the last flames of the "amalgam war" died away.

Born on August 3, 1836 near Winchester, Illinois, Greene Vardiman Black (Fig. 314) was not educated in a Dental College, but rather served an apprenticeship. In 1857 he opened a practice in Winchester, and in 1863 he moved to Jacksonville. Here he became known for experimental studies, leading to his being called in 1870 to the Missouri Dental College and to being offered a position as professor of pathology at the Chicago Dental College. In 1891 he exchanged the latter position for a professorship at Chicago's Northwestern University Dental School. In 1908, he published his principal work, a two-volume "Operative Dentistry," which was translated into German in 1914 by one of his students, Vienna's professor Hans Pichler, later a prominent oral surgeon, under the title of "Konservierende Zahnheilkunde." This most admired dental scientist of the United States died on August 31, 1915. His colleagues erected a monument for him in one of Chicago's parks[28].

It is Black's enduring and most important contribution to have established a system of cavity preparation. His demand of "extension for prevention" continues today to be impressed on every dental student of the world as an axiom of cavity preparation. Admittedly, it was the invention of a usable drilling engine that was the prerequisite for accomplishing this postulation, which seems a matter of course to us today. This device was invented in 1871 by Morrison, an American dentist[29], although Black himself and his students rejected it for removal of caries, preferring to continue the use of the excavator[30].

Black also engaged himself with all his authority to support the principle of the contact point. This claim was not fundamentally new in 1891, because as early as 1879 Safford Goodwin Perry, and in 1881 especially Marshall H. Webb of Pennsylvania had made similar suggestions at a meeting in London[31]. The latter had also invented an electrical hammer for condensing foil restorations.

Black also undertook to examine commercially available amalgams. Expressly for this purpose he constructed a "gnathodynamometer," with which the pressure exerted on the human tooth, and therewith on the filling material, too, could be measured. This was the first step in this direction since Borelli's attempt (Fig. 316)[32]. In experiments stretching over a period of years, he established an ideal metal mixture, one which was stable and did not discolor. Publication of his results led to standardization of the alloys, without his having any financial gain from the work. He also heated the preparations to avoid amalgam "aging," with its associated changes in working properties[33].

In 1859, the great scientist John Tomes in England[34] began to counter amalgam opponents and in 1862, according to his own experiments, he took a clear position: *With opposing opin-*

24 See p. 405, footnote 122
25 Townsend
26 J. D. White
27 Taft p. 89; Bogue
28 A. D. Black
29 See pp. 302 f.
30 Black II (a) p. 44; (b) p. 51
31 Perry; Webb
32 Black I (a) pp. 161 f.; (b) pp. 191 f. See pp. 171 f.
33 Black II (a) pp. 308 f.; (b) pp. 364 f.
34 See pp. 391 f.

ions and inconclusive results it is incumbent on those who regard the use of amalgam with unqualified disapprobation to show the grounds upon which their condemnation rests; . . . Dental surgery has arrived at that point when mere opinion, unless supported by clearly stated evidence, cannot be accepted as a guide for practice[35].

In 1859, a court dentist in Güstrow and manufacturer of copper amalgam, Georg Wilhelm Lippold, who deserves thanks for the introduction of this material to Germany, claimed that the preparation he had developed *had been introduced by a fictitious English firm namely one Dr. William Pilplod in London, mindful of the old German prejudice that the foreign was better than the home grown*[36]. In the same year, 1859, Tomes described a copper amalgam, *long known as "Sullivan's Cement"* in England, of which he criticized the black discoloration[37]. Similarly we read in *Dental Cosmos* in 1875 that copper amalgam dissolves most readily; *and that copper amalgam is not used in this country, though it is in Germany*[38]. Not least because of its *antiseptic properties*[39], already noted by W. D. Miller[40], the material has maintained its place up to the present day, especially in treatment of deciduous teeth.

In 1896, Miller's "Textbook of Conservative Dentistry" devoted 48 pages to gold restorations and only 6 pages to amalgam. However, he came to the conclusion that *excellent results can be attained with amalgam* if it is worked properly[41]. It should be noted explicitly that Miller's 412-page book was devoted entirely to tooth conservation, a subject with which earlier authors usually had dealt in only a few pages.

The last hesitations were abolished by the work of Adolph Witzel[42] concerning "Das Füllen der Zähne mit Amalgam" (The Filling of Teeth with Amalgam) published in 1899, a study resting on years of research. In more than 1000 microscopic and metallurgical experiments, he had examined the properties of a variety of amalgams under various conditions. It is remarkable that this is the first example of true "teamwork" in dentistry, because Witzel engaged a chemist and a physicist in his experiments beside his own assistants[43].

Especially because of the efforts of Black and Witzel, amalgam was established around the turn of the century all over the world, particularly as a material suitable for less well-to-do patients. Temporary uneasiness was elicited in 1926 through the publication of a German chemist, Alfred Stock, about "Die Gefährlichkeit des Quecksilberdampfes" (The Dangers of Mercury Fumes). Only after years of discussion the excitement ebbed. One came to the conclusion that those infinitesimal doses which might be expressed from amalgam fillings were not sufficient to harm a person's general well-being. Paracelsus' old sentence still holds true: *Dosis sola facit venenum (Only the dose makes the poison).*

Guttapercha, introduced to prosthetic dentistry by the younger Delabarre in 1848, had been used as early as 1847 according to Miller as a filling material by Bennett[44]. In 1848, "Hill's Stopping" appeared on the American market named after his inventor, the dentist Asa Hill from Norwalk, Connecticut[45]. It soon spread around the entire world. It consisted of guttapercha to which had been added caustic lime, quartz and feldspar (2 : 1 : 1). Only very much later one realized that this material was suitable exclusively as a temporary filling. Even Miller still recommended it in 1896 as a permanent restoration for places less exposed to friction[46].

After the middle of the century we find the first use of cements as restorative materials. We remember similar attempts, such as the mineral paste of Jaques Guillemeau in the 16th century, who used the material for the manufacture of prosthetic teeth, but also *to fill it in a hollow tooth*, and of the stone paste of Friedrich Hirsch, in 1796[47]. In 1802, Laforgue, with resignation, came to the conclusion that very flat hollow cavities which retained neither gold nor lead must be filled with a kind of putty which, unfortunately, was not available[48]. Prague's professor of dentistry, Franz Nessel, in 1840 praised the dental cement of Wolfsohn of Berlin as the best because of its rapid setting. The material consisted of Sandarac

35 Tomes (a) pp. 404 f.; (b) quotation
36 Lippold
37 Tomes (a) pp. 407 f.
38 Bogue
39 Miller (d)
40 See pp. 404 f.
41 Miller (c) p. 170
42 See pp. 313 f.
43 Witzel (c)
44 Miller (c) p. 53
45 Thorpe pp. 315—324
46 Miller (c) pp. 177 f.
47 See p. 234
48 Laforgue p. 150

resin, chalk and mastix dissolved in ether[49]. In 1851 Joseph Linderer mentioned, not from his own experience, a filling material made of chemically pure hydrate lime made into a paste with phosphoric acid. The first of these components was best obtained by grinding the enamel of teeth of carnivorous animals[50]. In 1855 an engineer, Sorel, brought out a phosphate cement in Paris, a material praised by the erudite Emile Magitot (see Fig. 414) because of its hardness and good color, while J. H. C. Weber, a practitioner in Paris, reported that he had never seen good and enduring results with it[51]. A year later we read, again in the not very original book of Nessel about a dental cement proposed by Ostermaier, which consisted of 13 parts finely pulverized caustic lime and 12 parts phosphoric acid. *The mixture is usable only within 1 to 2 minutes and cannot be stirred because of its easy crumbling*[52].

Truly usable was the "Cäment" recommended since 1858 by the Dresden court dentist A. Rostaing and the chemist Charles Sylvester Rostaing (father and son), a material that was already a zinc oxyphosphate cement[53]. Its composition was not made public. One obtained 12 ounces by remitting 20 pounds Sterling or 133 Taler to a Dresden banker. Lippold, too, complained about the severe terms of sale of another cement marketed by Süersen at approximately the same time, although in the same issue of *Der Zahnarzt*[54] an analysis appeared indicating that it consisted of 59 % zinc oxide and 31 % zinc chlorate, mixed with a solution of zinc chloride. This preparation soon disappeared because of its severe irritation to the pulp. The tortuous path of the "Os artificial" from Saxony to the USA is described poetically in 1860 in the first volume of *Dental Cosmos: It rose, as a bright star, far in the north of Germany, swept rapidly southward over Prussia, southern Germany, and France, and, like the German emigrant, scorning England's shores, struck boldly across the broad Atlantic to America, the father of dentistry, where it received a hearty welcome.* The prominent dentist of Philadelphia, Edwin Tyler Darby, ascertained in the same periodical in 1894, *that they have proven so much superior to those made in this country, that I rarely try any but those of German make.* But not for permanent fillings. *The ideal filling has not yet been discovered; but it will surely come, and it lies along these lines*[55].

According to his own reports, W. E. Driscoll of Manatee, Florida, combined the advantages of cement with those of amalgam by squeezing amalgam as a durable seal over a still plastic cement filling since 1874[56]. Independently, the Viennese dentist Salomon Robicsek introduced the same technique to Europe in 1894 as the "Doublir-Methode"[57].

Among the zinc oxysulfate cements the "Artificial Dentine", devised by the British dentist and manufacturer Thomas Fletcher, gained a foothold beginning in 1874. Initially mixed with water and later with gum arabic, the material was intended first as a liner and later found use as a temporary filling[58].

A new development came into the picture in the early years of the 20th century, especially for restorations of the anterior teeth, through the introduction of silicate cements. As early as 1878, Fletcher had been awarded a patent for "Translucent Cement" in England[59], but the material did not work out. In 1904 there appeared on the market in Berlin an "artificial dental enamel" developed by the chemist Paul Steenbock and tested clinically and manufactured by Hugo Ascher, a dentist. Because of the addition of aluminum, beryllium, calcium oxides, and silicic acid, it was harder and chiefly more transparent than cement but was nearly as easily workable. It was copied quickly around the world. Soon one learned to overcome the pulp damaging properties and low adhesion of the material by using cement liners and undercuts, and the material itself was vastly improved so that it continued to be used up to the present time for fillings of the anterior teeth. Only now has it been replaced frequently by the acrylic restorative materials.

The availability of usable cements was the prerequisite for the inlay technique, the insertion of mineral, metallic, and, recently, synthetic in-

49 Nessel (a) p. 327
50 Linderer (c) pp. 192 f.
51 Magitot (a) pp. 203 f.; Weber
52 Nessel (b) pp. 164
53 Rostaing. According to information (1968) from the Richter & Hoffmann firm (Harvard Cement), founded in Berlin in 1892. Rostaing's cement corresponded chemically to that used today. It had the disadvantage, however, that the acid was supplied in crystalline form and had to be heated or dissolved before use.
54 Der Zahnarzt. Berlin 14: 122—123, 1859
55 Roberts; Darby. See p. 276
56 Driscoll
57 Robicsek
58 Fletcher (a)
59 Fletcher (b and c); Coleman; Paffenbarger

lays prepared outside the patient's mouth after impressions were made of the properly prepared cavities. If we leave out of consideration the Indian inlays, made for purely cosmetic purposes[60], Linderer Sr. was the first to follow this principle with his veneer fillings, which he described explicitly as his method in his textbook published in 1834 in Berlin, claiming to have practiced the technique for 14 years. He prepared the cavities as nearly circular as possible, cut a walrus peg to size, cut threads into the peg and the cavity, and screwed it into place. When the cavities were not circular, he cut the walrus bone free-hand and forced it into place with the blow of a hammer or by using unslaked lime with turpentine or a strong fish-glue as cement[61]. His contemporary colleagues, however, were unable to agree with the assurances of his son Joseph when he stated in 1851, that *the tooth juices flowed into the peg*[62].

The first porcelain inlays may have been made by Professor Maynard[63] of Washington as reported in 1857 by the Bavarian-born Adelbert J. Volck of Baltimore[64]. He cut appropriately shaped pieces of porcelain teeth with carborundum stones and inserted them with gold foil into the cavity (Fig. 317). In 1862, New York's Barnabas Wood took up this idea again and fastened the porcelain inlays in place, at first with amalgam or guttapercha and later with cement. In the '80s, the S. S. White and Ash firms marketed porcelain cylinders with correspondingly shaped burs (Fig. 318).

In 1887/1888 Charles Henry Land took out a patent on his method to fire a porcelain inlay on a platinum foil, previously adapted to a cavity[65]. This technique did not widely come into use because of the difficult fusibility of the material. Furthermore, the shrinkage, characteristic of all porcelain masses, was a disadvantage. For this reason, Wilhelm Herbst, a dentist of Bremen, tried to introduce glass as a filling material in 1889. He used the milky glass of lampshades as the basic material, adding brown glass of drug bottles to color the mass. These glass mixtures were pulverized and melted in a plaster model made from a wax impression (Fig. 319)[66]. The problem was solved finally by an American, Newell Sill Jenkins, acting in Dresden as Royal Court Dentist. He compounded a low-melting porcelain material in 1897[67].

Slower was the development of the technique for inlays of gold, the material preferred at the present time. In the seventies and eighties, plaster models made from wax impressions, and later adapted gold foils, were flushed with gold solder and cemented into place as completely unprofiled metal products. In the United States Shepard W. Foster (1894) and Charles Lee Alexander (1896) made efforts to produce soldered contour-fillings. They made a wax model on the foil impression, coated this with gold foil, then embedded the whole in plaster, and let gold solder flow into it through a hole. Alexander was the first to use the term "cast filling" for the result, while Foster spoke of "laboratory fillings" in the discussion following Alexander's lecture. Each of these early inlays were given additional retention through pins, as one did not trust the cements yet (Fig. 320)[68].

The casting technique published in 1904 by Arthur Ollendorf, medical doctor of Breslau, brought an important advance for prosthetic dentistry. He fitted the wax model with a wide funnel, placed it into a clay pot filled with plaster which was fired in a furnace, and then poured the molten metal into it. In principle, this procedure is the same as described so impressively by the Florentine goldsmith Benvenuto Cellini as having been used in the cast of Perseus around 1550. Pressure was achieved by Ollendorf by pouring from a height and through the volume of the material. This technique also was made serviceable for cast fillings by the Parisian dentist Oskar Solbrig[69].

On January 15, 1907 the dentist William Henry Taggart from Chicago read a paper on "A New and Accurate Method of Making Gold Inlays" in New York. He had worked for 15 years on it, and it continues to be used up to the present time. He refrained from gold foil and made the model directly on the tooth with a special wax. Embedding and burnout of the wax proceeded as in Ollendorf's technique, but a much smaller sprue was applied as the casting was made in Taggart's special casting machine under pressure (Fig. 321). A nitrous

[60] See pp. 51 f.
[61] C. J. Linderer pp. 73 f.
[62] J. Linderer (c) p. 92
[63] See p. 313
[64] Denton
[65] See p. 276
[66] Herbst; Metcalf; Holtbuer pp. 35 f.
[67] Jenkins
[68] Foster; Alexander
[69] Ollendorf; Solbrig

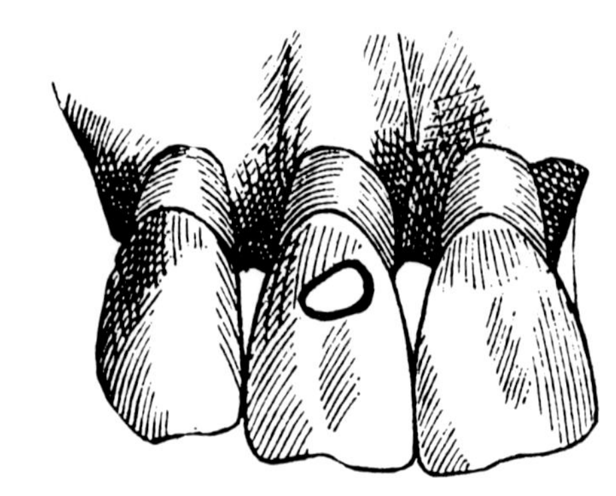

Fig. 317 *Volck: Porcelain inlay placed with gold-foil, before 1856*

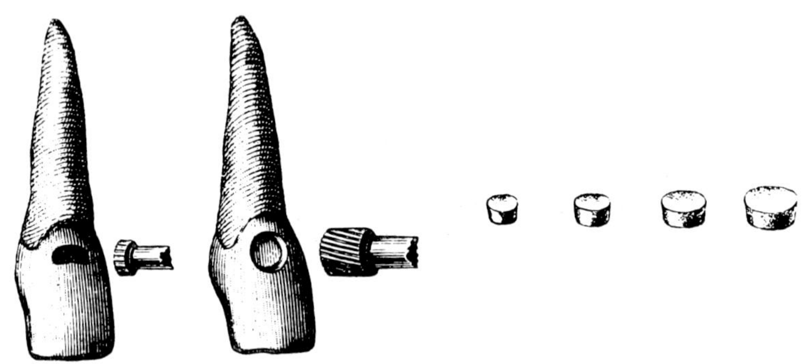

Fig. 318 *Pre-formed porcelain inlays with required burs, made by the S. S. White Co.*

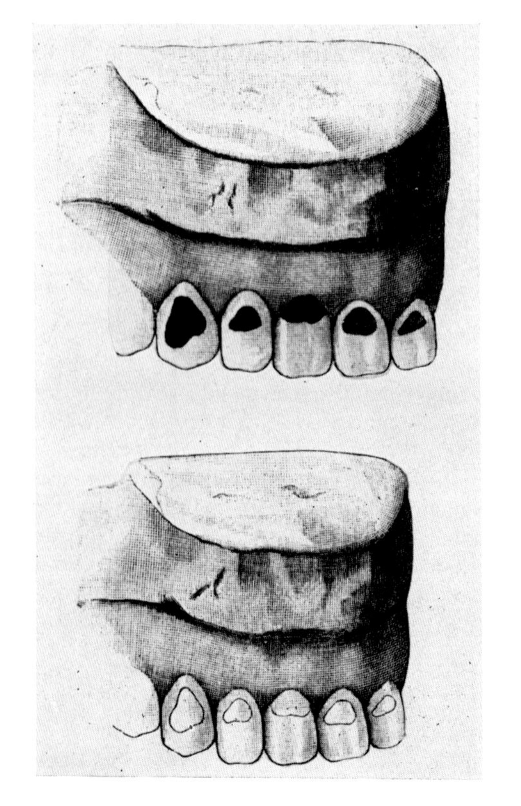

Fig. 319 *W. Herbst: Glas inlays made from wax impressions, 1889*

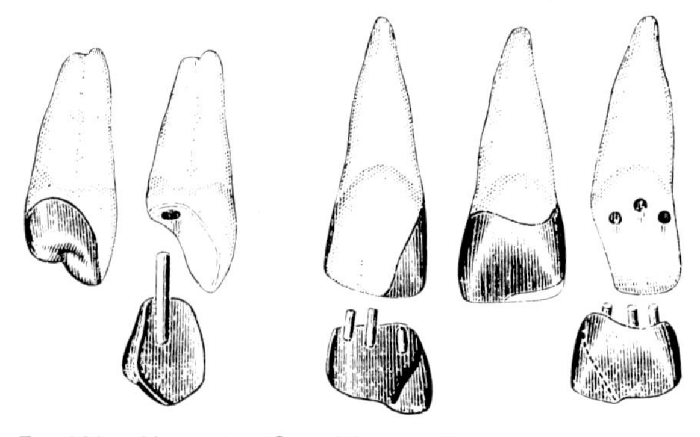

Fig. 320 *Alexander: Cast fillings, 1896*

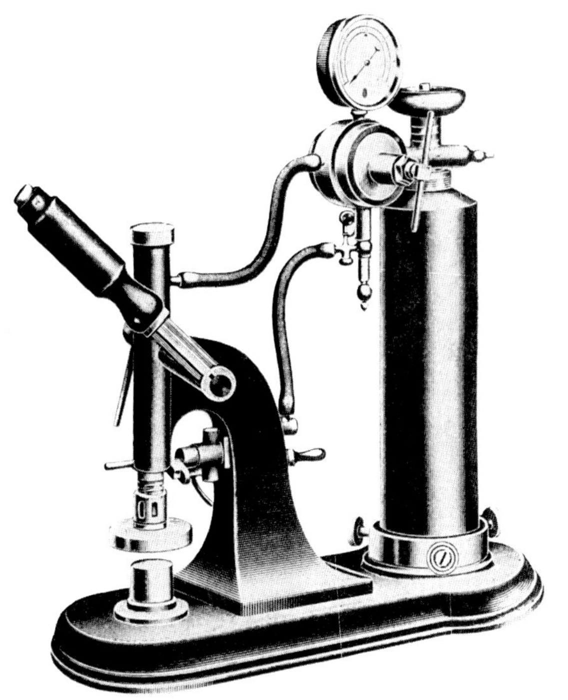
Fig. 321 *Taggart's casting machine*

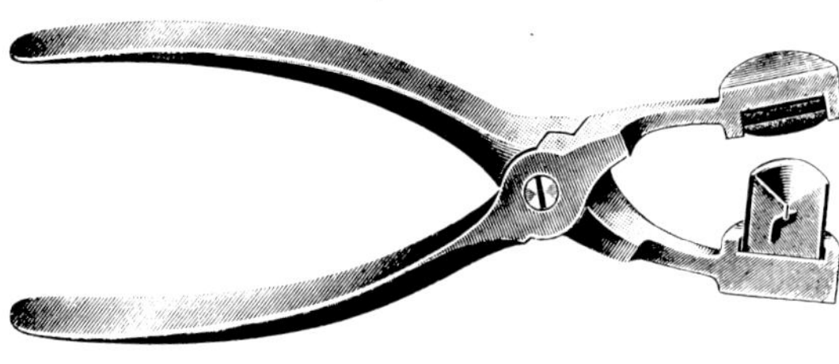
Fig. 322 *The Solbrig forceps*

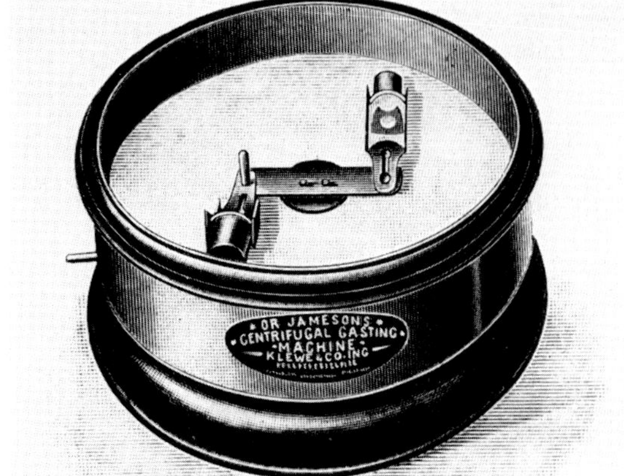

Fig. 323 *Jameson: Centrifugal apparatus*

oxide flame brought the metal on the casting flask to the melting point, then the cylinder was closed with a lever while laughing gas under pressure from a gas bomb forced the casting metal into the form[70].

Following announcement of this technique, a number of similar appliances, and others depending on the same principle, appeared. Among these the Solbrig forceps is startling because of its simplicity. A moist asbestos plate in one arm of the forceps produces steam at the moment of its closing which forces the casting gold into the form (Fig. 322)[71]. Since 1907 A. W. Jameson had used centrifugal force which proved an ideal agent (Fig. 323). Taggart, however, felt cheated of the financial fruits of his work and attempted to reserve the technique to the buyers of his quite expensive and slowly delivered machine. In a long trial, the last of its kind in the United States, it was possible to prove to him that B. Frederick Philbrook, a dentist of Denison, Iowa, had worked on gold casts under pneumatic pressure, and as early as 1897 had delivered a lecture to the Iowa State Dental Society, of which a copy was available. This event had been long forgotten, but in such a way the revolutionary procedure became the common property of dentistry since 1915[72].

With the perfection of the gold casting technique and the production of usable amalgams and silicate cements, these materials controlled restorative dentistry up to the present time, all other methods being kept in the background. Only most recently the experiments arising through the development of cold-curing acrylic resins have come to a satisfactory result in making them serviceable to restorative dentistry[73].

Development of the Dental Drill

The request, made at the end of the 19th century, for preventive cavity preparation would not have been able to be fulfilled without the invention of the foot powered dental drill

70 Taggart
71 Riechelmann
72 Philbrook; Bremner pp. 284 f.
73 See pp. 283 f.

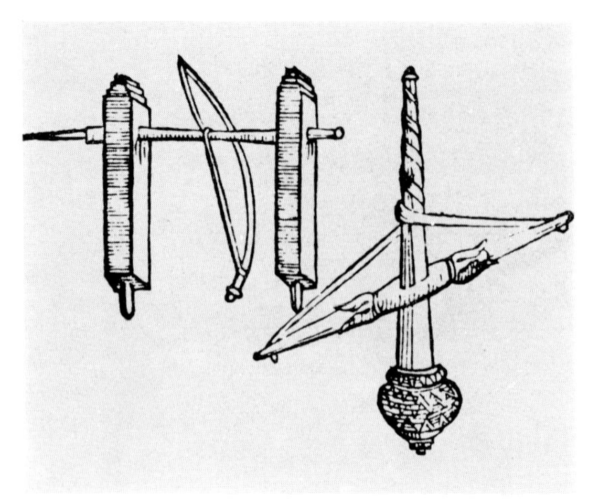

Fig. 324 *della Croce (de Cruce): Bow drill and string drill for preparation of skeletons, 1573 (1607)*

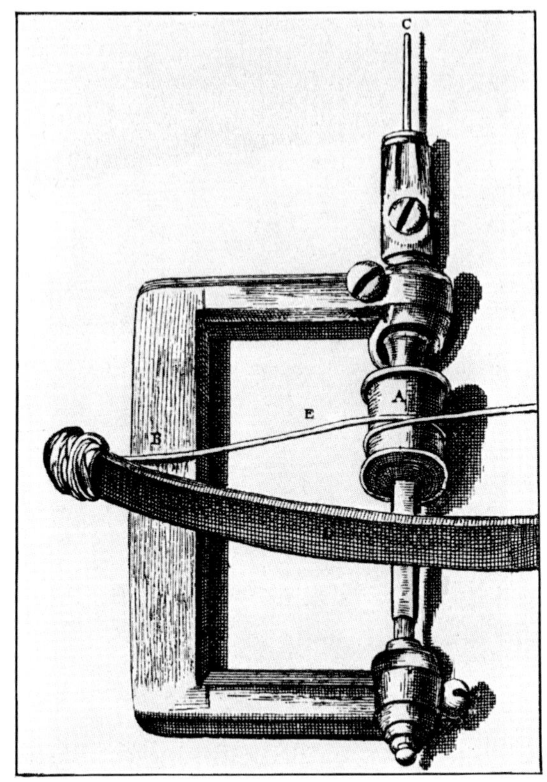

Fig. 325 *Fauchard: Bow drill for technical use, 1728*

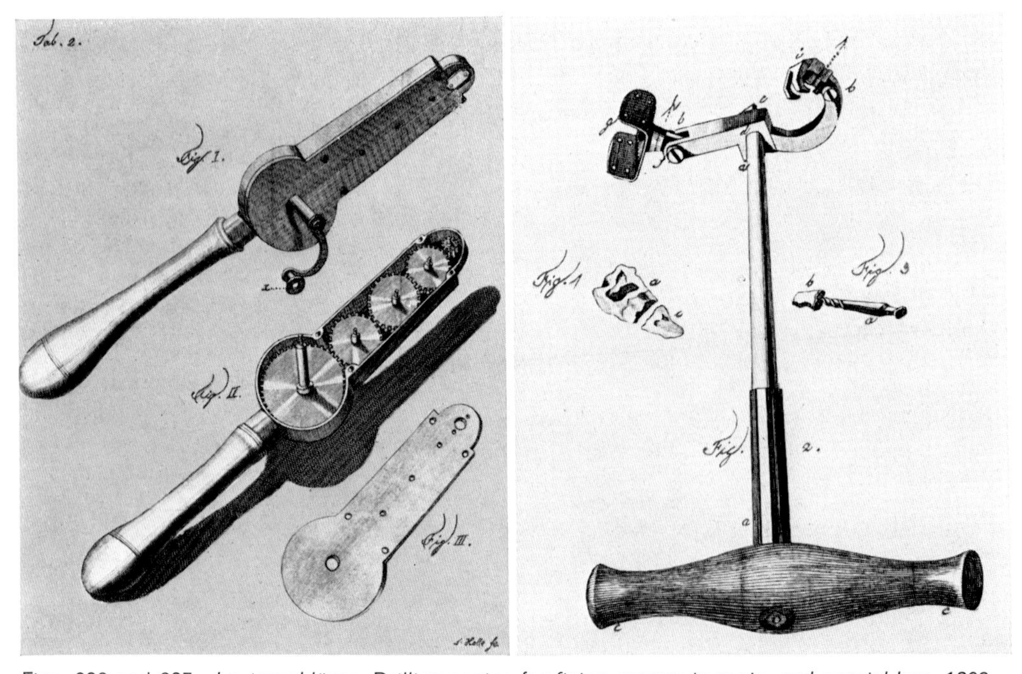

Figs. 326 and 327 *Lautenschläger: Drilling engine for fixing screws in roots, and special key, 1803*

by the American dentist Morrison, in 1871. A long road, rich in detours, had been travelled before the construction of this instrument which was to put restorative dentistry on a new foundation. We remember the hypothesis of the use of a drill for dental purposes in ancient Egypt. The first historical document is provided by Galen, in which it is noted that the Roman physician Archigenes had opened painful teeth with a fine trephine around the year 100 A.D.[74]. The same was suggested by the Veronese physician Giovanni d'Arcoli around 1450. How the rotary drilling instruments of that time may have looked is shown to us by the surgical textbook of the Venetian, della Croce, of 1573. The device had been used by him (and also by Vesalius in 1543) for drilling holes into the bones for the preparation of skeletons (Fig. 324). More than one hundred years later Cornelis Solingen smoothed rough edges of teeth with drilling tools[75].

It is amazing that the great Fauchard had not yet used the drill (foret) for therapeutic purposes. He used his appliance, driven by a violin bow, exclusively for the fabrication of dental prostheses[76] (Fig. 325). Only in the second edition of 1746 of his textbook he suggested that root canals which could not be probed with the finest needle should be enlarged with this device: *Then one will take up a fitting drill, mounted on a framework* (B) *which one holds in the left hand; and with the bow* (D) *in the right hand one opens the canal as much as necessary by following its direction*[77].

In the early 19th century, in the year 1803, the well-known court dentist Serre of Berlin[78] describes in the chapter of his textbook dealing with drilling of the teeth, that he turns a needle-like instrument between his thumb and index finger. He used it only on a tooth that had *an abscess inside, which often happens in abraded teeth.* Following drainage of the foul-smelling fluid the hole is closed with cotton wool[79]. As a whole, then, not much progress since Archigenes of the year 100 A.D.

The *pyramid-shaped* screw designed by its author is described in the same book. It is used to remove deeply embedded roots, by being screwed into them. Serre's screw was perfected in the same year (1803) by the court dentist Heinrich Lautenschläger of Berlin through a rather original drilling machine fabricated by Luckow, a mechanic. The canal of the resisting root was enlarged with the machine to provide room for a modified Serre-screw. This screw bore a crossbar to which could be attached an appropriate key, so that in this quite complicated manner the root could be pulled out of the alveolus (Figs. 326 and 327). As there were no means of advertising at that time, Lautenschläger declared in his publication of being ready *to deliver the instrument together with the necessary instructions against the fixed price of 1 Frederic d'or*[80].

Two years later, in 1805, the dentist Calmann Jacob, later Linderer, carried on a controversy against Lautenschläger's method of extraction and proposed, quite properly, the goat's foot elevator for root removal (Fig. 328). On the subject of a drilling machine he described a device already constructed by him in 1797. It consisted of a longish wooden box with an extending wheel on its side seen in figure 2, about which the string of a violin bow was wound (Fig. 6). A geared mechanism swung the impulse by 90° (Fig. 4) and transferred it to the drill proper. This violin bow drill was used on the patient only to widen roots for the insertion of pivot teeth but not for the removal of caries[81].

Much more dainty was the drill (porte-foret) depicted in 1830 by the Parisian dentiste Maury, *which one could drill holes into the teeth with even if they were quite in back of the mouth*[82] (Fig. 329). Another drilling instrument, also shown by Maury and many others, served exclusively technical purposes.

For the removal of caries one continued to use variously shaped excavators or rod-shaped burs rotated with the fingers (Figs. 330 and 331). More information about these instruments, which already served *to enlarge the entrances to cavities, to make even walls of the cavities so that at last some retention could be achieved for fillings,* is described for us by Anton Buzer of Meiningen in his "Handbuch der Zahnheilkunde" (Handbook of Dentistry) published in 1867: *All burs are best manufactured from a single piece because the effort of mounting*

[74] See pp. 23 f. and 74
[75] See pp. 133 and 184 f.
[76] Fauchard (a) II pp. 236 f. and 241; (b) pp. 82 f.
[77] Ibid. (a) I p. 171; (b) p. 64
[78] See p. 239
[79] Serre pp. 455 f.
[80] Lautenschläger. See p. 326
[81] Jacob
[82] Maury (a) pp. 321 f.; p. 507

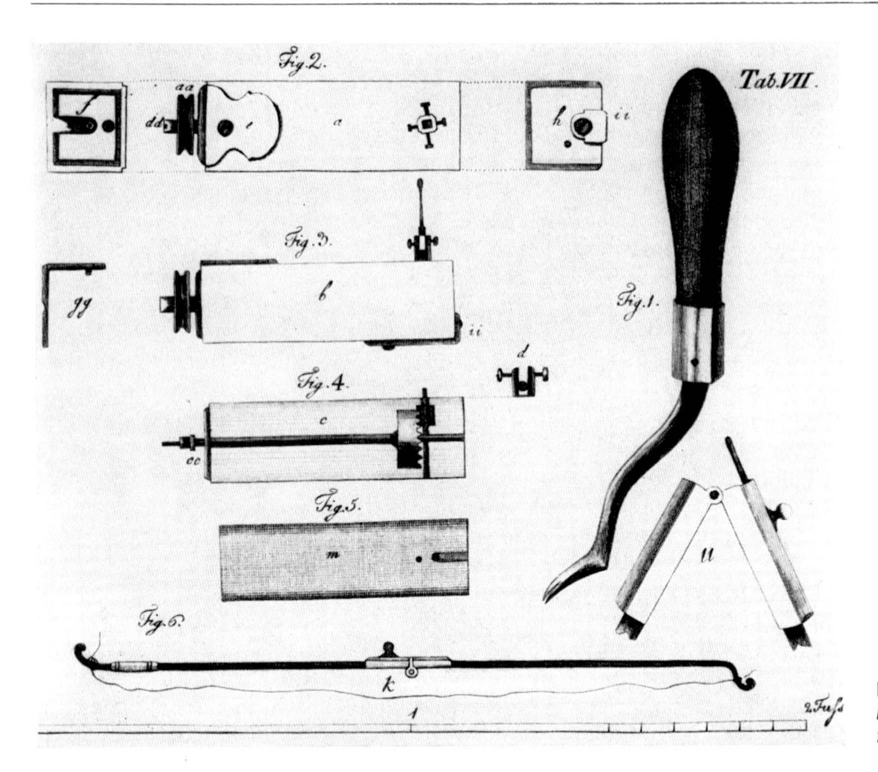

Fig. 328 *Jacob Linderer: Drilling engine, and goat's foot elevator, 1805*

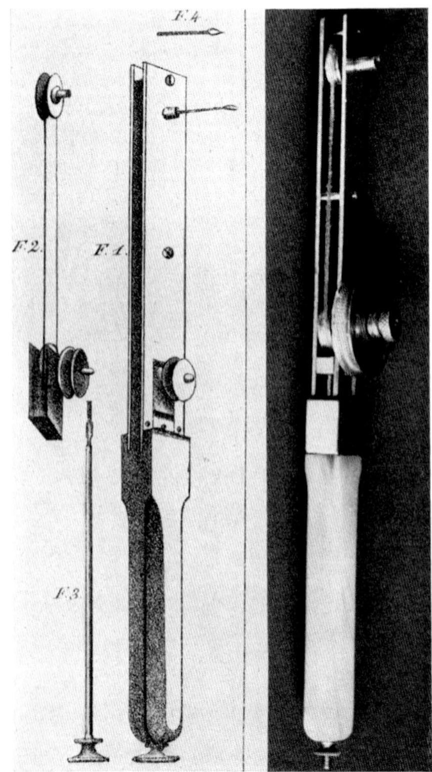

Fig. 329 *Maury: Porte-foret, 1830 (right side of picture: Forschungsinstitut für Geschichte der Zahnheilkunde, Cologne)*

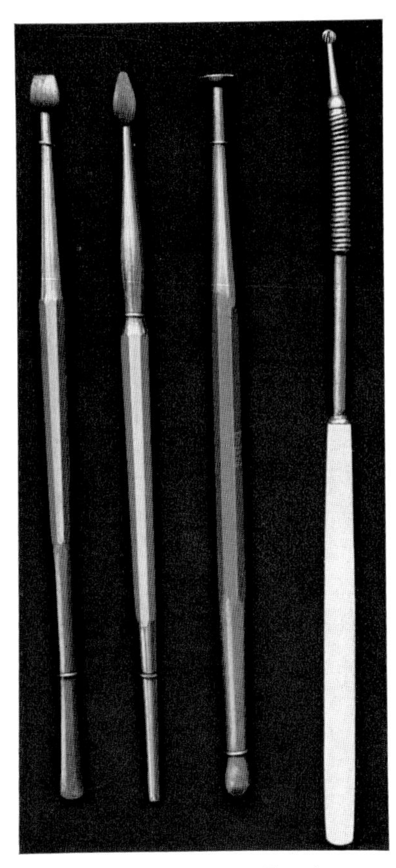

Fig. 330 *Hand drills (Forschungsinstitut für Geschichte der Zahnheilkunde, Cologne)*

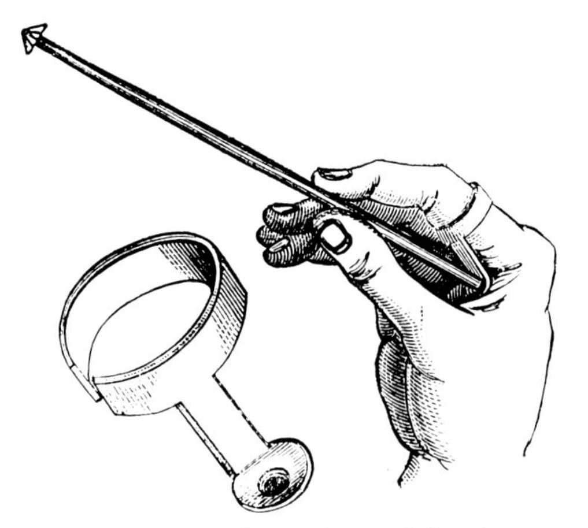

Fig. 331 *Westcott: Finger driven drill with supporting finger ring (from Taft, 1859)*

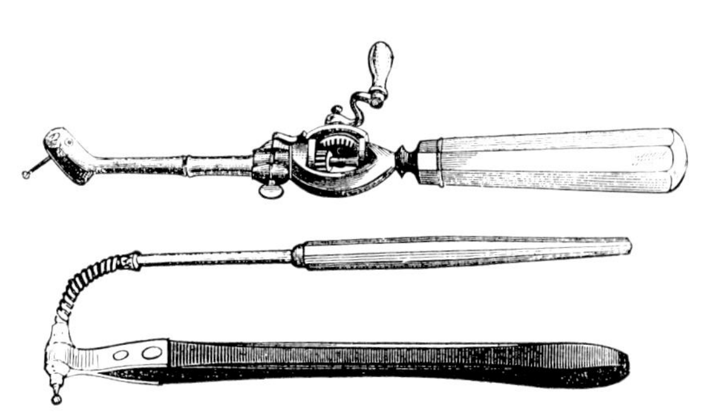

Fig. 332 *Drill-stocks of Chevalier and Charles Merry, St. Louis, 1858*

different drill tips on a hand holder appears to be time consuming in use. The hand holder is best 6- or 8-cornered because this shape is more securely turned in the hand than the cylindrical. The drilling machines devised by Chevalier, Merry, and others to simplify drilling are entirely superfluous[83].

Nonetheless, these designs (Fig. 332) from Taft's textbook of 1859 shall be shown. They shared the disadvantage that they required the use of both hands and worked fitfully because rotation was effected directly at the instrument. The same was true of an earlier (1838) device described by John Lewis (Fig. 333), the hand drill fitted with a ball joint offered by the Ash dental supply house in London (Fig. 334), the Mac Dowell apparatus which worked on the principle of the Archimedes screw, used in the '50s (Fig. 335), and one of Maynard in Washington[84] (Fig. 336). Thus one continued to resort predominantly to hand instruments.

One of the few who rose above the multitude of pure mechanically oriented tooth treaters in the New World following the end of the pioneer period was John Greenwood of New York, previously mentioned as a prosthetic dentist[85]. He was probably the first who, around the year 1790, used a foot pedal drilling machine (Fig. 337). His son, Isaac John Greenwood wrote about it to Jonathan Taft in 1860: *My father was the first to use the 'foot-drill' and he made it himself from an old spinning-*

[83] Buzer p. 128
[84] See p. 313
[85] See p. 258

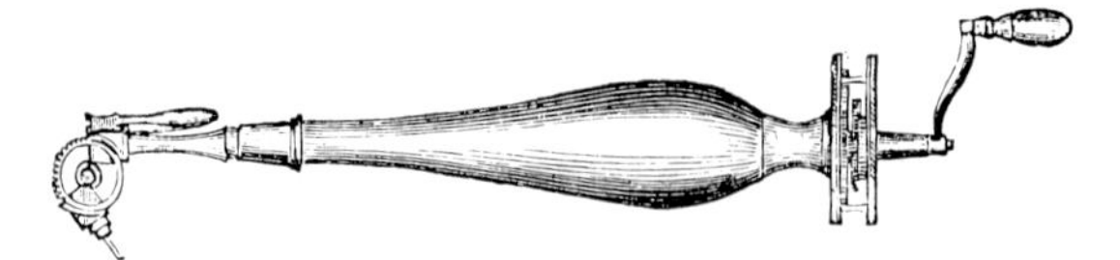

Fig. 333 *Drilling engine of Lewis, 1838*

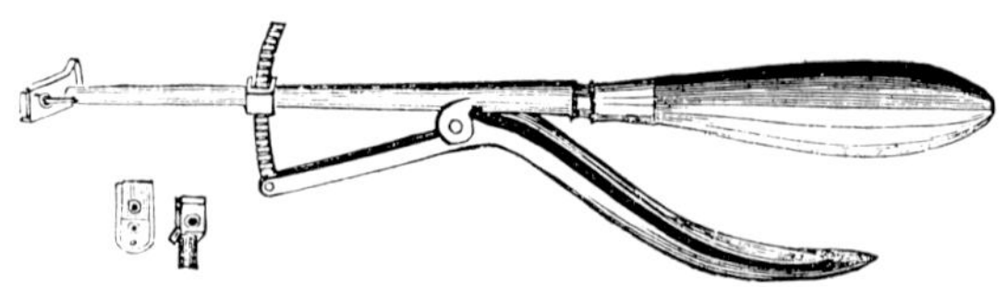

Fig. 336 *"Drill-stock, invented by Dr. Maynard" (from Harris)*

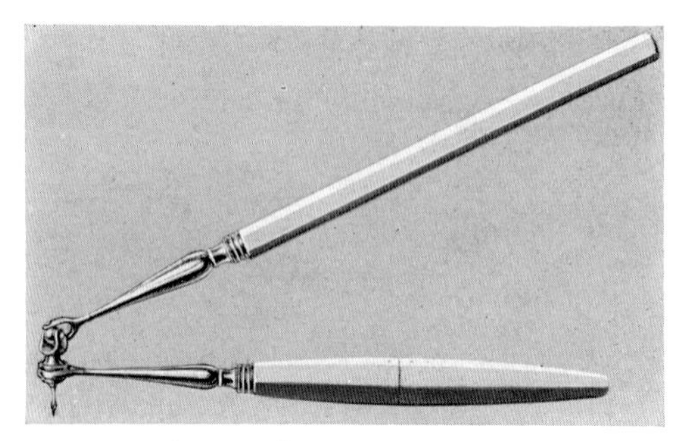

Fig. 334 *The Ash Company's drilling engine*

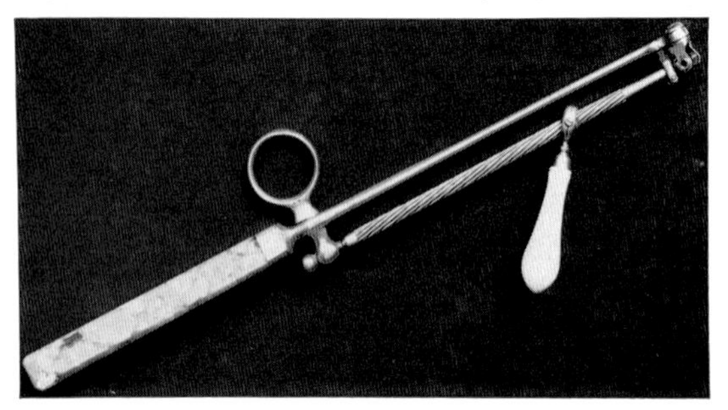

Fig. 335 *Drilling engine of MacDowell (Forschungsinstitut für Geschichte der Zahnheilkunde, Cologne)*

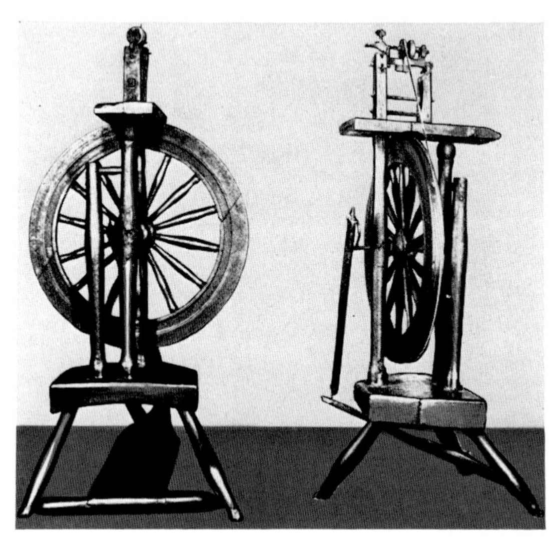

Fig. 337 *Greenwood's drill made from a spinning wheel, around 1790 (from Weinberger)*

*wheel of my grandmother's; and, since his death, I myself used it, the same one, altogether in my practice for twenty years, and I have it yet. I never had seen one before, and I know the hand bow-drill was always used before . . . This de-*vice, however, was only such as to drill *pieces of bone and ivory*. Above all, the younger Greenwood used the foot-drill *to make the hole to receive the pivot in the* (prosthetic) *tooth*[86].

It is amazing that this idea did not assert itself at that time. Only on February 7, 1871, as the bloody fighting between Germans and Frenchmen drew to a close, the dentist Morrison, to whom we also owe the first adjustable cast iron treatment chair, registered the patent for a foot-driven dental engine which already achieved 2,000 rpm (Figs. 338 and 339). The first device which reached the market in April, 1872 probably owed more of its design to the footpowered sewing machine than to the spinning wheel.

James Beall Morrison (Fig. 340) was the son of a carriage builder and nephew of a watchmaker of East Springfield, Ohio, in whose workshops he became acquainted with mechanical problems while still a child. During his dental training he soon attracted attention because of the precision of his gold technique, a skill that brought him first prize for a gold denture in 1852. In 1857 he established an office in St. Louis, went to Paris five years later for one year, and then to London for six more years, where he was associated for some time with John Tomes and Sercombe. Returned to the United States, he rendered the greatest

[86] Cf. Weinberger II pp. 254 f.

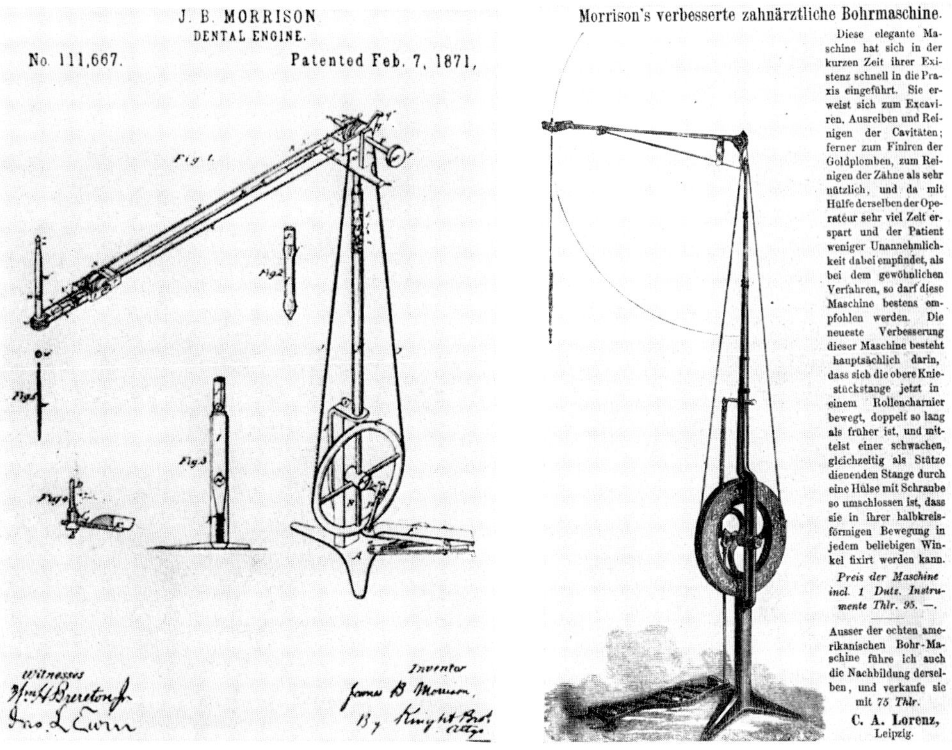

Figs. 338 and 339 *Patent for Morrison's dental engine, 1871, and the 1875 model (advertisement)*

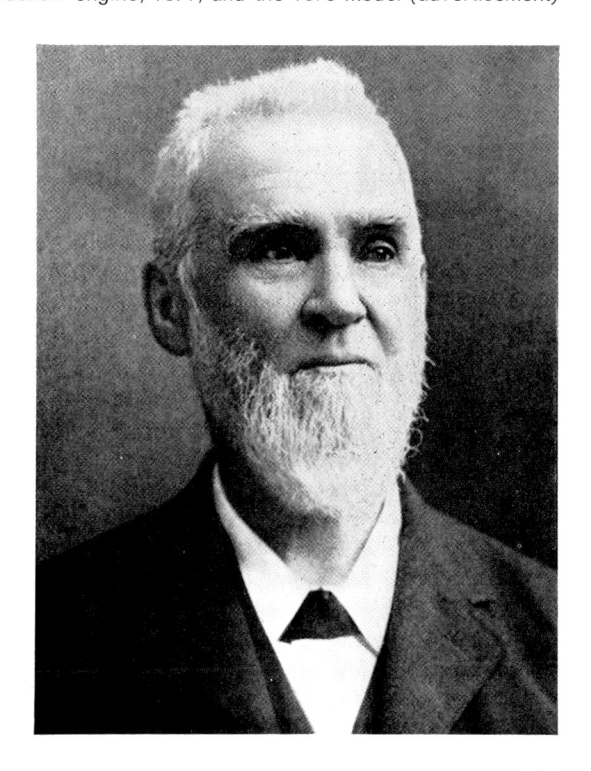

Fig. 340 *James Beall Morrison*

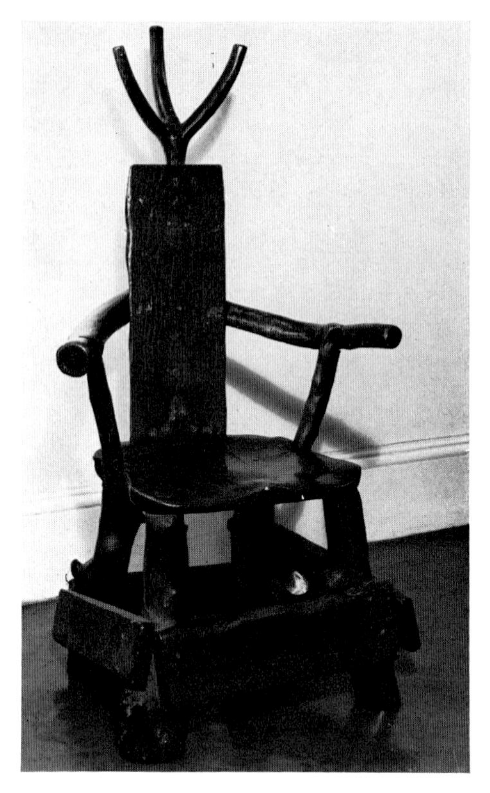

Fig. 341 *Wooden chair of unknown age from the east coast of England, which belonged to a "family of barbers" according to its buyer (British Dental Association, London)*

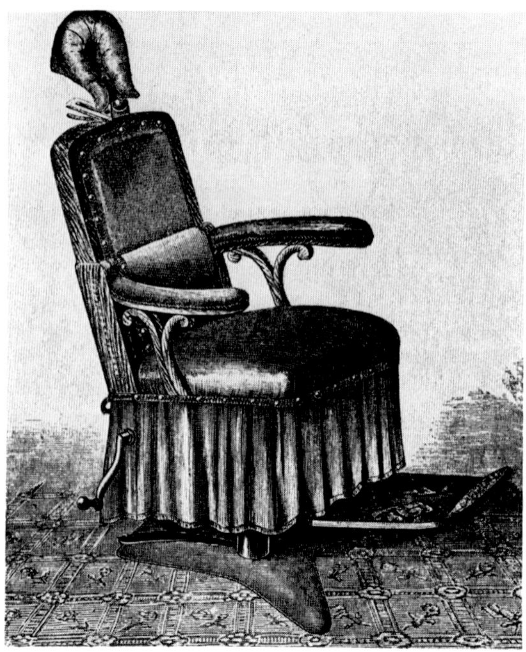

Fig. 342 *Morrison's adjustable treatment chair*

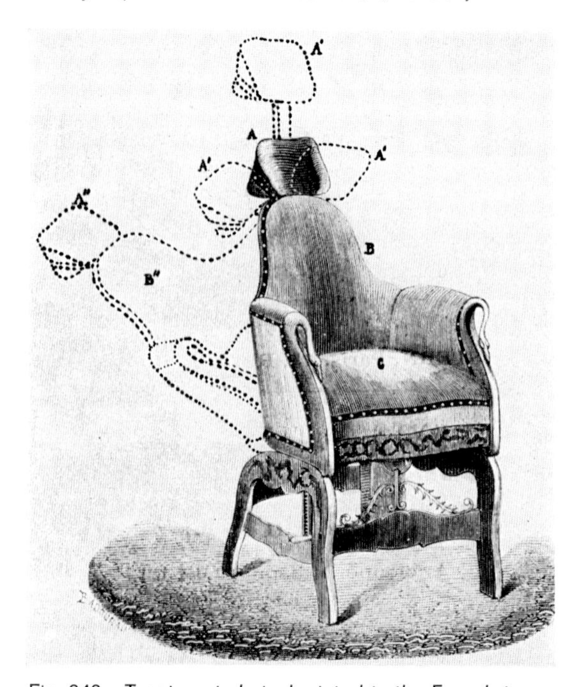

Fig. 343 *Treatment chair depicted in the French translation of the Harris and Austen textbook, advertisement, 1874*

service of his century to practical dentistry with his designs[87].
The chair constructed by Morrison was the first significant development of the old bathroom chair as we had come to know it in the 16th century in figure 138, and as is shown here in a sample of unknown age from the collection of the British Dental Association (Fig. 341). The Parisian chair of 1830, seen in figure 272, was still absolutely rigid, and improved designs of Harris and others offered only limited mobility (Fig. 342). Morrison's chair (Fig. 343) in contrast, could be adjusted in all directions, as evident in its 1869 description in the *Deutsche Vierteljahresschrift für Zahnheilkunde: The mechanism is of the kind that permits the operator to place his patient in any desired position, and the device for this purpose is so simple and so concealed to the eye that the most nervous patient does not become agitated at the sight of the chair. For this reason, the new chair . . . may properly be called one of the most pleasant inventions for contemporary dental surgery*[88]. Even more important for dentistry in general, however, was the manufacture of Morrison's pedal-powered drill, of which the first one was sold at a dental meeting in Binghamton, New York on April 17, 1872.
The news reached the Old World only slowly. Letters dating to the year 1872 are preserved, in which the later Professor and academic teacher in Zürich, Joseph Machwürth, then a dental student in Philadelphia, describes the advantages of the machine to his old teacher, Georg von Langsdorff of Freiburg im Breisgau, who also had been trained in America[89].
On April 7, 1873 the specialist for oral disease Heinrich Breslauer of Berlin (listed in the city's directory as "American dentist") demonstrated a bone resection machine especially designed for dental purposes, invented by Dr. Morrison of New York. He was very pleased with his impression on his patients of the new technique. *I operate with his machine for 4 weeks and coincidence would have it that among the patients were some quite nervous ladies for whom I have removed caries previously by manual excavation. Their judgement was unanimous that this type of operation, that is with the aid of this machine, is completely painless and relatively more pleasant than any other method of resection.*—In the same year Morrison's old partner in London, the dentist Edwin Sercombe, lectured to the Odontological Society of Great Britain about his one year of experience with the dental engine. He regarded the invention as the greatest gift to the profession since Barnum's rubber dam. *Dr. Morrison has also supplied a right-angled motion, which in some cases is most useful, . . . it is produced by an end being attached to the hand-piece, in which there is a double cog-action*[90].
Soon the foot pedaled dental engine began its victorious march into the "Ateliers" of dentists and dental-artists. The previously used hand-manipulated burs were adapted to the new machine, and the required supplementary instruments, such as handpieces and contra-angles were improved so that, as the advertisement shows, they were nearly identical to the principles of construction of today's instruments (Fig. 344).
Enamel was worked with corundum stones and disks introduced by Robert Arthur in 1872. In the last decade of the 19th century this material was replaced by the harder carborundum, an American invention too. Just at this time the first durable diamond grinding tools came out, consisting of copper wheels into the surface of which diamond powder was affixed by hammering. In 1932, the Drendel & Zweiling firm of Berlin developed cutting tools by galvanised bonding of the diamond grains of different size to the metallic surface.
Several wrong paths, however, were seriously discussed even after the Morrison dental engine was patented. Water-powered and pneumatically driven apparatuses were constructed, which consisted of a foot-driven bellows which emptied its air into a rubber hose. This transferred the pneumatic energy into a housing in which *draft screens, similar to those of a windmill, were found. A cannula is attached to these, for mounting the various drills.*—As curious and complicated as this construction, invented in 1868 by the S. S. White Co mechanic, George F. Green, may appear, it deserves our attention because it is the direct predecessor of today's air-driven dental turbine[91].
An entirely different attempt though predestined to failure, was shown by a Briton, George

[87] Morrison (c)
[88] Morrison (a)
[89] von Langsdorff (b)
[90] Morrison (b); Breslauer, Sercombe
[91] von Langsdorff (a); Black II p. 44; (b) p. 31

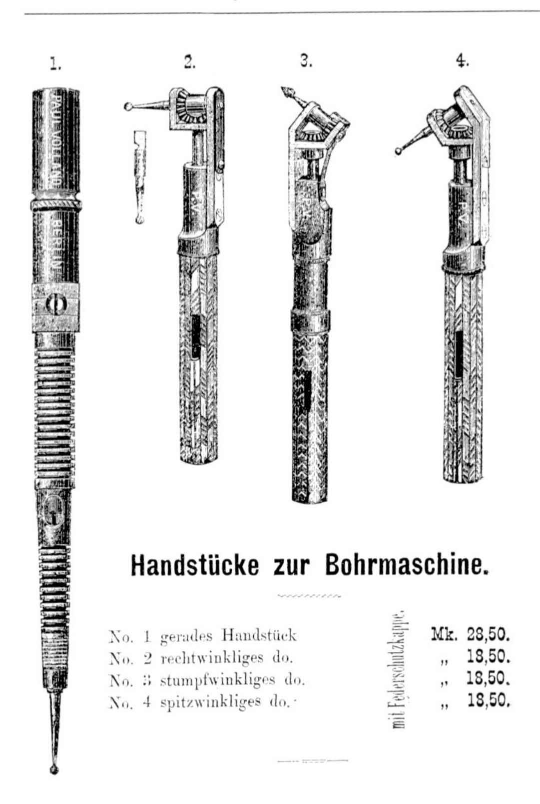

1.
2.
3.
4.
Handstücke zur Bohrmaschine.
No. 1 gerades Handstück Mk. 28,50.
No. 2 rechtwinkliges do. „ 18,50.
No. 3 stumpfwinkliges do. „ 18,50.
No. 4 spitzwinkliges do. „ 18,50.
mit Federschutzkappe.

Fig. 344 *Handpieces and contra-angles, advertisement, 1893*

Fig. 345 *Harrington's clockwork "Erado" drill, 1871*

Fellows Harrington, in his "Erado" (Lat: I scratch out). A graceful apparatus in appearance aside from its threateningly projecting bur, it appeared more like a snuffbox than a dental drill. As seen in figure 345, the apparatus was fitted with interchangeable handpieces and contra-angles. The key to wind up the clockwork was obviously the most frequently used component, because the spring action worked only for two minutes. Actually, this appliance of 1871 was revision of a model of 1865 that had failed to come into use because of its annoying noise. In a letter from John Tomes to Mac Quillen of Philadelphia in 1866 we find quite a negative evaluation: *We have just received, I believe in an incomplete form, an instrument to drill out diseased parts of teeth with burs, milling instruments, wheels, etc. The burs are fastened to a shaft which is driven by a strong watch spring*[92]. Harrington's "Erado" was soon cast aside through Morrison's more fortunate idea.

After the dental engine had made its entry into dental practices, one soon began to make it useful in the placement of gold hammered fillings. In an advertisement of 1892 a dentist with a mustache in the style of Napoleon III and arms somewhat too short looks greatly pleased upon an improved pneumatic hammer which can be attached to any drill engine (Fig. 346). It was undoubtedly a step forward when hammer blows no longer had to be delivered by hand although the pneumatic hammer as well as Bonwill's electric one, which was improved by Webb[93], soon were ousted by the mechanical models of Power and Bonwill. These latter were simply connected to the engine's flexible cable in place of the handpiece (Fig. 347).

Only very slowly electricity became the driving force of the dental engine in dental offices, although the first electric apparatus was devel-

[92] Miller (c) p. 65; Harrington; Campbell pp. 224 f.
[93] Dorn p. 3

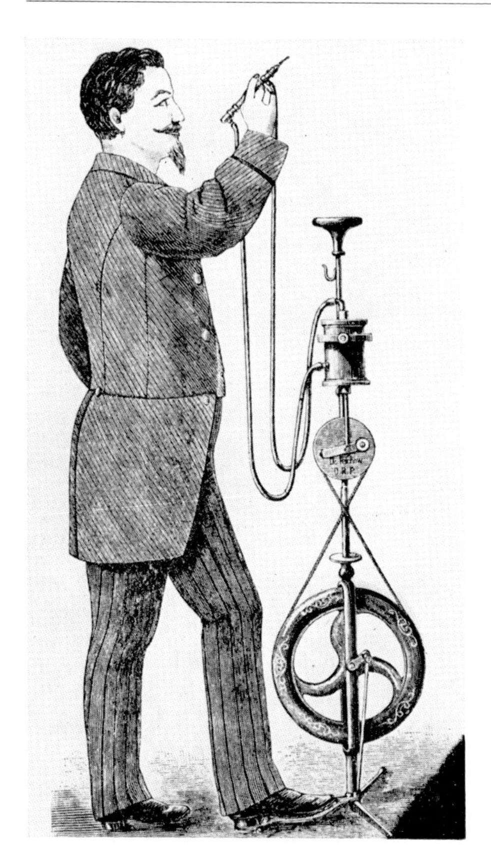

Fig. 346 *Pneumatic hammer*

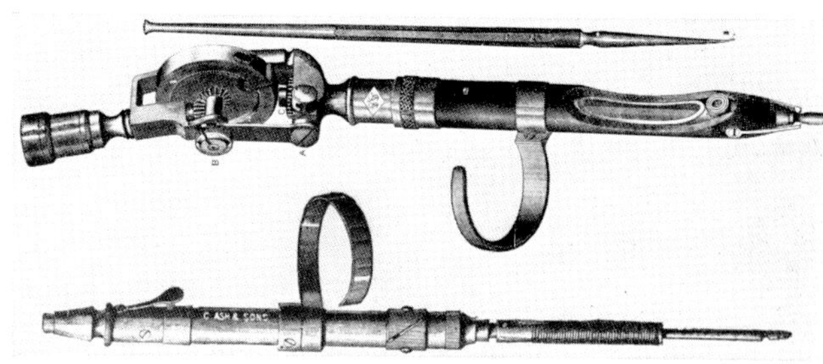

Fig. 347 *Power's and Bonwill's automatic hammer (Ash catalogue, 1898)*

oped nearly simultaneously with Morrison's machine. The previously mentioned George F. Green had demonstrated his electric burring engine as early as 1872 at the meeting of the American Dental Association in Niagara Falls. *This wonderfully effective little machine* ... *has,* we read in a booming advertisement of the S. S. White company, ... *attracted the attention of the busiest operators and has withstood the most careful examination and testing. The art of fencing lightning is developed to its fullest in this graceful, compact, portable dental drill.* Lest the lightning be too strong, one took the current from a storage battery which was empty after a few hundred hours of use. This instrument is also mentioned in the discussion of Sercombe's lecture in London. The speaker described it as *about eight inches long by three inches in each other direction ... The great objection to it was that the speed was not very controllable: it was too great, and liable to put the thing out of order,* he believed, however, optimistically that the use of electricity would some day eliminate the swaying standing on one foot[94]. The essential thing about this construction was that the motor and the drill were directly connected with each other without an intermediate transfer, a development to be taken up again only in 1965 with the advent of the micromotor (Fig. 348).

It is understandable that this clumsy device could not gain ground at the time against Morrison's invention. Only after a professor Griscome of a military institution in Washington inserted a flexible shaft between a Siemens induction motor and the actual drilling aggregate was a usable electric dental engine developed in 1883 that could be powered by a storage battery. This apparatus was bought and further developed by the S. S. White Co., who used a modified sewing machine motor as a driving power[95]. In 1887, the court dentist Fried-

[94] von Langsdorff (a); Sercombe
[95] Flörke; Dorn p. 3; Behne

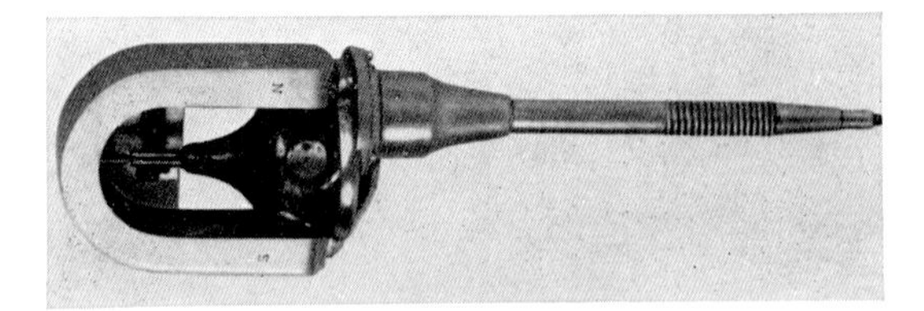

Fig. 348 *Green's electric drill, 1872*

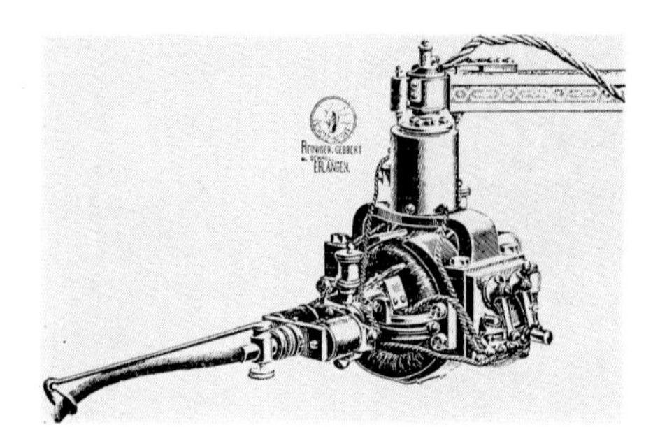

Fig. 350

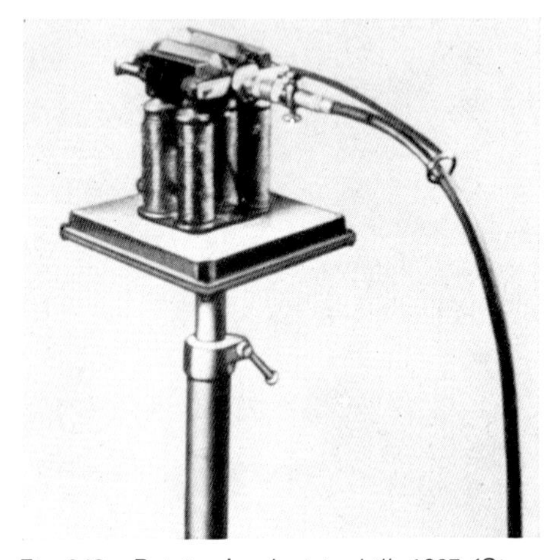

Fig. 349 *Reiniger's electric drill, 1887 (Siemens Archive)*

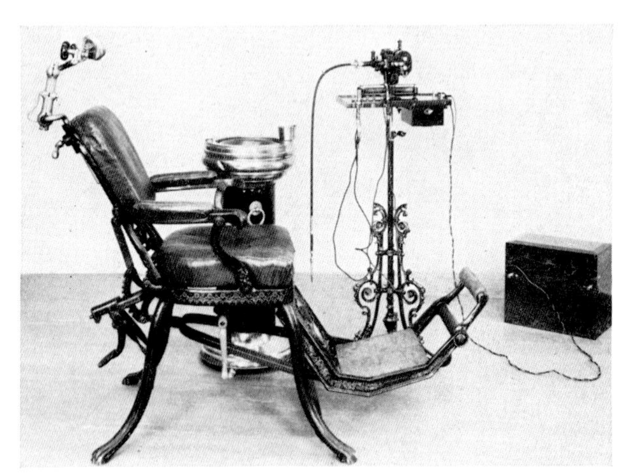

Figs. 350 and 351 *Mass-produced dental drill made by the firm of Reiniger, Gebbert & Schall, 1897 (Siemens Archive)*

rich Schneider of Erlangen was able to demonstrate a storage battery-powered apparatus (Fig. 349) for the first time in Germany at a meeting of dentists in Berlin. It was built by the former University mechanic in Erlangen, Reiniger, and was produced commercially beginning in 1891 (Figs. 350 and 351). In England the dentist Amos Kirby built a motor in 1889, in 1890 Cuttriss & Co. followed, and in 1894 W. G. Routledge, a dentist[96]. In the United States, two young German-Americans, the brothers Pieper of Philadelphia, offered their newly developed electric drill to Frank Ritter, another German immigrant, who was a cabinet maker specializing in dental furniture. Ritter immediately recognized the possibility of developing the apparatus, associated himself with the brothers Pieper in 1895, and began production in his factory in Rochester in the same year[97].

The foot-activated starter provided further progress. In the beginning this was a simple switch. In the advertisement of 1888 a resistance was already incorporated to permit selection of rotational speed (Fig. 352). Only a little later the motors were fitted with electromagnetic brakes to eliminate the tedious continued turning of the drill, caused by the momentum of the armature after the motor was switched off. In 1897, the previously unprotected motor was enclosed in a metal capsule (Fig. 353).

For decades thereafter, however, the foot-engine continued its service. Only when it had become possible to leave battery power behind at the turn of the century, when graceful mountings of motors on movable arms had been made,

[96] Behne; Donaldson
[97] Ritter

The Stand for carrying the Motor was devised with special reference to the convenience of dental practitioners. With it the operator controls the position of the Motor when in use. It is solid and easily adjustable, with an arm which can be raised or lowered or swung around at pleasure.

The Motor is placed at the end of the arm, giving the full advantage of the swing, which would not be available if an upright support alone was used. The conducting wires are carried up to the Motor on the inside of the upright column, thus placing them out of the way. The Stand was designed particularly for use with the S. S. White flexible arm, as affording superior advantages for motor use. The best position for it for most dentists is on the side of the chair opposite that on which they habitually stand in operating.

SWITCH-BOARD.

MOTOR STAND.

The Switch-Board, by which the speed of the Motor is controlled, is best placed handy to the foot of the operator, as the Switch is worked by a pedal. By a slight pressure of the foot, two, three, four, or six cells can be brought into service, giving the Motor any desired speed. Full illustrated directions for setting up the Battery and making the fluids supplied with each Battery.

It is our opinion that the dental outfit of the Detroit Motor Company is the best offered to the profession, and we have confidence in its efficiency.

PRICES.

Dental Motor, Battery, Stand, Switch-Board, and four yards of Cable, Hand-piece, Sleeve, and Cable, as per illustration $89.00

PARTS SEPARATELY.

Motor	$25.00	Hand-piece	$10.00
Motor Stand	15.00	Cable	1.50
Battery	25.00	Sleeve	2.50
Switch-Board	10.00		

No charge for boxing.

Red Fluid . . .	per gallon $0.60	White Fluid .	per gallon $0.10

Carboys or Jugs extra.

THE S. S. WHITE DENTAL MFG. CO.

Fig. 352 *Starter switch, S. S. White Co, 1888*

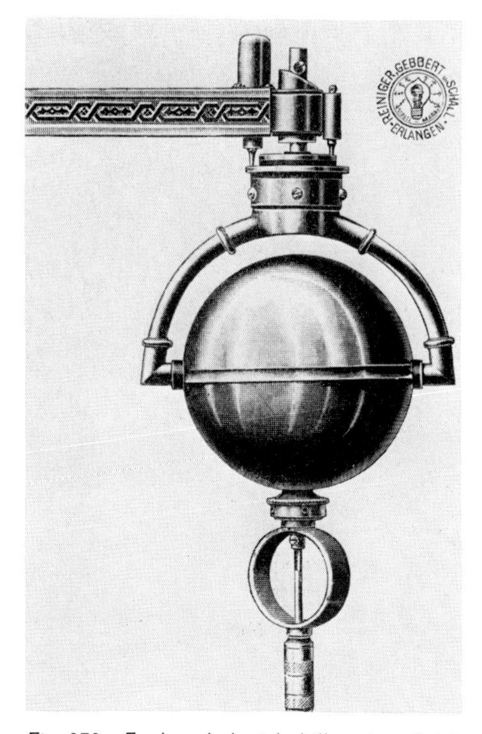

Fig. 353 *Enclosed dental drill motor, Reiniger, Gebbert & Schall, 1897 (Siemens Archive)*

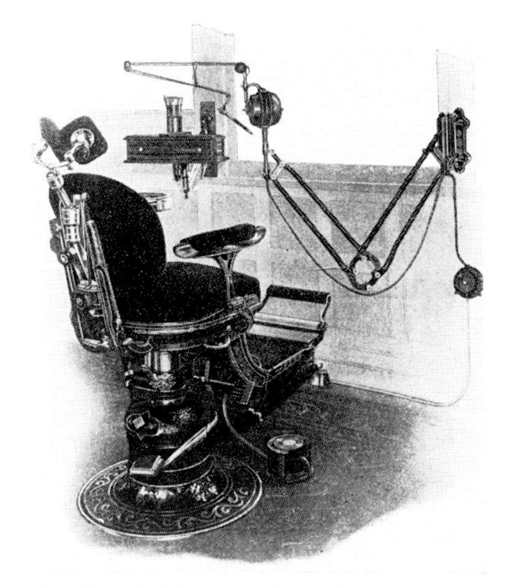

Fig. 354 *Folding bracket electric engine, Claudius Ash, 1910*

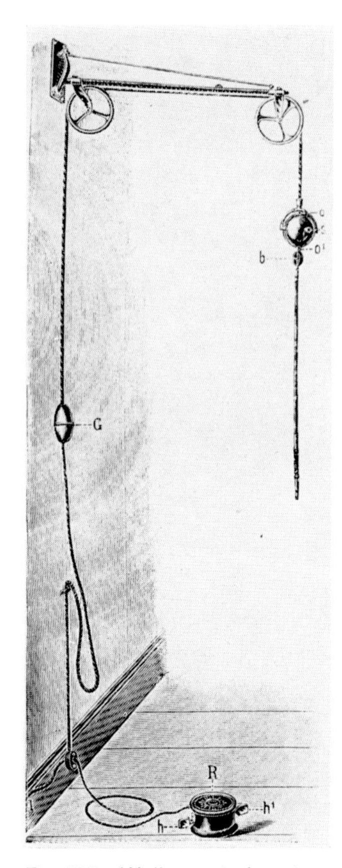

Fig. 355 *Wall-mounted engine*

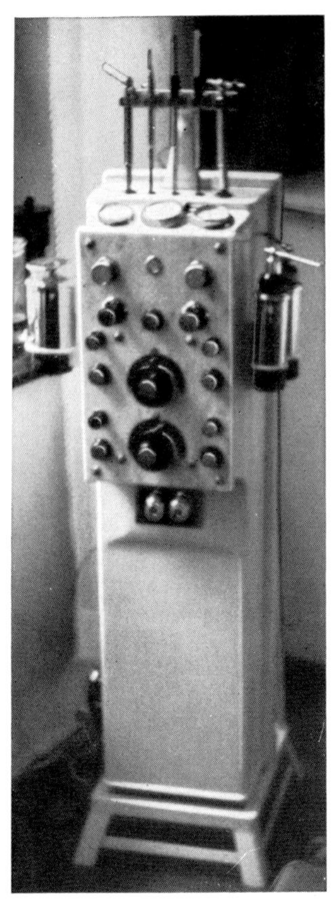

Fig. 356 *The Ritter electric switchboard, predecessor of the Ritter Unit, 1912*

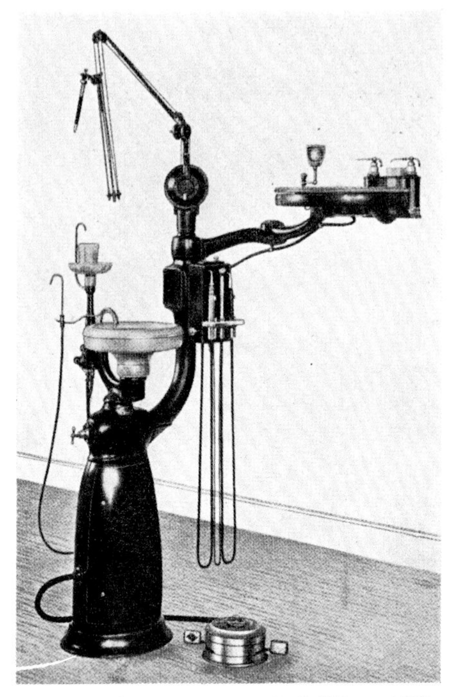

Fig. 357 *Equipment unit, S. S. White, 1931*

practicing dentists moved in a broad front to the electric machines (Figs. 354 and 355).
At the end of the '20s, the cord-driven Doriot arm began to be adopted. Designed by the Parisian dentist Constant Doriot to transfer the rotational power of the engine, it had been patented in Philadelphia as early as 1893 and was taken over by the S. S. White Co[98]. In 1917, the Ritter Co. in the United States combined treatment elements, such as the dental engine, spray, air blower, light sources, cuspidors, and cautery in a single unit, the so-called "Ritter Unit" soon produced by other firms, too (Figs. 356 and 357).
As early as 1911 the Belgian Emile Huet had developed an electric engine to rotate at a velocity of 10,000 rpm. He was not able, however, to interest a manufacturer in his construction, because handpieces at that time heated up and stopped at such a speed[99]. At first around 1936, the rotational speed of the motor was raised from 1200 to 3000 rpm, then to 6000 and later to 24,000 rpm through the incorporation of a high-speed gear. Again for decades the electric motor-driven dental engine was the most important tool of the dentist, until new developments were initiated through the airdriven turbine in 1957, and the micromotor in 1965.
These inventions, too, did not appear out of thin air. The beginning was made in 1948 by the "Dentalair" turbine of Ivar Norlén, a dentist from Stockholm. With a relatively high air requirement of 80 liters/minute, it reached a rotational speed of 140,000 rpm. In the following year the water turbine, developed at Washing-

[98] Personal communication S. S. White Co., May 18, 1966
[99] Huet

ton's National Bureau of Standards by Robert J. Nelsen came out. It contained a turbine power unit in the head of the anglepiece[100]. In the same year, the S. S. White Company turned up with a sand blasting device, developed at great expense. Although pain sensation was greatly reduced with the latter, quite unusual method, the device failed because it was impossible to aspirate the aluminum oxide cutting particles to any satisfactory extent. Furthermore, the sand blasting jet was able only to prepare unsharp cavity margins so that additional preparation was always necessary with the usual instruments. This shortcoming was shared by the White apparatus, the ultrasonic "Cavitron," a device introduced in the USA in 1955, and used today for the removal of calculus. None of these instruments were widely adopted. More success was achieved by insertion of an accelerating wrist joint in the Doriot-arms through which it was possible to increase the speed of grinding and drilling to 10,000 rpm. Such speeds required specially designed handpieces and contra-angles, presented on a congress in Hamburg as the "Imperator-System" in 1951. These included an automatic water cooling system, the Spraymatic. Hand in hand with this development came the production of above-mentioned diamond stones, and hard metal burs made of tungsten-carbide alloys.

During this time of a general search for new ways, one discovered almost coincidentally in the research laboratories of the U. S. Navy that Nelsen's water turbine idea could be made serviceable to air pressure. Building on that base, John Victor Borden, a Washington dentist, began to develop a dental air turbine, in 1946. His "Airotor" was the sensation of the International Dental Congress in Rome where it was introduced in 1957: *The climax was the Airotor, which was displayed by Amalgamated, Ritter, S. S. White, and others, and which was said to attain unbelievable rotational speeds, from 150,000 to 350,000 rpm. Even Pope Pius XII had the invention demonstrated in a special audience. Allegedly his treatment room was to be fitted with the new Airotor*[101].

The "unbelievable" velocity was attained by blowing condensed air loaded with oil-fog, approximately 28 liters/minute, on minute jet blades of a special contra-angle. Decisive in the process was the manufacture of ball bearings of such tiny dimensions. The unavoidable heat build-up of the instruments was compensated by continuous spraying with water. As much as the highest speed cutting and grinding simplified the work of the dentist in his preparation of enamel and dentin and in the removal of earlier fillings, he nonetheless continued to require the conventional drilling method for the removal of carious matter near the pulp until Kerr and Siemens offered him the handpiece-mounted micromotor in 1965. This device had been developed from a French design for the purpose of space navigation. Thus the dental unit finally lost its long accustomed appearance. Its noisy suspended motor and its troublesome arm disappeared in favor of totally new kinds of solutions, the final quality of which will be determined only after a longer period of clinical testing.

Pulp and Root Therapy

That which we define as pulp and root treatment, and which we summarize nowadays as "endodontics", a term taken from the Anglo-Saxon literature, was nothing more than the elimination of pain with the means and methods of ancient and medieval medical art until well into the 19th century. If we leave out of consideration the ultima ratio, the extraction of teeth, treatment of pulp and root consisted largely of trephination of the pulp cavity as had already been practiced by Archigenes, the application of the cautery according to the advice of Hippocrates and the Islamic physicians, or of cauterizing agents last heard of from Hunter. In the alternative, we might turn to luxation and reimplantation of the tooth after severance of the connecting vessel-nerve bundle, as once suggested by Dupont among others[102].

Laforgue of Paris had some justifiable scruples against this cruel treatment as early as in 1802: Frequently one experienced fracture of the root, mostly fistula formation occurred, and the teeth were lost anyway (true enough) after two to five years from *bone resorption* or *softening of their substance* (root resorption), and they also discolored. Maury, to the contrary, suggested the operation especially in youths for their premolars. Lefoulon drew back somewhat from the procedure in 1841, but it was

[100] Personal communication Norlén, October 24, 1971; Nelsen
[101] Vinski; Behne; Maretzky
[102] See pp. 220 and 188

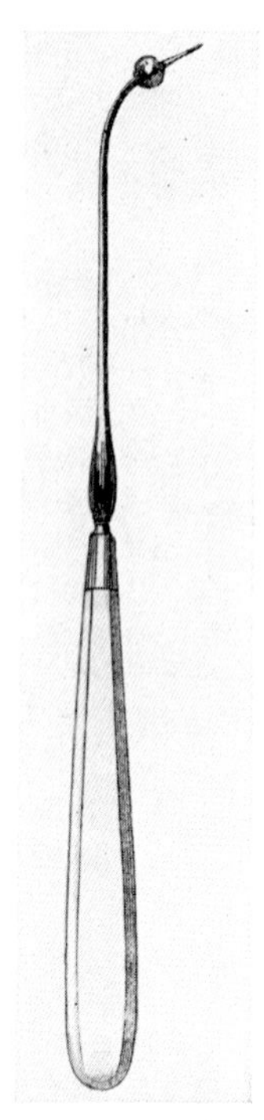

Fig. 358 *Lefoulon: Cautery for the contents of the root canal, 1841*

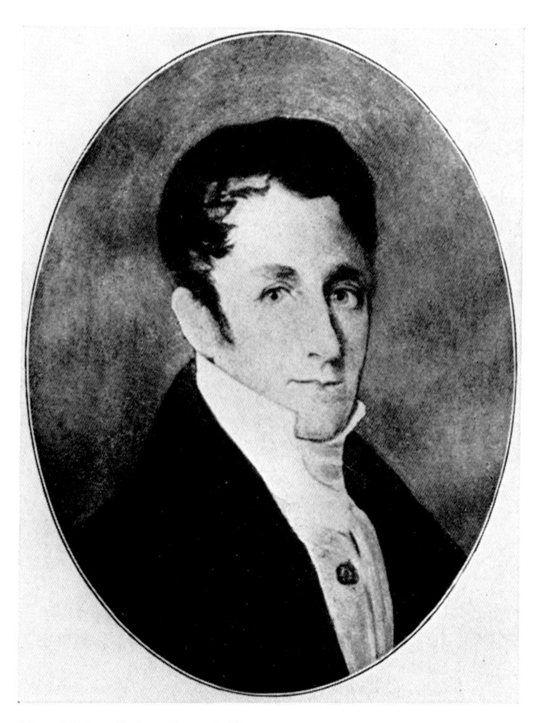

Fig. 359 *John Roach Spooner*

Désirabode who rejected with finality this robust procedure[103].

The burning iron, the "Cauterium actuale" of the Middle Ages, was used to dry out caries in the erroneous hope that a limit was thus put on its expansion, but especially to destroy the painful pulp. To reach the root canals, one constructed needle-like cauteries of platinum bearing small spheres as heat reservoirs (Fig. 358). Maury also used a kind of nerve-needle: several gold wires soldered to a rodlet, with which he sought to grasp and to extract the pulpal contents by turning it in the root canal. Alternatively, one cauterized the pulp with sulfuric and nitric acid or with silver nitrate.

It is to the credit of an American dentist working in Montreal, John Roach Spooner (Fig. 359) to have been the first to use arsenious acid to devitalize the pulp, if we disregard the Chinese healing arts and the prescriptions of antiquity and of the Middle Ages, which, however, found no resonance[104]. His brother Shearjashub Spooner made the discovery known in 1836 in his popular "Guide to Sound Teeth." Chapin Aaron Harris, the co-founder of the Baltimore Dental College[105], took up the idea, by mixing arsenic *with an equal quantity of sulphate of morphia.* In a later (1863) edition of Harris' work, J. R. Spooner's priority is explicitly noted[106].

Especially in Europe it took a long time before arsenic became commonly used among dentists. Désirabode in 1843 in Paris, J. Linderer in 1851 in Berlin, as well as Nessel in 1856 in Prague continued to prefer the cruel cautery, while Robinson in London in 1846 recommended at least a creosote-morphium mixture. In 1859, Tomes advised the use of arsenic in his textbook, and for Magitot in Paris in 1867 arsenious acid was *of sure and complete effect*[107].

In 1819 Ch. F. Delabarre described capping of an exposed pulp with a thin concave gold plate[108] just as Philipp Pfaff had proposed it

103 Laforgue pp. 112 f.; Maury (a) pp. 180 f.; Lefoulon pp. 267 f.; Désirabode pp. 413 f.
104 See pp. 43, 75, 95, and 110
105 See pp. 403 f.
106 Harris (a) p. 272; (b) 352 footnote
107 Magitot (a) p. 195
108 Delabarre pp. 61 f.

as early as 1756[109]. Delabarre says that he owed this new method to his father, the "Chirurgien Dentiste" of the Swedish Court. Later fillings were also arched over the pulpal perforations but Taft had improved this technique (1859) by protecting at first the defect with collodion or guttapercha dissolved in chloroform before inserting the gold cap or the filling[110]. W. D. Miller suggested that in the vicinity of the pulp the procedure ought to be as germ-free (sterile) as possible, and recommended antiseptic treatment with carbolic acid or sublimate solution before opening the pulp cavity. The wound of the pulp was closed with Fletcher's Artificial Dentine[111]. In the 1930s starting from this procedure were calcium hydroxide preparations developed successfully.

The authors of the early 19th century were already differentiating between pulpal pain and that of the periodontal membrane, as did Laforgue in 1802: *Nerves that can be touched with the probe leave no doubt whether they are the seat of pain . . . A percussion by a nail that shocks the tooth is often sufficient to reveal the site of the pain as the periosteum of the alveolus*[112]. Treatment usually consisted of tooth extraction. The American Simon P. Hullihen, who worked chiefly as an oral surgeon, proposed in 1852 that a drain be made for exudates at the cervix of the tooth, in principle just as the ancients had done by opening the pulp canal. Only in 1859 Taft suggested to attempt a therapy with drug-impregnated cotton inlays[113].

The first root canal filling is ascribed to Edward Hudson (Fig. 360), an Irish freedom fighter who emigrated to America in 1803 after long imprisonment and opened an office in Philadelphia. Robert Arthur reports of him in 1850 that he had extirpated the pulp since 1809 and that he had filled the roots of the anteriors up to the apex with gold foil. Hudson's charges from 1824/1825 appear to support this claim (Fig. 361).

Edward Maynard (Fig. 362), practicing in Washington and mentioned earlier in relation to his porcelain restorations, elevated this technique of root canal filling in 1838 to a method. As a practitioner of extraordinary manual skill, he made his own devices for root canal treatment, and was able to demonstrate his talents in Europe in 1845 when he was invited to treat the family of the Czar in St. Petersburg. Enticing invitations did not deter his return to his native land, where he received high honors and taught at several universities[114]. Taft described Maynard's technique in 1859 in his textbook with great exactness[115].

Europe was somewhat retarded in this respect. Gerhardt Paulson of Frankfurt am Main reported that gold root canal fillings as demonstrated by an American dentist passing through were completely new to him in 1862[116], and still in 1867 Magitot in Paris carried out devitalization and removal of the pulp followed by the final closure with gold, amalgam or cement without root filling[117].

In 1863/1864, American dentists such as Chauncey P. Fitch and John DeHaven White decisively rejected immediate placement of a filling on a dead pulp. The latter proposed that cotton soaked in creosote be inserted into the canal after removal of the pulp. It was the merit of Witzel who, in 1874, published a fundamental system of pulp treatment based—without doubt—on the influence of the antiseptic surgical techniques of Joseph Lister[118].

In Adolph Witzel, we meet one of the most important representatives of conservative dentistry (Fig. 363). Born on April 14, 1847 as the eldest of ten children of a barber in Langensalza, Thuringia, he studied in privation with Albrecht in Berlin[119] and settled in Essen in 1868 where he soon built up a respectable practice. At the Kassel meeting of the Central Society of German Dentists in 1874 he distinguished himself with a talk about "The Antiseptic Treatment of the Pulpal Diseases of the Tooth," followed by books about the same subject in analysis of pulp diseases that remains valid to this day, supporting it with histological illustrations. He indicated new therapeutic approaches with his antiseptic method of treatment. Following the study of medicine in Heidelberg, he was called to teach at the university of Jena in 1891 with the result that the institute

[109] See p. 231
[110] Taft (a) pp. 223 f.; (b) pp. 130 f.
[111] Miller (c) pp. 266 f.
[112] Laforgue (a) pp. 66 f.; (b) p. 59
[113] Taft (a) pp. 261 f.; (b) pp. 156 f.
[114] Thorpe pp. 217 f.
[115] Taft (a) pp. 253 f.; (b) pp. 151 f.
[116] Paulson
[117] Magitot (a) p. 200
[118] Since 1867 the surgeon of Glasgow, Lister, introduced with great success the antiseptic method into surgery.
[119] See p. 410

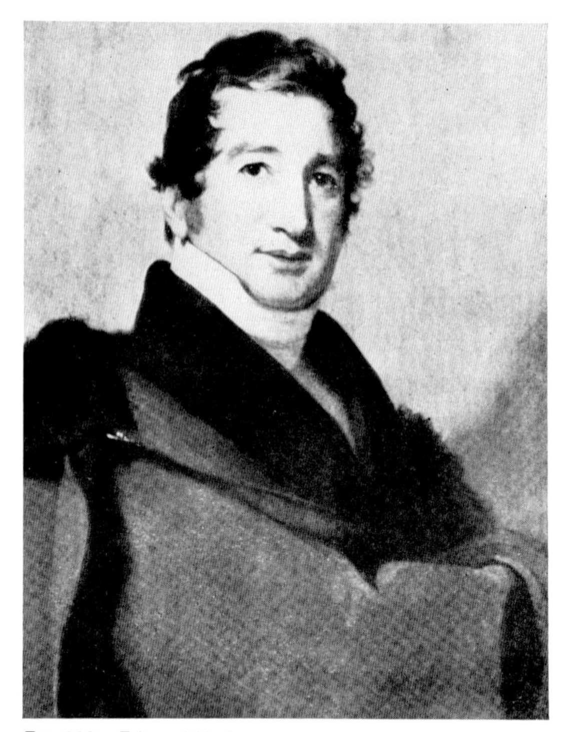

Fig. 360 *Edward Hudson*

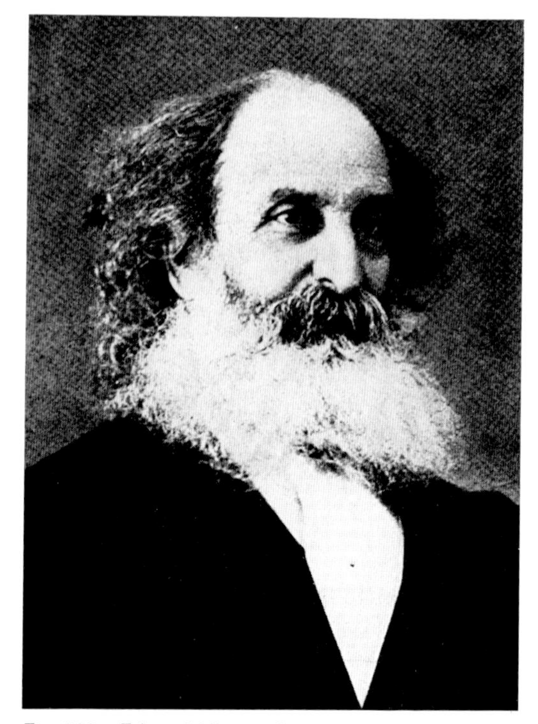

Fig. 362 *Edward Maynard*

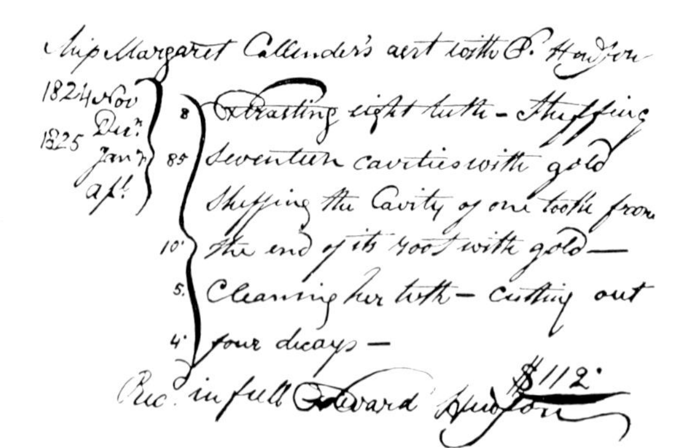

Miss Margaret Callender's acct with E. Hudson

1824 Nov
Dec
1825 Jan 7
ap!

8 Extracting eight teeth - Stuffing
85 seventeen cavities with gold
Stuffing the Cavity of one tooth from
10 the end of its root with gold —
5 Cleaning her teeth – cutting out
4 four decays –

Rec. in full Edward Hudson $112

Fig. 361 *Hudson's invoice for a root canal restoration with gold (from Thorpe)*

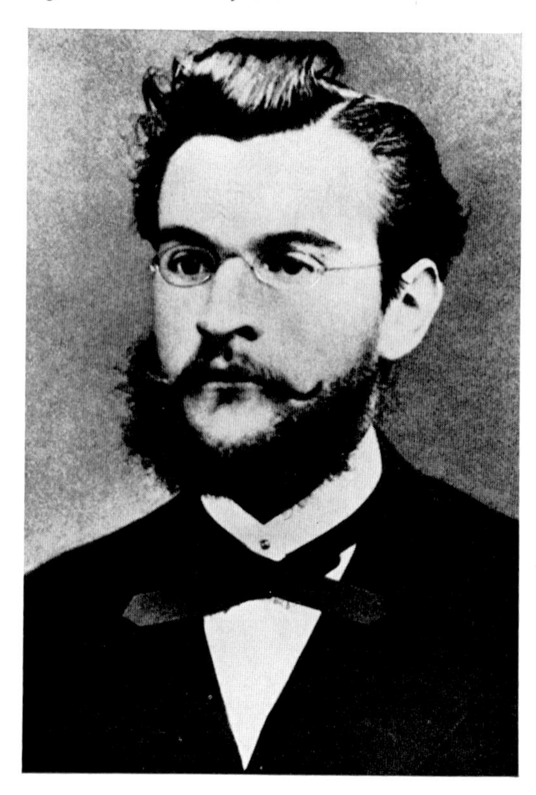

Fig. 363 *Adolph Witzel*

founded there by him soon became the third largest in Germany in the number of students. The period is marked by his studies of the amalgam problem[120]. In 1899 a cardiac disease put an end to his academic activity but he continued to devote himself to science from his retirement in Bonn, and the post-graduate courses which he held drew participants from ever widening circles until his successful life ended on July 12, 1906[121].

Adolph Witzel's antiseptic amputation technique consisted of removal of the coronal pulp previously devitalized with arsenic and replacing it initially with a paste containing phenol and later using sublimate or an iodoform cement. With this treatment the root-pulp shrank to the size of *antiseptic threads,* which made a far better filling *than the much praised but poor unsatisfactory root fillings of gold or tin.* In complete pulpitis the canals were cleansed with Arrington's nerve needle and filled with a cement paste that remained soft[122].

A further significant contribution to the pathology of dental diseases was made by the Hungarian physician Joseph Arkövy's "Diagnostik der Zahnkrankheiten" (Diagnosis of diseases of the teeth) published in 1885, in which therapy was excluded deliberately. Arkövy had founded a private institute of dentistry in Budapest in 1880, of which he was named the first director when it became a part of the university in 1890.

It is remarkable how many toxic materials were tried in the attempt to destroy the bacteria within the gangrenous pulp in the canals. While Witzel was satisfied with a 20 % solution of sublimate, Emil Schreier of Vienna proposed, in 1892, that a serrated neddle (as had been suggested by Robert Bruce Donaldson of Washington, and others) be used to insert metallic potassium or sodium into the moist root canal, where these would have reacted strongly and would have emulsified the remaining organic debris. Richard Schreiter, a dentist in Saxony, achieved the same purpose with caustic potash in 1894, and John Ross Callahan of Cincinnati published his method of widening narrow putrid canals with sulphuric acid in the same year[123].

In 1904, at the St. Louis International Dental Congress, John Peter Buckley of Hollywood described his careful studies of pulp gangrene and proposed a paste of tricresol and formaldehyde as disinfectant[124]. As a liquid this compound dominated the treatment of gangrene for several decades. In 1896, Miller suggested, that cotton impregnated with thymol, cement, guttapercha, gold foil, platinum, copper, or gold wires, wooden posts, and soft pastes of zinc oxide with iodoform, thymol, etc. ground up in oil of cloves be used as filling materials[125]. The latter, and a chloroform suspension of guttapercha (chloropercha) combined with nerve canal points of guttapercha asserted itself for root canal therapy in the beginning of the 20th century.

Periodontal Diseases

Although the technique of splinting loosened teeth and the removal of calculus was manifest in the oldest records[126], we find the first clear description of a condition known today as marginal periodontitis only in the second edition of Fauchard's book[127]. In 1757 Bourdet joined him with proposals for treatment of this disease which is not yet completely controlled. In 1770 Botot followed with the first specific report about this subject. Hunter, too, devoted several pages to it[128]. Little progress was made beyond Fauchard's definition and Bourdet's advice in the first half of the 19th century. Joseph Fox of London, who was the first to provide illustrations, spoke in 1806 quite generally of *an absorption of the sockets* (Fig. 364). Justifiably he noted that caries-prone individuals generally remained free of these symptoms[129]. In 1829, Thomas Bell perceived *premature old age, or an anticipation of senile decay,* which might occur even without local inflammation. He advised incision of the gingiva, and that general attention should be given to the stomach and that the blood should

120 See p. 293
121 Hesse
122 Witzel (a); (b) pp. 38 and 58 f.
123 Schreier; Schreiter; Callahan, his memorial, see p. 408
124 Buckley
125 Miller (c) pp. 342 f.
126 See pp. 25, 34, 99 f. See also p. 16
127 See p. 199. The Florentine goldsmith Benvenuto Cellini describes his loss of teeth as a 40-year-old during his long imprisonment in the Castle of San Angelo in Rome in 1539: "And my teeth began to die in my mouth and because they impinged on sound ones, they finally became quite loose in the chin and their roots would remain no longer in their sockets. When I noticed this I withdrew them as from a sheath, without pain and blood, and thus, sadly, I lost many of them."—On the basis of external circumstances, however, this may have been scurvy.
128 See pp. 214 and 220 f.
129 Fox p. 88

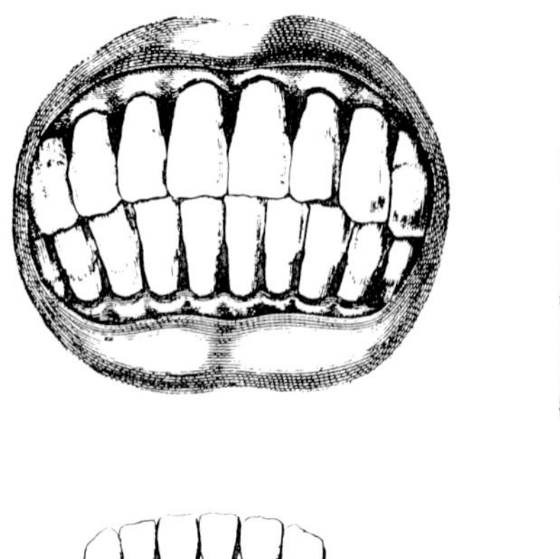
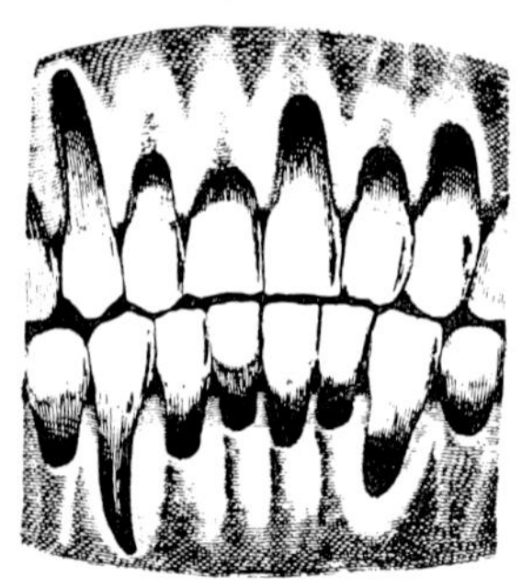
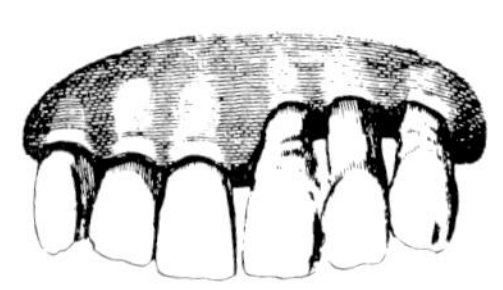

Fig. 364 *Fox: Periodontosis and periodontitis*

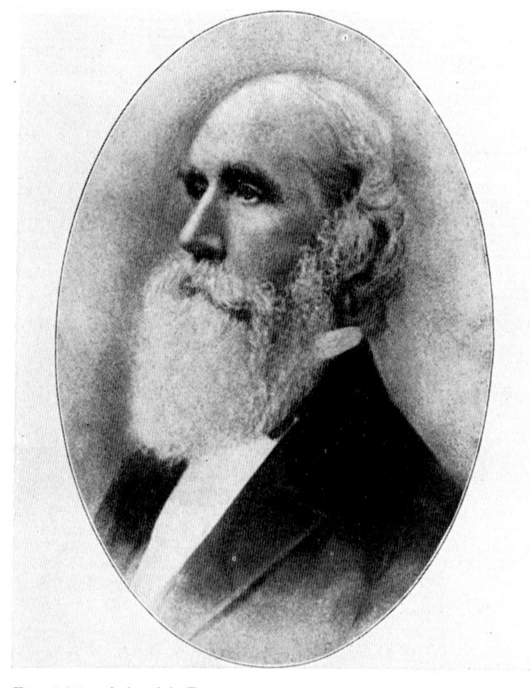

Fig. 365 *John M. Riggs*

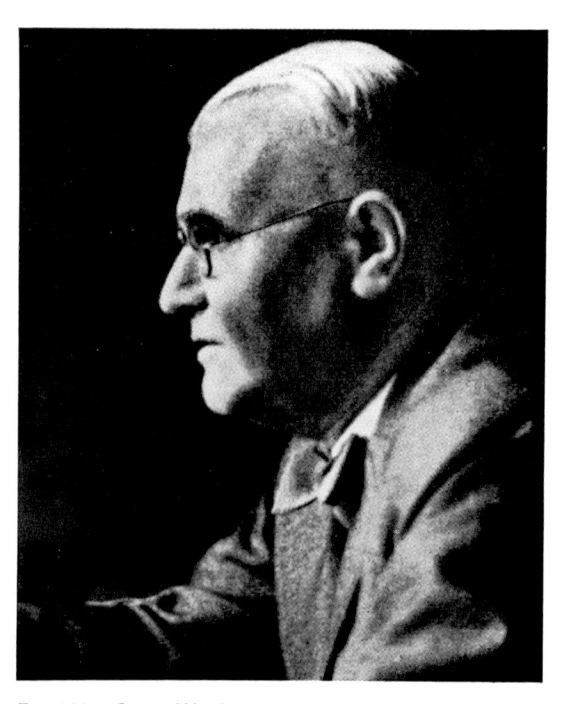

Fig. 366 *Oscar Weski*

be purified[130]. Désirabode in 1843 rejected Fauchard's scurvy theory of *pyorrhée interalvéolo-dentaire*[131] as did Bourdet, and ascribed responsibility to calculus and also to constitutional and hygienic factors as well as to skin diseases and syphilis. For general therapy he suggested bleeding and laxatives[132].

The Dresden physician Robert Ficinus made Leeuwenhoek's Animalcula responsible in his work of 1847 "Über das Ausfallen der Zähne..."(Concerning the Loss of Teeth...). These animals force their way into the fibers between gingiva and cement, loosen the former, and here form the tooth-loosening calculus[133].

That the younger Linderer differentiated already in 1851 between periodontosis and marginal periodontitis deserves attention. *The first of these diseases has been mistaken for chronic suppuration, but it is decisively different from it.* It is almost free of inflammation. The gingiva shrinks progressively so that the neck of the tooth is exposed. He furthermore described a hypertrophy of the gingival connective tissue, today called fibromatosis gingivae[134].

Despite serious efforts, John Tomes of London was unable to say anything positive about etiology. He proposed the removal of calculus, the use of a soft toothbrush, mild astringents and good oral hygiene as treatment[135].

In 1880 Magitot of Paris described the condition as a constitutional disease or one of primary damage to the periodontal membrane and to the cement caused by diabetes, albuminuria or gout, and which he named "Cemento-periostitis." In 1885, Arkövy, the Hungarian, in his textbook agreed with Magitot, with the restriction that *the primary site of the disease was the alveolar margin,* from which *caries alveolaris* proceeded to the periodontal membrane and cement[136]. W. D. Miller proposed in 1896 a synthesis of etiologic factors similar to Désirabode's for pyorrhea alveolaris: 1. predisposing factors such as *constitutional or local complaints, abnormal composition of the blood, digestive troubles, unfavorable hygienic conditions, etc.,* 2. local irritations as *tartar, food particles, or any other mechanical or chemical agents* and 3. bacteria. Rightfully, Miller rejected the idea of a specific etiologic agent, claiming that inflammation arose through the normal oral flora, *if the power of resistance of the peridental tissue be impaired by any one of above-mentioned local or constitutional causes. ... The prognosis is always unfavorable; in the front-teeth, however, a marked improvement, if not a complete cure, may be affected*[137].

While in Europe one maintained general etiologic and therapeutic factors, the pragmatic Americans directed their efforts more to the local symptoms. John M(ankey) Riggs (Fig. 365), a lifelong practitioner of Hartford, Connecticut, was the first one to give his undivided attention to pyorrhea alveolaris from 1856, a condition known thereafter in North America for a long time as "Riggs disease". His instruments consisted of six scalers with which he carefully penetrated into the soft tissue to remove every trace of calculus from the pockets. Then the teeth and roots were thoroughly polished with the dental engine. It is quite understandable that this first truly methodical therapy led to significant reduction of at least the inflammatory conditions[138].

As defender of antisepsis, Miller suggested that in the presence of gingival pockets, they be syringed additionally with an antiseptic solution[139]. True progress in the therapy of periodontal diseases was achieved when in 1901 the Viennese dentist Moritz Karolyi blamed shocks to the alveolar walls for pyorrhea alveolaris especially as they occur through tooth grinding at night. As a remedial measure, he suggested *grinding of the cusps and edges,* as is still done today, but especially the preparation of *bite plates, i. e., removable molar caps of gold* to be worn at night[140].

Proven as erroneous were later attempts in the Anglo-Saxon countries to treat pyorrhea alveolaris, which was considered as an infectious disease, with vaccines of microorganisms of the oral cavity, or with "ementin," an alkaloid of the ipecacuanha root which was used in general medicine to treat amebic dysentery, and which should now fight the harmless amebae in the mouth. In 1947 the bacteriologist, Heinrich

130 Bell pp. 202 f.
131 Introduction of the term "pyorrhea" is improperly ascribed to Alphonse Toirac by Geist-Jacobi (p. 190). Toirac, however, writes only descriptively of "suppuration alveolodentaire" in his "Dissertation sur les dents" of 1823. (Toirac p. 44).
132 Désirabode pp. 308 f.
133 Ficinus
134 J. Linderer (c) pp. 115 f.
135 Tomes (a) pp. 572 f.; (b) pp. 467 f.
136 Magitot (b); Arkövy pp. 230 f.
137 Miller (a) pp. 274 f.; (b) pp. 330 f.
138 Mills. Publication at first in 1878, after invention of the dental engine.
139 Miller (a) p. 278; (b) p. 334
140 Karolyi

Gins of Berlin, mistakingly considered the periodontal diseases as a specific infection with spirilla, i. e., a "spirillosis," acquired mostly in youth. He treated it with corresponding vaccines [141].

During the period between the two World Wars, two Swedes defended opposing theories of therapy: surgical removal of the pockets was the position taken by Leonard Widman in Stockholm, while Karl Elander of Göteborg and others preferred drug therapy for the pockets [142]. Both techniques were connected with thorough scaling of calculus, as had been requested already by Riggs and by W. J. Younger of San Francisco in 1880 [143], and for which improved special scalers have been developed continuously up to the present.

During this period, two Viennese dentists, Leo Fleischmann and Bernard Gottlieb, undertook histological examinations from which came extensive clarification of the pathological changes in tissue. In 1920, Gottlieb presented his important paper on "Epithelansatz am Zahne" (Epithelial Attachment on the Tooth)[144]. Later Gottlieb and his student, the Hungarian Balint Orban, emigrated to the United States.

A new method of research was initiated by Oskar Weski, a physician who had turned to the study of dentistry in Berlin in 1905 (Fig. 366). He opened an office in this city, where he zealously studied finely structured tissues and also carried out radiological research. In 1922, he realized that the designation "pyorrhea alveolaris" described only one symptom of the disease and that the periodontium, cement, bone and gingiva made up a functional system for which he coined the term "Paradentium." The diseases associated with tissue atrophy of this biological unit were named by Weski "Paradentosis" and "Paradentitis." From a diagnostic triad of the clinical-anatomic, the functional and the general state (of health), the therapeutic triad resulted consisting of local, relieving and general therapeutic measures [145].—In 1953, the term "Paradentium" with its corresponding derivations became changed to "Parodontium" only for philological reasons. The Anglo-American literature, however, did not adopt Weski's nomenclature. Here the term "periodontitis" is used in place of pyorrhea alveolaris.

Periodontology developed into a field of research in its own right. Eventually it was recognized on the side of internal medicine that there was no regular relationship between specific systemic diseases and the periodontological symptoms, so that today's therapeutic efforts are again concentrated more on the dental organ. Many problems in this field are awaiting clarification.

Caries Prevention

Early reports of practical measures intended to prevent dental caries have been found in certain Latin American Indian tribes, although it may be left open whether the touching-up practised there is done consciously for prophylactic reasons or ritually without conscious knowledge of prevention [147]. What little is available in the European and Islamic literature of the past centuries on this subject is limited in part to quite irrelevant dietetic suggestions doomed then as now to failure, e.g., prohibition of milk and milk products, mouthwash with urine, and later to the usual oral hygiene rules [148].

The Parisian court dentist Désirabode may have been the first one, in 1843, who considered caries prevention, even mentioning fluoride compounds: *Especially the fluorides, as is known, have the property of hardening the moistness* (caries), *as our studies have shown; but they have until now not met our hopes in any way: the stumbling block is the changeable nature of the saliva and the oral fluids which, alkaline, become acid so quickly, and vice versa. For all that, the following composition has shown that we are on the right track, because of its stability: silicate or fluorite and aluminum, dried and pulverized in equal parts with sufficient water. One makes a homogenous paste which one introduces into the carious tooth, and whose dehydration is promoted by the introduction of a hot plugger* [149].

Systematic administration of fluorides as an agent against caries began in the 20th century only starting from the United States although the district-physician of Baden, Erhardt, had

141 Goadby; Barrett (a and b); Gins
142 Elander
143 Sachs p. 155
144 Fleischmann and Gottlieb; Gottlieb
145 Weski
147 See pp. 56
148 See pp. 76, 92, and 198
149 Désirabode p. 409

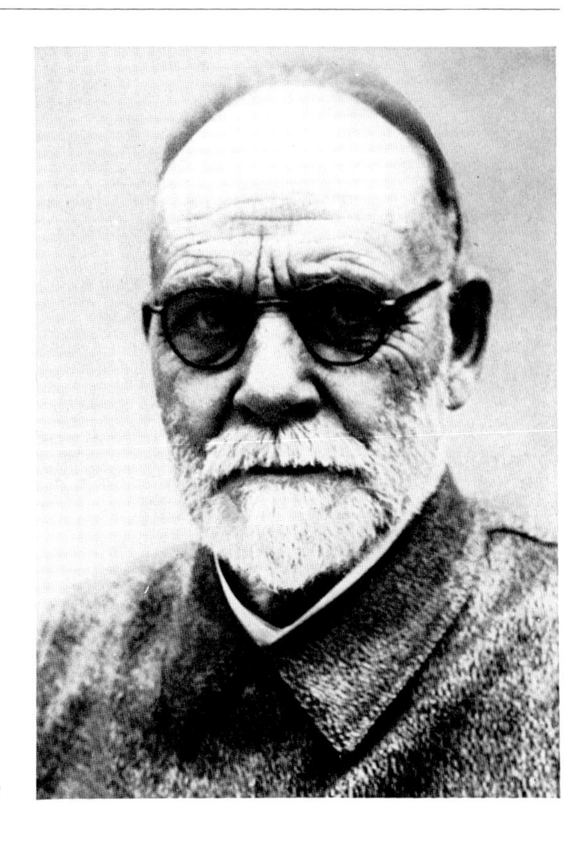

Fig. 367 *Carl Röse*

already recommended in 1874 that fluoride lozenges be given, *especially to children during eruption and in women during pregnancy for* several months. As he writes, he was given this suggestion from England, where *oral hygiene is known to be of a high standard* [150].

Here, Sir James Crichton-Browne in a lecture given to dentists in Cambridge (G. B.) in 1892, held responsible for the increasing attack of caries the lack of fluoride supply to the enamel and a soft diet, a nervous style of life, and urbanization. Enamel, however, is *to the tooth what its armour-plates are to a modern ship of war.* Fluorine would be best administered to pregnant women and to children in its natural form as a diet containing corn husks. Furthermore he recommended dental examinations *by a qualified dentist twice a year* on school ships, in reformatories, orphanages, and boarding schools [151].

In 1896 Albert Denninger, a chemist, addressed the Rhine Society for Natural Science on the topic "Fluorine, an Agent against Diseases of the Teeth." He believed that the principal cause of decay of the teeth of men was getting insufficient fluorine with the food, due to the high standard of cleansing agricultural products of sand. He recommended to compensate this lack by providing calcium fluoride. Pregnant women who took daily doses of fluorspar did not suffer the customary loss of teeth, and their children had teeth especially resistant to caries [152].

All these suggestions were almost completely lost to memory. New ways were sought and cast aside, e. g., prophylactic application of silver nitrate to the enamel practiced around the world at the turn of the century, but rejected as ineffective by the outstanding caries researcher,

150 Erhardt
151 Crichton-Browne
152 Hoffmann-Axthelm p. 8, on the basis of information from a granddaughter of Denninger. Under a misspelled name and without indication of the year, the Denninger paper was republished word for word in Dtsch. zahnärztl. Wschr. 10: 196—198, 1907, according to a reprint from the "Frankfurter Zeitung"

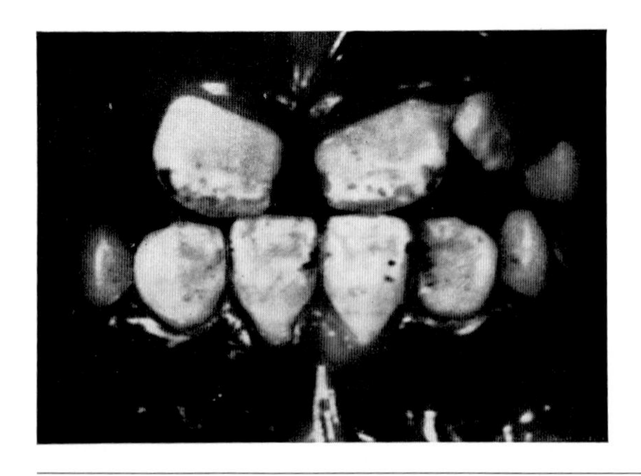

Fig. 368 *Dental fluorosis (Author's observation, 1952)*

W. D. Miller in his lecture in 1905 in London[153]. Whether Miller was entirely right remains an open question. In any event, the subsequent black discoloration of the teeth precludes its widespread use. Miller himself proposed the use of oral disinfectant solutions in addition to scrupulous oral hygiene[154].

In 1894 Carl Röse (Fig. 367), a physician, dentist, and recognized dental public health expert who enjoyed international esteem believed to have established that drinking of water rich in lime caused increased resistance to caries[155]. As the first lecturer on dentistry at the University of Freiburg im Breisgau he came to this conclusion on the basis of serial examinations of schoolchildren from lime-rich and lime-poor regions. To support his theory, he extended his researches assidiously, included larger population groups and was the first to collect comprehensive statistics on caries. His studies, which he began in 1900, included more than 220,000 subjects by 1906.

The work was carried out through the "Zentralstelle für Zahnhygiene" (Center for Dental Hygiene) in Dresden, of which he was appointed head, an institution founded and generously endowed by a manufacturer of mouthwash, Karl August Lingner. He furthermore wrote numerous scientific and popular articles making demands which seem obvious to us today but were fundamentally new at the time. Thus, he proposed among others long nursing periods, the consumption of coarse rye bread, and of milk[156], ideas that found little resonance at a time when Miller's school of thought prevailed that caries was predominantly a bacteriological problem. Poverty of natural minerals in the respective regions, he suggested, should be overcome by raising the degree of hardness of the drinking water[157].

In the meantime friction had built up between Lingner and the personally difficult Röse, in consequence of which the "Zentralstelle" was dissolved in 1909, thus pulling the ground from under further odontological research. Röse was supported at first by an international honorary fund of the dental world promoted by Jenkins, the discoverer of light-flowing porcelain, and others. In 1911 he settled in practice in Erfurt, turned to problems of nutritional physiology, and in 1913, embittered by the lack of resonance for his work, devoted himself completely to agriculture. He died, this pathfinder of nutritional prevention of caries, at the age of nearly 83 years, as a small farmer and gardener in needy circumstances in a village near Erfurt in 1947[158].

In 1911 Henry Percy Pickerill of New Zealand also sought to gain influence on caries through nutrition. He believed the cure to lie in remineralization of the enamel through secretion of saliva rich in calcium and sought to achieve this by promoting a "natural" diet rich in fruit. To this end he even demanded legal measures[159] as Röse, too, had sought similar measures to punish mothers who were capable of nursing but rejected this responsibility. It may be that this possibility of remineralization, or "rehar-

[153] Miller
[154] See p. 408
[155] Röse (a)
[156] Röse (a—c)
[157] Röse (c) pp. 449 f.
[158] Hertelendy-Michel; Romeick pp. 103 f.
[159] Pickerill pp. 292 f. See p. 400

dening" was first pointed out in 1910 by a Philadelphia dentist, Joseph Head[160].

An important contribution to the prevention of caries was made by pediatricians during the period between the two World Wars through the methodical prophylaxis of rickets. Sensible nutrition of the infant and the dispensing of vitamin D-preparations succeeded largely controlling the "English disease" and thus preventing its late sequela, described at length by Bunon in the 18th century as enamel hypoplasia of the permanent teeth[161]. These defects, rarely seen nowadays, are a site of predilection for caries, especially as mostly the first molars are affected.

In 1921 Bernhard Gottlieb of Vienna believed that he recognized a relation between the rate of caries and the degree of keratinization of the enamel cuticle and accordingly recommended strengthening of this "horny layer" through brush massage, intensive chewing, and tinctures containing tannic acid in analogy to the callous on a worker's skin[162]. Viggo Andresen of Copenhagen agreed and suggested prevention through preparations which had *mineralizing, keratinizing, and lanolinizing effects,* the latter because of his view that fats such as lanolin protected the enamel cuticle from dissolution by acids[163].

The protective properties of fluoride against caries were rediscovered through the roundabout path of recognition of enamel defects that occur as a result of excessive doses. These were perhaps first observed without knowledge of the causes by Magitot in northern Africa in 1867 (as H. Velu observed them there, especially in animals in 1931), then described in Italians of Pozzuoli by an American naval physician stationed in Naples, J. M. Eager, in 1901 who used the local terms "denti di Chiaie" or "denti scritti" (lettered teeth)[164].

In 1916 Greene Vardiman Black in a posthumous publication together with Frederick S. McKay called them "mottled enamel" as observed by him in various regions of the United States since 1908 (Fig. 368)[165]. Eager pointed to gases from volcanic sources, but Black properly made drinking water responsible for their occurence, even asking *the eminent investigator Dr. Carl Röse* about them, but the latter's numerous water analyses had never included fluoride content. The cause of the lower caries rate among the affected children was ascribed by Black to their general healthy living conditions *(a mild climate and almost continuous sunshine).* Thus the puzzle remained unsolved for the time being[166].

It was left to chemists to clarify the relation between the mottled enamel and the element fluorine and to demonstrate it: H. V. Churchill of the Aluminium Research Laboratories in New Kensington demonstrated in 1931 through spectographic drinking water analysis *that apparently the relative severity of the defect* (of the enamel) *in these various areas seems to follow the fluoride concentration*[167]. Demonstration of this relationship in animal experiments followed under the direction of the dentist A. E. Bard in the same year, by Margaret Cammack Smith and colleagues at the Agricultural Experiment Station of the University of Arizona[168].

The dentist H. Trendley Dean of the U. S. Public Health Service, in cooperation with numerous practicing colleagues in high fluoride regions, demonstrated through voluminous statistical material the relationship between the degree of fluoride ingestion and reduced caries susceptibility, and thus prepared the way for artificial enrichment of drinking water with fluoride compounds[169]. The direct stimulus for this was provided by the very careful animal experiments of Gerald J. Cox of Pittsburgh in 1939[170]. This path was followed with success in the United States, while in Europe one followed only very slowly although here, too, comprehensive experiments in naturally fluoridated areas yielded similarly unmistakable results as those in North America[171] (Fig. 368). Other means of transfer were suggested and more or less successfully studied, such as local application of fluoride solutions to the enamel[172], distribution of fluoride

160 Head
161 See pp. 208 f.
162 Gottlieb
163 Andresen
164 Velu; Eager. The occasional use, even by Eager, of the designation Chiaie after Prof. Stefano Chiaie of Naples rests, according to information received from Vincenzo Guerini (1916), on an error. This designation arises from a Neapolitan quarter, Chiala, in which the enamel spots are seen; see Dental Cosmos 58 (1916) p. 785
165 Black and McKay
166 McKay and Black; McKay
167 Churchill
168 Smith et al.
169 Dean
170 Cox et al.
171 E. g., Hoffmann-Axthelm pp. 28 f.
172 Knutson and Armstrong

tablets and the addition of fluoride to table salt, milk, or dentifrices[173].

More recent suggestions for prevention of caries have been made along the lines of altering the oral flora to reduce the number of *Lactobacillus acidophilus*, whose cariogenic effect pointed out by Russel W. Bunting already in 1928 is still uncertain[174]. Enzymatic interference also has been suggested, as has the sealing with resin of occlusal fissures to protect sites of predilection for attack.

Long-term results suitable for evaluation are available chiefly for drinking water fluoridation, and these speak an unambiguous language. But they also demonstrate that even life-long fluoride impregnation of tooth tissue does not make careful observation superfluous. The combination of individual conservative treatment with general preventive measures may be expected to provide the success-promising task of future dentistry.

[173] Wespi; Ziegler; Bibby
[174] Bunting et al.

References

Alexander, C(harles) L(ee)
Casting fillings and abutments for bridges. Dent. Cosmos 38 (1896) 850—860

Allan, George S.
The genesis of contour fillings. Dent. Cosmos 33 (1891) 465—473

Andresen, Viggo
Die Kolloidchemie der Zahnoberfläche. Dtsch. zahnärztl. Wschr. 27 (1927) 165—170

Arkövy, Joseph
Diagnostik der Zahnkrankheiten, Stuttgart 1885

Arthur, Robert
a) A treatise on the use of adhesive gold foil. Philadelphia 1857
b) Obituary. Dent. Cosmos 22 (1880) 437—439

Ash & Sons, Claudius
a) Katalog von künstlichen Zähnen, Instrumenten und Materialien . . . Berlin 1897/98
b) A century of dental Art. London 1921

Barrett, M. T.
a) The protozoa of the mouth in relation to pyorrhea alveolaris. Dent. Cosmos 56 (1914) 948—953
b) Clinical report upon amoebic pyorrhea. Dent. Cosmos 56 (1914) 1345—1350

Behne, E(rnst) A(ugust)
Die Entwicklung zahnärztlicher Bohrantriebe im Maschinenzeitalter. Verh. XX. Internat. Kongr. Gesch. Med. Berlin 1966. Hildesheim 1968, pp. 562—571

Bell, Thomas
The anatomy, physiology and diseases of the teeth. London 1829

Bibby, Basil G.
A test of the effect of fluoride-containing dentrifrices on dental caries. J. Dent. Research 24 (1945) 297—303

Black, Arthur D.
Operative dentistry: A review of the past 75 years. Dent. Cosmos 76 (1934) 43—65

Black, G(reene) V(ardiman)
A work on operative dentistry. 2 vols., Chicago, London 1908

Black, G(reene) V(ardiman) and Frederick S. Mc Kay
Mottled teeth: An endemic imperfection of the enamel of the teeth. Dent. Cosmos 58 (1916) 129—156

Bogue, E. A.
The physical properties and physiological action of dental amalgams. Dent. Cosmos 17 (1875) 118—133

Bremner, M. D. K.
The story of dentistry. Rev. 3rd ed., Brooklyn, London 1964

Breslauer, (Heinrich)
Die Anwendung einer Knochen-Resections-Maschine, insbesondere für zahnärztliche Zwecke . . . Korresp. bl. Zahnärzte 2 (1873) 155—161

Buckley, J(ohn) P(eter)
The chemistry of pulp-decomposition; . . . Dent. Cosmos 47 (1905) 223—229

Bunting, Russel W. et al.
Further studies of the relation of Bacillus acidophilus to dental caries. Dent. Cosmos 70 (1928) 1002—1009

Buzer, Anton
Handbuch der Zahnheilkunde. Berlin 1867

Callahan, John R(oss)
Sulfuric acid for opening root-canals. Dent. Cosmos 36 (1894) 329—331, 957—959

Campbell, J(ohn) Menzies
Dentistry then and now. Glasgow 1963

Christen, Arden G.
Sandford C. Barnum. Bull. Hist. Dent. 25 (1977) 3—9

Churchill, H. V.
Occurence of fluorides in some waters of the United States. Indust. Engin. Chem. News ed. 23 (1931) 996—998

Coleman, (Alfred)
Fletcher's white enamel. Trans. Odont. Soc. G. B. N. S. 5 (1873) 131—138

Cox, Gerald J., Margaret C. Matuschak, Sara F. Dixon, Mary L. Dodds, and W. E. Walker
Experimental dental caries. IV. Fluorine and its relation to dental caries. J. Dent. Research 18 (1939) 481—490

Crichton-Browne, Sir James
An address on tooth culture. The Lancet 70 (1892) Tome II, pp. 6—10

Cruce, Joanne Andrea de
Güldene Werckstatt der Chirurgy oder Wundt-Artzney . . . Franckfort 1607

Dagen, Georges
Documents pour servir à l'histoire de l'art dentaire en France . . . Paris (1926)

Darby, Edwin T(yler)
The relative merits of filling-materials. Dent. Cosmos 36 (1894) 175—181

Dean, H. Trendley
Fluorine and dental caries. Amer. J. Orth. Oral Surg. 33 (1947) 49—67

Delabarre, C(hristophe) F(rançois)
Odontologie, ou observations sur les dents humaines . . . Paris 1815

Denton, George B(ion)
Some interrelations between German and American dentistry, 1800—1914. J. Amer. Dent. Ass. 61 (1960) 587—598

Désirabode, (Malagou) A(ntoine)
Nouveaux éléments complets de la science et de l'art du dentiste. 2 vols., Paris 1843

Donaldson, J. A(rchie)
The development of the application of electricity to dental surgery up 1900. Brit. Dent. J. 109 (1960) 121—131

Dorn, Rudolf
Die Elektrizität und ihre Verwendung in der Zahnheilkunde. Leipzig 1898

Driscoll, W. E.
Fourteen year's recorded experience with alloy fillings. Dent. Cosmos 30 (1888) 602—603

Eager, J. M.
"Chiaie Teeth". Dent. Cosmos 44 (1902) 300—301

Elander, Karl
Eine medikamentöse Pyorrhoetherapie. Korresp. bl. Zahnärzte 46 (1920) 46—60

Erhardt
Kali fluoratum zur Erhaltung der Zähne. Memorabilien (Monatshefte für rationelle Ärzte), Heilbronn 19 (1874) 359—360

Fauchard, Pierre
a) Le chirurgien dentiste. Vol. II, 2nd ed., Paris 1746
b) The Surgeon Dentist. Transl. by Lilian Lindsay. London 1946

Ficinus, Robert
Über das Ausfallen der Zähne und das Wesen der Karies. J. Chir. Augenhk. Berlin 6 (1947) 1—43

Fitch, C(hauncey) P.
Alveolar abscess. Dent. Cosmos 5 (1863) 11—16

Fleischmann, L(eo), B(ernhard) Gottlieb
Beiträge zur Histologie und Pathogenese der Alveolarpyrrhoe. Österr. Zschr. Stomat. 18 (1920) 43—58

Fletcher, Thomas
a) On oxychloride of zinc, and the cements allied to it. Brit. J. Dent. Sc. 16 (1873) 97—99
b) Fletcher's patent porcellain cement. Brit. J. Dent. Sc. 21 (1878) 425—426
c) The chemical and physical effects of fillings upon teeth. Brit. J. Dent. Sc. 24 (1881) 505—507

Flörke, Emil
Welche Erfahrungen sind bislang über die Anwendung des electrischen Motors . . . gemacht worden? Korresp. bl. Zahnärzte 13 (1884) 319—322

Foster, S(heppard) W.
Some of the merits of contour fillings made in the laboratory. Dent. Cosmos 36 (1894) 720—721

Fox, Joseph
The history and treatment of the diseases of the teeth, . . . London 1806

Francis, C. E.
The rubber dam. Dent. Cosmos 7 (1866) 185—187

Gariot, J(ean) B(aptiste)
Traité des maladies de la bouche, Paris 1805

Gins, Heinrich A.
Die übertragbare Zahnfleischentzündung. Stuttgart 1947

Goadby, Kenneth Weldon
The mycology of the mouth. London 1903

Gottlieb, Bernhard
a) Der Epithelansatz am Zahne. Dtsch. Mschr. Zahnheilk. 39 (1921) 142—147
b) Ätiologie und Prophylaxe der Zahnkaries. Österr. Zschr. Stomat. 19 (1921) 142—147

Harrington's "Erado": Korresp. bl. Zahnärzte 2 (1872) 15—16

Harris, Chapin A(aron)
a) The principles and practice of dental surgery. 5th ed., Philadelphia 1853
b) Ibid. 8th ed., Philadelphia 1863

Head, Joseph
Enamel softening and rehardening as a factor in erosion. Dent. Cosmos 52 (1910) 46—48

Held, A(rthur)-J(ean); F. Piquet
Prophylaxie de la carie dentaire par les comprimés fluorés: prémiers résultats. Bull. Schweiz. Akad. med. Wiss. 10 (1954) 249—259

Herbst, Wilhelm
a) Glas as a filling material. (Ash's) Quart. Circ. (1889) 92—93
b) Methoden und Neuerungen auf dem Gebiet der Zahnheilkunde. Berlin (1895)

Hertelendy-Michel, Ingeborg
a) Carl Röse (1864—1947). Zahnärztl. Mitt. 53 (1963) 64—72; 101—104
b) Karl August Lingner-Dresden. Zahnärztl. Mitt. 55 (1965) 22—26; 111—114

Hesse, Liselotte
Die Gebrüder Witzel im Dienst der Zahnheilkunde. Med. Diss. Köln 1953

Hoffmann-Axthelm, Walter
Untersuchungen zum Fluorproblem . . . Leipzig 1959

Holtbuer, Fritz
Herbstsche Neuerungen. Leipzig o. J.

Huet, Emile
a) Amélioration à la technique opératoire par l'usage des moteurs à grande vitesse. L'Odontologie 50 (1913) 147—159
b) Fraises et fraisages. L'Odontologie 61 (1923) 145—158

Jacob (Linderer), Calmann
Bemerkungen über des Herrn Lautenschlägers Zahninstrument . . . J. Chir. Geburtsh. (Loder's J.) 4 (1805) 437—447

Jenkins, N(ewell) S(ill)
Porcelain in dentistry. Dent. Cosmos 47 (1905) 127—134

Karolyi, M(oritz)
a) Beobachtungen über Pyorrhoea alveolaris und Caries dentium. Österr.-ung. Vjschr. Zahnhk. 18 (1902) 520—526
b) Observations on pyorrhoea alveolaris and dental caries. (Ash's) Quart. Circ. (1902) 418—421

Knutson, John W.; Wallace D. Armstrong
The effect of topically applied sodium fluoride on dental caries experience. Pub. Health Rep., (I) 58 (1943) 1071; (II) 60 (1945) 1058—1090

Koecker, Leonhard
Principles of dental surgery, . . . London 1826

Laforgue, L(ouis)
a) L'art du dentiste . . . Paris 1802
b) Die Zahnarzneikunst . . . Transl. C. F. Angermann, Leipzig 1803

Langsdorff, Georg von
a) Neue zahnärztliche Operationsmaschinen. Dtsch. Vjschr. Zahnhk. 13 (1873) 284—287
b) Die zahnärztlichen Schulen in New York und Philadelphia. Dtsch. Vjschr. Zahnhk. 13 (1873) 297—300

Latimer, J. S.
Little things. Dent. Cosmos 6 (1864) 12—14

Lautenschläger, Heinrich
Nachricht von einem neuen Zahninstrument, . . . nebst Beschreibung eines dazu zweckmäßigen Bohrers. J. pract. Heilk., Berlin (Hufeland's J.) 17 (1803) 50—55

Lefoulon, (Pierre) (Joachim)
Nouveau traité théorique et pratique de l'art du dentiste. Paris 1841

Linderer, C(allman) J(acob)
Lehre von den gesamten Zahnoperationen . . . Berlin 1834 (See Jacob)

Linderer, Joseph
a) Handbuch der Zahnheilkunde. 2nd ed., Berlin 1842
b) Handbuch der Zahnheilkunde. Vol. II, Berlin 1848
c) Die Zahnheilkunde nach ihrem neuesten Standpunkte. Erlangen 1851

Lippold, (Georg Wilhelm F.)
Über einige zum Ausfüllen der Zähne zu verwendende Materialien. Der Zahnarzt, Berlin 14 (1859) 113—122

Maar, F. E. R. de
Wie introduceerde het zilveramalgaam in de tandheelkunde? Ned. tschr. Tandheelk. 75 (1968) 313—323; 395—404

Magitot, Emile
a) Traité de la carie dentaire. Paris 1867
b) Expulsive Gingivitis. Summary of Gaz. des Hôp. June 26, in: Dent. Cosmos 22 (1880) 559—560

Maretzky, Kurt
Ewiges Rom. Zahnärztl. Mitt. 45 (1957) 666—673

Maury, C. F.
Traité complet de l'art du dentiste. Nouv. éd. Paris 1833

McKay, Frederick S.
The establishment of the definite relation between enamel that is defective in its structure, as mottled enamel, and the liability of decay. Dent. Cosmos 71 (1929) 747—755

McKay, Frederick S. with G(reene) V(ardiman) Black
Mottled teeth: An endemic imperfection of the enamel of the teeth. Dent. Cosmos 58 (1916) 477—484; 627—644; 781—792; 894—904

Metcalf, Wm. H.
Vitreous fillings. Dent. Cosmos 33 (1891) 848—851

Miller, W(illoughby) D(ayton)
a) Die Mikroorganismen der Mundhöhle. Leipzig 1889
b) The micro-organisms of the human mouth. Philadelphia 1890
c) Lehrbuch der Conservirenden Zahnheilkunde. Leipzig 1896
d) Antiseptische Wirkung des Kupferamalgams. Zahnärztl. Wchbl. 2 (1889) Nr. 38, 4; Nr. 39, 2
e) Preventive treatment of the teeth, with special reference of silver nitrate. Dent. Cosmos 47 (1905) 913—922; Brit. Dent. J. 26 (1905) 641—652

Mills, George A.
Directions as to the treatment of the so-called Riggs Disease . . . Dent. Cosmos 20 (1878) 92—94

Morrison, James Beall
a) Morrison's Operationsstuhl. Dtsch. Vjschr. Zahnhk. 9 (1869) 236—238
b) Dr. Morrison's Bohrmaschine. Korresp. bl. Zahnärzte 2 (1873) 115—116
c) Obituary. Dent. Cosmos 60 (1918) 269—270

Nelsen, Robert J., et al.
Hydraulic turbine contra-angle handpiece. J. Amer. Dent. Ass. 47 (1953) 324—329

Nessel, Franz
a) Handbuch der Zahnheilkunde. Prag 1840
b) Compendium der Zahnheilkunde. Wien 1856

Ollendorf, (Arthur)
Eine neue Methode zur Herstellung von Zahnersatzstücken. Dtsch. Mschr. Zahnhk. 22 (1904) 657—664, 24 (1906) 110—111

Paffenbarger, Georg C., et al.
Dental silicate cements . . . J. Amer. Dent. Ass. 25, I (1938) 32—34

Paulsen, G(erhardt)
Erinnerungen eines alten Zahnarztes. Dtsch. Mschr. Zahnhk. 26 (1908) 369—392

Perry, Safford G(oodwin)
Management of proximate surfaces of bicuspids and molars. Dent. Cosmos 21 (1879) 242—254

Philbrook, B. Frederick
Obituary. J. Amer. Dent. Ass. 19 (1941) 313

Pickerill. H(enry) P(ercy)
The prevention of dental caries and oral sepsis. London 1912

Riechelmann, Otto
Die Solbrig-Zange, ihre Verwendung . . . Dtsch. Mschr. Zahnhk. 26 (1903) 289—299

Riggs, J(ohn) M.
Southern Dent. Ass., 4th annual session. Dent. Cosmos 24 (1882) 524—527

Ritter
1887—1962. Karlsruhe-Durlach

Roberts, Charles H.
Os artificial fillings. Dent. Cosmos 1 (1860) 573—575

Robinson, James
The surgical, mechanical, and medical treatment of the teeth . . . London 1846

Robicsek, S(alomon)
Über doublierte Plomben. Österr.-ung. Vjschr. Zahnhk. 8 (1892) 125—129

Röse, C(arl)
a) On the decay of teeth in the national schools. (Ash's) Quart. Circ. (1895) 1—11; 177—185
b) Die Verbreitung der Zahnverderbnis in Deutschland und den angrenzenden Ländern. Dtsch. Mschr. Zahnhk. 24 (1906) 337—354
c) Erdsalzarmut und Entartung. Dtsch. Mschr. Zahnhk. 26 (1908) 1—31; 131—149; 191—226; 244—275; 321—349; 445—458

Romeick, Dietrich
Die Erfurter Zahnärzte. Erfurt 1968

Rostaing, A., und C. S.
a) Über das unveränderliche und marmorharte Zahncäment von Rostaing. Der Zahnarzt, Berlin 13 (1858) 180—185
b) Patentanmeldungen. Korresp. bl. Zahnärzte 10 (1881) 67—69, 310—312

C(arl) Sauer
Die Rostaing'sche Cementplombe. Dtsch. Vjschr. Zahnhk. 18 (1878) 20—24

Sachs, Hans
Die Behandlung lockerer Zähne nach Younger-Sachs, Berlin 1929

Schneider, Friedrich
Über Zweckmäßigkeit der elektrischen und Wassermotoren. Dtsch. Mschr. Zahnhk. 5 (1887) 387—398

Schreier, Emil
Ein neues, auf chemischer Zersetzung beruhendes Verfahren, den jauchigen Inhalt von Wurzelcanälen unschädlich zu machen. Österr.-ung. Vjschr. Zahnhk. 8 (1892) 119—125

Schreiter, (Richard)
Kalium hydricum, ein empfehlenswertes Mittel . . . Dtsch. Mschr. Zahnhk. 12 (1894) 335—340

Sercombe, Edwin
Description of Dr. Morrison's Dental Engine. Trans. Odont. Soc. G. B. N. S. 5 (1873) 121—130

Serre, Johann Jakob Joseph
Praktische Darstellung aller Operationen der Zahnheilkunst. Berlin 1803

Smith, Margaret Cammack; Edith Lantz; Howard V. Smith
The cause of mottled enamel, a defect of human teeth. Univ. Arizona, Agricult. Exper. Station, Techn. Bull. No. 32, 1931. Ref. in: J. Dent. Research 12 (1932) 119—120

Solbrig, O.
Fabrication des blocs d'or coulés par la méthode de la cire perdue. Rev. Stom., Paris 14 (1907) 340—344, 357 f.

Stock, Alfred
Die Gefährlichkeit des Quecksilberdampfes. Leipzig, Berlin 1926

Taft, J(onathan)
A practical treatise on operative dentistry. Philadelphia 1859

Taggart, William H(enry)
A new and accurate method of making gold inlays. Dent. Cosmos 49 (1907) 1117—1121

Talma, (Amadée [Jules Louis] François)
Von den Gefahren der Anwendung des Silber-Amalgams . . . Der Zahnarzt, Berlin 1 (1846) 23—28

Thorpe, Burton Lee
History of dentistry. Ed. Charles R. E. Koch. Vol. III, Chicago 1906

Toirac, Alphonse
Dissertations sur les dents, . . . Med. Diss. Paris 1823

Tomes, John
a) A system of dental surgery. Philadelphia 1859
b) On certain conditions presented by amalgams used in filling faulty teeth. Trans. Odont. Soc. G. B. 3 (1861—63) 126—138

Townsend, Elisha
On the use of amalgam for filling teeth. Dent. News Letter 9 (1855) 35—40

Velu, H.
Dystrophie dentaire des mammifères des zones phosphatées (Darmous) et fluorose chronique. Compt. rend. Soc. biol. 10 (1931) 750—752

Vinski, Ivo
Two hundred and fifty years of rotary instruments in dentistry. Brit. Dent. J. 146 (1979) 217—223

Volck, Adelbert J.
Filling labial surfaces of upper incisors. Amer. Dent. Sc. 7 (1857) 322—324

Webb, Marshall H.
International Med. Congress: Restoration of contour, and prevention of decay. Dent. Cosmos 23 (1881) 593—596

Weber, J. H. C.
Bemerkungen über den Sorel'schen Kitt und das Kupferamalgam. Der Zahnarzt 14 (1859) 86—87

Weinberger, Bernhard Wolf
An introduction to the history of dentistry. Vols. I and II, St. Louis 1948

Weski, Oskar
Die "Alveolarpyrrhoe" auf der Leipziger Tagung des Zentralvereins. Zahnärztl. Rdsch. 31 (1922) 677—680, 32 (1923) 4—8

Wespi, Hans Jacob
Experiences and problems of fluoridated cooking salt in Switzerland. Arch. oral. Biol. 6 (1961) 33—39

White, J(ohn) D(eHaven)
Amalgam and the late Prof. Townsend. Dent. Cosmos 20 (1878) 351

Witzel, Adolph
a) Die praktische Behandlung exponirter und kauterisirter Pulpen. Dtsch. Vjschr. Zahnheilk. 14 (1874) 434—447
b) Pathologie und Therapie der Pulpakrankheiten des Zahnes. Hagen 1886
c) Das Füllen der Zähne mit Amalgam. Berlin 1899

Wood, B.
Enameling plugs and restoring the contour of defective teeth. Dent. Cosmos 4 (1863) 243—245

Ziegler, E(ugen)
Cariesprophylaxe durch Fluorierung der Milch. Schweiz. Med. Wschr. 83 (1953) 723—724

Chapter 13

Dental Surgery

Tooth Extraction

The earliest mention in our cultural sphere of the extraction of a tooth, offering relief from toothache with relative certainty of success, is surprisingly found only in the Hippocratic writings [1], and is followed with a minute description by the Roman Celsus in the first century A. D. [2]. Two centuries later Galen recommended medicamentous preparation—loosening the tooth with etching agents [3]—a method which was given preference more and more with the hemophobic Islamic physicians. Abulcasim alone represented an exception to this [4]. This etching therapy was adopted by the majority of physicians and surgeons in the Middle Ages. When any of them described the surgical extraction, however, from Guy de Chauliac, who was the first to mention the pelican [5], to Ambroise Paré [6], he adhered to the procedure described by Abulcasim. The actual performance of the procedure, however, until far into modern times remained in the hands of the tooth-drawers and lower barber-surgeons. In the 18th century, Fauchard gave a precise description of instruments used for extracting teeth [7] and the books of Jourdain, also in France, and of Bücking in Germany concerned themselves especially with dental surgery [8].

The 19th century had its beginning in this subject with the book, "Des accidents de l'extraction des dents" (Accidents in the Extraction of Teeth), published in 1802 by the Maître en Chirurgie and dentist Jacques René Duval, the biographer of Jourdain and author of a history of dentistry [9]. Endowed with a rich knowledge of literature, extending from Hippocrates to his own contemporaries, he described all possible complications in 93 well-organized pages, given mostly through quotations but also from personal experience, without anything essentially new. He arrived at the conclusion that accidents were not usually the fault of the well-trained dentist, but rather the result of external circumstances. Therefore the dentist need not have too great a fear of this procedure [10].

The preferred instruments of the first half of the century were pelicans, levers, keys, dental forceps, and curved-shank elevators, the first three of which extensively traumatized the tissue surrounding the tooth (Figs. 369 and 370). In order to eliminate this disadvantage, as already mentioned, almost all authors especially strove to improve the pelican. This instrument was so popular in Germany that in 1781 it served the former regimental medical officer Friedrich Schiller as a metaphor in his play "Die Räuber" (The Robbers) [11].

Mention of it is lacking, however, in the English language literature of the 19th century: Joseph Fox in 1806 limited himself essentially to the key, and Thomas Bell in 1826 restricted himself to the key, the forceps, and the lever [12]. Fox spoke of the "German key", while the surgeon Benjamin Bell claimed the instrument for his own country [13]. Regarding the nomenclature of this key we have been informed by the discussion of Johann Jacob Joseph Serre on page 240 of this book.

Added to this was the *pyramid-shaped root-screw,* also first described by Serre [14] in 1803, and named after him. Although it did not represent any real progress, it is still to be found in the catalogue of 1897 of the Ash Company. As figure 371 shows it is a matter of a dozen threaded screws which, depending on size, are screwed into the remainder of the root. Then, after a handle had been screwed on, it was pulled out much like a corkscrew [15]. The idea of this root-screw was passed along chiefly by Simon P. Hullihen in West Virginia in 1844 [16]. He

1 See p. 63
2 See pp. 70 f.
3 See p. 76
4 See p. 97 f.
5 See pp. 129
6 See p. 147
7 See pp. 201 f.
8 See pp. 214 f. and 232 f.
9 Larrey
10 Duval pp. 90 f.
11 II, 3: "Honesty quavers like a hollow tooth, you need only apply the pelican"
12 Fox pp. 144 f.; Bell pp. 288 f.
13 See p. 222
14 See p. 299
15 Serre pp. 93 f.
16 Hullihen (a)

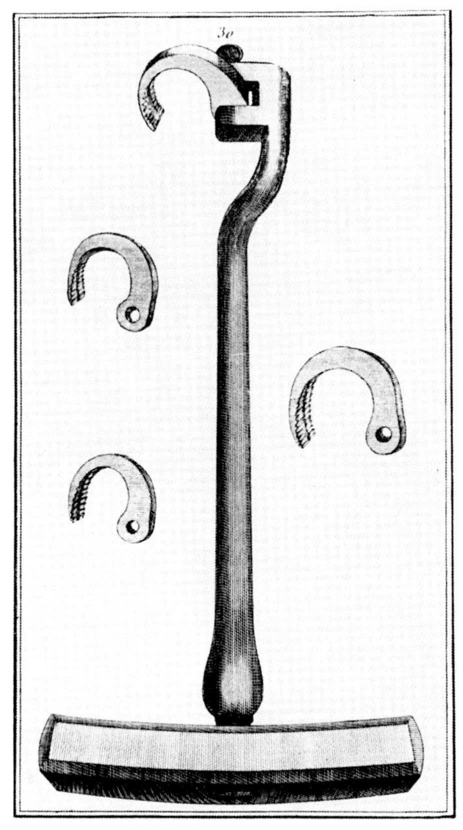

Fig. 369 *Laforgue: Key, 1802*

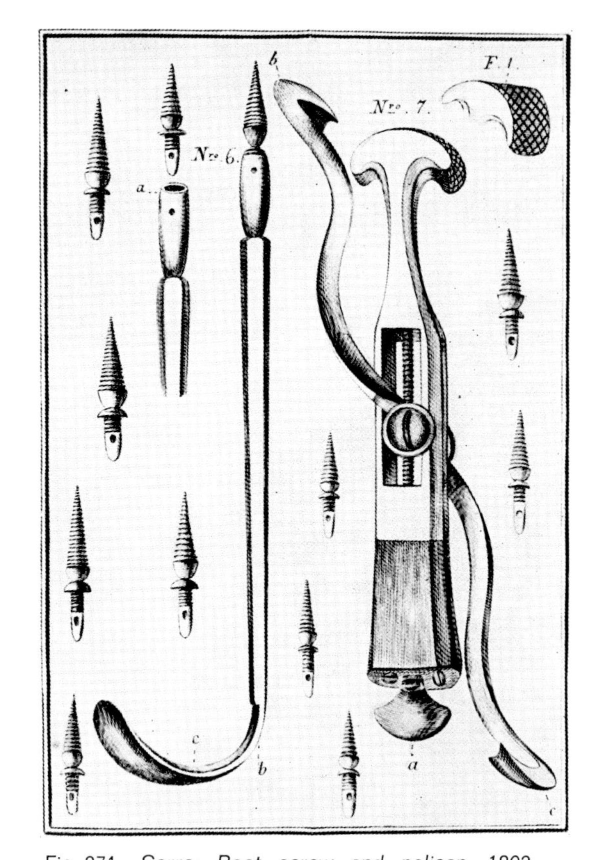

Fig. 371 *Serre: Root screw and pelican, 1803*

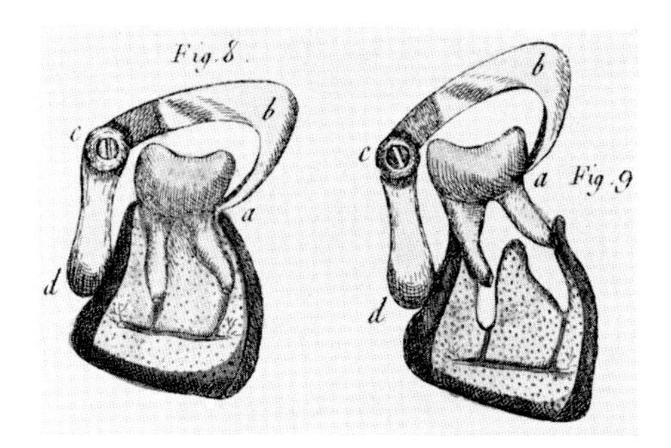

Fig. 370 *Delabarre: Mode of action of the key, 1815*

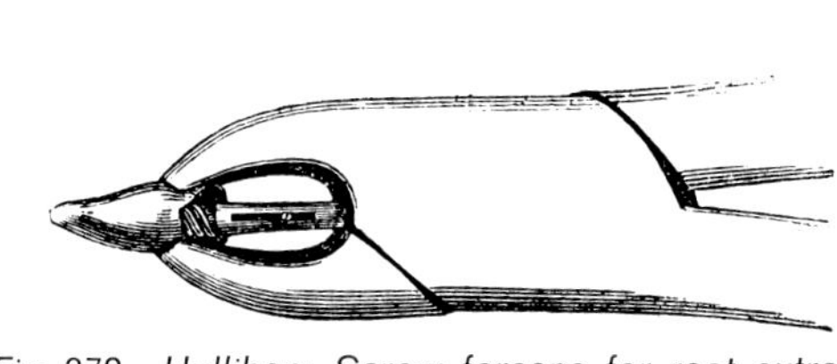

Fig. 372 *Hullihen: Screw forceps for root extraction, 1844*

was the first important oral surgeon in the modern sense (see Fig. 406). For the removal of the roots of maxillary anterior teeth, he combined a screw with a compound root forceps to avoid collapse of the root under the pressure of the forceps (Fig. 372). A combination between forceps and key was mentioned in an essay published in London in 1826 and in Leipzig in 1827 by de la Fons, a dentist active in London[17] (Fig. 373). In 1836 the Berlin dentist Eduard Blume pronounced the lever as antiquated and the pelican as indispensable[18]. Even in 1843 Désirabode

[17] de la Fons pp. 22 f.
[18] Blume p. 129

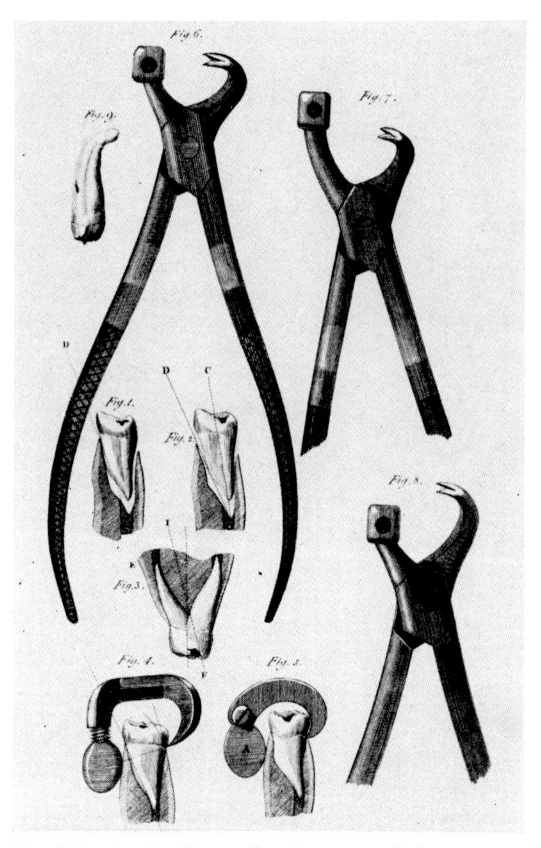

Fig. 373 *de la Fons: Combination of forceps and key, 1825*

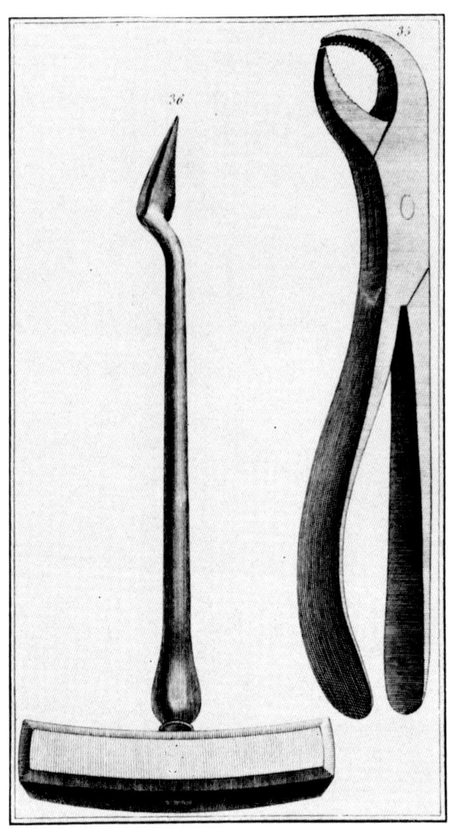

Fig. 374 *Laforgue: Elevator (from Lecluse) and forceps, 1802*

in Paris called the key (clef de Garengeot) the most widely used instrument, which he, however, had personally done without for a long time. The forceps (pince), straight or curved, is used essentially for the anterior teeth, the crow's bill (davier) for the molars, the goat's foot elevator (pied-de-biche) for the roots, and the lever of Lecluse (langue-de-carpe) for the third molars, in all cases in both maxilla and mandible. Désirabode believed that the pelican was no longer in general use except by a few practitioners and in northern Europe[19].

In the forties of this century dental surgery received new impulses on one hand through the introduction of anesthesia and on the other through the development of anatomically shaped forceps by John Tomes in London[20]. If we examine, for example, the forceps of Louis Laforgue of Paris from 1802 (Fig. 374), we see that this type of instrument had undergone few changes since the days of Ambroise Paré, some 250 years before (see Fig. 119).

In the June, 1841 issue of the *London Medical Gazette* Tomes published a paper on the correct construction and use of forceps. At first the contemporary set of instruments is described. As with Thomas Bell, the forceps are for the anterior teeth, the key is for the molars, and the elevator if all else fails. It is to be noted that Tomes decisively rejects the key. Especially, however, he finds the forceps insufficient. They should grip the tooth only, and the force should be brought to bear in the axis of the tooth. For each group of teeth, therefore, a forceps must be available which corresponds

[19] Désirabode (a) pp. 426 f.
[20] See pp. 391 f.

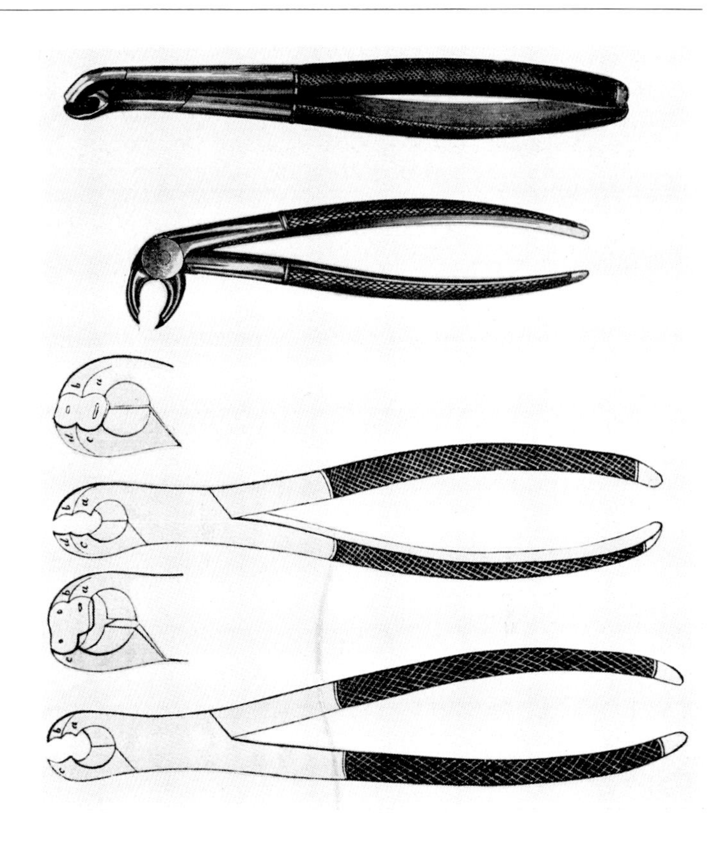

Fig. 375 *Tomes: Sketches and finished design of the forceps, 1841*

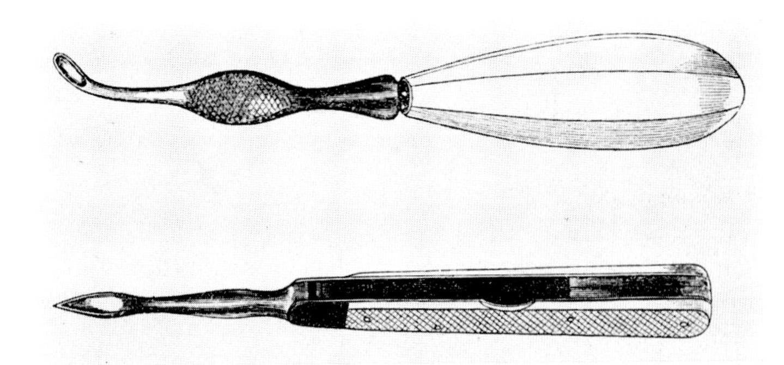

Fig. 376 *Tomes: Elevator, 1859*

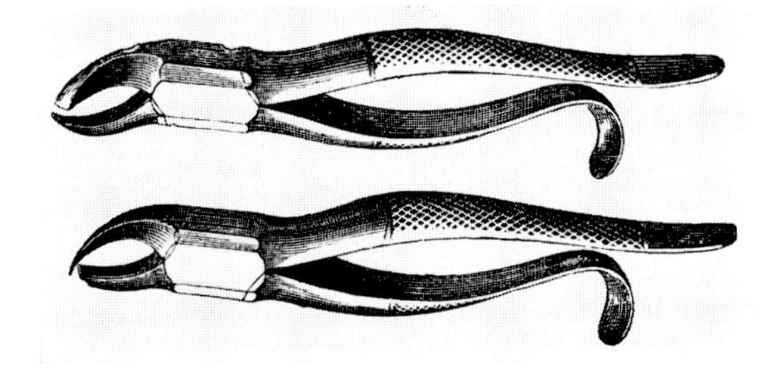

Fig. 377 *Forceps handles of Read (Ash catalogue, 1898)*

to their anatomical shape. *Forceps should be constructed and used upon the principle of lengthening the tooth for the extraction of which they are intended; thus enabling the operator to move it from side to side, or rotate it if the fang be single, and of a shape admitting of such motion. After these lateral movements have been produced the tooth may, unless the fangs have some peculiar position or shape, be raised in a perpendicular direction, leaving as little injury from its removal as the operation can admit*[21].

According to his own principles Tomes constructed a set of anatomically shaped forceps, and therewith elevated this device, which had been neglected up to that point, to dentistry's most important extraction instrument today (Fig. 375). It was a specially fortunate circumstance that he found a superb instrument maker in Jean-Marie Evrard, born in Toulouse and a former student of the famous Charrière in Paris who had been working in London since 1837. For the removal of roots Tomes later recommended the straight and curved levers in his textbook of 1859 (Fig. 376).

Tomes' forceps shapes retained their validity for the entire century. Recommended improvements, such as the bent-down handle, found no lasting acceptance (Fig. 377). After an even closer physical contact of the gripping devices on the cervix of the tooth was achieved (Berten 1905), the dental forceps had reached the form in which they have been used ever since.

Elimination of Pain

Thanks to local anesthesia, tooth extraction today has developed from a forced and by no means always completely performed procedure into a systematically planned operation generally performed independent of the reaction of the patient. It was precisely through this procedure, however, that general narcosis began with its dramatic attendant circumstances in the forties of the 19th century. The initiators of this idea, which was later to become far more important for general surgery than for dentistry, were two North American dentists.

To be sure, for millenia there had been no lack of attempts at least to limit the sensation of pain in operative procedures. Extracts from mandragora root, poppy juice, and alcoholic tinctures had already been administered in ancient times (Fig. 378), and since the early Middle Ages in the so-called sleeping sponges. As we have read, fumigation with henbane seeds served simultaneously for combating toothache and the toothworm (Fig. 379). The extraction itself, however, usually was carried out without anesthesia in accord with the minor extent of the procedure, and as a result consisted often enough only of breaking the tooth and leaving the root behind.

The agents used to achieve narcosis had been discovered long before. Ether is mentioned from the 16th century on, and laughing gas had been prepared in 1776 by the English chemist Joseph Priestley.

In England, the chemist Humphrey Davy had already ascertained the anesthetic effect of nitrous oxide and ether at the turn of the 19th century, as did his student, Michael Faraday, in 1818. In 1824 Henry Hill Hickman, an English surgeon, had operated on experimental animals painlessly in an atmosphere high in carbon dioxide, although the surgeons did not take advantage of this discovery. Ether and laughing gas reached the point of practical application via the detour of charlatans' exhibitions, and one of the first painlessly performed operations was, to the best of our knowledge, a tooth extraction.

In the United States, particularly in small towns and in the country, itinerant "chemistry professors" gave popular lectures about gases. These were followed by demonstrations of the enlivening effect of laughing gas, and more rarely, of the intoxicating effect of ether. Soon, this latter part became an end in itself: people amused themselves at "laughing-gas parties" and "ether frolics," which were, of course, appropriately publicized by the demonstrators (Figs. 380 and 381). Lyman reported in 1881 that William E. Clarke, a student of chemistry in Rochester, New York, had amused his fellow students with "ether entertainments" in 1839, a performance he continued later as a student at Berkshire Medical College. After returning to Rochester, he performed the first ether narcosis on the basis of his experiences: in January of 1842 he laid a towel soaked with ether over the face of a young woman, one Miss Hobbie, whereupon Elijah Pope, a dentist, was able to remove a tooth painlessly[22].

[21] Tomes (a); (b) pp. 547 f.; Cope p. 21
[22] Lyman p. 6

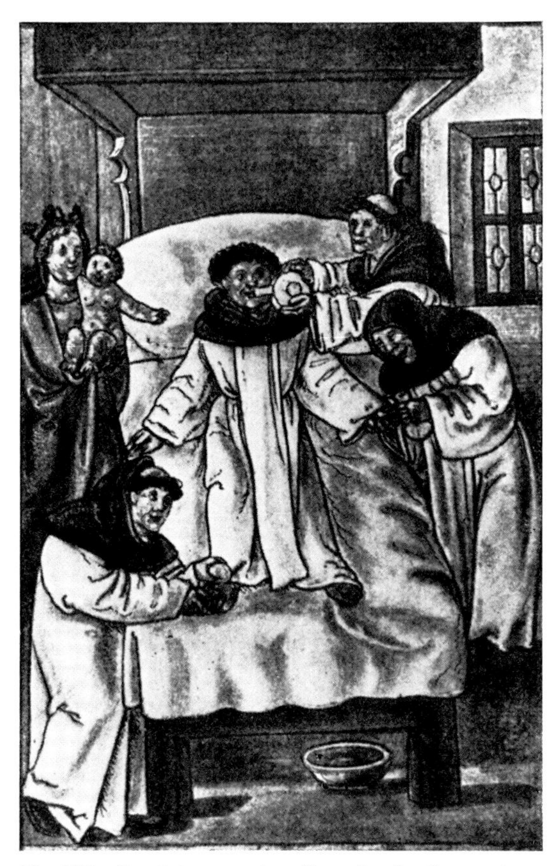

Fig. 378 *Dominican monks offer a lay brother a sleeping potion (Lucerne 1593)*

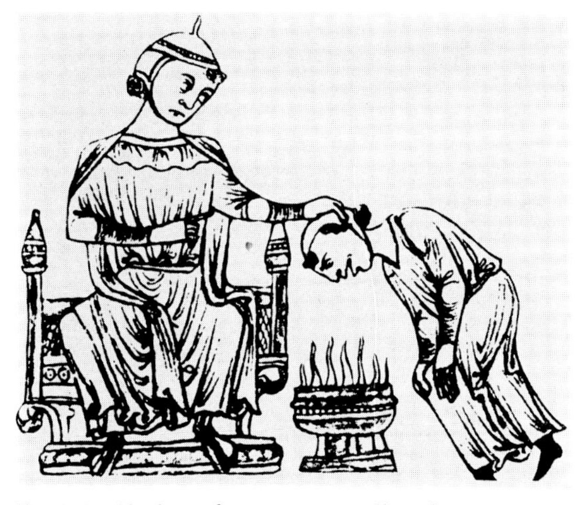

Fig. 379 *Henbane fumigation in a French commentary of the 13th century (Cambridge, Trinity College Ms. 0, I 20; see Figs. 89 to 91)*

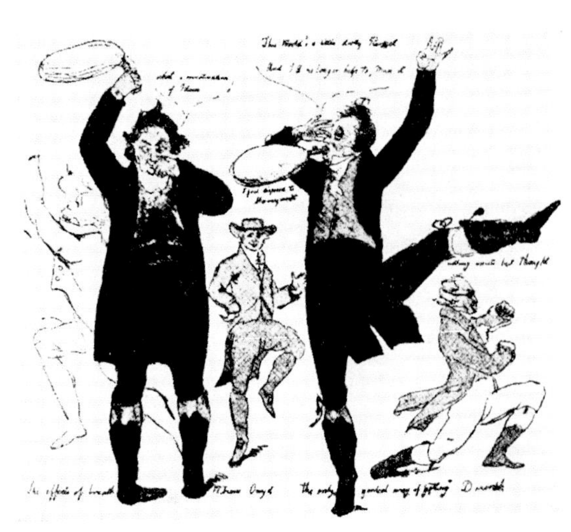

Fig. 380 *Laughing gas party*

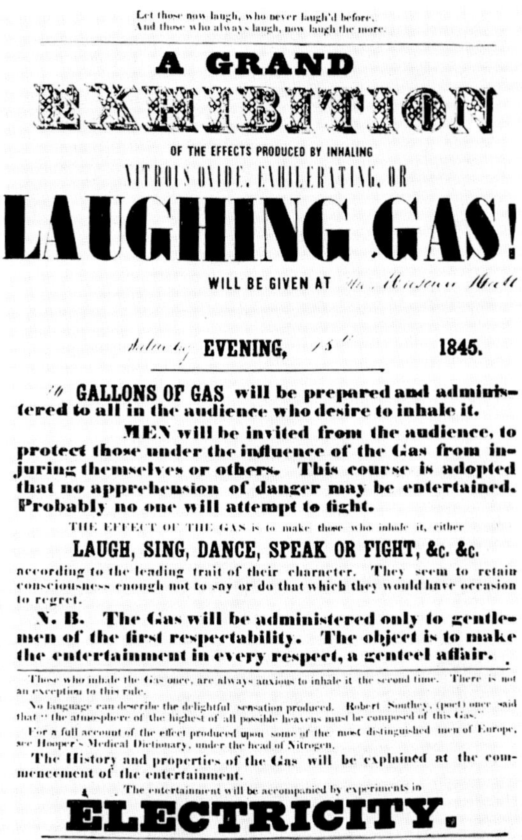

Let those now laugh, who never laugh'd before,
And those who always laugh, now laugh the more.

A GRAND

EXHIBITION

OF THE EFFECTS PRODUCED BY INHALING

NITROUS OXIDE, EXHILERATING, OR

LAUGHING GAS!

WILL BE GIVEN AT

EVENING, 1845.

GALLONS OF GAS will be prepared and administered to all in the audience who desire to inhale it.

MEN will be invited from the audience, to protect those under the influence of the Gas from injuring themselves or others. This course is adopted that no apprehension of danger may be entertained. Probably no one will attempt to fight.

THE EFFECT OF THE GAS is to make those who inhale it, either

LAUGH, SING, DANCE, SPEAK OR FIGHT, &c. &c.

according to the leading trait of their character. They seem to retain consciousness enough not to say or do that which they would have occasion to regret.

N. B. The Gas will be administered only to gentlemen of the first respectability. The object is to make the entertainment in every respect, a genteel affair.

Those who inhale the Gas once, are always anxious to inhale it the second time. There is not an exception to this rule.

No language can describe the delightful sensation produced. Robert Southey, (poet) once said that "the atmosphere of the highest of all possible heavens must be composed of this Gas."

For a full account of the effect produced upon some of the most distinguished men of Europe, see Hooper's Medical Dictionary, under the head of Nitrogen.

The History and properties of the Gas will be explained at the commencement of the entertainment.

The entertainment will be accompanied by experiments in

ELECTRICITY.

ENTERTAINMENT TO COMMENCE AT 7 O'CLOCK.

TICKETS CENTS,

For sale at the principal Bookstores, and at the Door.

Fig. 381 *Announcement of a laughing gas party, 1845*

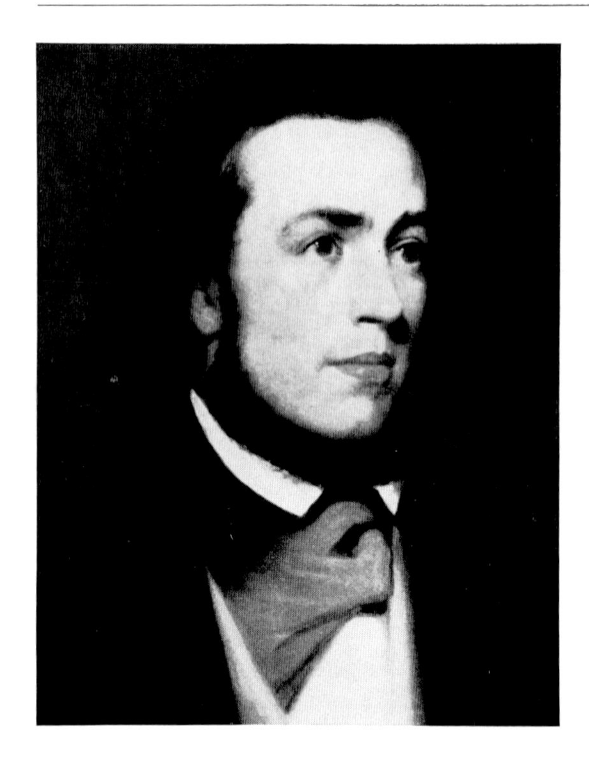

Fig. 382 *Horace Wells (anonymous painting, Hunt Memorial Medical Society, Hartford, Connecticut)*

The next ether narcosis was carried out two months later—totally independent—on March 30, 1842 by Crawford William Long, a physician in Jefferson, Georgia, who removed a tumor on the neck. This narcosis, too, was inspired by an "ether frolic," in which not Long, but the patient had participated [23].

Neither Clarke nor Long recognized then the significance of their discovery. Long, who had undertaken several other operations under the effect of ether, reported it, but only in 1849, after ether narcosis had become widely known.

In 1844, two years after these first anesthesias, a dentist in Hartford Connecticut, Horace Wells (Fig. 382), was present at a "laughing-gas party" given with nitrous oxide by Gardner Quincy Colton, an unsuccessful medical student. He noticed that a friend who had been actively inhaling the gas, was led by the intoxication to run into a bench. Then, however, he was animated by the trauma without feeling the certainly considerable pain, and sat down next to him again. Wells suddenly saw the light and visited a former student, Riggs, who was later a periodontal specialist [24]. He made an appointment with him for the next day for the extraction of one of his own teeth under the influence of laughing gas. In the presence of the demonstrator Colton, who provided a pouch of gas, the man who had hurt himself and two further witnesses, Riggs painlessly extracted an upper left molar from his colleague on December 11, 1844. When Wells awoke, according to Riggs' description of 1885, he cried out, *A new era in tooth-pulling!* [25] Wells successfully repeated the process in numerous cases, but when friends advised him to claim a patent he is said to have answered: *No, let it be free as the air* [26].

Another student and former associate of Wells, William Thomas Green Morton (Fig. 383), who was working in Boston, is said to have arranged a demonstration for Wells before the outstanding surgeon of Boston, John Collins Warren. The fact is that this failed, because the patient was apparently resistent to narcosis. The highly

23 Keys p. 22
24 See p. 317
25 Riggs
26 Bremner p. 185

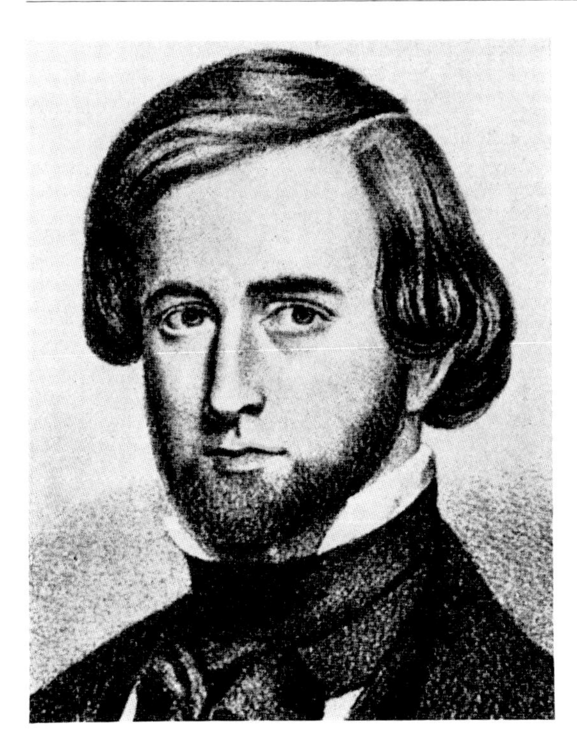

Fig. 383 *W. G. T. Morton*

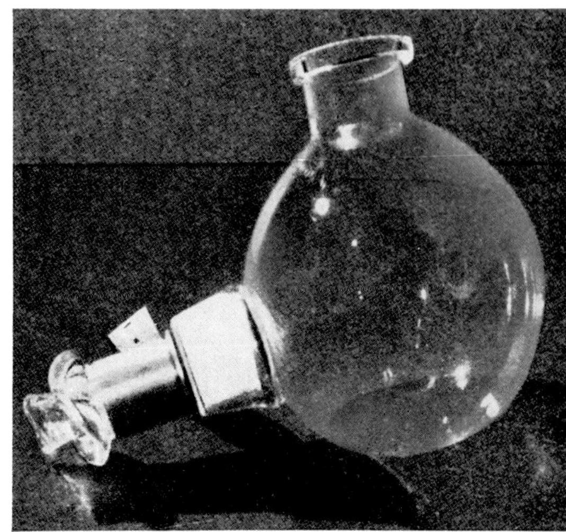

Fig. 384 *Morton's anesthesia apparatus*

sensitive Wells could not recover from this misfortune and the scorn and mockery that resulted from it. He worked fanatically on the perfection of nitrous oxide anesthesia, not only on patients but also through experiments on himself. In this way he became addicted, exhausted himself in his struggle for complete recognition of his priority, and finally, under the most unlucky circumstances, ended his own life in a New York detention cell: under a chloroform narcosis which he had induced himself, he severed his tibial artery on January 24, 1848, leaving behind a moving farewell letter to his wife [27].

Morton did not abandon the idea of eliminating pain, particularly since Wells' successes were by no means unknown to him. Also present at the unsuccessful demonstration was the geologist and chemist Charles Thomas Jackson, who is said to have recommended to Morton the use of ether as confirmed by Riggs in 1885. Morton tested this narcotic agent immediately and successfully on September 30, 1846, during a tooth extraction. As he was of a completely different disposition than Wells he applied for a patent together with Jackson in Washington on October 27. This was not, however, granted because despite all possible aromatic additives his mysterious "Letheon" was immediately recognizable as ether. Further supported by Jackson he undertook experiments on animals, patients, and himself. In place of the handkerchief soaked in ether used until that time, he constructed a first anesthesia apparatus, a glass balloon with a mouthpiece, in which pieces of sponge saturated with the medication were placed (Fig. 384). The demonstration before Warren in the Boston Hospital on October 16, which the students expected to be as amusing as the one by the unfortunate Wells, was a complete success. Warren removed a tumor of the neck, without the patient emitting the usual cry of pain, and then, in the silent pause which followed, said *Gentlemen, this is no humbug!* [28] (Fig. 385). A newspaper report in the *Boston Daily Advertiser* by an eyewitness, Henry J. Bigelow, sent by his father, reached London on December 17, 1846. On the 19th of December, the dentist James

[27] Raper (a) p. 123
[28] Raper (a) p. 92

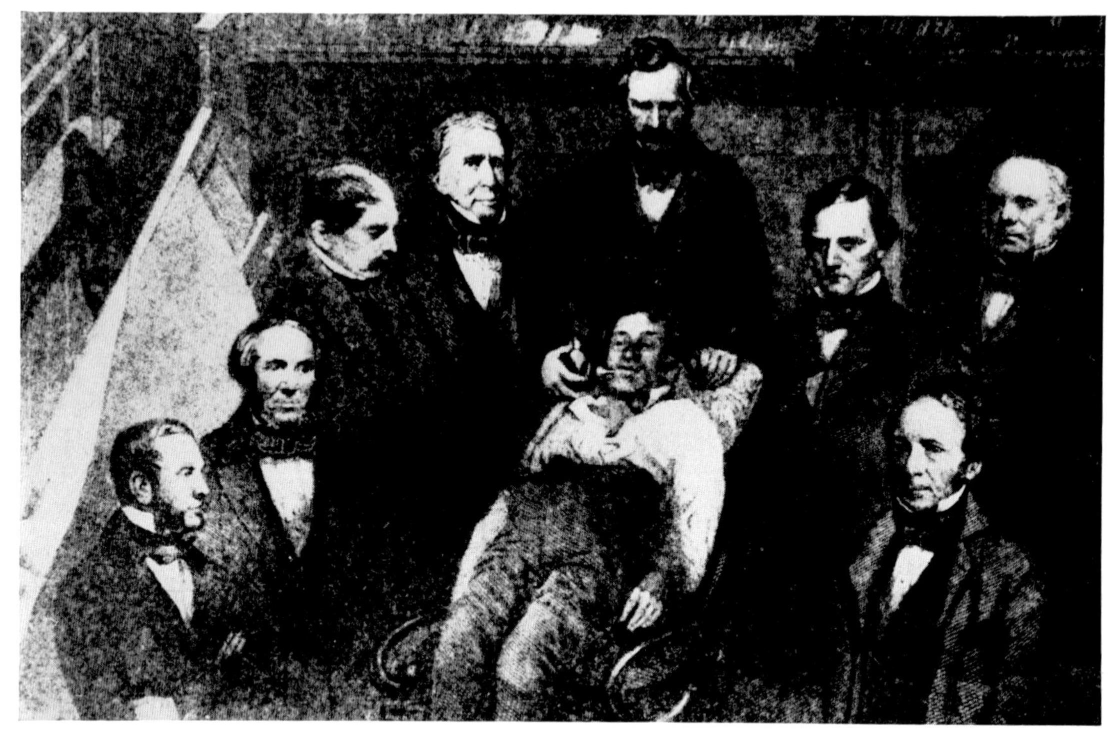

Fig. 385 *Morton's ether anesthesia, 1846; left of Morton, acting as anesthetist, is the surgeon, Warren; Bigelow far left*

Robinson (Fig. 386), who had just published his textbook[29], there extracted a molar from a Miss Lonsdale in what was the first European anesthesia[30]. Two days afterwards Robert Liston, a London surgeon, undertook a femoral amputation and evulsion of the great toe nails, *one of the most painfull operations in surgery,* with ether narcosis. The Parisian surgeon Malgaigne was the first to follow on the continent, and he was followed in turn by physicians in Bern, Erlangen, Vienna, and other cities, all at about the same time, in January of 1847[31].

After the surgeons came the dentists. In 1847, the Berlin professional journal, *Der Zahnarzt* (The Dentist) reported on the extraction of a molar under the influence of ether on January 24, by two physicians in Leipzig, and then, in the April edition, on four patients treated by one dentist in Berlin. We read of a complete freedom from pain, *although complete unconsciousness did not occur in any of these cases*[32]. The procedure had thus been performed, as it still occurs when ether is used today, in the first (analgesic) stage. In an appendix to his 1848 textbook, the dentist Joseph Linderer already described in considerable detail the *Anesthesia with sulphuric ether,* and shows his apparatus, which also worked with pieces of sponge[33] (Fig. 387). In 1856, Friedrich Turnovsky, a physician and dentist of Budapest, who had been a student of Carabelli, showed a picture of what, according to him, was the first anesthetic apparatus developed in Hungary[34] (Fig. 388).

In the meantime a bitter struggle over priority between Morton and Jackson waged with all possible means, in which Horace Wells also took part timidly until his death. As a result of this Morton became a poor man. His colleagues incomprehensibly opposed both the principle of narcosis and him. Many physicians joined this movement, and clerical circles damned the man who had dared to eliminate

[29] See p. 263
[30] Robinson (a)
[31] Walser
[32] Der Zahnarzt 2 (1847): 95 and 128
[33] Linderer (a) p. 484 f.
[34] Turnovsky p. 69

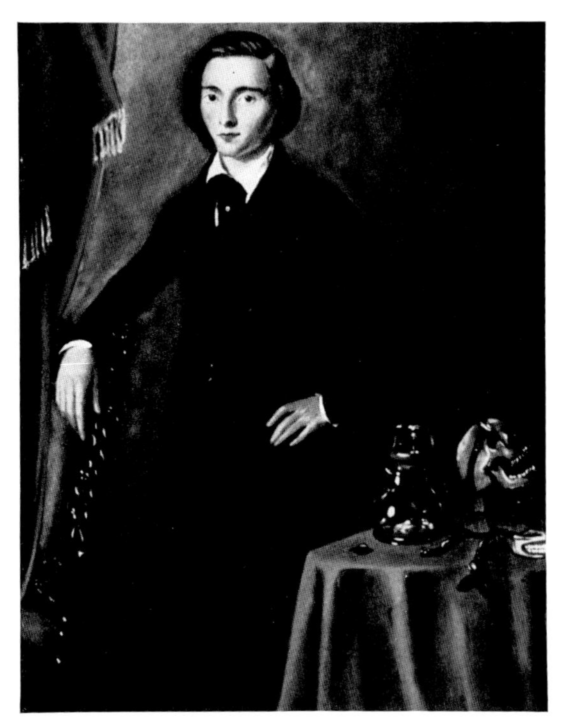

Fig. 386 *James Robinson with his anesthesia apparatus, 1849 (Painting by Alexander Richardson, Meibauer Collection, New York; from Proskauer and Witt)*

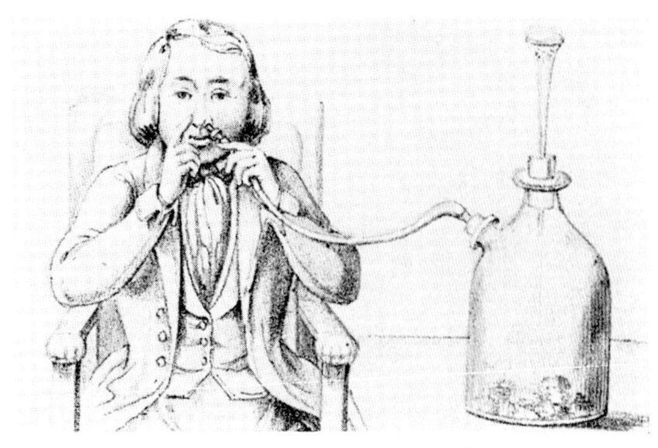

Fig. 387 *Joseph Linderer: Ether ancsthesia apparatus, 1848*

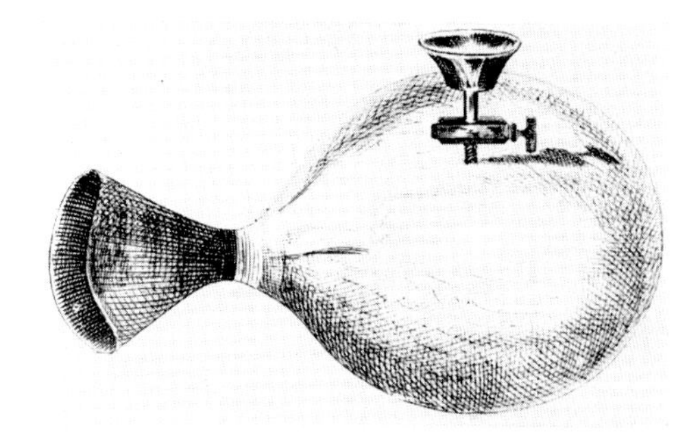

Fig. 388 *Turnovsky: Ether anesthesia apparatus made of a steer bladder, 1856*

the "pain ordained by God." Thus, he was found dying in New York's Central Park on July 15, 1868 [35]. His opponent, Jackson, died in 1880 after years of residence in an insane asylum, while the first user of narcosis, Long, had already passed on in 1878 of paralysis. In London also, James Robinson, the personal dentist to the Prince Consort Albert, who had first tested ether narcosis in Europe, also died under unusual circumstances: in 1862, while working in the garden, he injured himself in the thigh with a knife that slipped and bled to death on the following day [36].

In November of 1847, the Edinburgh gynecologist James Young Simpson introduced chloroform, which was considerably faster and more pleasant in effect as a narcotic agent. Soon, however, the first deaths occurred, and the dangers of the new agent were recognized in dental circles too. Therefore, despite the many advantages, chloroform did not completely eliminate ether, which was advocated chiefly by Warren in Boston. In 1851, Linderer wrote that chloroform *has completely displaced ether for now,* but advised against its use in persons *who have a defect of the lungs or heart.* Like many of his contemporaries Linderer also used chloroform as a local anesthetic through application of cotton saturated with it to both sides of the tooth. *It really seems that the sensitivity is less in many cases,* a point on which we completely agree with him, not because of the local effect, but rather as a result of the chloroform inhaled in the process [37].

Not until 18 years after Wells' unfortunate demonstration was the relatively harmless laughing-gas introduced, just by the same Colton (Fig. 389) who had indirectly provided the stimulus for Wells' self-experiment. Meanwhile Colton had continued to offer his entertainments and had always told the story of the painless tooth extraction. As a result an elderly lady in New Haven, Connecticut, was motivated to have some of her teeth removed while under the influence of nitrous oxide in

[35] Raper (a) p. 179
[36] Robinson (b)
[37] Linderer (b) p. 175 f.

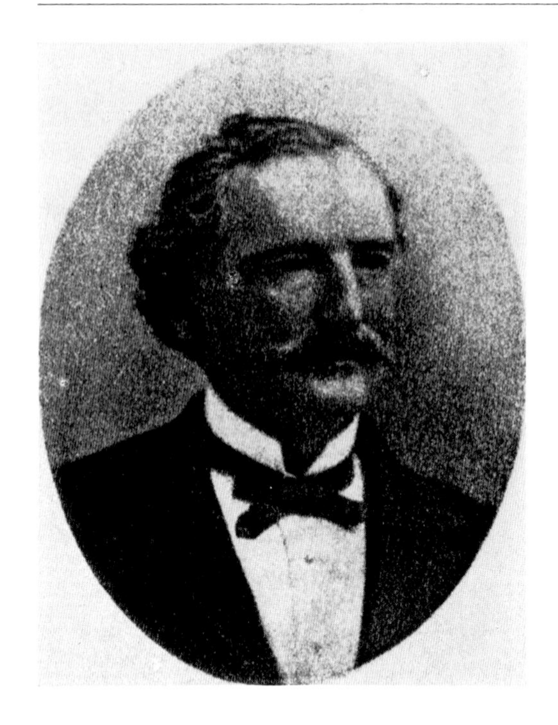

Fig. 389 *Gordon Quincy Colton*

1862. The experiment succeeded completely, and Colton thereafter included tooth extractions in his program. Soon people came in hordes, simply to have their teeth pulled painlessly. Recognizing the opportunity, he opened *an institution in New York, which is still flourishing today, in which Colton gave the gas and his assistants extracted teeth* (as reported in 1896 [38]). Colton died at the age of 85 in 1898 in Rotterdam, while on a European journey [39]. In 1877 it was reported that he and his co-workers had administered the gas to 92,000 persons without incident [40]. After the construction of repeatedly improved apparatuses, nitrous oxide slowly succeeded as the leading anesthetic in dental practice, particularly in the United States. Still, European dentists as well, including, for example, the prominent Parisian dentist Pierre-Apollonie Préterre [41], who was the co-founder of the first French dental journal, *Art dentaire,* in 1857, also were engaged in it (Figs. 390 and 391).

The development of endotracheal narcosis was of decisive importance, especially for modern oral surgery, because of the elimination of the danger of aspiration in operations in the oral cavity. The Leipzig surgeon Friedrich Trendelenburg in 1871 was the first to introduce a tube through a tracheal incision into a person's trachea for the purpose of narcosis. The tube was wrapped in an inflatable rubber sleeve to seal it off against infiltrating blood (Fig. 392). It is said that the Englishman John Snow, who had been working as a specialist in anesthesiology in London since 1847 and who, near the end of his life, had reported about 867 chloroform narcoses for tooth extractions [42], had carried out animal experimentations in this manner. In 1878, after preparatory experiments on corpses, William MacEwen, a surgeon in Glasgow, used the path through the oral cavity [43]. Intubation narcosis first became feasible in 1903, when Franz Kuhn, a surgeon in Kassel, developed a flexible tube made of metal spirals, which was inserted into the trachea with a mandrel through the mouth or nose (Fig. 393). After the lumen was packed and sealed around the

38 Geist-Jacobi p. 182
39 McNeille
40 Macintosh p. 7; Colton
41 Préterre pp. 158 f.
42 Snow p. 314
43 MacEwen

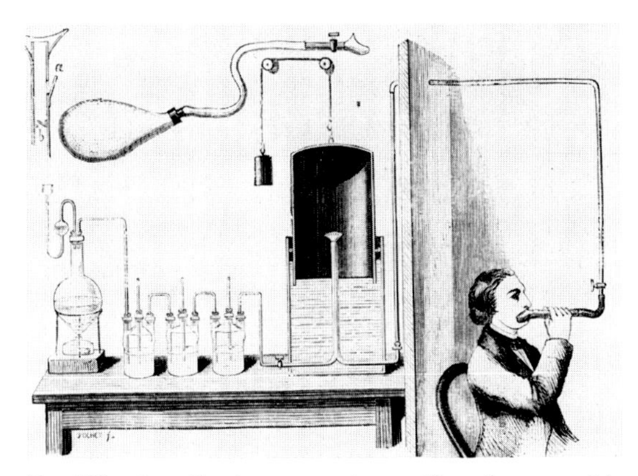

Fig. 390 *Anesthesia apparatus with nitrous oxide generator (from Préterre, 1872, p. 245)*

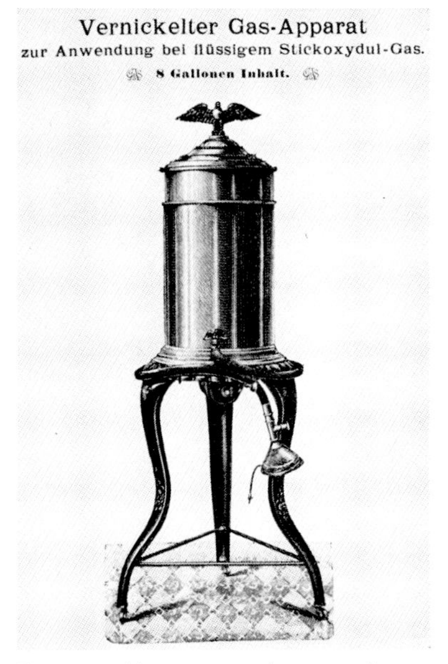

Fig. 391 *Nitrous oxide anesthesia apparatus (Ash catalogue, 1898)*

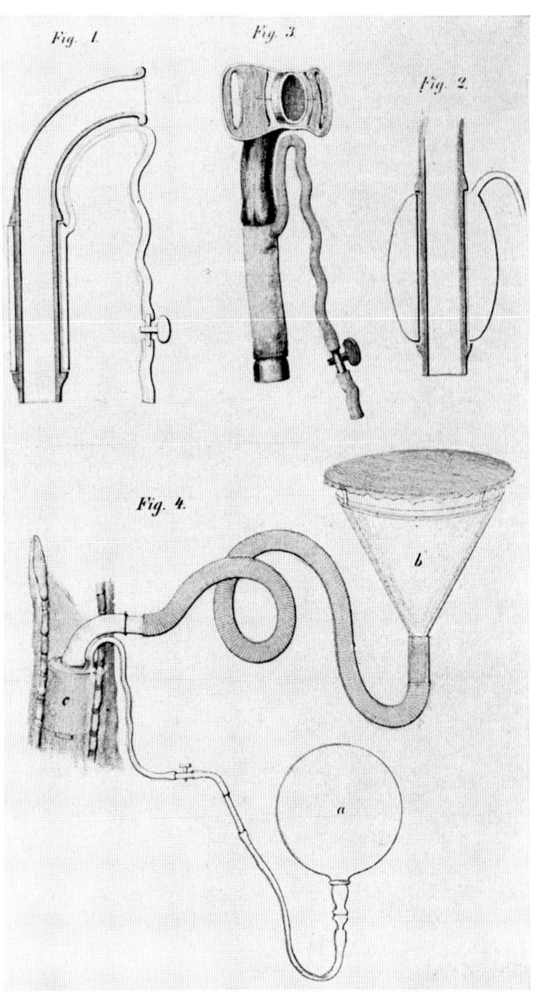

Fig. 392 *Trendelenburg: Endotracheal anesthesia via a tracheal incision, 1871*

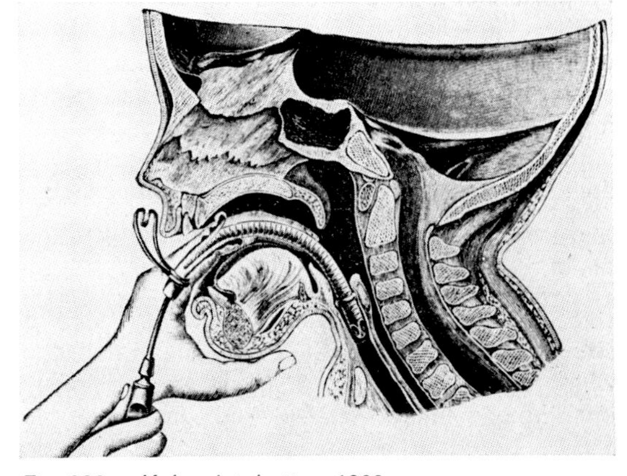

Fig. 393 *Kuhn: Intubation, 1903*

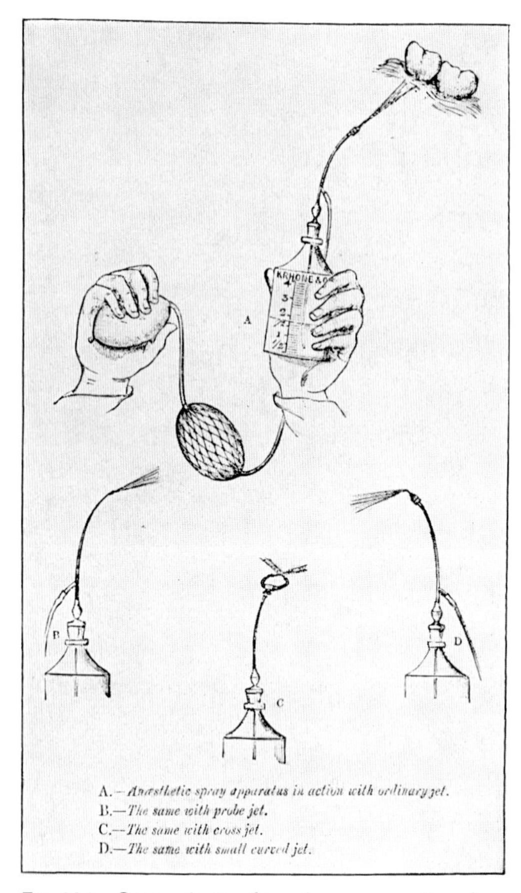

Fig. 394 *Spray device for ether evaporation, from Richardson, 1866*

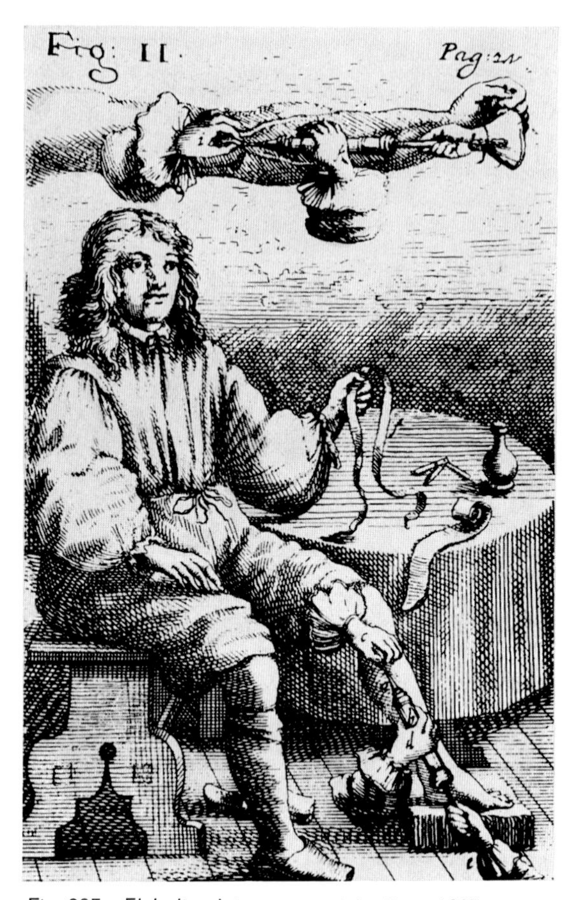

Fig. 395 *Elsholtz: Intravenous injection, 1667*

tube extensive procedures such as resections of the maxilla could then be performed without danger under a deep narcosis [44].

In the eighties ethyl bromide and ethyl chloride were introduced; they are only suitable for short-term narcoses, however. Because of its rapid effectiveness ethyl chloride came into vogue as a preliminary for ether narcosis, while dentists availed themselves of its intense cold of evaporation, which had been recommended by Camille Redard, the first professor of operative dentistry at Geneva's Ecole dentaire, since 1888. Ethyl chloride quickly induces a circumscribed freezing of the mucus membrane which allows, for example, an almost painless opening of submucosal abscesses. Previously, in 1866, Benjamin Ward Richardson in London had tried with less success to develop a freezing anesthesia with an ether spray and had recommended an appropriate apparatus for the purpose [45] (Fig. 394).

This search for new ways originated primarily from the fact that a relatively large number of untoward incidents were occurring in tooth extractions, particularly under chloroform narcosis. This was therefore, justifiably regarded, as too dangerous a manipulation for such a trivial procedure. In the meantime, however, the basis for modern local anesthesia had been created through the construction of suitable injection syringes and the development of corresponding drugs.

[44] Trendelenburg; Kuhn
[45] Richardson

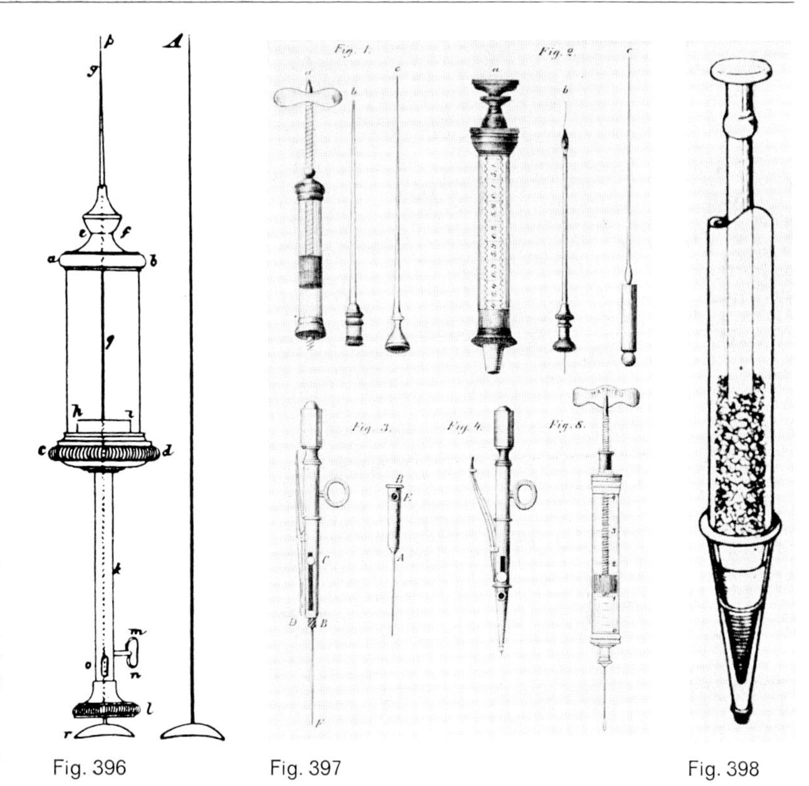

Fig. 396 *Neuner: Stylet syringe, 1827*

Fig. 397 *1: Syringe, from Pravaz; 2: Luer syringe; 3 and 4: Rynd syringes; 8: syringe from Mathieu*

Fig. 398 *Ferguson's syringe, approximately 1850*

Fig. 396 Fig. 397 Fig. 398

Initially, the injection syringe was nothing more than a dainty variation of the enema syringe which had been well-known for a long time. We find it represented in 1667 in the book "Clysmatica nova," by Johann Sigismund Elsholtz, the personal physician in Berlin to the Great Elector. He was preceded in 1656 in London by the builder of the Cathedral of St. Paul, Sir Christopher Wren, whose experiments on animals were performed with an animal's bladder and a quill as an injection instrument. Elsholtz had been performing intravenous injections and transfusions from man to man with a syringe for medical purposes since 1664 [46] (Fig. 395). In 1667 he was followed by Jean Baptiste Denis in Paris, and by Carlo Fracassati in Pisa. Experiments of this nature were, of course, made possible only through Harvey's discovery of the blood-circulation (1628).

In 1827 we find a "Stiletto syringe" which already seems quite functional, pictured in the *Journal der Chirurgie* by the Chief Physician of Darmstadt, A. Neuner (Fig. 396). He had constructed it for the *production of cataracts in dead eyes* [47].

In 1853, the Lyon surgeon Charles Gabriel Pravaz publicly announced a syringe with a screw for measured injections, which became so popular that in the 19th century people generally mentioned only the Pravaz syringe. The manufacturer of this syringe is said to have been the German instrument maker Luer, who was working in Paris, and later introduced under his own name a product with a graduated cylinder and no screw (Fig. 397). The first subcutaneous injections for the relief of pain may have been performed by the Irish physician Francis Rynd in 1845 and in 1853 by the Scot Alexander Wood with a syringe constructed in London by a Mr. Ferguson [48] (Fig. 398). Both of them administered morphine solutions to eliminate pain of neuralgic problems, whereby Wood soon observed that the alleviation of

[46] Elsholtz pp. 21 f.
[47] Neuner
[48] Artelt (a)

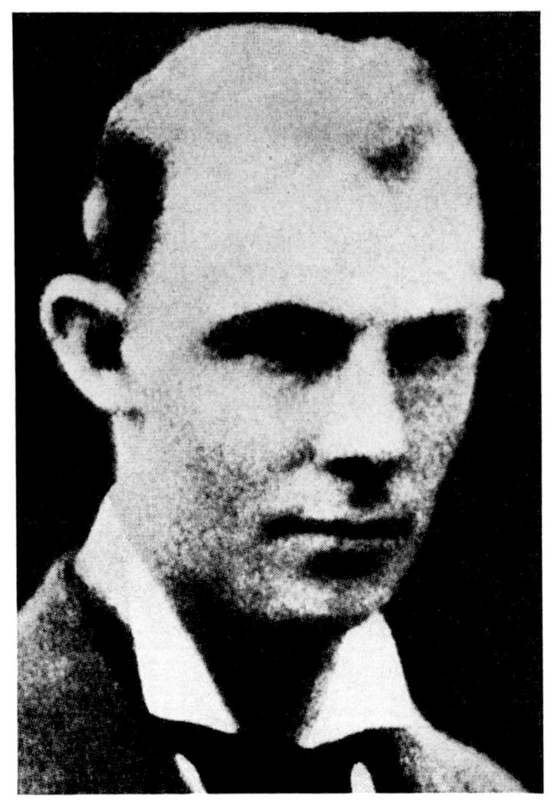

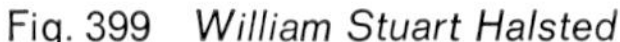

Fig. 399 *William Stuart Halsted*

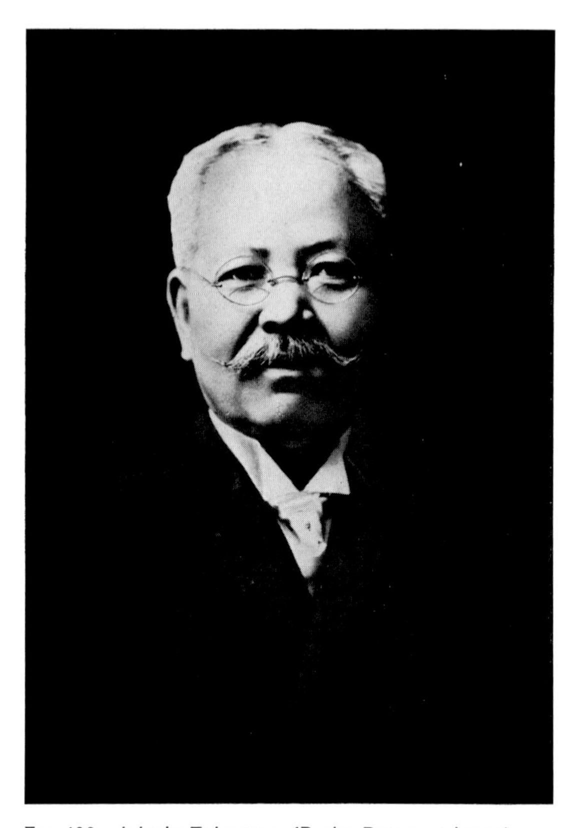

Fig. 400 *Jokichi Takamine (Parke-Davis archives)*

pain was caused not by the local effect on the trunk of the nerve, but rather by the overall effect on the central nervous system. In the sixties, after extensive experimentation and discussion, dentists also recognized that local morphine injections for tooth extractions had not fulfilled their expectations.

Meanwhile a young chemist in Göttingen, Albert Niemann, had isolated the principal alkaloid of the South American coca bush from its leaves in 1860, as the result of a dissertation assigned to him by Friedrich Woehler, the discoverer of urea synthesis. Niemann suggested the name "Cocain" for it[49]. In 1868 the Peruvian General Surgeon Thomas Moréno y Maiz believed to recognize a certain anesthetic effect, but not until 1884, after many probing experiments, the Viennese ophthalmologist Carl Koller made this highly effective remedy available to the practical use. Koller had received the suggestion from Sigmund Freud, who had occupied himself initially with research into the known but poorly evaluated cocaine, but was then devoted completely to psychoanalysis. When the instillation of a 2 % cocaine solution into the conjunctival sack of the eye was demonstrated at the Ophthalmological Congress in Heidelberg on September 15, 1884[50], it stimulated especially the American surgeons and dentists to reexamine the agent. As early as October 20, the dentist of New York J. Morgan Howe was inserting a 2 % cocaine solution with varying success in cavities to be prepared. In the beginning of November, the application of cocaine proved to be effective in the hands of Milwaukee Dentist John Carmichael in the opening of a submucosal abscess and in the fitting of coronal rings. A previously neglected publication in 1880 by the physiologist Vasili Con-

49 Niemann p. 508
50 Koller

stantinovich von Anrep of Würzburg also was rediscovered[51]. According to this, he had obtained a temporary *insensitivity to relatively sharp needle punctures* after injecting a weak cocaine solution (0.003-0.05 %)[52].

In November of 1884, William Stuart Halsted (Fig. 399) and Richard J. Hall, surgeons at the Roosevelt Hospital in New York, already had achieved loss of feeling in the extremities through cocaine injections in the immediate vicinity of nerve trunks. On November 26, Hall had one of his upper central incisors prepared and filled without the slightest pain by the dentist Charles A. Nash after the injection of a cocaine solution next to the infraorbital foramen. Hall reported this in a letter to the *New York Medical Journal*, and Nash described it in almost the same words to the publisher of the *Dental Cosmos*[53]. On December 1, Hall added to his letter a report on the first mandibular anesthesia, which is given here in part: *This evening, Dr. Halsted gave me an injection of seventeen minims, the needle being introduced along the internal surface of the left ramus until it touched the inferior dental nerve, causing a sharp twinge along the whole line of the lower teeth. In three minutes there was numbness and tingling of the skin, extending from the angle of the mouth to the median line, and also of the left border of the tongue. In six minutes, there was complete anaesthesia of the left half of the lower lip, on both the cutaneous and the mucous surfaces, extending from the median line to the angle of the mouth and downward to the inferior border of the jaw. A pin thrust completely through the lip caused no sensation whatever. There was also complete anaesthesia of the posterior surface of the gums and of the lower teeth on the left side, exactly to the median line; hard blows upon the teeth with the back of a knife caused no sensation . . .*[54].

In a conduction anesthesia of the upper and lower jaw arranged by Halsted, the dentist Edward H. Raymond performed restorative treatment on a friend in December of 1884, about which he made a presentation before the New York Odontological Society on January 20, 1885. He also reported on the successful application of a 4 % solution to an exposed part of the dental pulp[55].

These discoveries only slowly reached Europe, although the complete development had taken its course from Heidelberg. Not even the American in Germany, W. D. Miller of Berlin, knew anything yet about the injection of the drug in his publication of 1885, "Über die Anwendung des Cocain" (On the Application of Cocaine). Understandably, he was not satisfied by the results of inserting even a 30 % solution in cavities[56].

Soon the other side of the medication was also recognized, in the danger of addiction. As a result of experiments on themselves numerous physicians and dentists had succumbed to the drug. Halsted himself was able to get rid of the addiction by a vigorously followed withdrawal cure and was still able to contribute further to operating technique through the invention of the rubber glove in 1890.

Cocaine seemed to Professor Robert Baume, a Berlin dentist, *too much a waste of time* (since the solution had, to be prepared by himself) *and, because of the after-effects (weakness, periostitis), not satisfying over the long run. I have therefore returned to nitrous oxide*, although he still used cocaine as a topical anesthetic[57]. This return to laughing-gas took piace most completely in the United States. In Europe it was recognized that more extensive procedures could be performed through injection of lower concentrations of cocaine; this view was supported in the nineties especially by Paul Reclus in Paris and Carl Ludwig Schleich in Berlin.

In 1901 the hormone adrenalin was isolated from the adrenal medulla by the Japanese Jokichi Takamine (Fig. 400) in the USA, and in the same country, but entirely independently, by Thomas Bell Aldrich. Only a little later the surgeon Heinrich Braun in Leipzig (Fig.401) had the idea of mixing this vessel-contracting agent with the cocaine solution. After the first experiment on himself he recognized *that a new era had dawned for local anesthesia!*[58]. In 1904 adrenalin became the first hormone ever to be synthesized by a chemist at the "Farbwerke Hoechst," Friedrich Stolz (Fig. 402), under the trade name of "Suprarenin."

[51] Howe; Carmichael; e. g., Dental Cosmos 27 (1885): 53 f.
[52] von Anrep p. 47
[53] Nash
[54] Quoted by Artelt (b)
[55] Raymond
[56] Miller
[57] Baume p. 839
[58] Braun (a); (b) p. 156

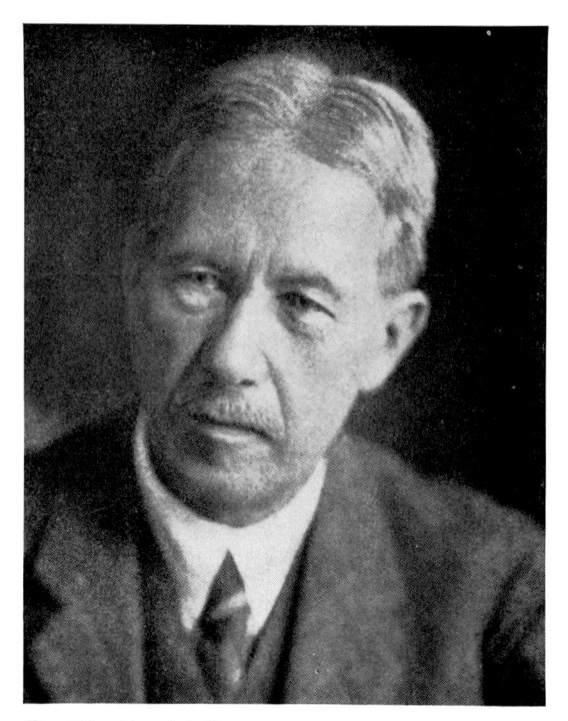

Fig. 401 *Heinrich Braun*

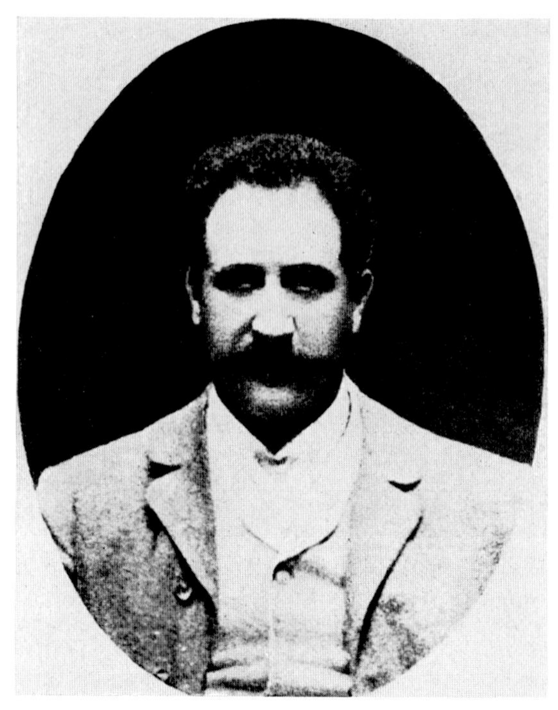

Fig. 403 *Alfred Einhorn (Farbwerke Hoechst archives)*

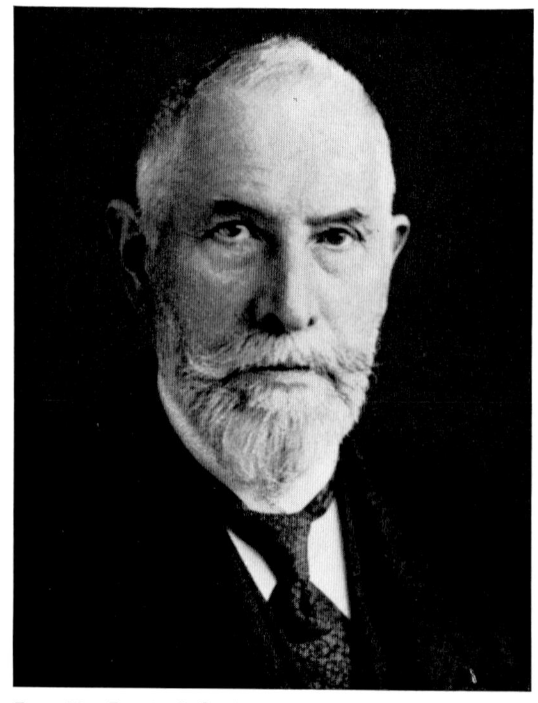

Fig. 402 *Friedrich Stolz*

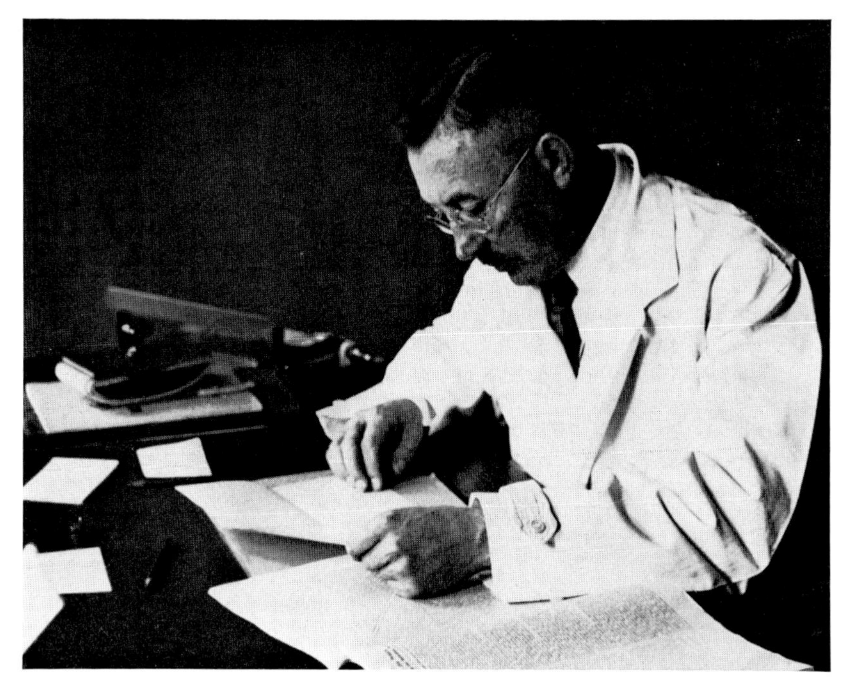

Fig. 404 *Guido Fischer*

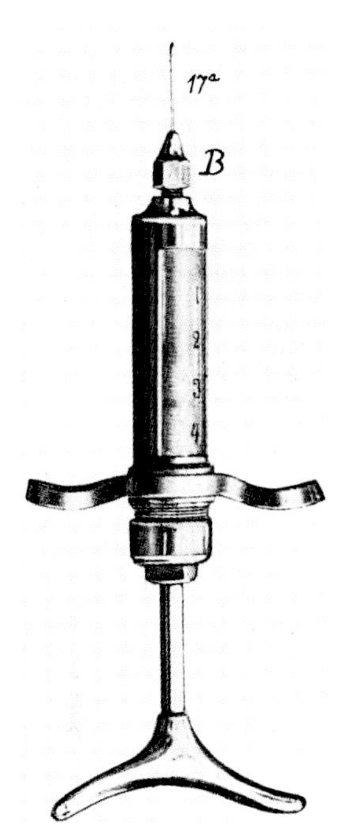

Fig. 405
The Fischer syringe

Another step into the new era of local anesthesia was taken when the chemist Alfred Einhorn (Fig. 403) together with Richard Willstätter developed procaine in Munich in 1905. Too, it was manufactured by the "Farbwerke Hoechst" under the name "Novocain." Procaine, which was significantly less toxic than cocaine, was introduced in surgery by Braun and soon established itself in conjunction with synthetic adrenalin[59] as the leading local anesthetic for dental procedures in Europe, particularly after it was offered in tablet form. From these a germ-free solution was easily made by boiling them with the required quantity of distilled water to which the vasoconstrictor could be added.

The local anesthetic "Nirvanin" had already been developed by Einhorn in 1898 but was later dropped in favor of "Novocain." Nirvanin was a chemical first step to lidocaine preparations produced first in Sweden after the second World War.

Guido Fischer, the director of the Dental University Institute at Greifswald and later a professor in Marburg and Hamburg (Fig. 404), indefatigably promoted local anesthesia with "Novocain-Suprarenin" through lectures and articles from 1906 on[60]. He visited Moscow and St. Petersburg (Leningrad), and also the New World in 1910 at the invitation of six universities. He succeeded in this lecture tour to establish local anesthesia in the United States over laughing-gas narcosis[61]. Fischer constructed the special syringe named after him, which exposed several disadvantages of the Pravaz syringe, the then dominant instrument which had been developed in 1906. Because of insufficient sterilizability, however, it is now outdated (Fig. 405). In 1917 the cylinder ampule was developed by the North American physician Harvey Samuel Cook while he was an army surgeon during the first World War. It was called a "cartridge" according to the principle of a cartridge in a gun barrel and has always been up-to-date.

59 Braun (c)
60 Fischer (a)
61 Bremner p. 205; Lyons. An earlier mention of Novocain-Suprarenin is found in the American literature in Dental Cosmos 48 (1906): 882; more extensively in Dental Cosmos 50 (1908): 821—827

Cook had cut the glass tubes himself and produced the pistons from eraser rubber.

The problem of eliminating pain in dentistry was herewith principally solved in the first quarter of our century. Further improvement was provided by refined anesthetic and vasoconstrictive drugs developed after the second World War. Furthermore the aimed use of antibiotic and chemotherapeutic preparations, the introduction of which is associated with the names of Sir Alexander Fleming (1928) and Gerhard Domagk (1932), allowed troubling postoperative pain to be greatly reduced. In oral surgery, perfected apparatuses made possible endotracheal narcosis almost free of problems. As a result, almost every procedure affecting the jaws and mouth can be performed today under conditions which seem optimal, both the operator and the patient.

Oral Surgery

The field of clinical oral surgery, which is so extensive today, was founded in the forties of the last century by Simon P. Hullihen (Fig. 406), who established the first specialized clinic for the field in Wheeling, West Virginia. According to his notes he had operated *about 150 hare-lips and cleft palates, 150 cancers, 200 antrum cases, 25 cases of making new noses, 50 new lips, and 10 underjaws,* but also 300 cases of cataract and strabism and 200 cases of general surgery. Well known is his report on the surgical elimination of an alveolar protrusion of the mandible through mobilization and repositioning of the anterior part of the alveolar process including the teeth, and all this alone in the last ten years of his short life[62]. On methodology he reported in dental journals. In 1857 he died at the age of 47.

James Edward Garretson (Fig. 407), who practiced in Philadelphia and whose clinic was associated with the Dental College there (Fig. 408), soon followed Hullihen's path. Through his success in operations, but mainly through his work "A Treatise on the Diseases and Surgery of the Mouth, Jaws and Associate Parts," which was published in 1869 and which underwent six editions through 1895 under the title "A System of Oral Surgery," he established jaw surgery as an independent field.

It was proved very quickly that men such as Hullihen and Garretson, who were skillful dentists and physicians, had obtained operative results completely different from those of the general surgeons. Their familiarity with intraoral work and their knowledge of dental technique made it possible for them to construct the auxiliary apparatuses necessary for surgical procedures on the jaw.

Within the scope of this book, we can only concern ourselves with the systematic development of specialized out-patient dental surgery. Besides local anesthesia, which was coming gradually into general use in the nineties, the discovery by Wilhelm Conrad Röntgen in Würzburg of the phenomenon of X-rays on November 8, 1895, was of decisive importance[63]. The first photographs of teeth were made already on the 2nd of February 1896 by the Frankfurt physicist Walter König and also, probably only a few days later, with the help of a physicist there, Friedrich Giesel, by Otto Walkhoff, a dentist then still practicing in Braunschweig. The first radiographs of teeth in the United States followed one year after Röntgen's discovery by the dentist C. Edmund Kells, who became one of the many martyrs to this diagnostic aid. Because of an X-ray cancer originating from his fingers and continually recurring, he parted from life. *He shot himself*[64].

What had been achieved previously in dental surgery were acts of individual virtuosity by surgically talented dentists more than therapeutic methods of general importance. Nevertheless, these pioneer deeds ought not to be underrrated because they formed the basis for dentistry to develop from the exclusively practiced tooth extraction to a standard far beyond the limits of thousands of years.

The first description of a procedure called the "apicectomy" in English, "Wurzelspitzenresektion" in German, and in French "résection apicale" belongs to this development. We find an early mention of it in a report from 1880 on a lecture given by John Nutting Farrar in New York[65]. Four years earlier he had recommended treating chronic processes at the apex

[62] Hullihen (b); Goldwyn

[63] Albert v. Koelliker proposed, on January 23, 1896, in Würzburg, to call the X-rays "Röntgen rays"

[64] Hauser; Raper (b)

[65] It is incorrect to ascribe priority to Désirabode. Only once (1858) did he sever the nerve connection to a maxillary premolar at the apex from the oral vestibule; Désirabode (b). The chapter "De la résection des dents" in his text (Désirabode [a] pp. 416 f.) deals with the severance of the crown

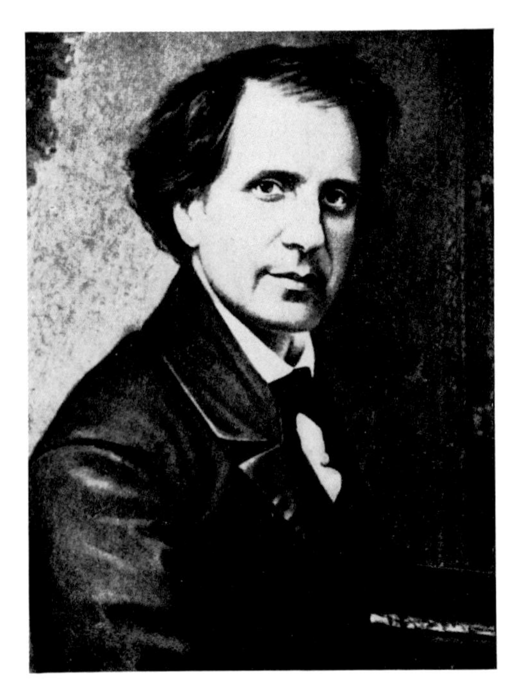

Fig. 406 *Simon P. Hullihen*

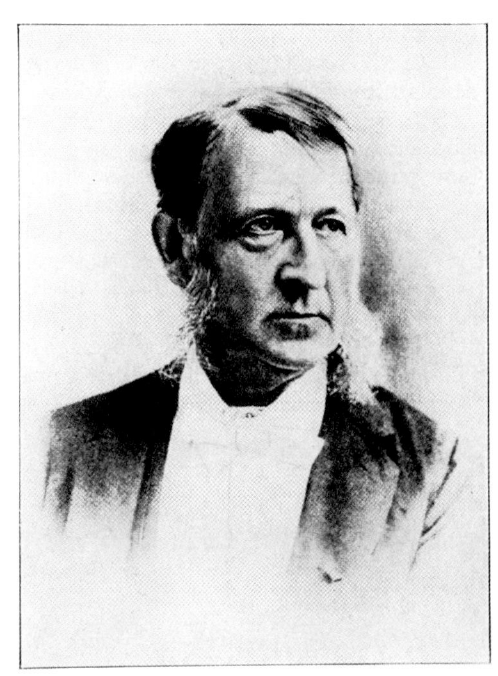

Fig. 407 *James Edward Garretson*

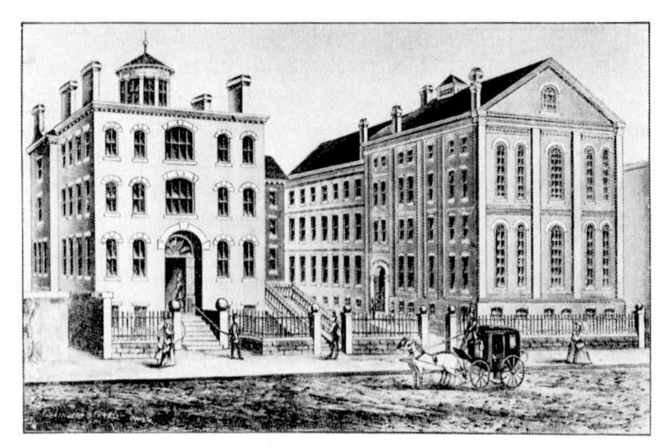

Fig. 408 *The new building of the Philadelphia Dental College and the Oral Surgery Clinic*

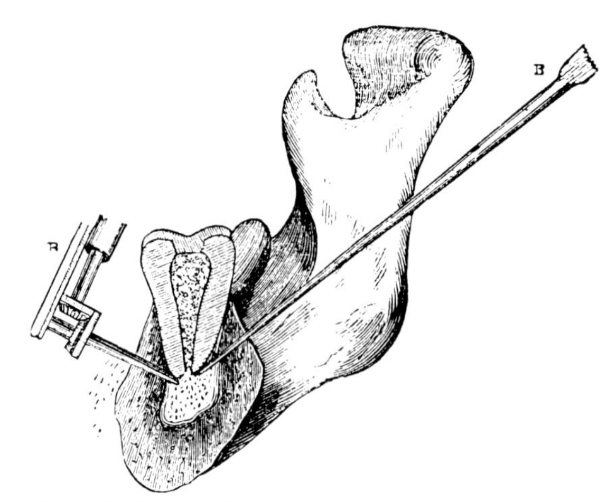

Fig. 409 *Farrar: Surgical exposure of an apical inflammation, 1880*

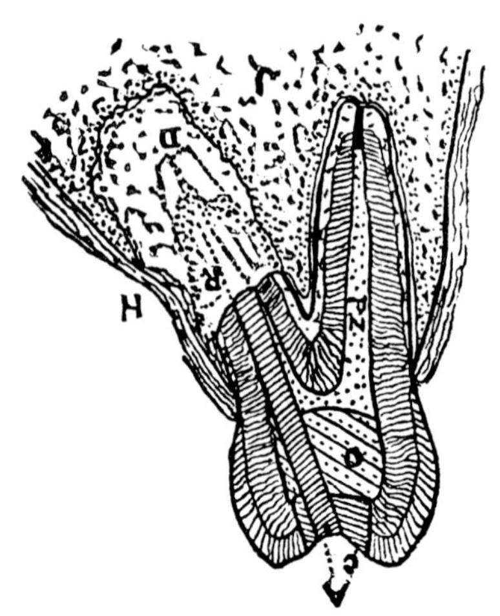

Fig. 410 *Farrar: Apicectomy of a molar root, 1884*

by means of injections through it. He still advised this method for the anterior teeth or if a fistula was present, but for the inaccessible molars he recommended penetrating with a drill from the oral vestibule to the apical site of inflammation to create an artificial fistula, a method which, although seldom used today, is called "apicotomy"[66] (Fig. 409). Then, in 1884, Farrar published on the basis of nine years of experience his *radical and heroic* method of amputating more or less large parts of the root or even of the whole root of a molar with simultaneous filling of the root canal[67] (Fig. 410). At about the same time similar suggestions were made by Charles William Dunn, Claude Martin, and chiefly by Meyer Louis Rhein in New York in 1890[68].

The credit for the methodical development of apicectomy under cocaine anesthesia in the years 1895 to 1899 belongs to the professor of the University of Breslau, Carl Partsch (Fig. 411), a surgeon who had turned to dentistry[69]. The Viennese professor Rudolf Weiser joined him and propagated Partsch's method at the IIIrd International Dental Congress in Paris in 1900[70]. At about the same time Partsch introduced the curved incision named after him, which is still predominantly used today. It was not until 1908, however, that he recommended closing the wound with silk thread[71] (Fig. 412).

Partsch also earned particular credit in the field of cyst operations. We remember the treatment of Scultetus, Fauchard, Runge, and Jourdain of such hollow tumors[72], which they took mostly for an abscess.

In 1829 a report from the surgical clinic at the Hôtel Dieu in Paris, then under the direction of Guillaume Dupuytren, mentioned bone cysts (kystes osseux) in the jaw region as if it was a matter of course in discussing a case from 20 years before. Through pressure on the tumor, Dupuytren produced *a light crepitation, a feeling similar to that of paper rumpled between the fingers, or, even better, very dry parchment,* . . . (which is) *according to M. Dupuytren the pathognomonic indication for this affliction.* This symptom still bears the name today of this great surgeon, who was one of the first who dared to perform a mandibular resection. As further diagnostic aid the exploratory puncture was used. The therapy consisted in a wide opening and removal of the edges of the bone, irrigation with etching substances and packing in order to destroy the membrane of the sinus by infection. In the case of recurrences he employed the cautery to pull up *everything by the roots*[73].

While Baron Dupuytren always called the cysts tumors (tumeurs), even prominent dentists such as Taft and Tomes regarded these hollow growths as alveolar abscesses still in 1859. The cyst shown by Tomes, which fills the maxillary sinus, bears the footnote: *An upper jaw in which the effect of alveolar abscess in excavating the bone is shown*[74] (Fig. 413). In 1870 Carl Wedl and Moriz Heider[75] in Vienna declared with resignation that *the theory of bone cysts is still a long way from being settled*[76]. From the pen of Magitot in Paris two comprehensive works on this topic were published in 1869 and 1872.

Emile Magitot (Fig. 414) made a significant contribution to the development of scientific odontology in France. As son of a dentist at first he received all manner of encouragement during his medical studies, but his turning away from practical to scientific dentistry as a student threatened to deprive him of his parental support. He became acquainted with researchers such as Legros and Broca through the histologist Charles Robin, for whom he worked as a dissector. His first works were devoted to odontogenesis, and his dissertation of 1857 also dealt with this theme[77]. In collaboration with Robin a comprehensive work on the development of the dental follicle[78] followed publications about comparative anatomical topics such as periodontal pathosis[79]. His classification of cysts (1869) as follicular and periosteal or alveolodental (today radicular) has retained its importance to the present day. In 1877 his "Traité des anomalies du système dentaire chez l'homme et les mammifères" (Treatise on Anomalies of the Dental Sys-

[66] Farrar (a); (b) Vita Farrar, see p. 374
[67] Farrar (c)
[68] Martin (a); Riethmüller; Rhein
[69] Partsch (b); (c)
[70] Weiser
[71] Partsch (d); (e) p. 50
[72] See pp. 181, 199, 229, and 215
[73] Dupuytren (a and b)
[74] Taft pp. 297 f.; Tomes (b) p. 557
[77] Magitot (a)
[76] Wedl/Heider
[77] Magitot (a). See p. 396
[78] Robin
[79] See p. 317; Magitot (d)

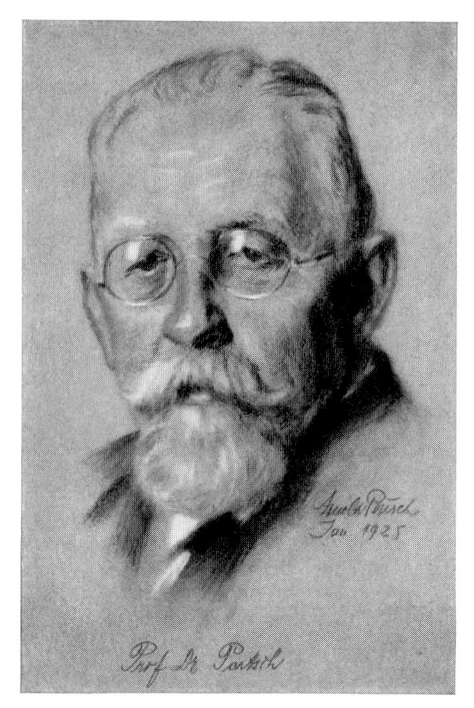

Fig. 411 *Carl Partsch*

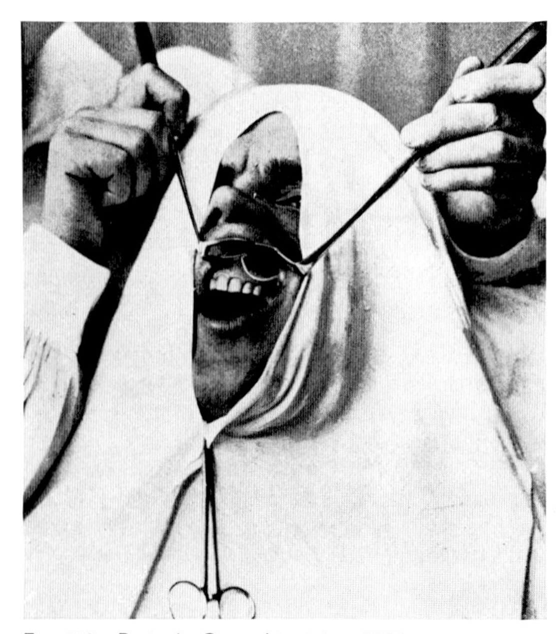

Fig. 412 *Partsch: Curved incision, 1905*

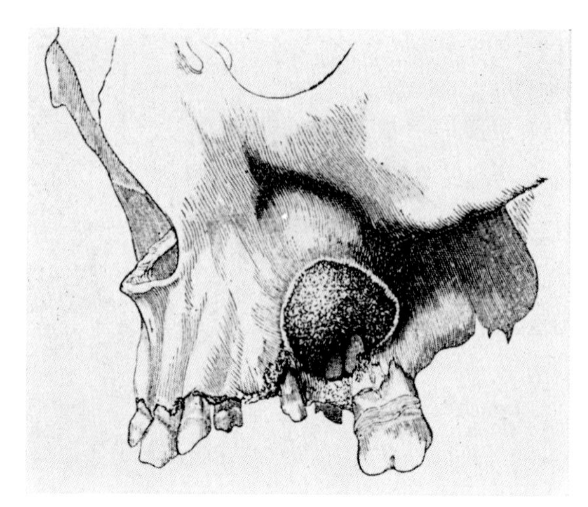

Fig. 413 *Depiction of a cyst in Tomes (1859) with the footnote: "An upper jaw in which the effect of alveolar abscess in excavating the bone is shown."*

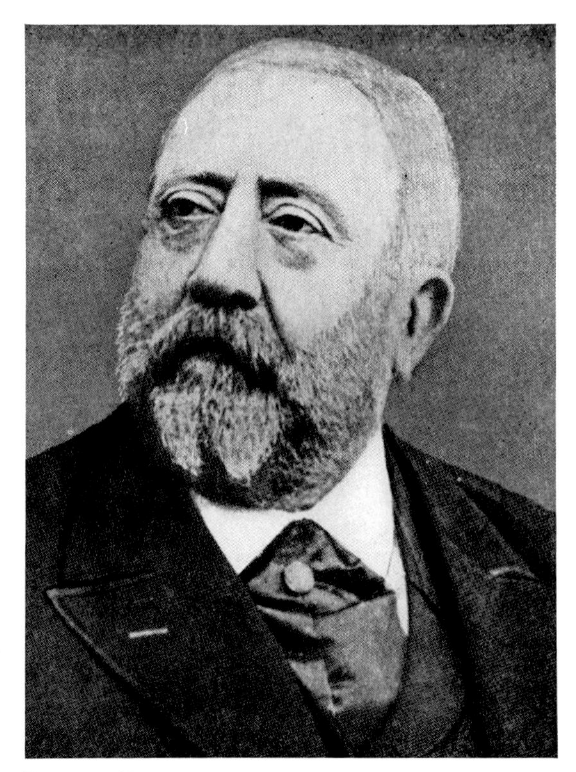

Fig. 414 *Emile Magitot*

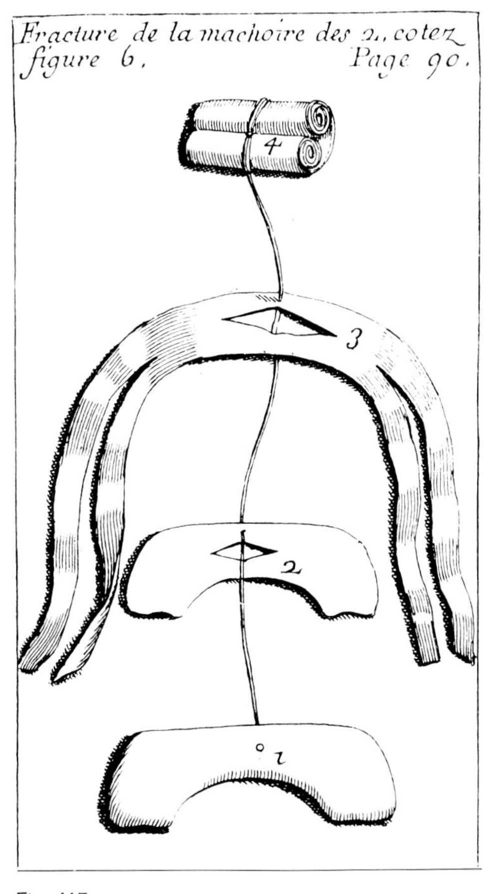

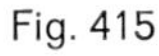
Fig. 415

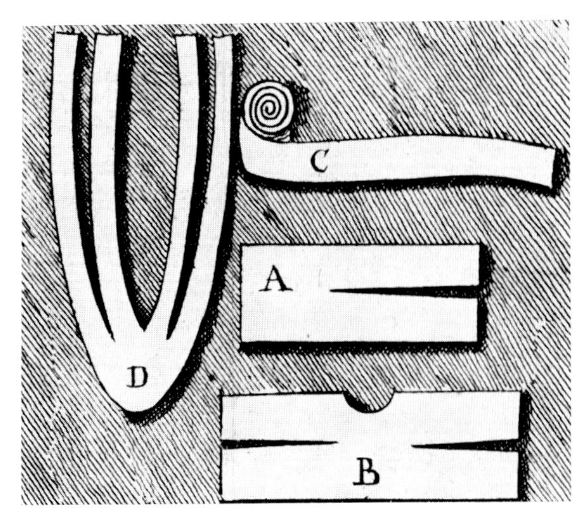

Fig. 416

Figs. 415 and 416 *Dressing materials for treatment of jaw fractures, by Le Clerc (1700) and Petit (1723)*

tem in Man and the Mammals) was rewarded with a prize of 10,000 francs upon the recommendation of the Academy of Science. In the field of industrial hygiene he fought against the use of phosphorus in match factories because it had the dreadful result of causing phosphorus necrosis of the mandible, which was then quite a frequently ocurring occupational disease. In 1888 he founded the "Société de Stomatologie," an organization of stomatologically acting physicians, and in 1894 he issued the journal *Revue de Stomatologie* which still comes out today. However, as a physician, he opposed the legalization of dentistry as a separate profession[80]. Magitot could have become for France what Sir John Tomes still represents for the field of British dentistry, but by prejudice he turned his back on the aspiring group whose intellectual leader he should have become, and left this task to the Parisian dentist Charles Godon (see Fig. 456).

Magitot's theories on the formation of cysts have proved true only in part. While he maintained the hypothesis that the epithelium of the cyst arose from an irritation of the root canal through the periodontal connective tissue, the Parisian surgeon and pathologist Louis Charles Malassez confronted him in 1885 with the hypothesis, accepted today, that it develops from "epithelial rests" (débris or amas épithéliaux paradentaires) within the periodontal membrane of the root sheath, provoked by a stimulus

[80] Cruet; Sauvez; Jost p. 37

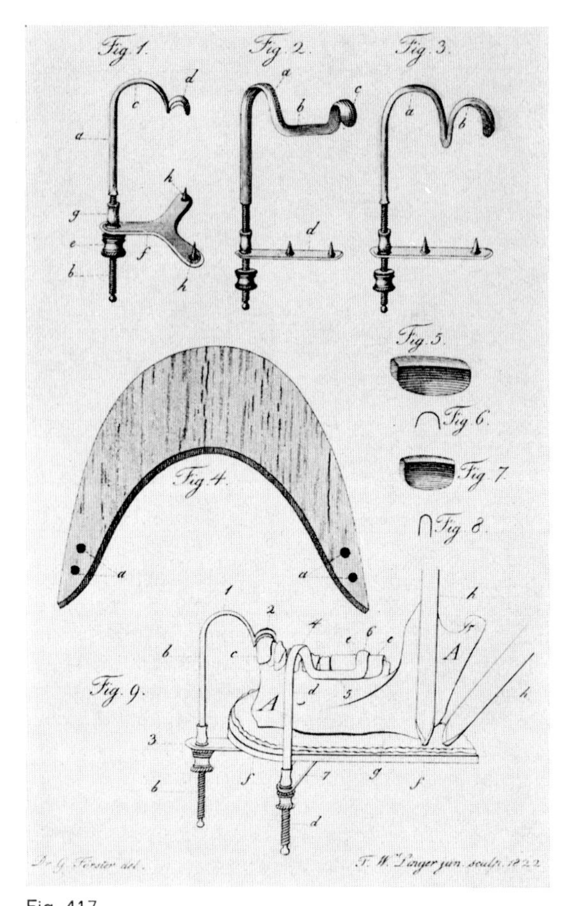

Fig. 417

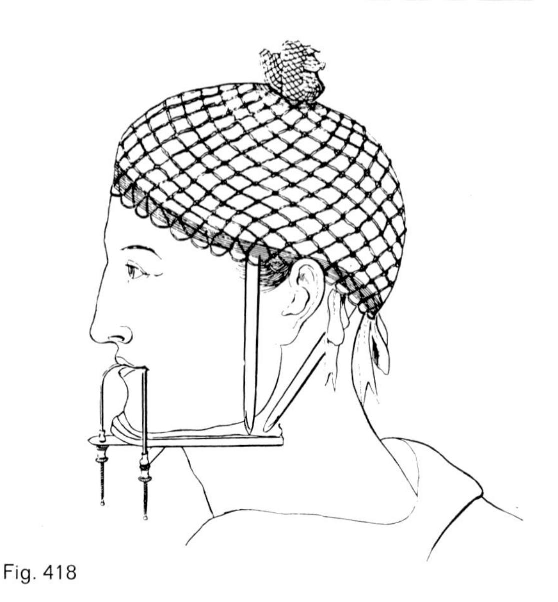

Fig. 418

Figs. 417 and 418 *Rütenick: Apparatus for splinting a mandibular fracture, exploded view and in place, 1799*

from the root canal [81]. There are extensive discussions on this theme transmitted to us, in which we must support the arguments of Magitot's opponents [82].

Let us now return to therapy: in 1892 Partsch recommended that cysts lined with epithelium be included in the oral cavity through removal of the facial cyst wall [83], a procedure which Garretson had already described in a similar manner, but which seemed to him too involved and painful [84]. Not until 1910 Partsch recommended the method, which he had previously rejected, of stripping smaller cysts of their follicles and suturing the wound immediately with silk thread. Both ways have stood the test to the present day; in German-speaking areas they are named in honor of the author, "Partsch I" and "Partsch II." The surgeon Partsch justifiably took credit for having *pressed the scalpel into the dentist's hand* [85].

Treatment of Fractures of the Jaw

Taking care of fractures of the jaw, the first diagnoses and prognoses of which are found in an Egyptian papyrus, lay unequivocally in the hands of the surgeons until after the middle of the 19th century. Particularly with regard to the mandible, it had hardly progressed at the end of the

81 Magitot (d and e); Malassez (a and b)
82 Magitot (f) pp. 12 f.
83 Partsch (a)
84 Garretson p. 831
85 Partsch (e) p. 44

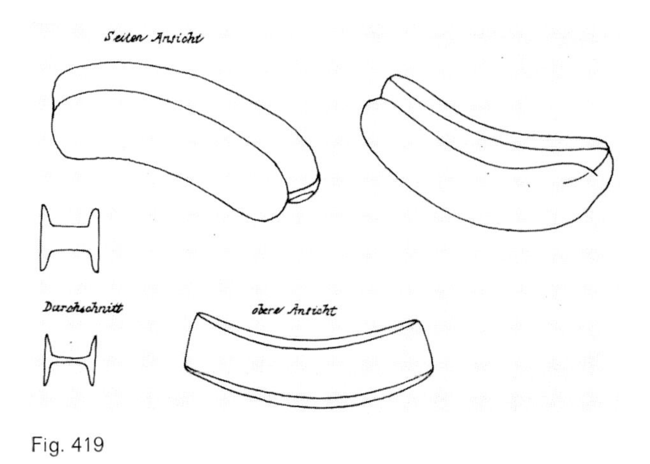

Fig. 419

Fig. 419 *Späth: Horn splints for mandibular splinting, 1836*

Fig. 420 *Robert: Lingual metal plate held in place by wire ligatures, 1852 (according to the author, the absence of wire anterior to the dental arch is an error in drawing)*

Fig. 421 *Morel-Lavallée: Fixation of the mandible with guttapercha, 1855*

18th century beyond the theories of Hippocrates and Celsus, Abulcasim and Wiliam of Saliceto: after resetting the teeth neighbored to the fracture line were joined by ligatures, and the corpus mandibulae was held immobile by a chin sling [86]. Later this method is found pictorially represented in woodcuts by Brunschwig and Ryff (See Figs. 142 and 147).

In the 18th century the capistrum was recommended by the Parisian surgeons Charles Gabriel Le Clerc and Jean Louis Petit as an aid to healing. While Le Clerc in 1700 used a "carton" formed to fit the chin [87] (Fig. 415), which was also done by Brunschwig in 1497 and also by Heister in 1718, the famous Petit limited himself to bandages only in 1723. This was a generally observed regression during the 18th century and heedless of Hippocrates' warning against the dislocating affect of bandages. The illustration shows it in a slightly different manner [88] (Fig. 416). In 1788 Andreas Bonn in Amsterdam also represented typical maxillary and mandibular fractures in his atlas of bone diseases, but in his text there are neither the attempt to systematize nor any therapeutic recommendations [89].

Around the turn of the century the Parisian surgeons Chopart and Desault [90] (1779), the Prussian regimental physician Rütenick (1799), the Englishman Francis Bush (1822) and the dentist of Braunschweig, Fr. Hartig (1830) [91] constructed complicated, but in principle similar, apparatuses for the extra-oral fixation of the mandible. The one by Rütenick consisted of splints from sheets of silver (Fig. 417 and 418, No.'s 5—8), wrapped in linen, which were laid over the rows of teeth at the site of the fracture and fastened under the chin by a hooked screw joint (No.'s 1—3), with the help of a wooden plate (No. 4) like Le Clerc's "carton." He went beyond his colleagues in the use of a head cap for relief [91]. According to contemporary reports (e. g., from Malgaigne [92]) all of these apparatuses, despite numerous variations, could be worn only for a short period of time because of the sores they caused.

In his "Leçons sur les maladies des os" (Lectures on Diseases of the Bones), which was published in Paris in 1803, the surgeon Alexis Boyer recommended a kind of intraoral splinting. After application of the customary bandages he put particular emphasis on absolute immobility: *An opening might also be preserved by introducing two pieces of corc, one on each side, between the teeth* [93]. Presumably the mandible was fixed in this situation by a capistrum. In 1836 the chief surgeon in Nürtingen, Württem-

86 See pp. 63 f., 72, 100, and 117
87 See pp. 164 f.
88 Le Clerc pp. 82 f.; Heister pp. 161 f.; Petit (a) II pp. 52 f.; see pp. 63 f.
89 Bonn pp. 2 f.; Tab. IV—VII
90 Chopart/Desault pp. 216 f.
91 Branco (Rütenick); Hartig
92 Malgaigne p. 395
93 Boyer I p. 93

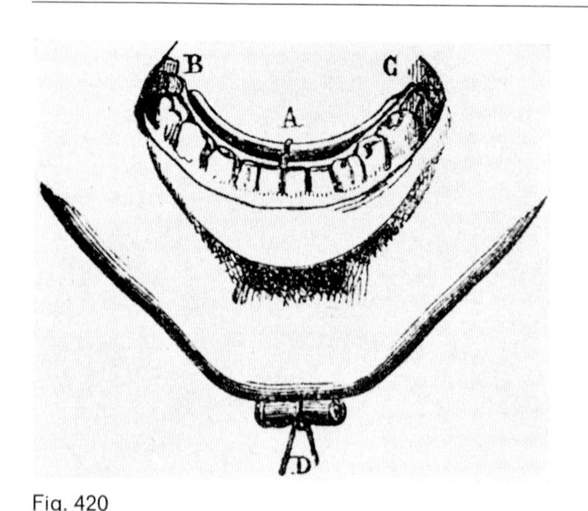

Fig. 420

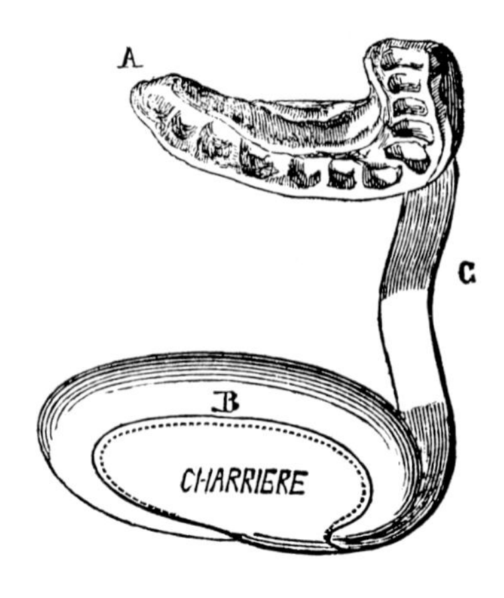

Fig. 421

berg, Johann Paul Spaeth, claimed that this material was too soft and smelled badly. Therefore he had a turner produce two doubly grooved horns for him, one for the sick and one for the healthy side [94] (Fig. 419).

In 1840 the military surgeon Jean-Baptiste Baudens presented in Paris the case of an oblique fracture of the corpus mandibulae, immobilized by threads brought through the skin on both sides of the bone with a needle and knotted over the crowns of the teeth [95], an anticipation of circumferential wiring. This Alphonse Robert performed in Paris in 1852: he looped a silver wire over the row of teeth and over a lead plate (later zinc) which was lingually adapted to the teeth, and knotted it under the chin over a tampon [96] (Fig. 420). This way the wire served to hold the metal plate in place, and therefore only indirectly adjusted the fracture. An early wire suture, perhaps the first, between two holes drilled next to the fracture line was already publicized in 1847 by Gurdon Buck, a surgeon at the New York Hospital [97].

Victor Morel-Lavallée's methods were important for further development. In 1855 he advised after repositioning and immobilization by wire ligatures to press softened guttapercha over the row of teeth until the occlusal surfaces were covered by only a thin layer of it. In special cases he employed a kind of impression tray (moule) as an aid, which was fastened under the chin by a spring and a plate soldered to this (Fig. 421). This method may have formed the basis for the later development of the hard rubber splints [98].

In 1855, the same year as Morel in Paris, Frank Hastings Hamilton of Buffalo, who was later a medical inspector during the Civil War, informed the American Medical Association of a similar procedure. He softened two pieces guttapercha and with them wrapped *the back teeth on each side of the mouth; taking care, of course, that on the fractured side the splint extends sufficiently far forwards to traverse thoroughly the line of fracture.* Thereupon he applied the four-tailed capistrum described by himself. Later, in 1857, he had a kind of impression tray (silver cap) made for him by a dentist, which he filled with guttapercha [99].

The first mention of arrangements for maxillary fractures comes from the personal surgeon to three English kings, Richard Wiseman, in his case reports of 1676, "Severall chirurgicall treatises." This "British Paré" was called to a youth, *his face being beaten in and the lower jaw sticking out* from the blow of a hoof. He inserted his finger behind the uvula and pulled the body of the maxilla forward; when it was released, however, it immediately returned to its former position. Then, he *formed an Instru-*

[94] Späth
[95] Baudens
[96] Robert
[97] Hamilton pp. 127 f.; Schwartz
[98] Morel-Lavallée (a—c)
[99] Hamilton pp. 130 f.

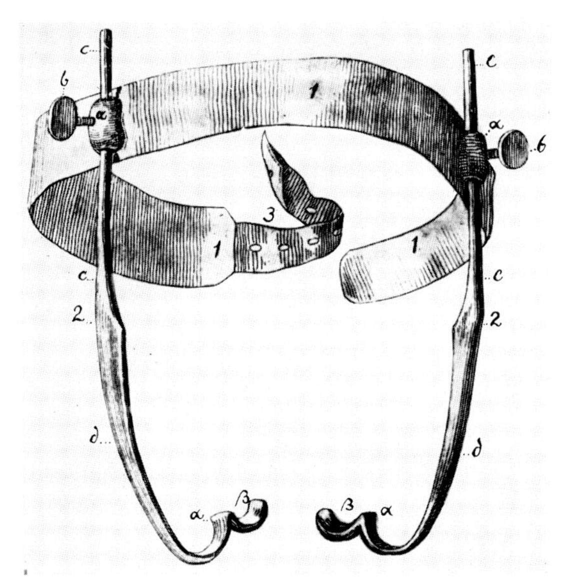

Fig. 422 *C. F. Graefe: Maxillary fracture splint, 1822*

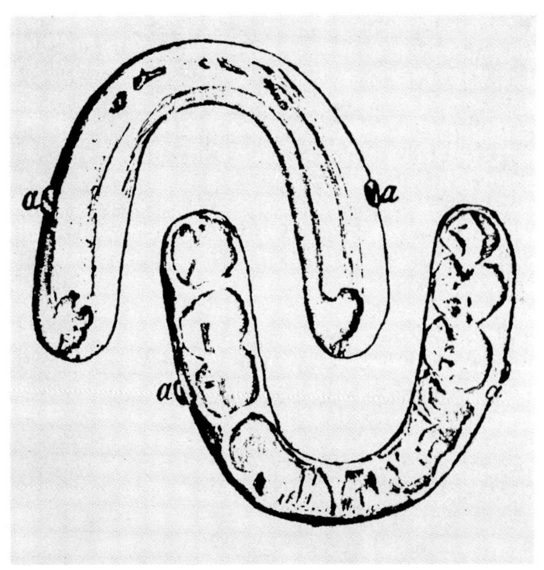

Fig. 424 *Gunning: Interdental splint of vulcanized rubber, seen from above and below, 1864*

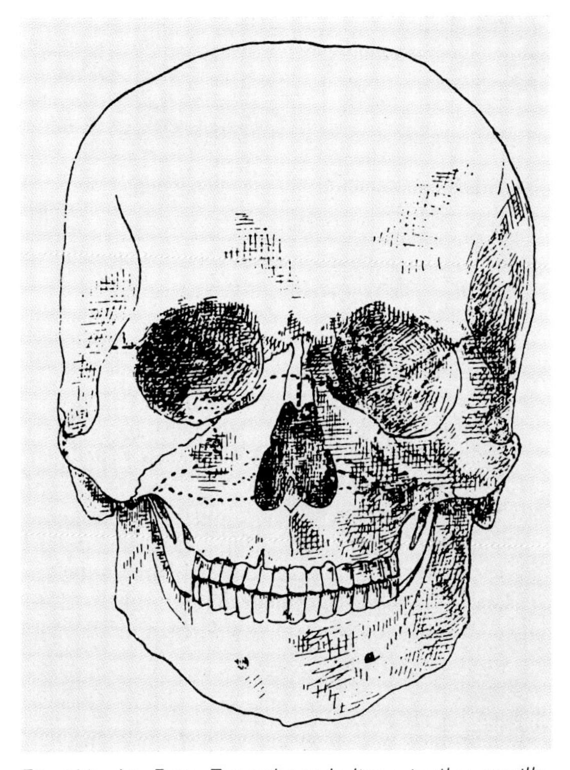

Fig. 423 *Le Fort: Typical weak lines in the maxilla, 1901*

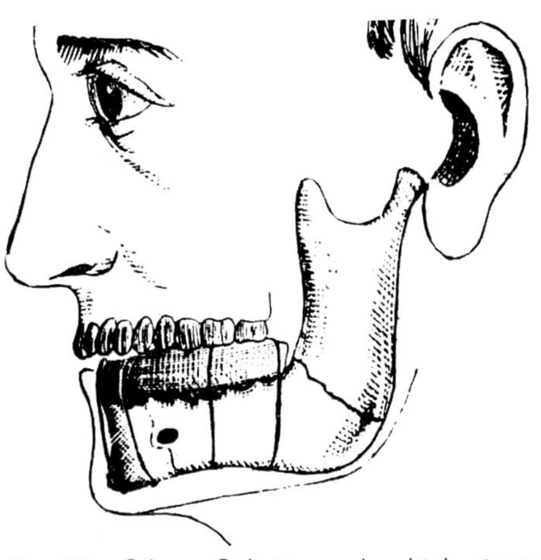

Fig. 425 *Gilmer: Splinting and multiple circumferential wiring, 1881*

ment bended up at one end, which he called *my Extender,* but *the fractured body returned back again.* Then Wiseman made an improved instrument, with which the fragment was held in place alternately *by the hand of the Child, his Mother, and my Servants* until callus had formed [100].

Treatment of a partial fracture of the maxilla was described probably for the first time in 1731 by the important Parisian surgeon, Henry-François Le Dran: Four distal upper molars (he did not yet differentiate between molars and premolars) of an old man were tipped palatally with their alveoli when he was run over. The mandible was fractured in several places in the region of the chin. To secure the shaky maxillary fragment, Le Dran had the Dentiste du Roi (court dentist), Jean François Caperon, bind the four teeth still firm in their alveoli to a fifth tooth with slings of thread. After application of a chin cap the six mandibular anteriors were ligated similarly. As soon as ten to twelve days later, the thread ligatures fell away, but the fragments had become firm—an early example of dental and surgical cooperation [101].

In comparison with these rather primitive attempts, it was a significant advance when, in 1822, the Berlin surgeon Carl Ferdinand (von) Graefe—who also performed the first successful surgical closure of a palatal cleft in 1817—had his doctoral candidate, Reiche, describe an apparatus, which was similar to the Rütenick attachment on the head in another form to immobilize the fractured maxilla. An upholstered steel forehead band bore two adjustable arms to support the fragment in the correct position [102] (Fig. 422).

Morel-Lavallée modified his guttapercha methods also for the maxilla. Thereafter, in the second half of the century, one supported the fractured maxilla with a splint of hard rubber bearing two wire bars called "deer antlers." This was an application of the Kingsley apparatus from 1880 (see Figs. 429 and 430), but for the maxilla. Later it was connected elastically with rubber bands to a head cap.

With regard to the taxonomy of maxillary fractures, two French surgeons are particularly deserving of credit. In 1866, Alphonse Guérin in Paris described the horizontal separation of the tooth-bearing portion of the maxilla without dislocation which bears his name. Subsequently, in 1901, the surgeon René Le Fort of Lille stated that *the fracture without dislocation is the rule.* This knowledge, which presumbly had been responsible for the lack of interest until then in fractures of the middle third of the facial skeleton, he had gained from 35 cadaver heads which he had subjected to various traumas and, after maceration of the soft parts, dissected. He found chiefly in his investigations those typical weak lines which result in three principal groups of fractures on the facial section of the skull and which still bear his name today [103] (Fig. 423).

In the dental textbooks of the first half of the 19th century jaw fractures are mentioned only peripherally as an incident in tooth extraction. If an author, such as Désirabode, devoted several pages to its therapy in 1843, the recommendations consisted only of quotations from surgeons, whereby Baudens' procedure was rejected as too painful [104].

The transfer of the treatment of jaw fracture into the hands of dentists took place in the second half of the century as a result of the use of hard rubber as a splinting material which dentists in particular knew how to manipulate. Its introduction in 1864 probably stems from two American dentists, the London-born Thomas Brian Gunning and James Baxter Bean. According to Gunning in New York, the mandible was first reduced and held in this position with wire loops so that an impression could be taken from both halves. A hard rubber splint enveloping both rows of teeth in the approximate position of occlusion was vulcanized from the models and fastened with screws to holes previously drilled in the molars of the mandible (Fig. 424). The first patient treated after this principle was the author himself, who had been thrown from a horse [105].

With regard to Bean the former Medical Inspektor Covey (in the defeated Confederate Army of the American Civil War, 1861—1865) reports that Bean had taken care of mandibular fractures in the last months of the war with an "interdental splint" of hard rubber. Bean took wax impressions of the single

100 Wiseman pp. 472 f.
101 Le Dran I pp. 9 f.
102 Reiche pp. 20 f.; Graefe; Michaelis. Graefe was not raised to peerage until in 1826
103 Guérin; Le Fort
104 Désirabode (a) pp. 530 f.
105 Gilmer (a); Sands; Kingsley pp. 384 f.; Fraser-Moodie

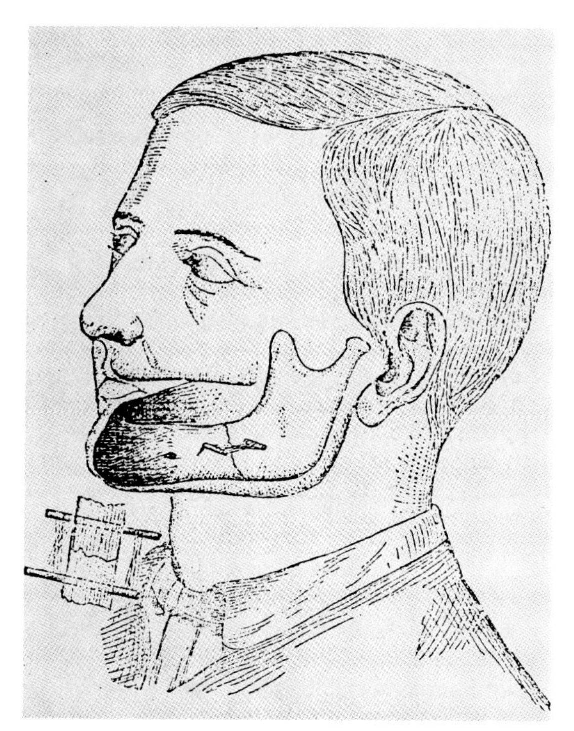

Fig. 426 *Gilmer: Percutaneous osteosynthesis in an edentulous mandible, drawing by G. V. Black in 1881*

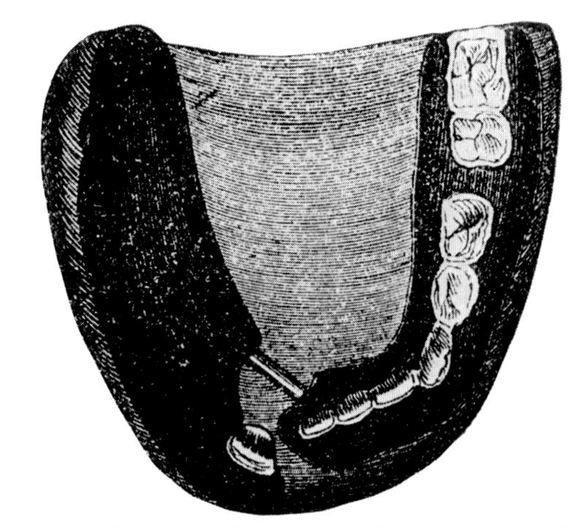

Fig. 428 *Süersen: Separation of dislocated healing fragments with swelling hickory posts, 1871*

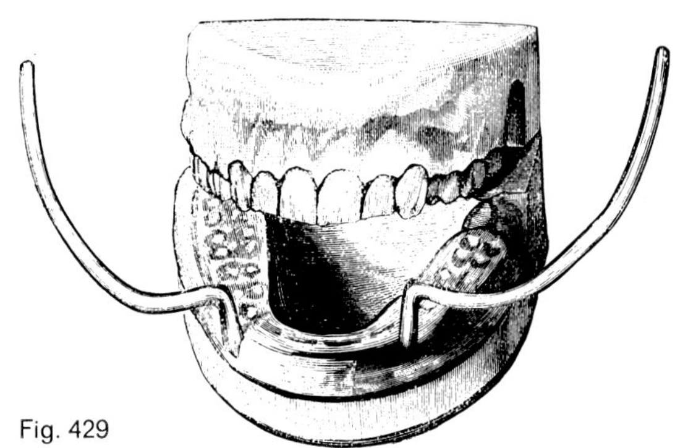

Fig. 429

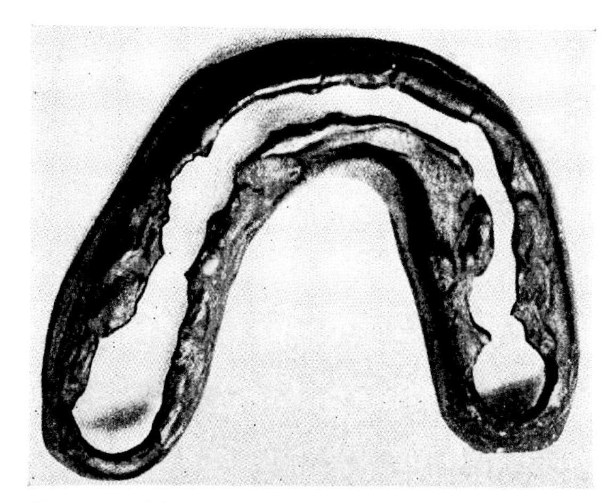

Fig. 427 *Vulcanized rubber splints that have been worn, from Weber and Haun (illustration from Hauptmeyer)*

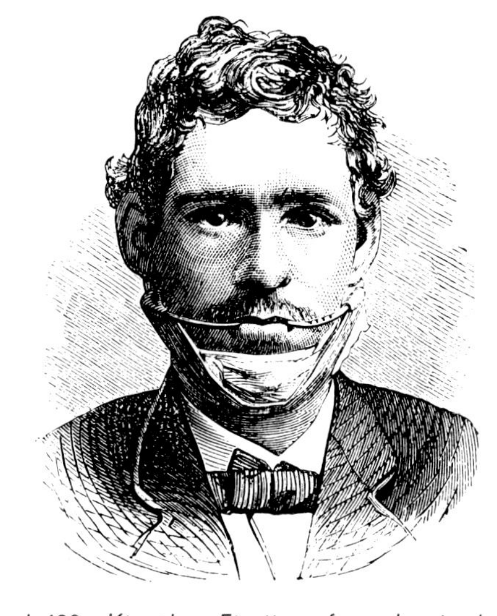

Fig. 430

Figs. 429 and 430 *Kingsley: Fixation of a vulcanized rubber splint by side bars attached to a chin bandage, 1880*

fragments, and placed the separated plaster casts in occlusion with the maxilla. The splint, which enveloped both maxilla and mandible, was held in place by a chin sling [106].

In 1881 a dentist in Quincy, Illinois, Thomas Lewis Gilmer, who was later a co-founder of the Dental School at the Northwestern University in Chicago, reported on the fastening of "Gunning's splint" by twisting wire around the edentulous mandible (Fig. 425), as had already been recommended in Paris by Robert in 1852. We also have to thank Gilmer for probably the first description of a percutaneous osteosynthesis: two pins were inserted in holes drilled next to the fracture line, and the two ends, the lingual one and the one protruding through the outer skin, were tied together with wire (Fig. 426).

Even more important is Gilmer's suggestion of fastening the broken mandible to the maxilla. He treated a bilateral fracture first on one side by wire osteosynthesis and laced all remaining teeth of the maxilla and mandible singly with iron wire. *The ends of each wire were brought together and twisted, fastening it securely to the teeth. This being done, the teeth of the lower jaw were exactly articulated with those of the upper and the wires of the lower teeth secured to those of the upper by bringing them together and twisting, thus firmly lashing the lower to the upper jaw.* Herewith we have for the first time the reapparance of a method which had already been indicated but not actually described in an early print of William of Saliceto in the 15th century [107].

In 1865, at a dentist's meeting in Leipzig, J. H. C. Weber, a dentist working in Paris, was the first European to demonstrate a modified hard rubber dressing. He took an impression *while trying to hold the fractured pieces in the best position.* His splint comprised only the lower arch of teeth, the cutting edges and occlusal surfaces of which were left exposed, so that according to his statement, the patient was soon able to begin to chew (in contrast to the interdental splint), and *complete healing seemed to have taken place after three weeks* [108]. Carl Haun, a dentist in Erfurt, proceeded according to the same principle in combination with gutta-percha in 1867 [109] (Fig. 427). In treating the wounded of the Franco-Prussian war (1870—1871), Süersen discovered Bean's impression method quite independently and presented it to his German colleagues in Berlin in 1871. He also had the idea of forcing apart mandibular fractures which had healed with contraction by squeezing increasingly longer hickory pins between two hard rubber splints which individually enclosed each fragment [110] (Fig. 428).

Extraoral splinting of mandibular fractures was further developed in 1858 by Henry Hayward in London, who, after taking an impression, stamped an encircling metal plate and provided it with extraoral wire bars. This method was perfected by Kingsley in New York by the use of hard rubber plates, the upper sides of which he formed as occlusal surfaces (Figs. 429 and 430). The bars were then held in place by a chin bandage [111].

Claude Martin (Fig. 431), the Médecin-Dentiste and teacher at the Ecole du service de Santé militaire in Lyon, made special efforts towards further developing the encircling plate splint. Born on May 17, 1843 in St. Etienne as the son of a ribbon weaver Martin began as an apprentice to a lacemaker in Lyon. A dentist, struck by his adroitness, took him in as his apprentice and then sent him to Paris to his brother's practice. He was taken into lectures and clinical demonstrations by medical students whom he had befriended. Afterwards he studied for many more years under severe hardships in Paris and Lyon, where he settled as a dentist in 1873. Léopold Ollier, the well-known surgeon introduced him to the clinics where he took an interest in jaw fractures and especially in the field of surgical prosthetics. Here he advocated the necessity of an immediate insertion of the protheses, he had prepared for jaw resections (prothèse immédiate), in order to counteract the traction by the scar tissue. He published his experiences, based on a considerable amount of clinical material, in 1889 in a comprehensive work in which he described the prosthetic reconstruction of the nose and other parts of the face, as well as the preparation of obturators [112]. Martin died a highly respected man on January 30, 1911 in Lyon, the city where he had worked [113].

106 Covey
107 Gilmer (a and b). See p. 117
108 Weber
109 Haun
110 Süersen. See Fig. 266
111 Kingsley pp. 398 f.
112 Martin (c). See p. 231
113 Martin (d)

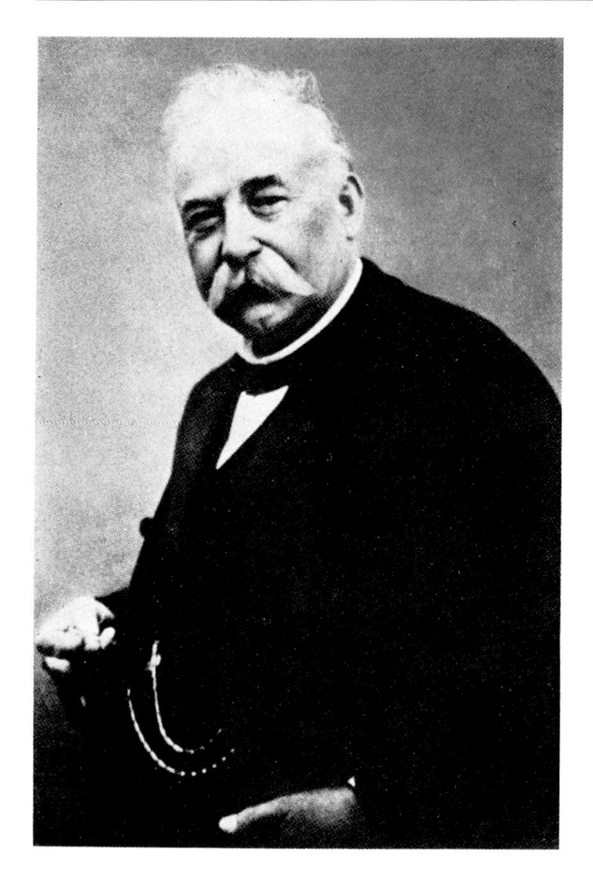

Fig. 431 *Claude Martin*

His method for splinting mandibular fractures, which he discussed in 1887 in a special book, was based on the principle of Morel-Lavallée (see Fig. 421). He used hard rubber instead of guttapercha, and instead of the simple pelotte on the apparatus from 1855 he used a plate adjusted to the outer edge of the mandible, into which was fitted a steel spring (Figs. 432 and 433). The outer plate bore hooks for rubber bands which were fastened to a head cap, so that the splint and the upper arch of teeth were pressed against each other[114]. Martin saw the advantage of this quite complicated apparatus in the fact that the patient could open his mouth to eat, an advantage which was soon eliminated by the intramaxillary rubber lacing of the wire splints.

The first description of an arch bar as we know it today probably stemmed from the London dentist Gurnell E. Hammond, while working with the wounded in besieged Paris in 1871. He bent an iron wire on a model which he passed over the teeth and fastened it with tying wire[115] (Fig. 434). This procedure was perfected independently by a method of the dentist Carl Sauer from Berlin who divided the bar, which was made preferably of spring-action gold wire, and joined it by lingually attached shells (Fig. 435). The final reposition he left to the effects of springforces which proved particularly effective with older fractures where callus formation had already begun[116]. In 1887 Sauer recommended soldering an inclined plane to the arch bar in the case of defective fractures[117] (see Fig. 439), and in 1889 he advised the use of an iron bar, adapted to the arch of teeth only on the labial side, as an emergency splint. It was bent previously by hand in the mouth to the

114 Martin (b) pp. 41 f.
115 Hammond
116 Sauer (a)
117 Schnoor

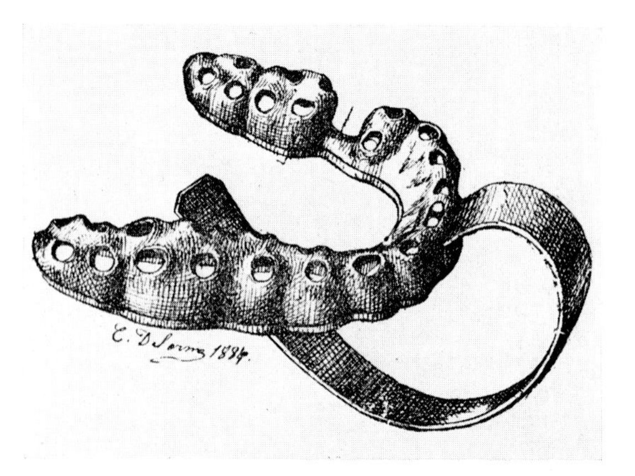

Fig. 432

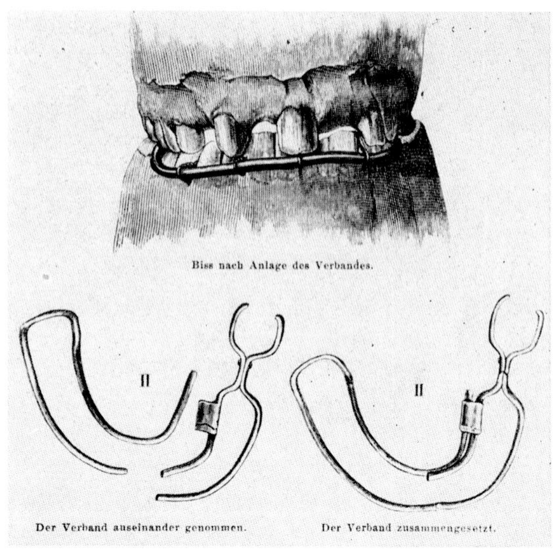

Fig. 435 *Sauer: Circumferential spring bar, 1881*

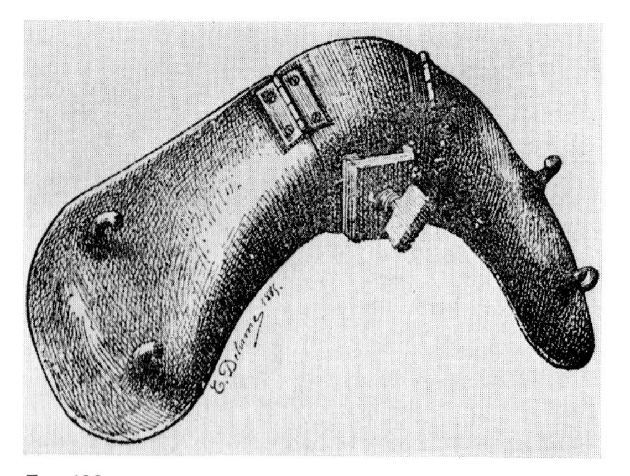

Fig. 433

Figs. 432 and 433 *Martin: Mandibular splinting devices, 1887*

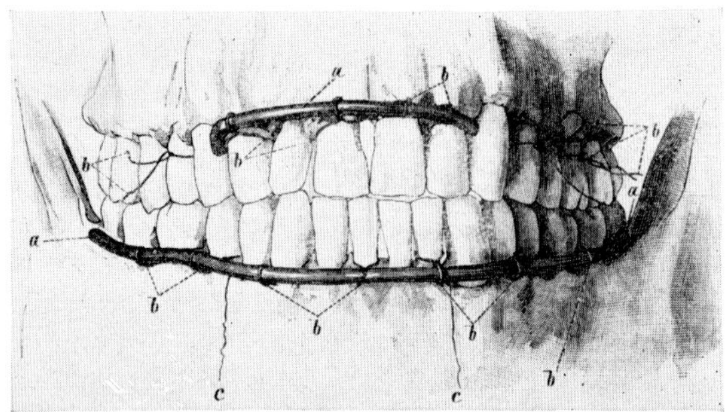

Fig. 436 *Sauer: Emergency arch bar of iron wire, 1889*

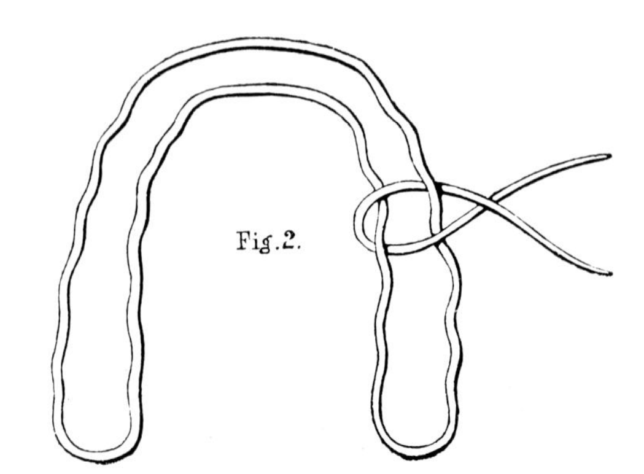

Fig. 434 *Hammond: Circumferential arch bar, 1871*

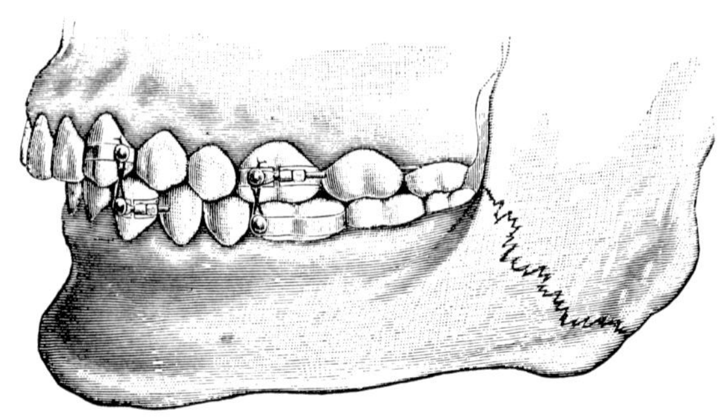

Fig. 437 *Angle: Fixation of the fractured mandible with orthodontic bands*

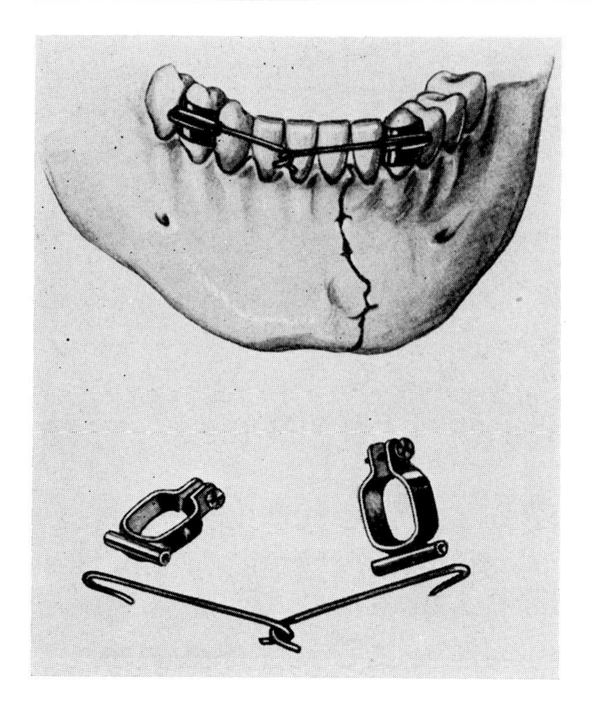

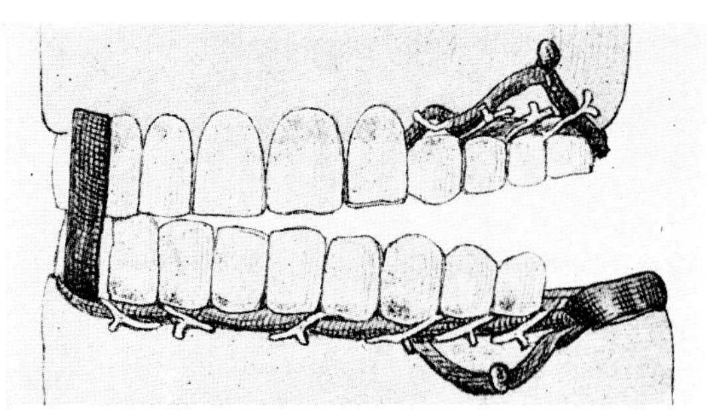

Fig. 439 *Heitmüller: Upper supplemental splint for the attachment of rubber bands, 1897 (Sauer's inclined plane at left)*

Fig. 438 *Löhers: Annular nut device to secure splints, 1893*

ideal position, and the reduction was achieved through systematic tightening of the ligatures [118] (Fig. 436).

In the USA Angle attempted in 1890 to make his orthodontic system useful in the treatment of fractures; his procedure, however, was a step backwards because with the help of ligaments he rigidly tied the repositioned mandible to the maxilla, as Gilmer had done before [119] (Fig. 437). Heinrich Löhers, a dentist in Heidelberg, possibly stimulated by this method, used the ligaments for securing Sauer's arch bar with his own annular nut device in 1893 [120] (Fig. 438).

It is difficult to ascertain by whom the intermaxillary traction with rubber rings, introduced into orthodontics by Tucker in 1852 [121], were first applied to the treatment of fractures of the jaw. In German literature Karl Heitmüller in Göttingen recommended the application of an auxiliary bar to the maxilla in 1897, from which he pulled the depressed mandibular fragment into the occlusal position with rubber bands (Fig. 439). Independently, in 1923, the dentist of the US Navy, W. L. Darnall, proposed the use of intermaxillary rubber bands for the first time in the United States [122].

Both of the systems whose evolutions are described here, the encircling plate and the tied-in arch bar, have undergone a parallel development in numerous variations up to the present time. The arch bar which could be produced without the help of a laboratory, proved particularly valuable in emergency cases and for military surgery. When nowadays the latter is enveloped by a cold-curing acrylic after being applied [123], it means, in general, a union of both methods of treating jaw fractures in which the advantages of both are to a great extent preserved.

Increasingly, surgical (osteosynthetic) methods are being used today for difficult fractures. A presentation of such purely clinical measures, however, lies beyond the scope of this book.

118 Sauer (b)
119 Angle pp. 285 f.
120 Röse pp. 48 f.; Löhers did not publish about this device, but left it to Carl Röse, then working in Freiburg im Breisgau. See p. 320
121 See p. 373
122 Heitmüller; Thoma
123 Schuchardt

References

Angle, Edward H(artley)
Treatment of malocclusion of the teeth and fractures of the maxillae. Philadelphia 1900

Anrep, B. (= Vasili Konstantinowich) von
Über die physiologische Wirkung des Cocain. Arch. Physiol., Bonn 21 (1880) 38—77

Artelt, Walter
a) Glas und Heilkunde in ihren geschichtlichen Wechselbeziehungen. Glastechn. Ber. 25 (1952) 231—341
b) Die deutsche Zahnhk. und die Anfänge von Narkose und Lokalanästhesie. Zahnärztl. Mitt. 54 (1964) 566—569, 671—677, 758—762, 853—856

Baudens, (Jean Baptiste Lucien)
Communications verbales. Bull. de l'académie royale de médecine (1844), pp. 230—231, 341 f.

Baume, Robert
Lehrbuch der Zahnheilkunde. 3rd ed., Leipzig 1890

Bell, Thomas
The anatomy, physiology and diseases of the teeth. London 1829

Berten, J(akob)
Über die Konstruktion eines neuen Satzes Zahnextraktionszangen. Österr.-ung. Vjschr. Zahnhk. 21 (1905) 129—153

Bleichsteiner, A.
Kieferbrüche. In: Handb. d. Zahnhk., ed. Julius Scheff. Vol. II, Wien 1892, pp. 77—90

Blume, E(duard)
Der praktische Zahnarzt . . . Berlin 1836

Bonn, Andreas
Tabulae ossium morbosorum. Amstelaedami 1788

(Boyer, Alexis)
The lectures of Boyer upon diseases of the bones. 2 vols., arr. by A. Richerand, transl. by M. Farrell, London 1807

Branco
Über die Fraktur des Unterkiefers nebst Beschreibung und Abbildung der Rütenickschen Maschine. (Rust's) Magazin ges. Heilk. 18 (1825) 3—59

Braun, Heinrich
a) Über den Einfluß . . . und über die Bedeutung des Adrenalins für die Localanästhesie. (Langenbeck's) Arch. klin. Chir. 69 (1903) 541—591
b) Die örtliche Betäubung, . . . 6. Ed., Leipzig 1921
c) Über einige neue örtliche Anaesthetica . . . Dtsch. med. Wschr. 31 (1905) 1667—1671

Bremner, M. D. K.
The story of dentistry . . . Rev. 3rd ed., Brooklyn, London 1964

Brunn, Ruth von
Die Entdeckung der Anästhesie. Ciba Zschr., Basel 11 (1952) 4776—4782

Buess, H(einrich)
Die Entwicklung der Injektionsgeräte. Ciba Zschr., Basel 9 (1946) 3637—3642

Carmichael, J. P.
The practical use of cocaine chloride in dental surgery. Dent. Cosmos 27 (1885) 78—81

Chopart, (François), (Pierre Joseph) Desault
Traité des maladies chirurgicales, . . . Vol. I. Paris 4 (de la république = 1795)

Colton, G(ardner) Q(uincy)
Nitrous oxide gas an anaesthetic. Dent. Cosmos 5 (1864) 490—493

Cope, Zachary
Sir John Tomes. London 1961

Covey, E. N.
The interdental splint. Brit. J. Dent. Sc. 19 (1866) 145—153

Cruet, Ludger
Magitot et son œuvre. Revue Stomatologie, Paris 24 (1922) 65—83

Désirabode, (Malagou) A(ntoine)
a) Nouveaux éléments complets de la science et de l'art du dentiste. Paris 1843
b) Eine neue Art, einen Zahn zu operieren. Summary in: Der Zahnarzt, Berlin 13 (1858) 283—285

Dingmann, Reed O., Paul Natwig
Surgery of facial fractures. Philadelphia, London 1964

Dupuytren, Guillaume
a) Kystes osseux développés dans l'épaisseur de l'os. Lancette française 2 (1829) 133—134
b) Leçons orales de clinique chirurgicale faites à l'Hôtel Dieu de Paris. 2nd ed., vol. II, Art. VII, pp. 129—148. Paris 1839

Duval, J(acques) R(ené)
Des accidents de l'extraction des dents. Paris 1802

Elsholtius, Jo(hann) Sig(mund)
Clysmatica nova: . . . Coloniae brandenburgicae (Berlin) 1667

Eulenburg, Albert
Die hypodermatische Injektion der Arzneimittel, 2nd ed., Berlin 1867

Farrar, J(ohn) N(utting)
a) Radical treatment of alveolar abscess. Dent. Cosmos 18 (1876) 582—584
b) Idem. Dent. Cosmos 22 (1880) 376—383
c) Radical and heroic treatment of alveolar abscess by amputation of roots of the teeth. Dent. Cosmos 26 (1884) 79—81, 135—139

Fischer, Guido
a) Beiträge zur Frage der lokalen Anästhesie. Dtsch. Mschr. Zahnhk. 24 (1906) 305—336
b) Die Technik der lokalen Injektionsanästhesie. Dtsch. zahnärztl. Wschr. 12 (1909) 486—489

Fons, J. P. de la
A description of the new patent instrument for extracting teeth; also of a patent method of fixing. London 1826

Fox, Joseph
The history and treatment of the diseases of the teeth, . . . London 1806

Fraser-Moodie, W.
Mr. Gunning and his splint. Brit. J. Oral Surg. 7 (1969) 112—115

Garretson, James E(dward)
A system of oral surgery. 3rd ed., Philadelphia 1869

Geist-Jacobi, G(eorge) P(ierce)
Geschichte der Zahnheilkunde. Tübingen 1896

Gilmer, Thomas L(ewis)
a) Fractures of the inferior maxilla. Ohio State J. Dent. Sc. 1 (1881) 309—320; 2 (1882) 14—25, 57—104, 112—122
b) A case of fracture of the lower jaw with remarks on the treatment. Arch. Dent. 4 (1887) 388—390

Goldwyn, Robert M.
Simon P. Hullihen: pioneer oral and plastic surgeon. Plast. Reconstr. Surg. 52 (1973) 250—257

Graefe, Carl Ferdinand (von)
Jahresbericht. J. Chir. Augenhk., Berlin 4 (1822) 692—693

Guérin, A(lphonse)
Des fractures du maxillaire supérieur. Arch. gén. méd., Paris, 6. série, 8 (1866) 5—13

Gurlt, E(rnst)
Handbuch von der Lehre von den Knochenbrüchen. Part II, Hamm 1864

Hamilton, Frank Hastings
A practical treatise on fractures and dislocations. Philadelphia

Hammond, Gurnell E.
New treatment of fractured maxillae. Monthly Rev. Dent. Surg. 1 (1872/73) 547—550

Hartig, Fr.
Beschreibung eines neuen Apparates zur Retention des Unterkiefers. J. Chir. Augenhk., Berlin 14 (1830) 496—506

Haun, C(arl)
Mittheilung über einen Verband, die Körperbrüche des Unterkiefers zu heilen. Dtsch. Vjschr. Zahnhk. 7 (1867) 213—222

Hauptmeyer, Friedrich
Die Behandlung der Brüche des Unter- und Oberkiefers mittels Zahnschienen. Handb. d. Zahnheilkunde, Vol. I, pp. 104—145, Wiesbaden 1917

Hauser, Paul
Die Bedeutung Frankfurter Forscher für die Einführung der Röntgenologie in der Zahnheilkunde . . . Verh. XX. Internat. Kongr. Gesch. Med. Berlin 1966. Hildesheim 1968, pp. 553—561

Heister, Laurentius
Chirurgie, . . . 2nd ed., Nürnberg 1724

Heitmüller, (Karl)
Die Verwendung des elastischen Gummibandes bei Kieferbrüchen, . . . Dtsch. Mschr. Zahnhk. 15 (1897) 523—529

Howe, J. Morgan
Hydrochlorate of Cocain, . . . Dent. Cosmos 26 (1884) 710—716

Hullihen, Simon P.
a) Compound root forceps. Amer. J. Dent. Sc. 4 (1844) 245 f.
b) Case of elongation of the under jaw . . . Amer. J. Dent. Sci 9 (1849) 157—165

Jost, Johann
Die Entwicklung des zahnärztlichen Berufes und Standes im 19. Jahrhundert. Med. Diss. Zürich 1960

Keys, Thomas E.
The history of surgical anesthesia. New York 1963

Kingsley, Norman W.
A treatise on oral deformities. New York 1880

Koller, Carl
Vorläufige Mittheilung über locale Anästhesierung am Auge. Berichte Dtsch. Ophtal. Ges. 1884, 60—63

Kuhn, Franz
Die perorale Intubation. Berlin 1911

Laforgue, Louis
L'art du dentiste. Paris 1802

Larrey, (Félix Hippolyte)
Zum Gedächtnis an Duval. Der Zahnarzt, Berlin 9 (1854) 314—320

Le Clerc, (Charles Gabriel)
L'appareil commode en faveur des jeunes chirurgiens. Paris 1700

Le Fort, René
Etude expérimentale sur les fractures de la mâchoire supérieure. Revue de Chir., Paris 23 (1901) 208—227; 360—379; 479—507

Liaudet, Ph.
Über die Anwendung von Chloroform bei der Extraktion kranker Zähne. Der Zahnarzt, Berlin 4 (1849) 33—35

Linderer, Joseph
a) Handbuch der Zahnheilkunde. Vol. II, Berlin 1848
b) Die Zahnheilkunde nach ihrem neuesten Standpunkte. Erlangen 1851

Lyman, H(enry) M.
Artificial anesthesia and anesthetics. New York 1881

Lyons, Chalmers J.
The history of oral surgery and its influence on the profession of dentistry. Dent. Cosmos 76 (1934) 26—40

MacEwen, William
Introduction of tracheal tubes by the mouth instead of performing trachotomy or laryngotomy. Brit. Med. J. 2 (1880) 122—124

Macintosh, Robert R., Freda B. Bannister
Essentials of general anesthesia. 3rd ed., Oxford 1943

McNeille, C. S.
Obituary Dr. Gardner Quincy Colton. Dent. Cosmos 40 (1898) 874

Magitot, E(mile)
a) Etude sur le développement et la structure des dents humaines. Thèse méd., Paris 1857
b) Traité de la carie dentaire. Paris 1867
c) Traité des anomalies du système dentaire chez l'homme et les mammifères. Paris 1877
d) Essay sur la pathogénie des kystes et abcès des mâchoires. Gâz. Hôp., Paris 42 (1869) 245—246; 250 f.
e) Mémoire sur les kystes des mâchoires. Arch. Gén. Méd. 20—21 (1872/73) 399—413; 681—699; 154—174; 437—486
f) Die Cysten des Oberkiefers . . . Transl. B. Manassewitsch, Berlin, Neuwied 1888

Malassez, L(ouis)
a) Sur l'existence d'amas épithéliaux autour des dents chez l'homme adulte et à l'état normal (débris épithéliaux paradentaires). Arch. physiol., Paris 3. Série (1885) pp. 139—148 Sur le rôle des débris épithéliaux paradentaires. Idem pp. 309—340; 379—449
b) Über die Existenz epithelialer Massen um die Wurzeln der Zähne (paradentäre Reste). Transl. C. Redard and K. Walz. Arch. et Rev. Suisses d'Odontologie 2 (1888) 264—280; 304—321; 350—364; 388—404; 442—444; 483—497; 3 (1889) 19—36; 62—76; 113—123

Malgaigne, J(oseph) F(rançois)
Traité des fractures et des luxations. Vol. I, Paris 1847

Martin, Claude
a) De la trépanation des extrémités des dents . . . Assoc. franç. pour l'avancement des sciences (1881). Paris 1882, 865—866
b) Du traitement des fractures du maxillaire inférieur par un nouvel appareil. Paris 1887
c) Prothèse immédiate appliquée à la résection des maxillaires. Paris 1889
d) Obituary Dr. Claude Martin. Dent. Cosmos 53 (1911) 497—498

Michaelis, Heinrich
Beschreibung der neuerdings angegebenen Maschinen zur Heilung der Kinnladenbrüche. J. Chir. Augenhk., Berlin 5 (1823) 346—355

Miller, W(illoughby) D(ayton)
Über die Anwendung des Cocain. Korresp. bl. Zahnärzte 14 (1885) 297—299

Morel-Lavallée, (Victor Auguste François)
a) Nouvel appareil pour les fractures des mâchoires. Gaz. hôp., Paris 28 (1855) 404
b) Gaz. hôp., Paris 33 (1860) 576
c) Appareil en gutta-percha pour les fractures des mâchoires . . . Bull. gén. thérap. 63 (1862) 246—248, 352—358, 398—399

Nash. Charles A.
To the editor of the Dental Cosmos. Dent. Cosmos 27 (1885) 63—64

Neuner, A.
Über die künstliche Erzeugung von Cataracten in todten Augen . . . J. Chir. Augenhk., Berlin 10 (1827) 480—492

Niemann, Albert
Über eine organische Base in den Cocablättern. Med. Diss. in: Vjschr. pract. Pharmacie 9 (1860) 489—524

Partsch, C(arl)
a) Über Kiefercysten. Dtsch. Mschr. Zahnhk. 10 (1892) 271—304
b) 3. Bericht der Polikklinik für Zahn- und Mundkrankheiten . . . Breslau. Dtsch. Mschr. Zahnhk. 14 (1896) 492—496
c) Über Wurzelresection. Dtsch. Mschr. Zahnhk. 17 (1899) 348—367
d) Die Aufklappung der Schleimhautbedeckung der Kiefer. Dtsch. Mschr. Zahnhk. 23 (1905) 593—611
e) Die chronische Wurzelhautentzüdung. Dtsch. Zahnhk. 6 (1908)
f) Zur Behandlung der Kiefercysten. Dtsch. Mschr. Zahnhk. 28 (1910) 252—256

Petit, (Jean Louis)
a) Traité des maladies des os. Paris 1767
b) A treatise of the diseases of the bones. London 1726

Préterre, A(pollonie)
Les dents. Traité pratique des maladies de ces organes. 3rd ed., Paris 1872

Raper, Howard Railey
a) Man against pain. New York 1947
b) Notes on the early history of radiodontia. Oral Surg. 6 (1953) 70—81

Raymond, E(dward) H.
Hydrochlorate of cocaine as a local anesthetic in dental surgery. Dent. Cosmos 27 (1885) 207—216

Reiche, Carol(us) Frid(ericus) Guilelm(us)
De maxillae superioris fractura. Med. Diss. Berlin 1822

Rhein, M. L.
Amputation of roots as a radical cure in chronic alveolar abscess. Dent. Cosmos 32 (1890) 904—905

Richardson, (Benjamin Ward)
A new method of producing local anesthesia applicable to dental surgery. Trans. Odont. Soc. G. B. 5 (1866) 45—68

Richter, Adolph Leopold
40 lithographierte Tafeln nebst Erklärung und Erläuterung derselben . . . Berlin 1828

Riethmüller, Richard H.
Root resection in chronic dento-alveolar abscess. History. Summary in: Dent. Cosmos 57 (1915) 397

Riggs, John M.
The discovery of anesthesia. South. Dent. J. 4 (1885) 281—283

Robert, (Alphonse)
Nouveau procédé de traitement des fractures de la portion alvéolaire de la mâchoire inférieure. Bull. gén. thérap., Paris 42 (1852) 22—25

Robin, Ch(arles); E(mile) Magitot
Mémoire sur la genèse et le développement des follicules dentaires . . . J. physiol., Paris 3 (1860), 1—51, 300—322, 663—684

Robinson, James
a) A Treatise on the inhalation of the vapor of ether, . . . London 1847
b) Obituary James Robinson, Esq. London Dent. Rev. 4 (1862) 189—191

Röse, Carl
Über Kieferbrüche und Kieferverbände. Jena 1893

Rowe, Norman Lester
The history of the treatment of maxillo-facial trauma. Ann. Roy. Coll. Surg. England 49 (1971) 329—349

Sands, Austin L.
Fracture of lower jaw, treated by infra-dental splints. Dent. Cosmos 5 (1864) 124—127

Sauer, C(arl)
a) Herstellung eines neuen Verbandes bei Unterkieferbrüchen. Dtsch. Vjschr. Zahnhk. 21 (1881) 362—375
b) Nothverband bei Kieferbrüchen aus Eisendraht. Dtsch. Mschr. Zahnhk. 7 (1889) 381—392

Sauvez, E.
Obituary Dr. E. Magitot. Dent. Cosmos 39 (1897) 680—681

Schnoor, Gustav
Professor Sauer's Anwendung der schiefen Ebene . . . Dtsch. Mschr. Zahnhk. 5 (1887) 217—219

Schröder, Hermann
Frakturen und Luxationen der Kiefer. Berlin 1911

Schuchardt, Karl
Ein Vorschlag zur Verbesserung der Drahtschienenverbände. Dtsch. Zahn-Mund-Kieferhk. 24 (1956) 39—44

Schwartz, Laszlo L.
The development of the treatment of jaw fractures. J. Oral Surg. 2 (1944) 193—221

Serre, Johann Jacob Joseph
Praktische Darstellung aller Operationen der Zahnheilkunst. Berlin 1803

Snow, John
On chloroform and other anesthetics. Ed. Benjamin W. Richardson, London 1858

Späth
Komplicirte Fraktur des Unterkiefers. Med. Corresp.bl. würtemb., ärztl. Verein 6 (1836) 276—277

Süersen, W(ilhelm)
Über Verletzungen resp. Fracturen des Ober- und Unterkiefers. Dtsch. Vjschr. Zahnhk. 11 (1871) 261—273

Taft, J(onathan)
A practical treatise on operative dentistry. Philadelphia 1859

Thoma, Kurt H
A historical review of methods advocated for the treatment of jaw fractures, . . . Oral Surg. 2 (1944) 399—504

Tomes, John
a) On the construction and application of forceps for extracting teeth. London Med. Gaz., N. S. Vol. II (1841) 424—430
b) A system of dental surgery. Philadelphia 1859

Trendelenburg, (Friedrich)
Tamponade der Trachea. Arch. klin. Chir. 12 (1871) 121—133

Turnovsky, Friedrich
Handbuch der Zahnheilkunde . . . Pesth 1856

Walser, Hans H.
Zur Einführung der Äthernarkose im deutschen Sprachgebiet im Jahre 1847. Aarau 1957

Wassmund, Martin
Frakturen und Luxationen. Berlin 1927

Weber, (I. H. C.)
Adhäsionsgebisse und über Unterkieferbrüche. Dtsch. Vjschr. Zahnhk. 5 (1865) 285—292

Wedl, Carl; Moriz Heider
Anatomischer Befund über eine Cyste des Oberkiefers nebst klinischen Bemerkungen über Cysten. Dtsch. Mschr. Zahnhk. 5 (1865) 1—6

Weiser, Rudolf
Die Resultate der radicalen Behandlung des Alveolar-Abscesses und der Zahnwurzelcyste bei Conservierung des Zahnes. Österr.-ungar. Vjschr. Zahnhk. 16 (1900) 2456—2471

Wiseman, Richard
Severall chirurgicall treatises. London 1676

Chapter 14

Orthodontics

The field of orthodontics—called in the English speaking countries "Orthodontia" during the 19th century, in France then frequently "Orthopédie dentaire", and in Germany of the 20th century "Kieferorthopädie" (jaw orthopedics)—was added to the three traditional specialities: prosthodontics, dental surgery, and conservative dentistry as a speciality in its own rights.

The earliest mention of anomalies of the jaw is found in Hippocrates, and the first orthodontic advice is to be read in the Roman Celsus, around the time of Christ [1]. The recommendation of Celsus that persistent deciduous teeth should be extracted, and that permanent teeth which erupt in the wrong direction ought to be corrected by finger pressure, dominated the therapy in this area up to the 18th century. As an example, a page is shown from the third chapter of the "Artzney Buchlein", the oldest dental textbook of 1530 [2], in which Celsus' advice is repeated, although in a more circumstantial manner (Fig. 440). In 1728 Fauchard described the first orthodontic appliances, and in 1757 we find an early recommendation of serial extraction by his intellectual successor, Bourdet [3]. In London Berdmore gave some advice, and the theoretical foundations of orthodontics were clearly defined there by John Hunter in 1778 [4]. In 1803 the court dentist in Berlin, Serre, had already prepared plate appliances which were not described in more detail and fashioned by a goldsmith from an impression [5]. Otherwise, however, he preferred forceful straightening because of its more rapid results, for which he quotes his colleague Brunner, who had been his contemporary when he worked in Vienna [6]. All these efforts were directed exclusively at the cosmetic effect.

Herewith we come to the 19th century, during the first decades of which the advice of an influential student of Hunter, Joseph Fox in London (1803), prevailed. He saw the only effective treatment for prevention of occlusal anomalies in a measure which was thoroughly misleading: in the serial extraction of the primary teeth, particularly the second deciduous molars, even before they had loosened: *When the second temporary molares have been removed there remain no other obstacles in the way of the completion of the second dentition* [7].

To eliminate an anterior crossbite Fox employed an arch of gold or silver which had two small ivory chocks as bite blocks (Fig. 441). The teeth were labially drawn toward the arch with silk threads which were to be adjusted every three days [8]. In the second part of the work of 1806 a leather head-chin cap is shown. It served the exclusive purpose, however, of making a tooth extraction free of complications possible for patients suffering from jaw luxation [9] (Fig. 442).

No original thoughts on this subject are found by the Parisian dentists of the early 19th century, such as Laforgue (1802) and Gariot (1805). C. F. Delabarre was the first to bring forth new ideas in his "Odontologie" which appeared in 1815 [10], and which was followed in 1819 by a detailed presentation in the specialized work, "Traité sur la seconde dentition" (Treatise on the Second Dentition). He sharply and justifiably rejects the premature extraction of deciduous teeth which was preferred by Fox, and proves in the text and the illustrations the value of the "dents temporaires" as space maintainers. His method is the *natural method,* that of supervising the natural growth. Man only has to *help Nature, when she cannot complete her tasks alone* [11]. The physician should only act under special circumstances, when there are obstacles to the development of the jaw bones.

Delabarre was one of the first to strive for a certain systematization of occlusal anomalies,

[1] See pp. 62 and 71 f.
[2] See pp. 159 f.
[3] See pp. 200 f. and 212 f.
[4] See pp. 218 and 221 f.
[5] See p. 241
[6] See p. 237
[7] Fox (a) p. 56
[8] Fox (a) pp. 67 f.
[9] Fox (b) pp. 169 f.
[10] Delabarre (a) pp. 46 f.
[11] Delabarre (b) p. 130

Es pflegt ſich oft zu begeben das den kindern nach ſyben Jaren/wenn die zeen beginnen auß zufallē/andere zene wachſen neben den yhenigen die do außfallen ſolden / derhalben ſal man den alden zan der außfallen ſal neben welchen der newe erſcheynet von dem zanfleiſche wol reinigen vnnd offt wackeln/ alſo lange baß er ſich leth außzihen / darnach ſal man den newen alle tage an den orth do der forige geſtanden hat trucken/vnnd lencken/alſo lange baß er ahn den rechten orth do der forige geſtanden hat komme/vnd den andern gleich werde/Denn wenn mans vor ſihet ſo bleibet der alde ſtehen vnd wirdt ſchwartz/ der Junge vorhindert das er nicht fein gerade kan gewachſen/ vñ darnach mit keinerley weiſe an ſeinen rechten orth gebracht werden.

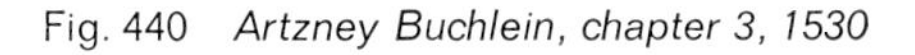

Fig. 440 *Artzney Buchlein, chapter 3, 1530*

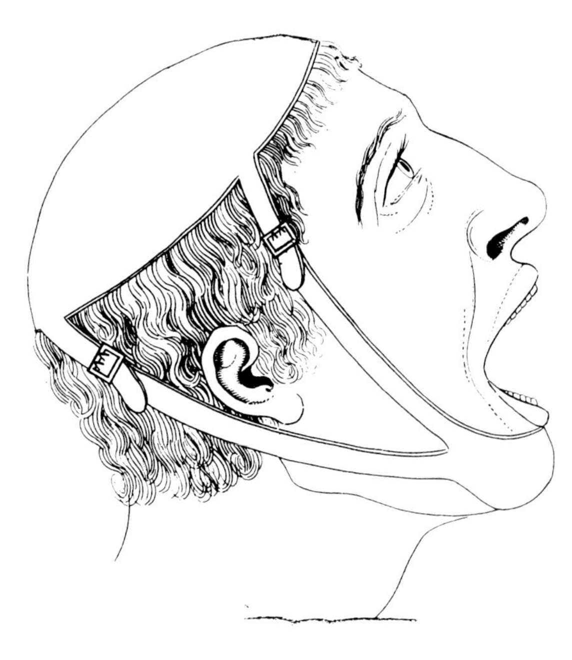

Fig. 442 *Fox: Chin cap to prevent luxation of the jaw, 1803*

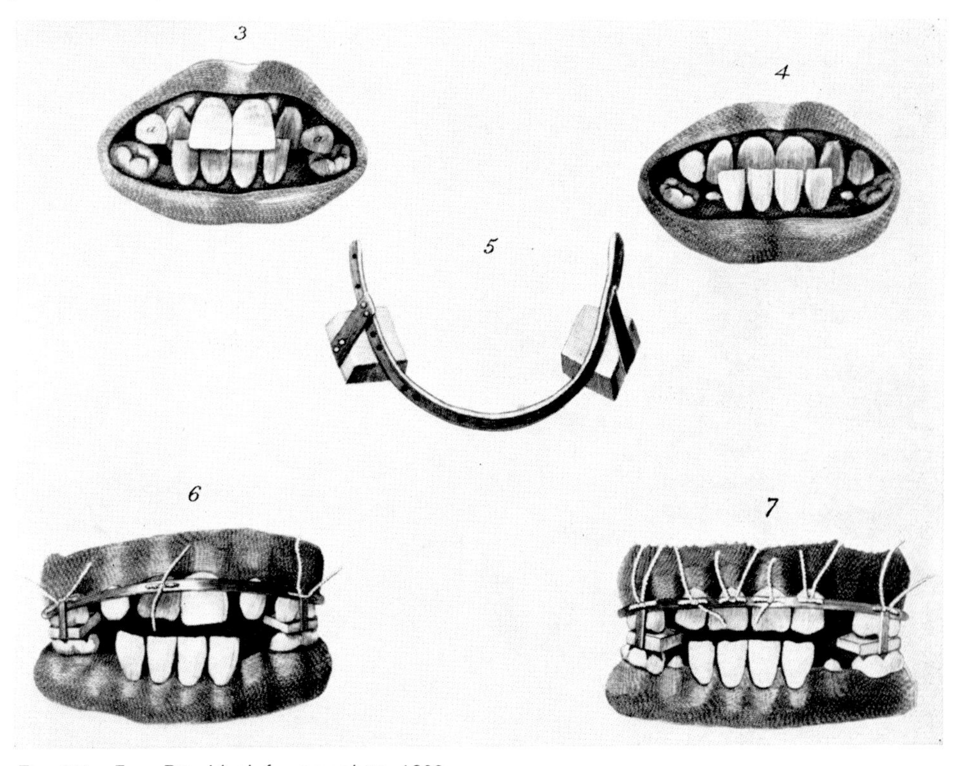

Fig. 441 *Fox: Bite block for crossbite, 1803*

through description and illustration of the individual kinds. He also discussed critically the appliances of his predecessors since the time of Fauchard, and presented them as illustrations. Here Fox's construction (baillon de Fox) and also the inclined plane of his Parisian colleague L. J. Catalan in 1808 were both rejected because the unsupported bar sank into the gingiva and was torture for children (Fig. 443). He achieved bite block through a wire screen put in place in the area of the mandibular molars. The teeth were then arranged with silk threads without an inclined plane, a method which was probably the least unsatisfactory of the means available to him (Fig. 444). First of all we find in Delabarre an early description of a kind of band appliance fixed to a tooth turned on its axis, a procedure which, in principle, is still used today[12] (Fig. 445). He separated crowded teeth by means of swelling threads placed between them or, following the recommendation of Pierre Auzeby of Lyon, *in a work full of errors* from 1771, with similarly swelling wooden wedges[13].

A classification of malocclusions, which formed a precedent in France, is encountered under the heading "Dent (pathologie)" from the "Dictionnaire de Médecine" which appeared from 1832 to 1839, of which we have on hand the second edition from 1832 to 1845. The author, Jean-Nicolas Marjolin, starts by differentiating between obliqueness (obliquité) of the teeth and anomalies of the dental arch. In the former, there are anterior, posterior, and lateral types, and one from rotation around the axis of the tooth. He attributed the lack of space as the cause and unfortunately recommended as therapy first of all the old premature serial extraction of the primary teeth. If this does not help, space must be provided by filing the teeth to make them narrower, or with the forceps. He knew of the use of ligatures and metal bands only from hearsay, and he viewed forceful straightening with suspicion.

The anomalies of the dental arch are classified as "proéminence," i. e., an oblique protrusion of the upper, of the lower, or of both rows of anterior teeth, and "rétroition," i. e., an oblique position of the front teeth to the inside, and as "inversion," today's mesial occlusion[14]. For "proéminence" the therapy consisted of the extraction of a pair of premolars followed by the application of a labial arch and insertion of a palatal plate through which the outer arch is pulled back together with the protruding front teeth by means of ligatures. In "rétroition" the file should be employed. Mesial occlusion, however, he regarded as incurable which was then undoubtedly the case. If only a few upper incisors hook behind the lower ones he advises the use of Catalan's inclined plane. Maury in his handbook essentially adhered to the insights of "professeur Marjolin" whom he quotes frequently, but he also furnished illustrations[15] (Fig. 446).

Christopher Starr Brewster, an American dentist working in Paris, recommended the spiral spring as the first elastic means of treatment in 1840. Unfortunately this was only a vague description, with no illustrations. With a gold palatal plate which carried a *system of spiral springs* he was able in less than three months, to close a severely open bite with a distal position through a *progressive and constant pulling* of the crooked teeth towards an approximately normal position[16].

In 1841 Lefoulon adopted Marjolin's classifications. He rejected the forceful straightening with the greatest determination but on the other hand, the inclined plane was to him infallible. He was, justifiably, a little doubtful whether Delabarre had actually ever tested this auxiliary means of treatment which he had rejected[17]. It is worthy of note that Lefoulon had already taken the step from orthodontist towards jaw orthopedist: . . . *the vault of the palate and, to an even lesser extent, the dental arches are not unchangeable in their dimensions, as was believed for a long time* . . .[18]. Therefore, even with crowded teeth the first premolars need not be removed. Rather a spring-action gold arch should first be placed within the row of teeth which was designated as a *passif spring*. If individual teeth point outwards they should be tied with silken ligatures which have the effect of an *active spring (ressort aktif)* . . . *One of the greatest advantages of this completely new method is that it is neither painful nor annoying*[19]. His lingual arch, how-

12 Ibid. pp. 148 f.
13 Ibid. pp. 140 f.; Auzeby: Traité d'Odontalgie, Lyon 1771, Paris 1772
14 Marjolin p. 452 f.
15 Maury (a) p. 54 f.; (b) p. 78 f.
16 Brewster
17 Lefoulon p. 234 f.
18 Ibid. p. 190
19 Ibid. p. 194; see pp. xxx and xxxi

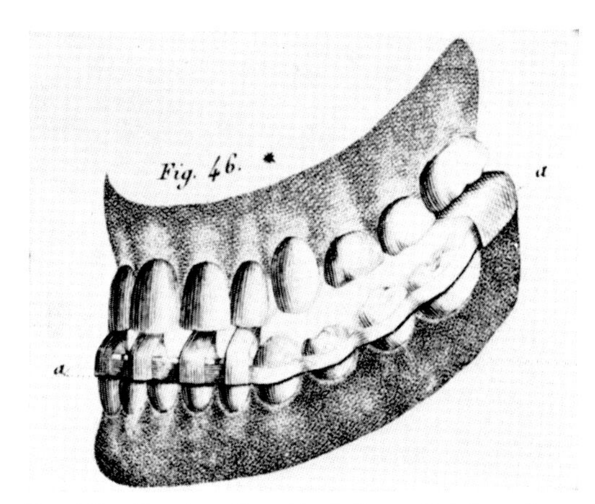

Fig. 443 *Catalan: Bite block (from Delabarre)*

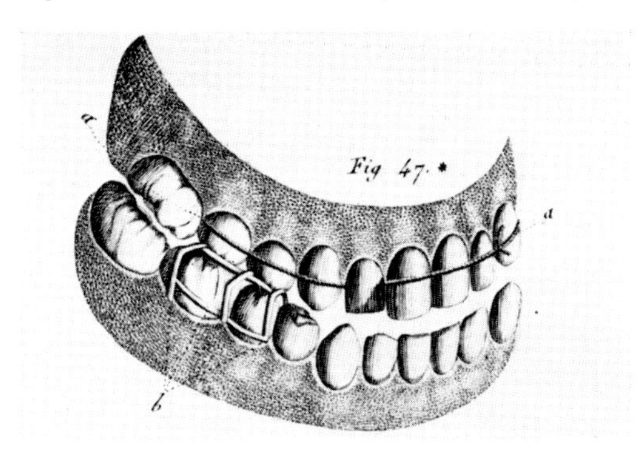

Fig. 444 *Delabarre: Bite block and repositioning of an incisor with silk ligatures, 1815*

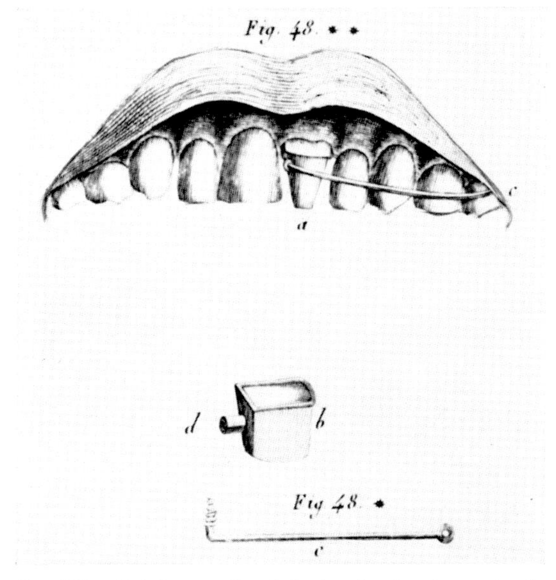

Fig. 445 *Delabarre: Band device for turning a tooth, 1815*

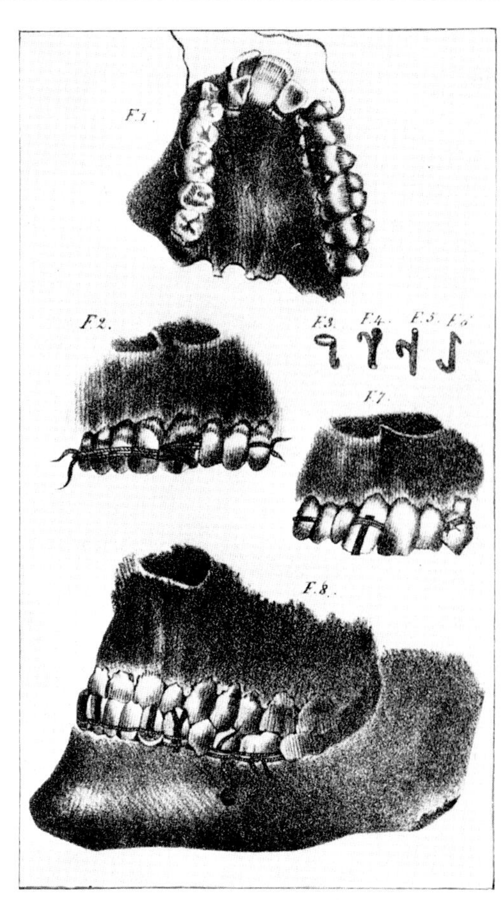

Fig. 446 *Maury: Orthodontics with silk ligatures, 1830*

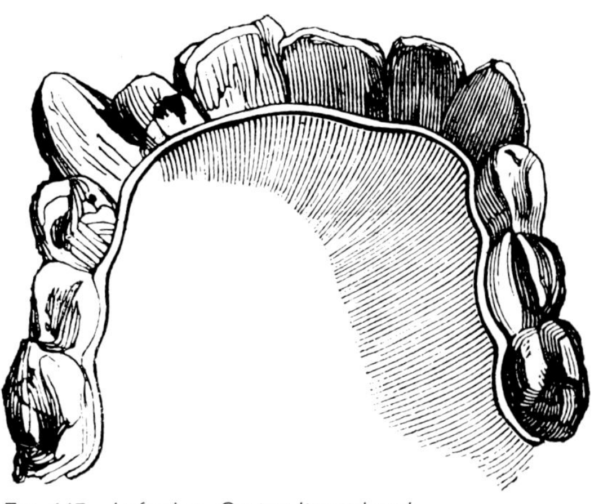

Fig. 447 *Lefoulon: Spring lingual arch*

ever, presumably because of the lack of a permanently elastic material and durable means of fastening, was not able to establish itself at that time (Fig. 447).

Lefoulon's idea was independently reintroduced in the United States by Jackson in 1887 and, with special success, by Mershon in 1909. As is evident in his case reports, he combined it with the inclined plane. The inventor of the lingual arch headed this chapter of his textbook with the title "Orthodontosie," although in keeping with J. Linderer he had already published an article in 1839 under the title of "Orthopédie dentaire" [20].

In 1841, the same year as Lefoulon's book, a special work came out in Paris, a "Précis sur le redressement des dents" (Outline of the Straightening of the Teeth), by J. M. Alexis Schange, of which a third edition and a German translation had been printed in 1842. His classification of occlusal anomalies, too, is similar to that of Marjolin. This is not so, however, as regards the appliances. As is shown in figure 448 (top), a protuding lateral incisor is pulled into the row of teeth through a ligature which is anchored on the molars of the other side. Schange hoped to eliminate gaping protrusion through silk threads attached to a plate, as is shown in the lower half of the picture. He achieved the same thing by means of a labial arch from which he then worked with silk threads, or small screws for traction or pulling, according to choice (Fig. 449). Herewith we have an early recommendation of the screw [21]. Further he also made use of a rubber band, which is probably the first use of elastic rubber in orthodontics (Fig. 450): *The length of this strip of rubber stretched over the anteriors need only be about half as long as the area which it should cover.* According to Schange this force always allows the straightening of protruding teeth especially with young persons, as long as there is enough room [22].

In order to shift the central incisors toward the lingual side while simultaneously shifting the canines to the labial side, Schange constructed a screw which did not, however, live up to his expectations. A band appliance served for rotating individual incisors. As seen in the picture it also appears to have been fastened with a screw (Fig. 451).

The most important idea of Schange is his demand that the pulling arrangement be anchored principally on several molars which are generally bound together with a gold clamp, and that a mechanical immobilization of what had been achieved so far be carried out *for a long time*. This seems all the more necessary in light of the fact that the "cures" hardly required more than a quarter of a year then. For this purpose the aid shown in figure 450 is employed: *I use for this purpose a small band of hard rubber, which is attached on both ends to molar clasps. This small apparatus which I have Dr.* (Claude) *Lachaise to thank for, and to which I will return* (see above) *has perfectly achieved the aim which I had intended* [23].

In 1843 we find practically nothing new in Désirabode's corresponding chapter of his unillustrated book headed under the title of "Hygiène et Orthopédie." He rightly distrusted the long silk ligatures. Therefore he attached immobile labial and lingual bars to the two most distal molars from which he then effected the movement with silk or platinum wire. *This apparatus is, in fact, the only one that we use, because it is more certain by far than the simple threads* [24]. He had nothing to say for the expansion method of his countryman Lefoulon and created space in the old manner through the removal of the first premolars or through filing of the teeth into a narrower shape.

The first specialized orthodontic work ever was the essay, "Der Schiefstand der Zähne" (The Oblique Position of the Teeth), by Friedrich Christoph Kneisel, a court dentist in Berlin. This work, which comprises 21 pages and appeared in 1836, is written in two languages, German and French. He classified the *anomalous positions* as general and partial obliqueness, whereby the former includes both the maxillary and mandibular anterior mesiocclusion as well as edge-to-edge occlusion. He considered the causes to be hereditary factors, nursing difficulties, and insufficient exercise of the jaws in childhood. This latter cause *appears very frequently, unfortunately, in the upper classes, where the children mainly receive everything cut into small bites* [25]. He is not as decidedly against

[20] J. Linderer (d) p. 473. See pp. 376 and 378
[21] See p. 368
[22] Schange p. 128 f.
[23] Ibid. pp. 104 f.
[24] Désirabode p. 187
[25] Kneisel pp. 9 f.

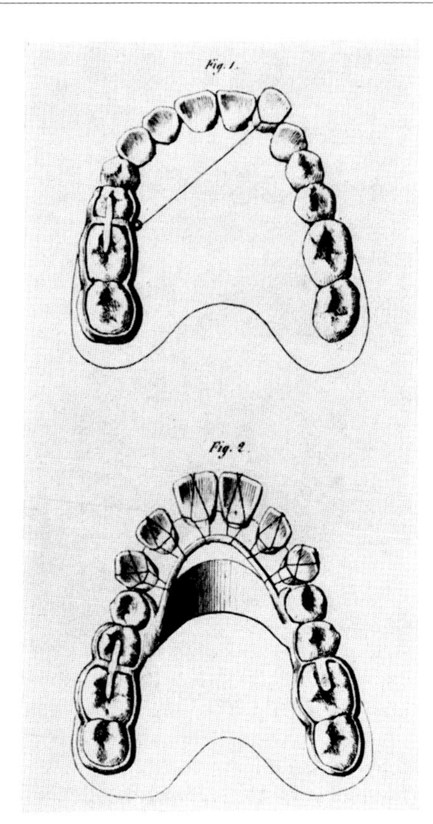

Fig. 448 *Schange: Repositioning a lateral incisor and treatment of protrusion, 1841*

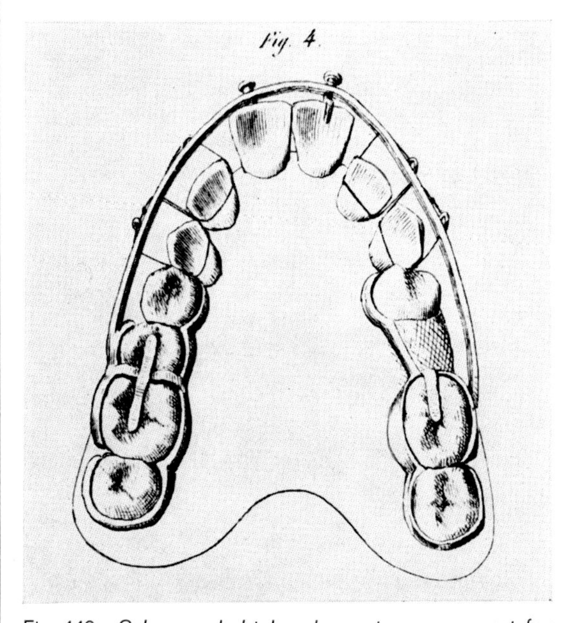

Fig. 449 *Schange: Labial arch serving as support for secondary elements, 1841*

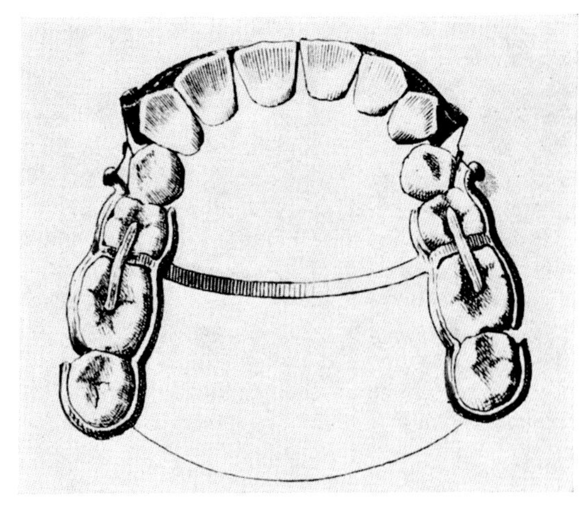

Fig. 450 *Schange: First use of a rubber band, applied labially in treatment of protrusion, 1841*

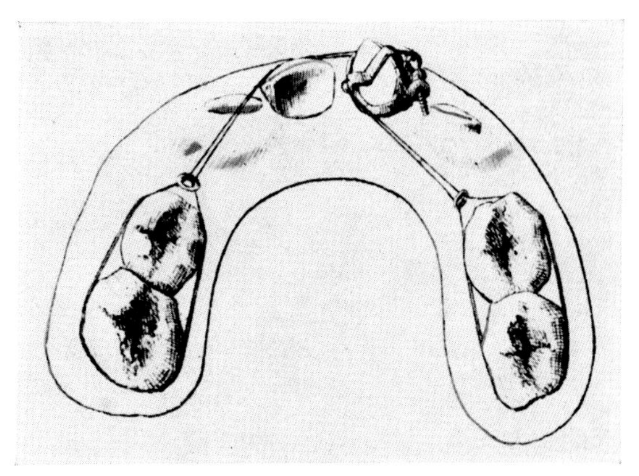

Fig. 451 *Schange: Screw-retained band device, 1841*

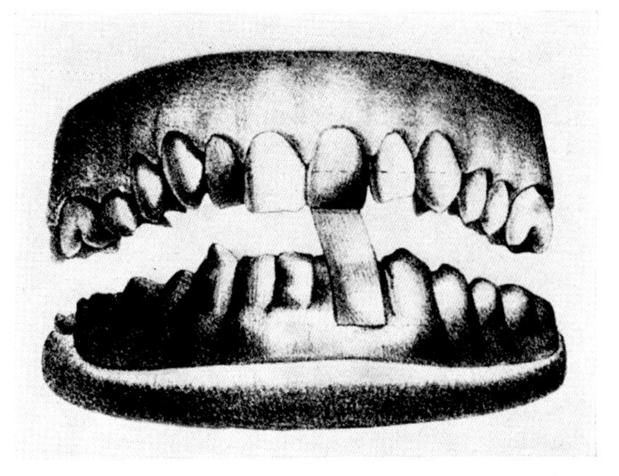

Fig. 452 *Kneisel: Gold spring as an inclined plane, 1836*

the premature removal of the primary teeth as is Delabarre.

Luxation with the pelican, the "redresser" of Fauchard, is strongly rejected as being too dangerous for the tooth. In the use of ligatures, the tooth serving as the point of support also changes its position. Therefore, Kneisel advises covering the mandibular arch with a capsule (unfortunately not recognizable from the illustration) constructed from a model to which a gold spring is soldered (Fig. 452). This modification of the inclined plane marks the limits of his orthodontic therapy, if we neglect his recommendation that *a linen cloth* be wrapped around head and chin at night *for a stronger pressure of the mandible against the maxilla,* and that *its shifting be prevented by the wearing of a cap with ear flaps*[26]. His concept that the teeth serving as fulcra had to have attained a certain firmness already, *or else the tooth crowns will be twisted by the pressure brought to bear on them, while the roots of same remain in one position ...* seems curious[27]. This lapse was already pointed out to Kneisel by Nessel in Prague in 1840[28].

Kneisel's little book induced his colleague from Berlin, Berthold Alexander Lomnitz, to write a likewise small "Lehre vom Schiefstand der Zähne" (Instruction on the Malposition of the Teeth) in 1840. Quite well-versed in professional literature he proves to his predecessor that his inclined plane had already been described by Hunter, Fox, Catalan, and others. This small book of 40 pages, which is extremely modest in appearance in comparison to Kneisel's essay, is thoroughly anti-Kneisel, yet still brings forth no new ideas.

We have to thank the Viennese professor Georg Carabelli, a scientifically important man, for the first useful nomenclature of the kinds of occlusion, published in 1842. It took root in German-speaking areas for a rather long time[29]. He based his classification *of the various positions of the incisors and canines*[30]: 1. the normal occlusion (mordex normalis), 2. the straight (edge-to-edge) occlusion (mordex rectus), 3. the open occlusion (mordex apertus, Fig. 453), 4. the protruding occlusion (mordex prorsus, maxillary and mandibular protrusion), 5. the retruding occlusion (mordex retrosus, inversion), and 6. the zig-zag occlusion (mordex tortuosus, cross bite). The seventh and eighth points, the (partially toothed) *senile occlusion* (Greisengebiß), and the (edentulous) *senile mouth* (Greisenmund, mordex senilis and os senile) have no significance here. The uncommon Latin term "mordex" was taken by the author from a comedy of the Roman poet Plautus.

Carabelli, too, is in favor of keeping the primary teeth for a long time, not, however, from indications as clear as Delabarre's. He feared that if too long an interval existed between the extraction and the eruption, so much *bone mass* would form that the replacing tooth might not be able to penetrate it, and thus either grow in incorrectly or even not at all[31]. As the therapy volume remained unwritten we find his therapeutic recommendations only in the "Handbuch der Zahnheilkunde" (Handbook of Dentistry) of 1840 by his student Franz Nessel, who had represented dentistry since 1828 as the first professor of the subject at the University in Prague. The device of his master, which he described and illustrated, consists of a labial arch which had a threaded screw for depressing the tooth, and a gear shaft for pulling[32] (Fig. 454). A year later, in Paris, Schange likewise considered the use of the screw's effect[33].

Both Linderers in Berlin, father and son[34], also occupied themselves with the *straightening of the teeth.* In the 1834 textbook by the father there is hardly anything new, but he is still at the pinnacle of his time[35]. In the collaborative work of 1842 the recommendation is made for *obliquely positioned teeth,* i. e. a protrusion with gaps, of a *special plate flexing to the rear,* a labial bar which is supported by the incisal edges and is pulled distally by silk threads anchored on the molars (Fig. 455). In the case of prognathic crowding, which is called appropriately *rabbit mouth,* the transverse strut, described by Hunter, is advised for expan-

[26] Ibid. p. 19. Weinberger justly sees the first orthodontic use of the head-chin cap for orthodontic purposes here. The cap of Fox (Fig. 442) had a different indication (Weinberger pp. 220 and 240. See pp. 362 f.

[27] Kneisel p. 11

[28] Nessel p. 170

[29] See pp. 397 f.

[30] Carabelli pp. 126 f.

[31] Ibid. pp. 77 f., footnote

[32] Nessel pp. 169 f.

[33] See p. 352. Delabarre had used the screw only as a retention device for bands in 1819 (see Fig. 445)

[34] See pp. 272 f.

[35] C. J. Linderer pp. 101 f

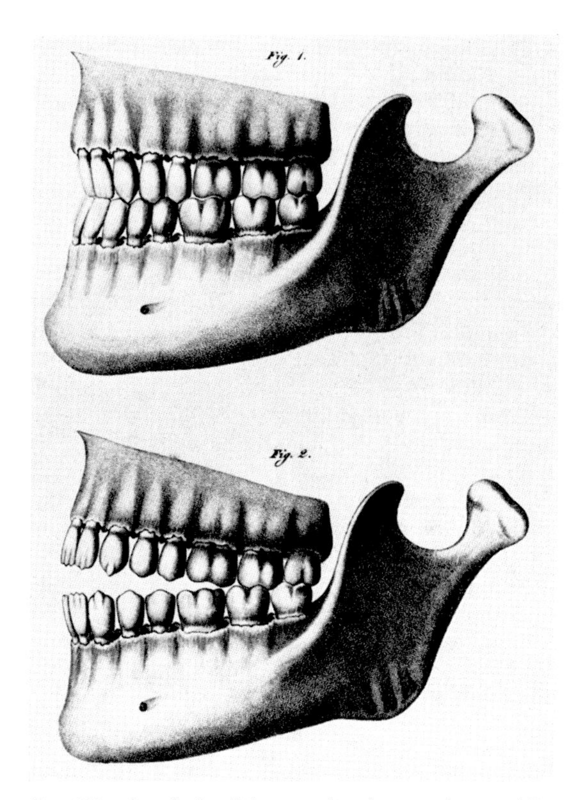

Fig. 453 *Carabelli: Edge-to-edge bite and open bite, 1842*

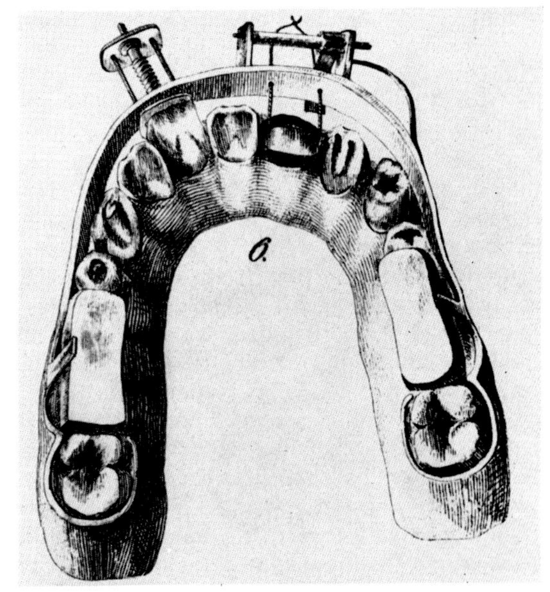

Fig. 454 *Carabelli: Labial arch with a threaded screw and spindle to move single teeth (from Nessel, 1840)*

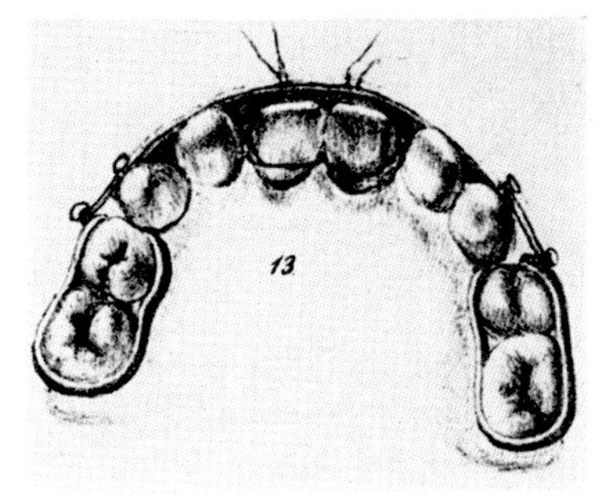

Fig. 455 *Linderer: Labial arch, 1842*

sion after removal of the first premolar[36]. This device separates the posterior teeth by means of a screw with a bolt[37].

In his last work dating from 1851, Joseph Linderer, self-critically, acknowledged that *this important matter had been discussed far too little in his handbook*[38]. The first recommendation here is, once again, that of Celsus' finger pressure. Furthermore he recommended an *expansion machine for the maxilla* which had at this time already been used by Robinson in London: he constructed a gold plate to the edge of which he attached "Federharz" (spring resin), i. e., vulcanized rubber. This was to *induce the pressure on the gingiva and the processus* (alveolaris), thus, here also a jaw orthopedic procedure[39]. With this Linderer foregoes the removal of the first premolars. The *open mouth* (bite) was treated, as is occasionally still done today as a last resort by extraction of the molars.

In London, which we had left with Fox in 1806, Leonhard Koecker, who had emigrated from Philadelphia in 1822[40], and who was known for being an enthusiastic tooth-extractor, still knew nothing of the inclined plane in 1826. His

[36] See pp. 221 f.
[37] J. Linderer (a) pp. 471 f.
[38] J. Linderer (c) p. 179
[39] Ibid. pp. 228 f.
[40] See pp. 273 f.

urgent recommendations were limited to the serial extraction of the first molar, even before the age of twelve [41].

In 1829 Thomas Bell justifiably deplored the influence of such a respected author as Fox, because his guidelines in the removal of the primary teeth were adopted without question. His text often adheres quite closely to Delabarres's "Seconde dentition," but he maintains in an eulogy to the Frenchman that he had already come to hold the same opinions before having read his work [42]. Bell's procedure for treatment of anterior cross-bite is the same in principle as that of Fox, except that instead of a gold bar he uses one of cast brass which extends to the premolars and fits tightly to the anterior teeth on the labial side. He achieves a bite block through gold crowns set on each molar on both sides: *The cap should extend as far as the neck of the tooth on each side, and should be accurately adapted to all the irregularities of the surface, by being stamped between a brass cast of the tooth and a hollow cast of lead. It is made of gold, containing such a portion of alloy as to render it hard and elastic.* The edge is bent in somewhat, so that it grips the neck of tooth firmly through the effect of the spring [43]. It is surprising that Bell did not use this *gold cap* also for the preservation of damaged teeth, but cement probably still needed to be invented for that.

In 1839 William Robertson in Birmingham recommended a modified inclined plane (Fig. 456) and repeated Fox's views on the removal of the deciduous teeth [44]. James Robinson, on the other hand, who devoted thirty pages of his textbook to the "Irregularity of the Teeth," regarded the maintainance of the deciduous teeth as the best preventive measure. For therapy he used several original appliances and also used chiefly the one recommended in 1840 by Brewster in Paris [45] and the spiral spring introduced in England in 1845 by Sir Edwin Saunders, the dentist of Queen Victoria [46]. For expansion of the jaw a plate was fitted with a hinge at its center, and two traverse springs pressed the dental arch and the alveolar process apart (Fig. 457). For treatment of protrusion Robinson used "Indian rubber": he attached a horseshoe-shaped plate encompassing the incisors to a plate cut from bone. He squeezed rubber between a labial arch and the teeth, as Linderer did later, and thereby forced the incisors toward the oral cavity [47] (Fig. 458).

The serial extraction of the four permanent first molars, already recommended by Bourdet (1757) and Koecker (1826) among others, was thoroughly substantiated for the first time in 1857 by Samuel Maclean, a dentist in London: *(1.) The prevention and correction of the similar forms of irregularities . . ., without the aid of mechanical means. (2.) The promotion of a healthier state of the remaining teeth. (3.) The prevention of distressing and in some cases even very serious symptoms, which frequently accompany the development of the wisdom teeth in over-crowded arches* [48] (abbreviated).

John Tomes, whose orientation was more of an odontological and surgical one, referred in his textbook of 1859 essentially to his friend William Anthony Harrison, who worked with ivory plates and had achieved shifting of the teeth through (swelling) wooden wedges forced between the plate and the tooth as had already been recommended by Saunders in 1845. Tomes preferred metal plates on the base of his own experience. If the vertical dimension is to be increased, then these cover the molars also (Fig. 459). The halves of the plate are connected by a labial arch, from which the individual motion is carried out with silk ligatures, or, as Tomes particularly recommended, with vulcanized rubber (that means rubber bands) [49]. He tried to eliminate the open bite with a head-chin cap. For a twisted incisor room is created by a spring soldered to the plate (Fig. 460).

The Paris-born Amadée-François Talma, who was working as court dentist in Brussels, and was a nephew to the great tragedian, devoted forty pages in his 1852 textbook to the chapter "Orthopédie dentaire." [50] He discerned the causes of occlusal deviations in anomalies of the jaw, the alveolar process, and the shape of the tooth, as in outside influences such as pressure by the tongue and lips,

[41] Koecker pp. 191 f.
[42] Bell pp. 92 f.
[43] Ibid. p. 100
[44] Robertson pp. 46 f.
[45] See p. 364
[46] Robinson pp. 48 f; Saunders
[47] Robinson pp. 45 f.
[48] Maclean
[49] Tomes pp. 173 f. See pp. 391 f.
[50] Talma (b) pp. 69 f.; Cohen

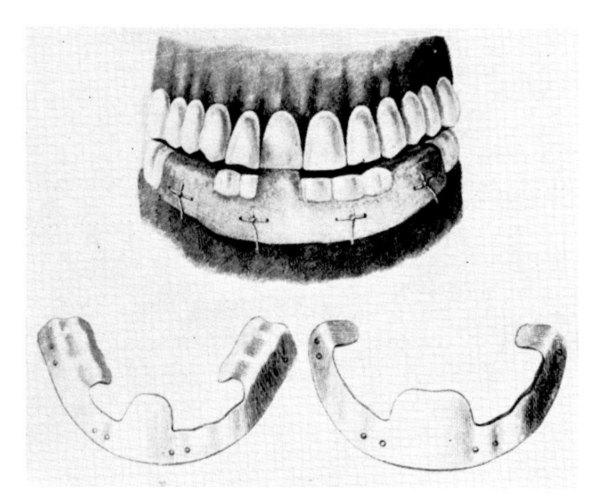

Fig. 456 *Robertson: Inclined plane, 1839*

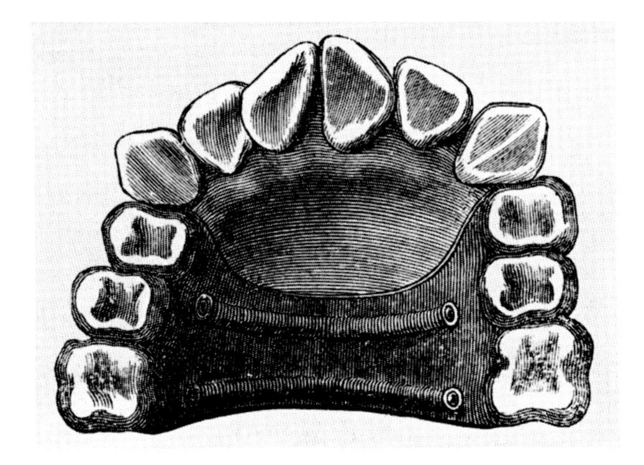

Fig. 457 *Robinson: Expansion of the jaw with a spring plate, 1846*

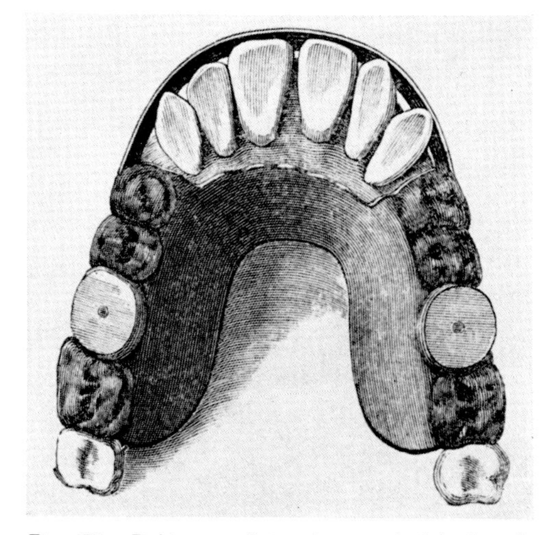

Fig. 458 *Robinson: Bite plane with labial arch, 1846*

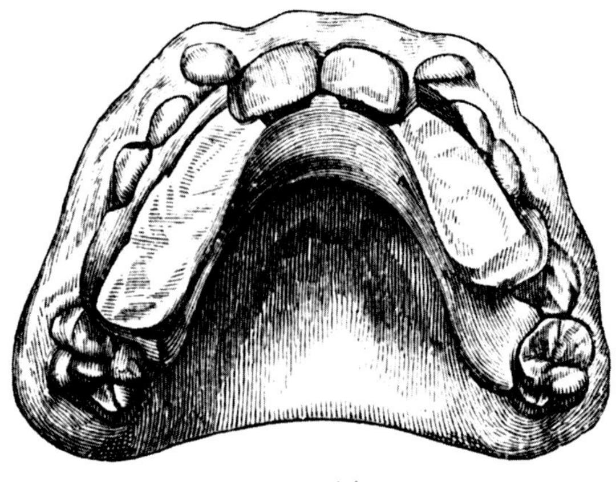

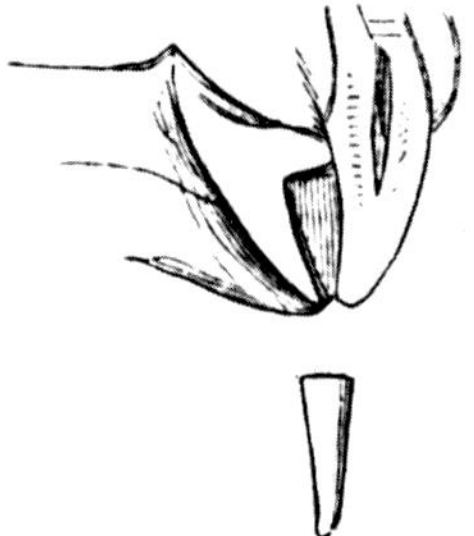

Fig. 459 *Tomes: Tooth movement through wooden posts, 1859*

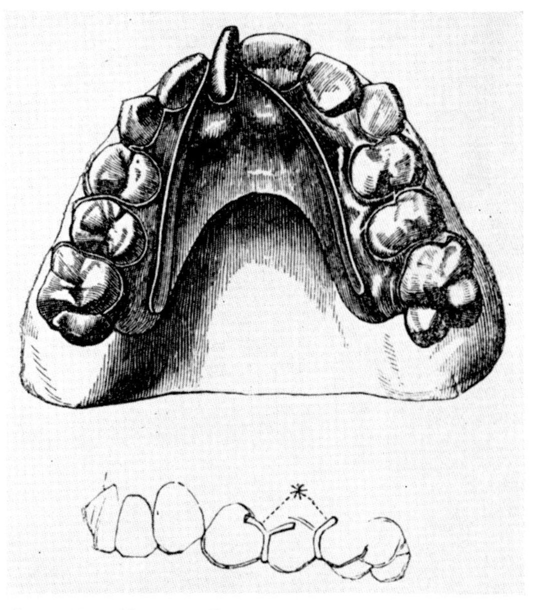

Fig. 460 *Tomes: Tooth rotation with plate-borne springs, 1859*

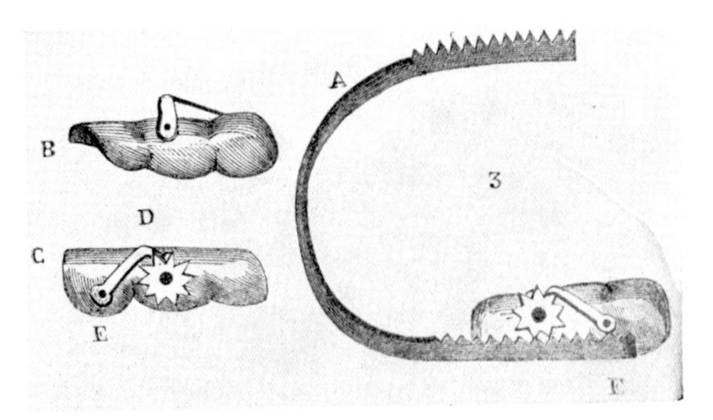

Fig. 461 *Rogers: The "Régulateur," geared design to move protruded anteriors, 1845*

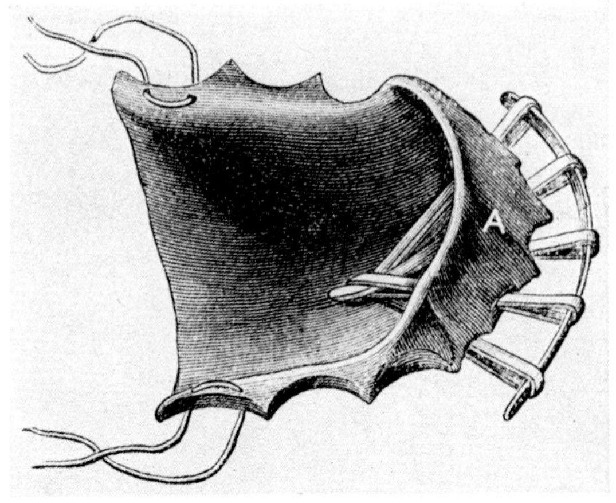

Fig. 463 *Kingsley: Bite plane for "jumping the bite," 1880*

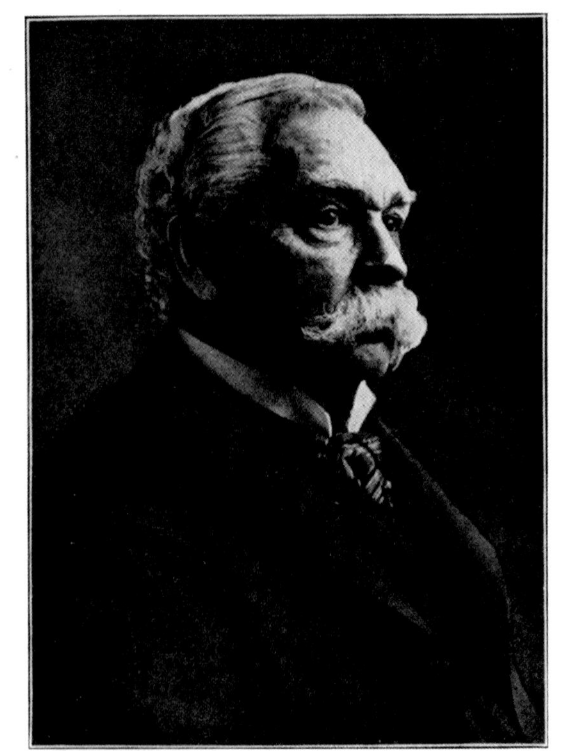

Fig. 462 *Norman William Kingsley*

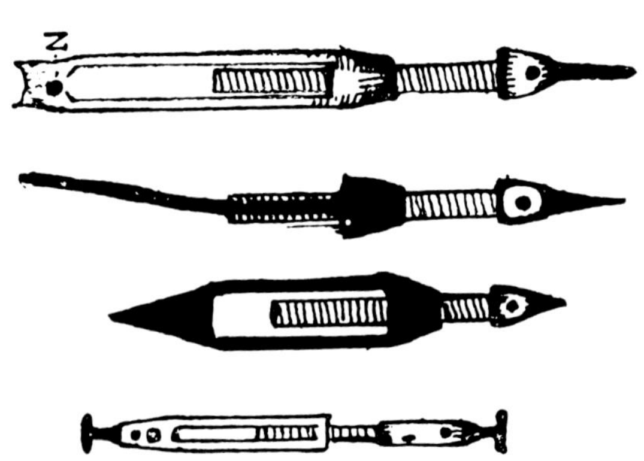

Fig. 464 *Dwinelle: Jackscrew, 1849*

and sucking of the tongue and thumb, and others. Otherwise he worked with the methods of his predecessors, and used springs, bands, rings, and hard rubber wedges but rejected silk threads. A system of his own he did not develop. Talma, however, was one of the first to recognize the necessity for a governmentally controlled school dental service, and was already demanding it in 1843 in his essay "Mémoire sur la Conservation des Dents."[51] It was not until 1902 that the first municipal school dental clinic in the world was founded in Strassburg, Alsace, by an unsalaried university lecturer, Ernst Jessen[52].

In the United States the older authors limited themselves to pages-long word-for-word repe-

[51] Talma (a)
[52] Jessen

titions of Fox's teachings mentioning his name. Two examples are Levi Spear Parmly, who, during his five years of residence in London, published his "Lectures on the Natural History and Management of the Teeth" simultaneously there and in New York in 1820[53], and Samuel Sheldon Fitch, who presented his "A System of Dental Surgery" in 1829[54]. In 1844 Amos Westcott recommended the head-chin cap described by Fox for the treatment of luxations for the first time for maxillary orthopedics, if Kneisel's use of a linen cloth is disregarded[55].

After Brewster had introduced the spiral spring, and Lachaise and Schange had introduced the elastic rubber band to orthodontics, Elisha Gustavus Tucker made public the use of rubber rings in 1852 which he had cut from home-made *rubber tubes of different sizes and thicknesses*[56]. The framework of gold or silver was fitted with small hooks which allowed the pulling rings to perform their task.

Numerous other appliances were also constructed especially by the North American dentists, most of which, however, disappeared just as quickly as, for example, the "Régulateur" by William Rogers, working in Paris in 1845: a gear construction fastened to the molars activated a correspondingly serrated labial arch appliance in a distal direction, and was supposed to pull back the protruding front teeth this way[57] (Fig. 461). The development of orthodontics which began in the second half of the century in the United States by leaps and bounds passed lightly over such ephemeral inventions. This upswing is fundamentally connected with the names of Kingsley, Farrar, and especially of Angle.

Norman William Kingsley (Fig. 462), who is often called the "father of orthodontia" in American professional literature, was born on October 26, 1829, in Stockholm, New York. At first, he acted as a retail salesman, then he received a meagre dental education from his uncle. Nonetheless, his natural talent soon asserted itself. In 1852 he went to New York, where he worked at first as an associate, and then successfully in his own practice. Here, he improved the shapes of porcelain teeth, which won him gold medals at the world fairs in New York and Paris. In 1859 he constructed an artificial soft palate[58], and about the same time he turned to orthodontics. In his early essays he had already propagated *jumping the bite,* the abrupt repositioning of the mandible from a distal bite to a normal "occlusion by putting in a bite plane," a protrusive plate with an inclined plane (Fig. 463).

Kingsley's use of quickly effective forces necessitated a discussion with Tomes' (correct) conception, that movements of the teeth produce absorption of the bone in the direction of the pressure followed by a corresponding build-up on the other side[59]. Kingsley, on the other hand, found the explanation of the process in *that the vascularity of the alveoli permits an elasticity which allows the teeth to be moved outwardly, carrying the external processes along with them*[60].

In Kingsley's "Treatise on Oral Deformities as a Branch of Mechanical Surgery" which, appearing in 1880, constituted the first specialized American work we recognize his absolutely eclectic orientation. Bound to no particular method, he used in every case the means of treatment which seemed to him the most suited. Among these he considered as the most important one the jackscrew (Fig. 464), invented by his countryman William Henry Dwinelle and by Charles Gaine in Bath, England, both in 1849[61]. The screw was inserted into appropriately sawed hard rubber plates by Kingsley[62]. He used Tucker's rubber rings to pull back protruding incisors, attaching them to a plate, as hard rubber plates were, in general, the treatment devices he preferred. He obtained expansion of the maxilla through hickory wedges pressed into the interdental spaces. Later he preferred hard rubber in connection with an immobilization plate (1880). He used inclined planes in appropriate cases, although he had rejected them initially, and also recommended the head-chin cap.

It speaks well for the author that he, according to the preface, had worked for more than ten years on this book, and it is even more praiseworthy, that with true professionalism he ac-

[53] Parmly pp. 81 f.
[54] Fitch pp. 111 f.
[55] See p. 362 and 368
[56] Quoted by Weinberger p. 347
[57] Rogers p. 389
[58] See p. 279
[59] Tomes pp. 155 f.
[60] Kingsley p. 60
[61] See Weinberger p. 387. Gaine was the author of the first specialised British book, "On certain Irregularities of the Teeth", in which he published his invention.
[62] Kingsley pp. 69 f.

knowledges as such all efforts by others[63]. Kingsley became a co-founder of the New York College of Dentistry, and received an honorary doctorate from the Baltimore College of Dental Surgery in 1871. Numerous other honors were conferred on him. In addition to his profession, and later, at his seat of retirement, Warren Point, near the town where he had worked, he occupied himself with sculptures, paintings, and the newly burgeoning photography. He died there a highly respected man at the age of 84 on February 20, 1913.

A contemporary of Kingsley in San Francisco, Emerson Colon Angell described for the first time in 1860 the procedure of palatal suture splitting which is still employed today in cases of extreme crowding. This came out in the newly founded journal, *Dental Cosmos*. The appliance, which consists of a bar equipped with a threaded screw, transversely spans the palatal arch and is joined to the palatal side of the premolars on both sides (Fig. 465):

... the patient was provided with a key and instructed to keep the shaft as uniformly firm as possible. Those directions were industriously followed, and at the end of two weeks, the jaw was so much widened as to leave a space between the front incisors, as indicated in diagram No. 2, showing conclusively that the maxillary bones had separated[64]. The editor of the journal rejects this procedure in an introduction, because he doubted the possibility of separating the maxilla: *Even admitting the impression of the writer to be correct, it would be a very strong argument against the use of such an apparatus; for surely the irregularity of the teeth is a trifling affair compared with the separation of the maxilla, which could not take place without inducing serious disturbance in the surrounding hard and soft parts.* In this instance, the *Dental Cosmos* was in error.

The next person of great importance for orthodontics after Kingsley was John Nutting Farrar who practiced in the Borough of Brooklyn in New York City. He was born on April 24, 1839 in the state of Massachusetts, and studied dentistry in Philadelphia; then, until 1874, he studied medicine. One year afterwards, in 1875, Farrar read his first orthodontic paper, in which he investigated the physiological and pathological tissue alterations which take place in *regulating the teeth*. He summarized his results in four points: 1. the force must be intermittent, and may not exceed certain established limits; 2. rubber tensioners are to be rejected as unscientific, while screws and bolts, on the other hand, yield favorable results; 3. movements of 1/240 of an inch every morning and evening caused no trouble, and therefore, 4. here is the limit between physiological and pathological stress of the tissue[65]. He described his methods and apparatuses in numerous articles in the *Dental Cosmos* which appear to us today to be exceptionally mechanistic (Fig. 466). He compiled his results in his "Treatise on the Irregularities of the Teeth and their Correction" which came out in the years 1888 to 1897 in two volumes. Here we read that Luther Dimmick Shepard claimed to be the first who attached bands by cement in 1867[66].

It is surprising that Farrar, who had published such a plethora of interesting works in the *Dental Cosmos*, was not found worthy of an obituary, as had been his professional opponent Kingsley who had died a few months before him. There appeared only a concise report of his death in New York on June 12, 1913. If only on the basis of his warning against excessive stress on the periodontium from orthodontic measures as also for his pioneer achievements in surgery[67] he had truly deserved praise.

The British dentist Henry Clay Quinby also employed screws, but chiefly he introduced wide flat springs of gold, which he fastened to an encircling hard rubber plate (Fig. 467). The publication was made in 1883 in London in his general textbook, "Notes on Dental Practice."[68]

The next step forward also came from England: in 1871 at a meeting in London Walter Harris Coffin announced an expansion appliance of a new design, which is still named after him today, although Bonwill claimed to have used it already in 1862[69]. He vulcanized a spring-action piano wire, bent into the shape of a "W" into a hard rubber plate, separated the plate in the middle and activated the spring, so that the halves of the plate pressed the alveolar processes to the outside[70] (Fig.

[63] See also p. 279
[64] Angell
[65] Farrar (a)
[66] Farrar (b); (c) p. 1229
[67] See p. 344 f.
[68] Quinby p. 102 f.
[69] Bonwill
[70] Coleman

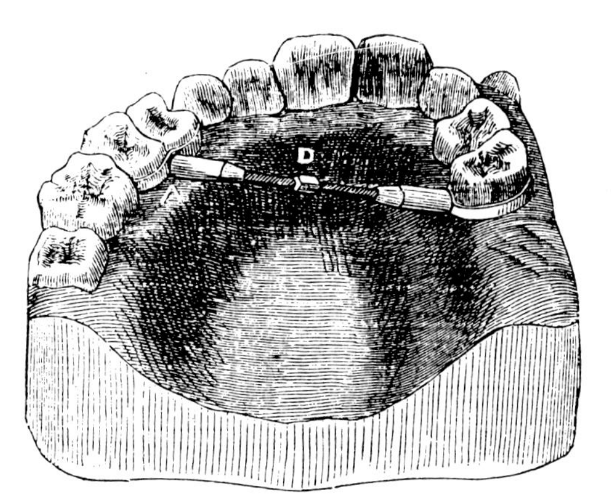

Fig. 465 *Angell: Screw spindle for breaking the palatal suture, in situ, 1860*

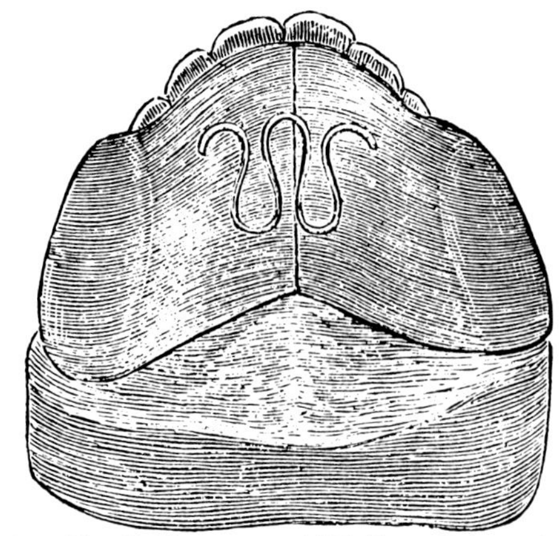

Fig. 468 *The Coffin spring, 1871 (from Coleman)*

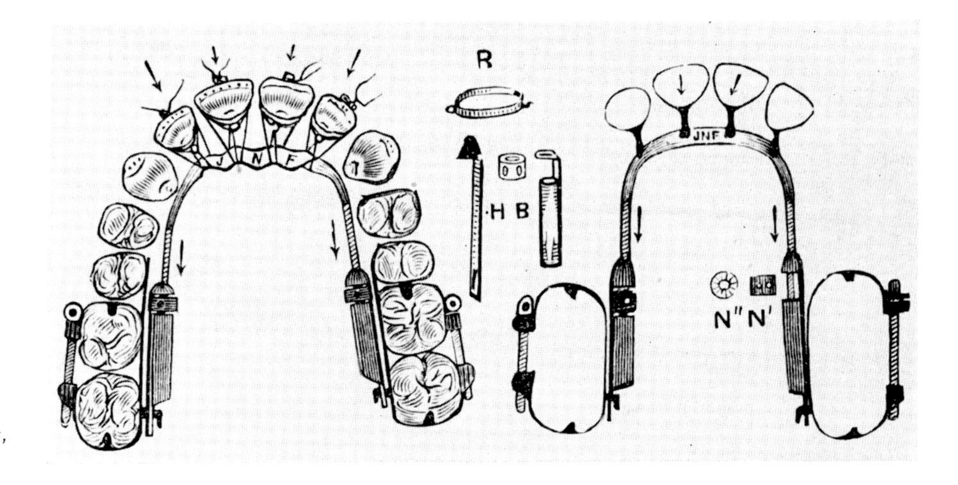

Fig. 466 *Farrar: Screw appliances, 1886*

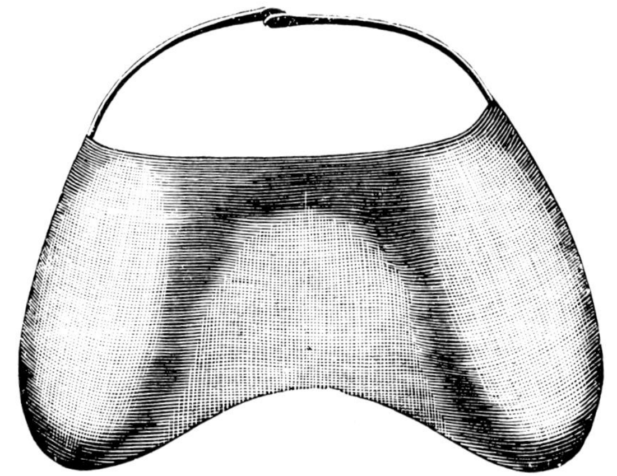

Fig. 467 *Quinby: Plate device activated by band springs, 1883*

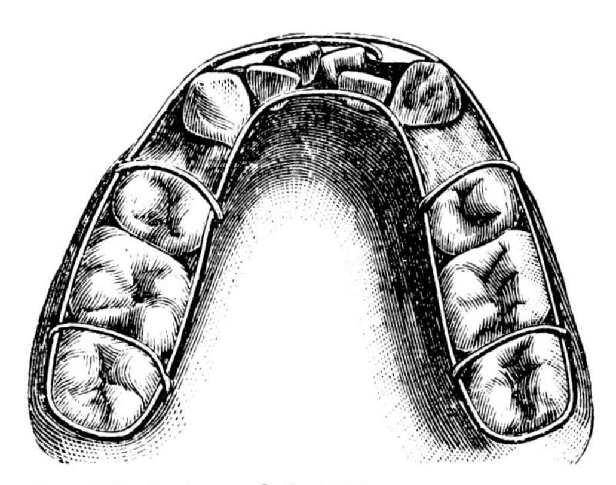

Fig. 469 *Jackson: Crib, 1887*

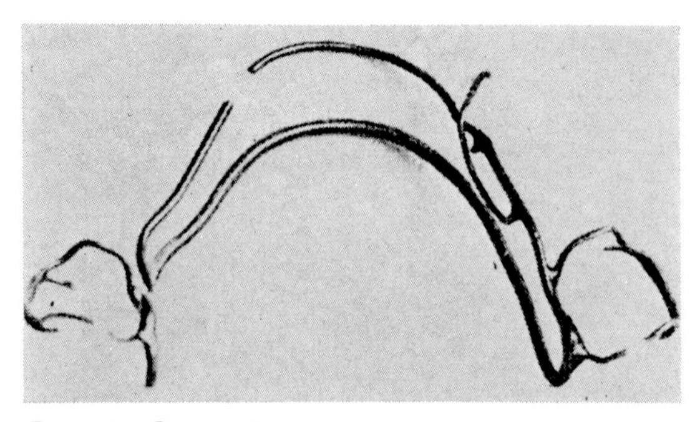

Fig. 470 *Crozat: Removable labio-lingual wire appliance, 1920*

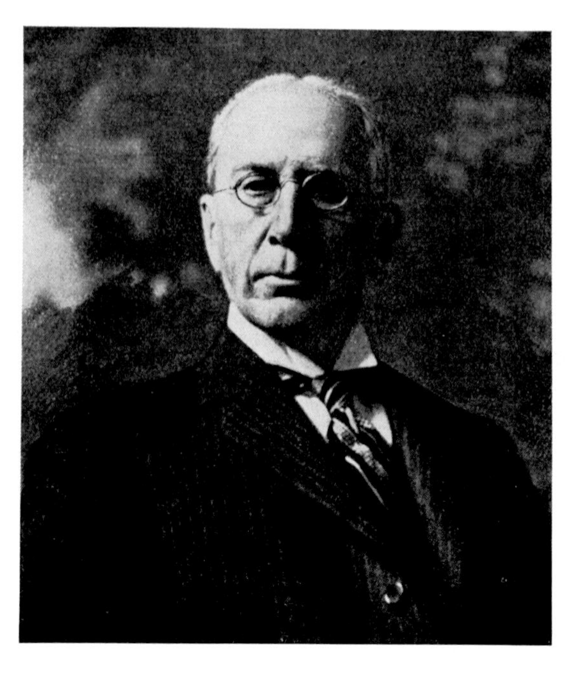

Fig. 471 *Edward Hartley Angle*

468). Expansion plates of this type are used up to the present day, although now the spring is usually replaced by a dilatation screw because its effect can be controlled more precisely.

Victor Hugo Jackson, in New York, used only round spring-action platinum-iridium wire for his treatment aid, designated as a "crib." He reported on it in 1887 and gradually developed it into a universal tool[71]. The appliance was fastened with wire clasps which overlapped the interdental space between the crowns of the premolars and molars, in order to be joined then to the neck of the tooth on the buccal side (Fig. 469). Just as it had in orthodontics, this kind of anchoring had taken root in prosthetics. For individual motions, the author soldered auxiliary springs to the wire bar, which was his other contribution also still valid today. In 1920 George B. Crozat, an orthodontist in New Orleans, resumed the principle evolved by Jackson with a finer detachable lingual arch appliance named after him[72] (Fig. 470).

The credit for having put orthodontics on a scientific foundation and for having delineated it as an independent speciality of the profession, belongs unquestionably to Edward Hartley Angle (Fig. 471). He was born on June 1, 1855 in Herrick, Pennsylvania, and at first settled in Towanda after his training at the Pennsylvania Dental College. Then, after two years of life in the country because of a tubercular infection, he settled in Minneapolis, where he turned to orthodontics. In 1886 he was appointed to the professors's chair for this subject at the University there, and in the following year, gave his epochal lecture at the 9th International Medical Convention, "Notes on Orthodontia, with a New System of Regulation and Retention." Through supplementary American and German reports of the meeting we are fairly well informed about the lecture and the rather vehement discussion which followed[73]. Among the means available at the time, Angle particularly acknowledged the screw spindle (from Dwinelle) and the piano wire (from Coffin). He was against the intermittent action in Farrar's system and emphasized the importance of retention. He made the following requests for the appliances: cleanliness, continuous wear, non-contact with the palate (thus, no plates), stability, and limitation to as little space as possible. In the discussion Farrar was the first

[71] Jackson (a)—(c)
[72] Crozat
[73] Angle (a)

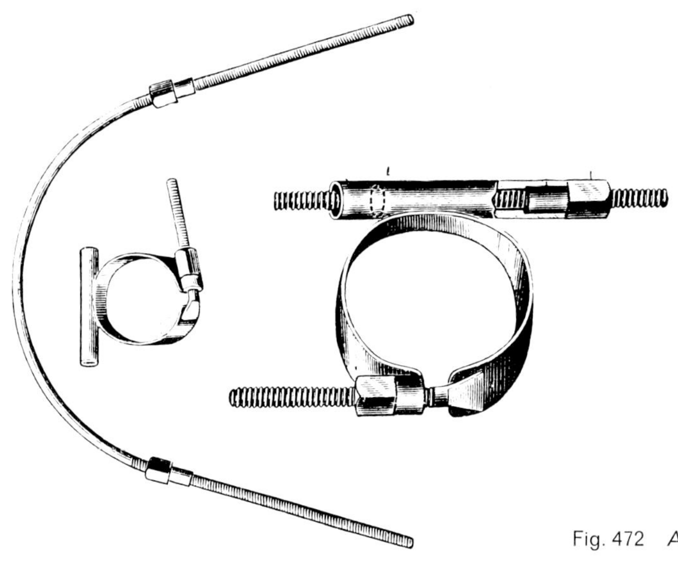

Fig. 472 *Angle: Expansion arch and clamp bands, 1899*

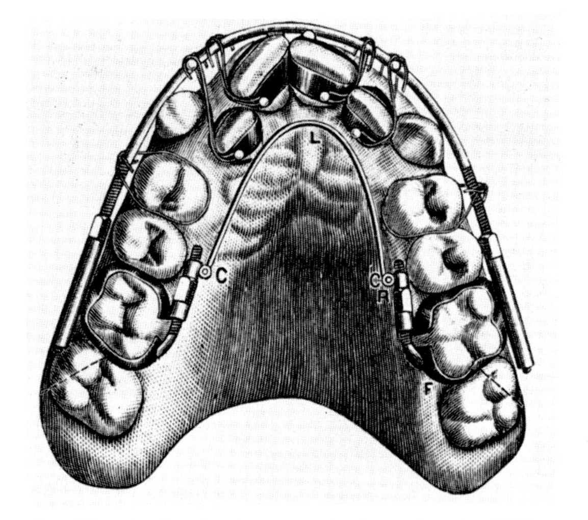

Fig. 473 *Angle: Appliance with clamp bands, 1899*

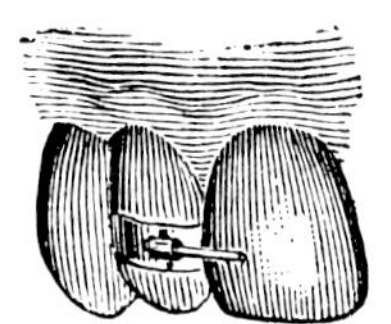

Fig. 474 *Angle: Retainer*

to take a stand against rejection of the intermittent effects, while others doubted the originality of his apparatuses.
The significance of Angle's devices was their simplification and standardization. While previously every appliance represented a more or less complicated new construction, henceforth every practitioner could assemble a mechanism appropriate to the case from prefabricated (and patented) elements in a kind of building block system. The base was an elastic arch which was attached to the first molars with screw bands. The teeth to be moved were fastened to it with wire ligatures (Fig. 472). The teeth were fitted with a band having a soldered little tube through which a pin could be inserted after the "regulation" was complete for the purpose of "retention" (Figs. 473 and 474). Uncompromisingly Angle rejected any extraction of teeth. He worked until the end of his life on the perfection of this system which soon conquered the entire world. His book came out in seven repeatedly revised editions until 1907, and was translated into almost all European languages.

In 1899 Angle published his "Classification of Malocclusion."[74] Unlike all his predecessors he did not make the position of the anterior teeth in relation to each other as a base, but rather the occlusal relation between the upper and lower first molars. The neutral or normal occlusion was ranked in Class I, a distal position of the mandibular molars, and therewith of the mandible, was put in Class II, and a mesial relation in Class III (Fig. 475).

In 1893 Calvin Suveril Case at the Chicago Dental College had drawn attention to the fact that a bodily movement of the tooth as a whole including the root and not merely a tipping had to be undertaken, in order to avoid recurrences, and he also devised proper treatment aids for it[75] (Figs. 476 and 477). Angle took up this challenge, and developed first the pin and tubes appliance in 1913 which was exceptionally difficult to manipulate, then the ribbon arch, and then, in 1928, as *the latest and best in orthodontic mechanisms,* the edgewise arch. This arch rested in a groove of small hooks attached to the tooth with bands, so that a movement of the tooth through tipping was avoided[76] (Fig. 478). In 1931 this device was supplemented by the twin wire arch of Joseph E. Johnson (Fig. 479). There is a direct line from these devices to the multiband and lightwire appliances of today.

In 1897 Angle went to St. Louis, where he opened the Angle School of Orthodontia in 1900. In 1901 he founded the American Society of Orthodontia, and in 1907 he started the journal, *American Orthodontist.* About 1914 he moved to his place of retirement in Pasadena, California, at the age of sixty, but was persuaded by his students to be president of the "Angle College of Orthodontia" founded for him there in 1922.

Angle's appliance was supplemented by George Cook Ainsworth, a professor at the Harvard Dental School in Boston in 1904, through a combination of the expansion arch with two lingual bars fitted closely to the canines and the lateral adjacent teeth (Fig. 480). Through bands anchored on the first premolars, or in expansion in the mixed dentition on the first primary molars, this expansion appliance is effective mainly in the canine region, where the expansion arch's effect is insufficient[77].

The reintroduction of Lefoulon's spring-action lingual arch by John Valentine Mershon in Philadelphia meant a significant step forward in 1909. It had delicate springs for individual movements, and was anchored with a special lock to the molar bands[78] (Figs. 481 and 482). The importance of this new aid was found in the fact that now the movements of the teeth were not induced any more by the jerky pulling force of tightened ligatures and screws, but rather could be effected through the continuous pressing force of dainty springs, with significantly less trauma to the tissue. Combined with the high labial arch which extends through the oral vestibule and also carries fine finger-springs or spring loops[79] (Fig. 483), constructed by Angle's student Lloyd Steele Lourie in Chicago in 1918, the Mershon-Lourie appliance became a superb unified device, upon which almost all later wire appliances are based.

As Angle and his adherents could not bring themselves to support this progressive method, American orthodontics was divided into two feuding camps. This situation prevailed until August 11, 1930, when the great pioneer Angle fell victim to a heart attack during his vacation at Monica Beach, California, at the age of 75, working until the end and, in the opinion of his opponents, intolerantly fighting for his system. Also here we have another instance of the often observed tragedy of genius: at first a revolutionary, then an autocrat, and in old age, a block to further progress.

In Europe, Angle's system was instituted and defended chiefly by Alfred Körbitz, who founded an institute for further education in Berlin in 1902 which soon came to enjoy a reputation throughout the continent. His early expansion apparatus from 1910[80] which reminds of Ainsworth's one was further developed by his student and successor as head of the institute, Paul Wilhelm Simon, into the spring-beam apparatus in 1928[81] (Figs. 484 and 485). This was manufactured from stainless steel, then introduced into dental prosthetics, and therewith showed the way to less expensive regulation of malocclusion for the masses.

Extraction therapy, which had initially found

[74] Angle (c)
[75] Case (a and c)
[76] Angle (d—f)
[77] Ainsworth
[78] Mershon (a and b)
[79] Lourie
[80] Körbitz
[81] Simon (c and d)

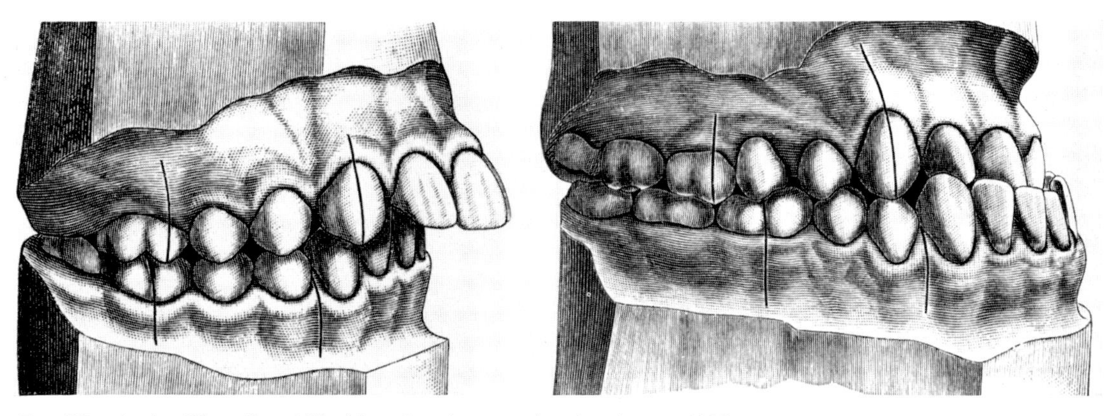

Fig. 475 *Angle: Class II and III of his classification of malocclusion, 1899*

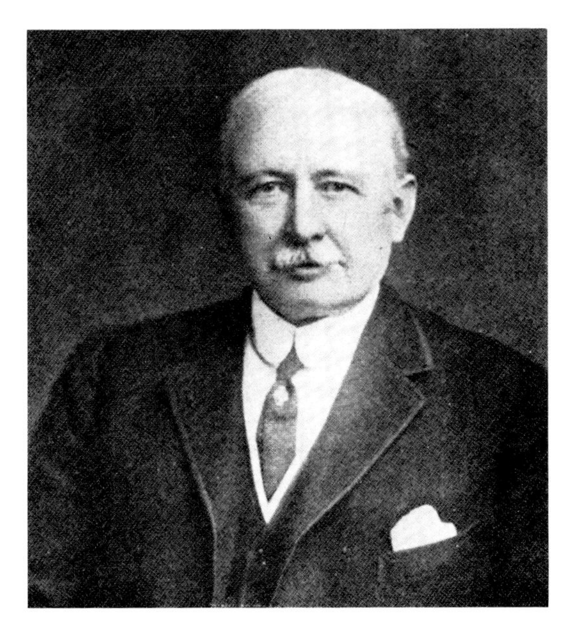

Fig. 476 *Calvin Suveril Case*

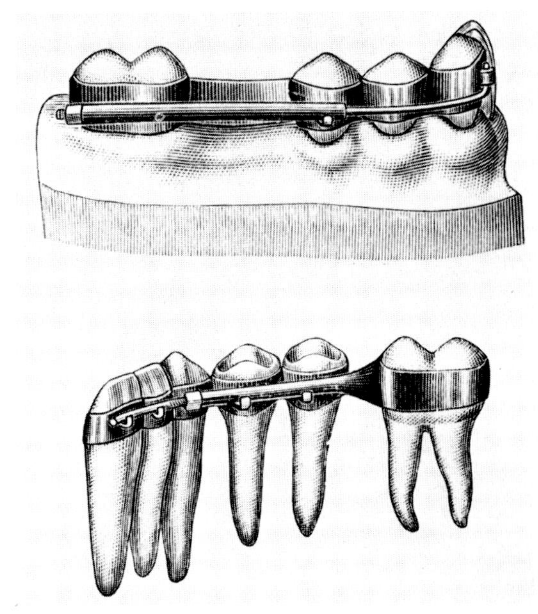

Fig. 477 *Case: Bodily movement, 1893*

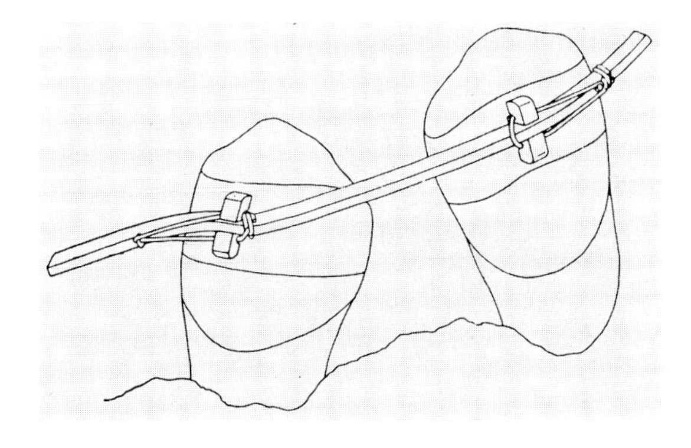

Fig. 478 *Angle: Edgewise arch, 1928*

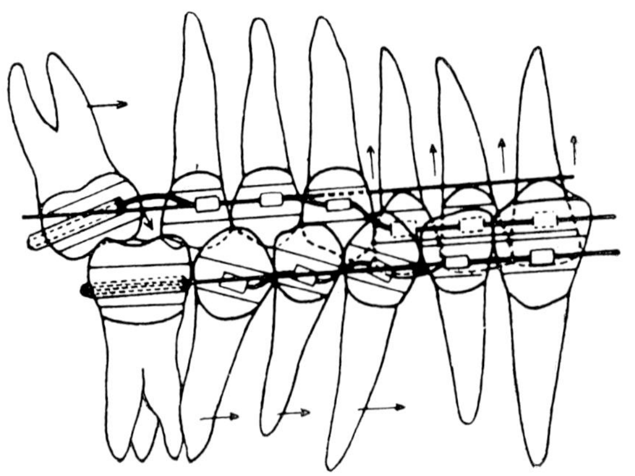

Fig. 479 *Johnson: Twin wire arch, 1931*

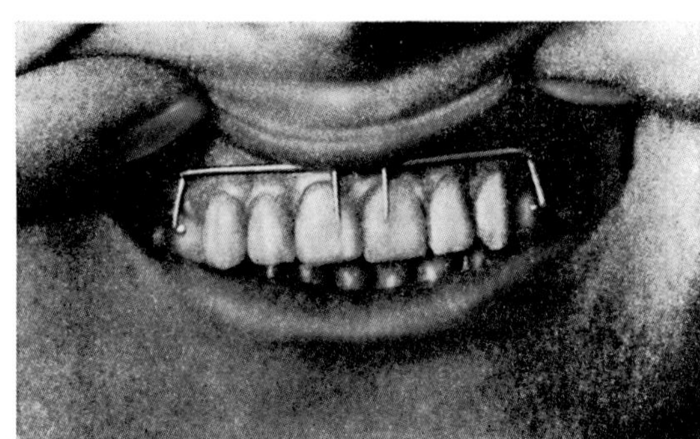

Fig. 483 *Lourie: High labial arch with spring extensions, 1918*

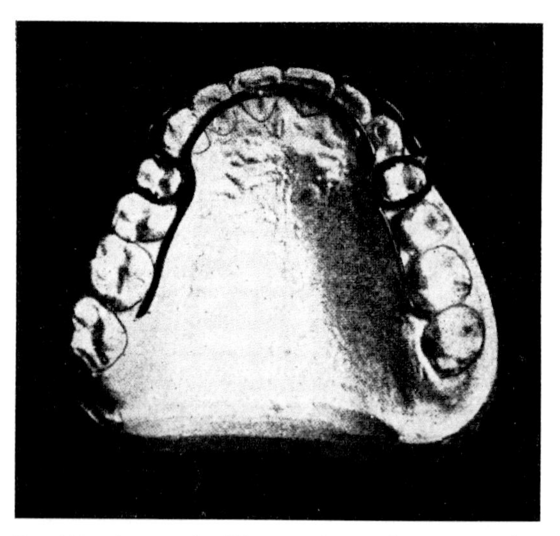

Fig. 480 *Ainsworth: "New appliance for moving dislocated teeth into position," 1904*

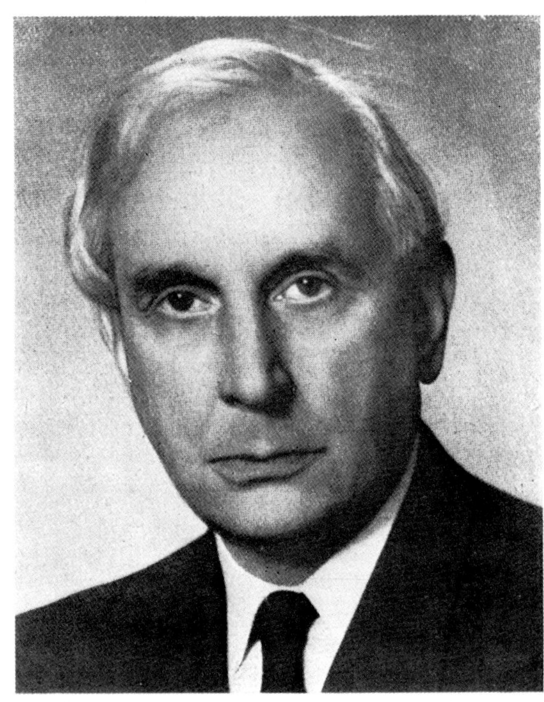

Fig. 484 *Paul Wilhelm Simon*

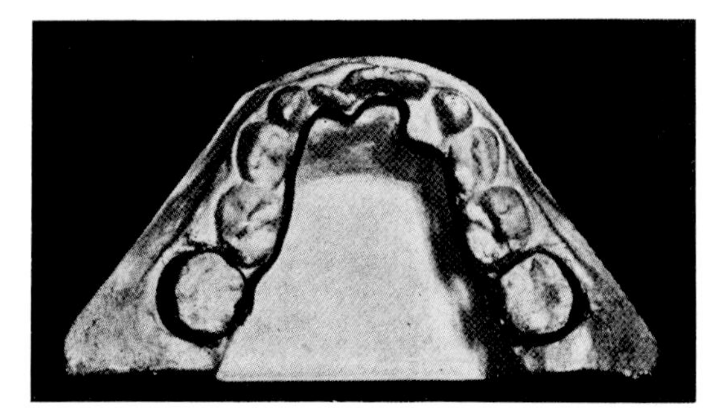

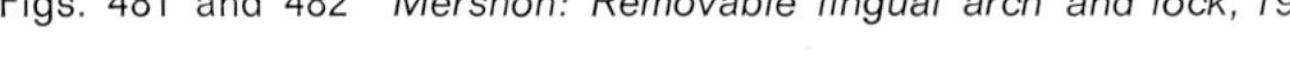

Figs. 481 and 482 *Mershon: Removable lingual arch and lock, 1918*

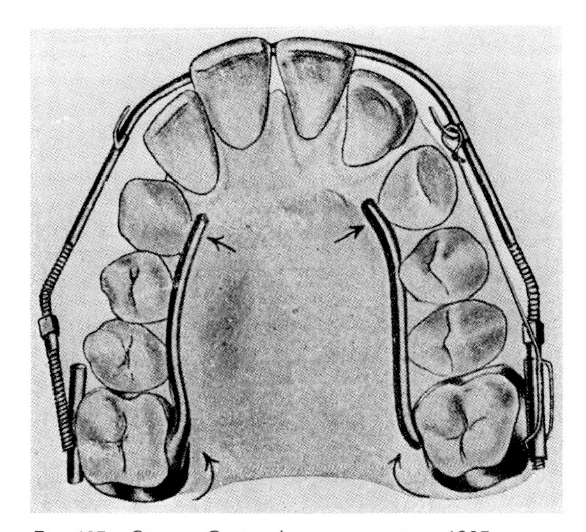

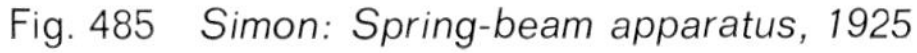

Fig. 485 *Simon: Spring-beam apparatus, 1925*

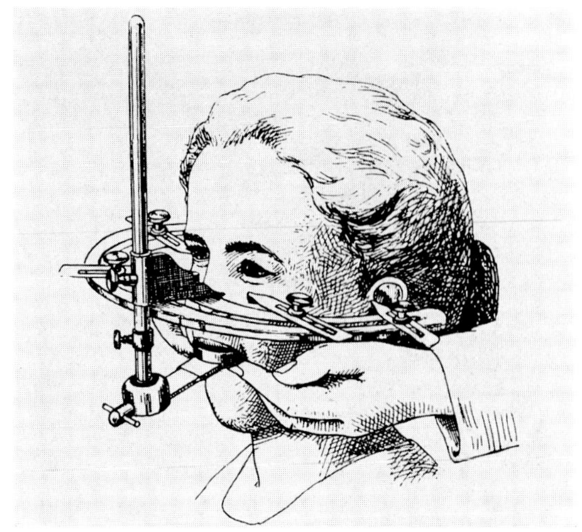

Fig. 486 *Simon: Gnathostatic impression, 1914*

many adherents, was forced for decades completely into the background because of Angle's rejection, although prominent orthodontists such as Case had advocated it[82]. Only when Axel Fredrik Lundström, in his dissertation at the University of Stockholm on the connections between malocclusion and apical base, had supported extraction scientifically as a therapeutic measure in orthodontics in 1923 it found the recognition it deserved which has lasted to the present day.

Angle's classification of the types of occlusion remained unshaken up to the first half of the 20th century, in contrast to most of its short-lived antecedents. Beyond the nomenclatures known to us of Marjolin (1829), Kneisel (1836), Carabelli (1842), and Linderer (1851), others were published by the anatomist Hermann Welcker in Halle in 1862, by Carl Wedl in Vienna in 1870, and by Magitot in Paris in 1872, and further classifications by Josef Iszlai, lecturer at the University in Budapest, in 1881 and 1891. To give an example, our present-day mesial occlusion was called "inversion" by Marjolin, "allgemeiner Schiefstand" (general oblique position) by Kneisel, "mordex prorsus" by Carabelli, "Greisenkinn" (senile chin) by Linderer, "Opistognathie" by Welcker, "antéversion" by Magitot, "Hundemaul" (dog's mouth) by Wedl, and "Epharmosis" by Iszlai[84].

Until Angle, everyone had oriented himself exclusively by the position of the anterior teeth, and often only to those of the maxilla. Gradually, however, it was recognized, stimulated especially by Angle's great opponent Case, that even the position of the molars did not provide the sole valid key to correct diagnosis, and efforts were made toward a realignment with measuring points on the skull. The beginning of this movement came in 1916 from J. A. W. van Loon, a Dutchman who had been trained by Körbitz. He was able, with the help of a facial mask, to adjust the impressions in relation to the skull as in life[85]. This considerably circumstantial method was simplified by Simon in 1919 with his "Gnathostat," an apparatus which, while the impression was being taken, was adapted to the Frankfort horizontal plane by means of a face bow with four pointers to the measuring points (Fig. 486). The base of the casts obtained corresponds then to this plane. Two vertical lines erected on it determine the orbital (frontal) plane, and the median-sagittal plane is derived from two points on the palatal suture. This method has been extended by the photostatic recording process, borrowed from criminology, which by means of a fixed head position,

[82] Case (b)
[83] Lundström
[84] Welcker p. 48; Wedl p. 80; Magitot p. 300; Iszlai
[85] van Loon

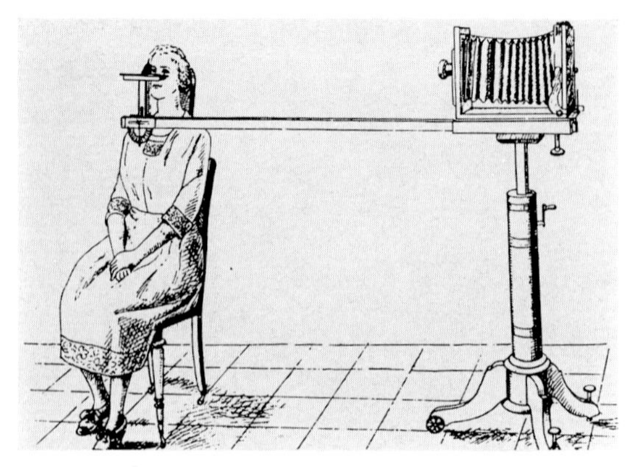

Fig. 487 *Simon: Photostatic diagnosis, 1919*

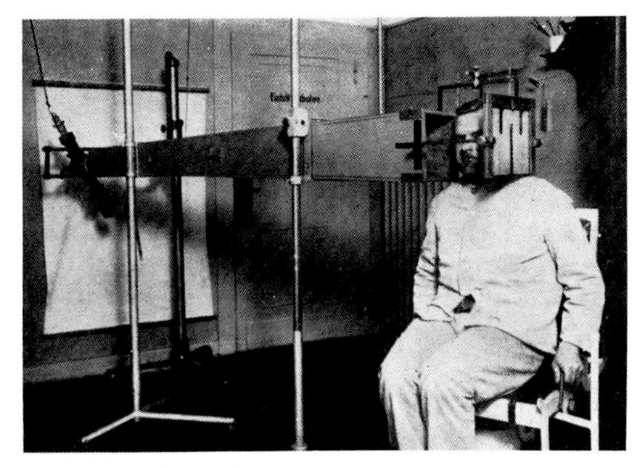

Fig. 488 *Hofrath: Cephalometric radiography, 1931*

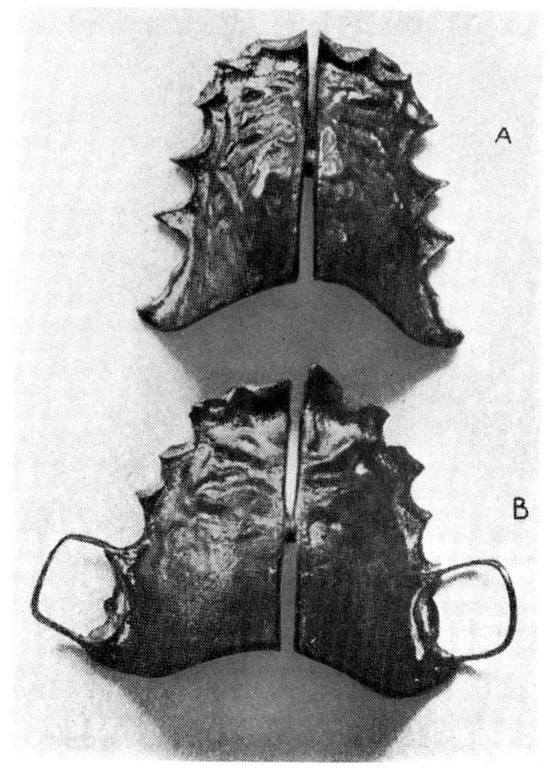

Fig. 489 *Nord screw, 1928*

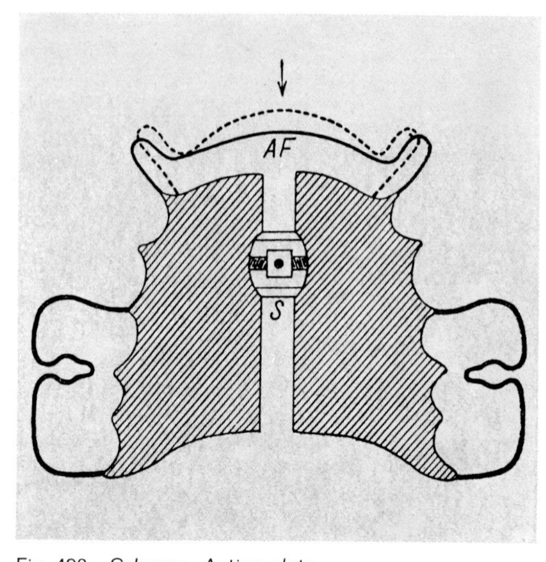

Fig. 490 *Schwarz: Active plate*

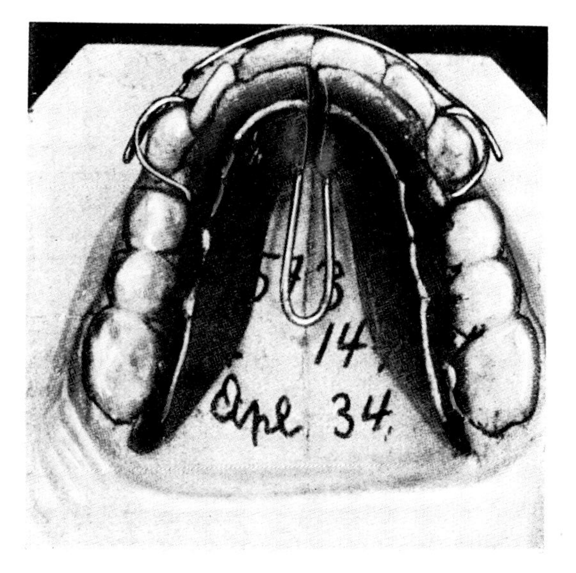

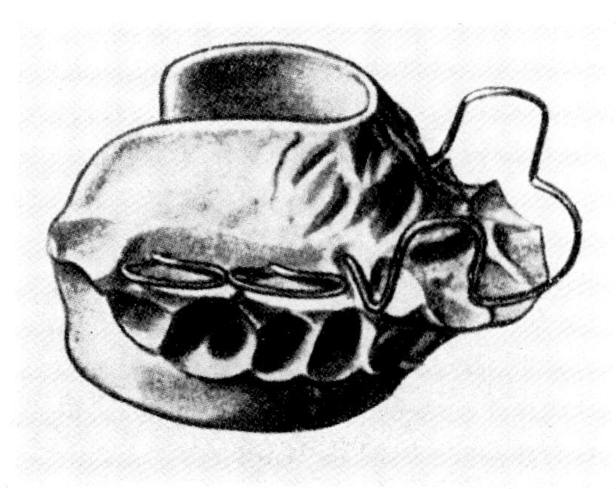

Fig. 491 *Andresen: Activator, 1936, and later depiction by L. Petrik*

yields symmetrical frontal and profile pictures[86] (Fig. 487).
The dental arch index, which was developed in 1907 by Albéric Pont, the founder and later the director of the École dentaire in Lyon, has been introduced as a further diagnostic aid. apical base, had supported extraction scientifically as a therapeutic measure in orthodontics in 1923[83] it found the recognition it deserved, which has lasted to the present day.
Cephalometric radiography was the result of a further consequent development of Simon's "Photostatic," and it is around this that present-day orthodontics is largely oriented. It was developed to the point of practical use at about the same time by Herbert Hofrath in Düsseldorf, published in 1931 (Fig. 488), and in 1932 by Birdsall Holly Broadbent in Cleveland[88]. While methods of this type were achieved in the twenties with great effort especially in Europe, they took the USA by storm. In Angle's last year of life he had already distanced himself a little from the *Dogma of the constancy of the molars,* and, after his death, the new ways came to America with hasty steps, and were significantly developed there by important orthodontists such as Charles Henry Tweed, Herbert I. Margolis, Wayne A. Bolton, and others.
The histological investigations of the Viennese School before and after World War I signified great progress in the scientific elucidation of periodontal tissue alterations during tooth movements. In this respect, Albin Oppenheim in Vienna, a student of Angle's, is particularly deserving of credit. In the end of the twenties, Albert H. Ketcham of Denver, Colorado, demonstrated by means of systematic X-ray examinations that tooth damage is the result of forced procedures. Now the importance of a biological measuring of the forces effective on the teeth and the periodontium, to which Farrar was probably the first to make reference, is generally recognized[89].
Practitioners of the New World have remained faithful to fixed appliances up to the present day, while in Europe a gradual transition began to removable plate devices. Some milestones of this development are: the dilatation screw inserted into a plate by the Dutchman Charles Frederick Leopold Nord in 1928 (Fig. 489), by means of which the force can be measured out more precisely than with Coffin's spring[90], and the "active plate" by Arthur Martin Schwarz in Vienna in the middle of the thirties (Fig. 490). This was developed with guided screws and clamps of a new

[86] Simon (a and b)
[87] Pont
[88] Hofrath; Broadbent
[89] Oppenheim; Ketcham; see p. 374
[90] Nord. See p. 374

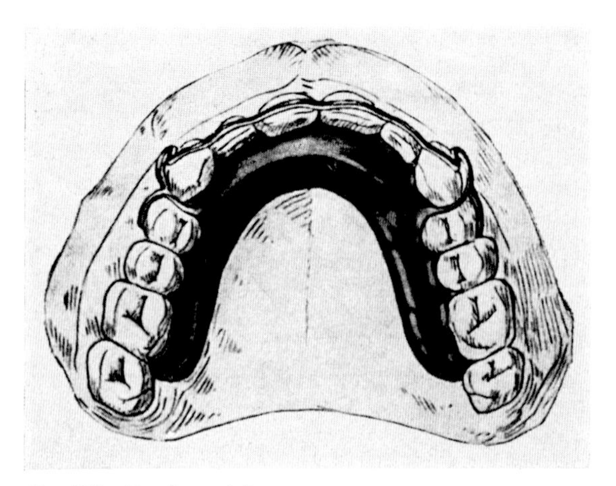

Fig. 492 *Hawley retainer*

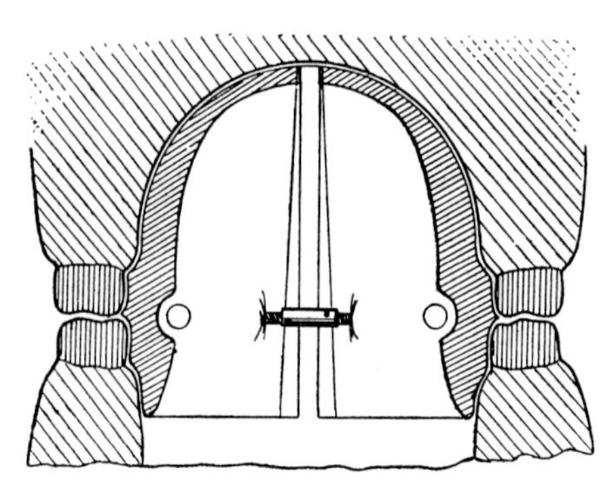

Fig. 493 *Robin: Monobloc, 1902*

design into an extremely versatile device by this jaw orthopedist, who was as creative as he was ingenious [91].

With the transition from Angle to Mershon and Lourie, and further to the new plate devices, an important step had already been taken from purely mechanical orthodontics to biological methods. In the thirties the phenomenon of "functional adaptation" developed in 1895 by the anatomist in Halle, Albert Roux, began to be employed even for the elimination of occlusal anomalies. This path had already been taken successfully in general orthopedics, even though mechanical aids in that area had by no means proved superfluous.

The "Norwegian System of Functional Gnatho-orthopedics" was devised in Oslo and presented in Berlin in 1935 by the Dane Viggo Andresen [92], and scientfically grounded and promoted by Karl Häupl. It works with a passive plate device which spans the maxilla and the mandible, and is activated, according to the theory of its authors, by the normal function of the musculature of mastication, the tongue, and the cheeks. The device, which therefore is called the "Activator" (Fig. 491), was developed from the "Retainer" of an American, Charles Augustus Hawley (Fig. 492), through the addition of side wings for the mandible. It has the task of transmitting the muscle action, which occurs chiefly at night as a functional stimulus, to the region of the masticating apparatus to be altered. It corresponds in principle to the "Monobloc" invented by Pierre Robin in Paris as early as 1902, but had remained unknown in the orthodontic literature [93]. At that time Robin had been unable to assert himself against the prevailing Angle system (Fig. 493).

Muscle training in the way of mandibular stretching exercises with the head bent-back in order to eliminate the distal bite had been recommended in 1918 by Alfred Paul Rogers of Boston, who had pondered the problem for as long as a decade. However, the results did not meet his high expectations [94]. Today these ideas of myofunctional therapy are being resurrected in eastern Europe for preventive and early treatment in nurseries and kindergardens.

After functional jaw orthopedics had found wide recognition, particularly in central European regions efforts were made to alter the activator, its "biomechanical apparatus," in such a fashion that it could be worn during daytime, too. This was to have the effect of a shortened period of treatment and to increase the certainty of success. These endeavors gave rise to numerous succeeding devices which were in part capable of performing even more extensive treatments. Today, however, the European dentists, too, are increasingly turning to the fixed appliances, which have meanwhile developed in the USA into extremely refined, but very sophisticated devices.

[91] Schwarz; Schwarz and Gratzinger
[92] Andresen
[93] Robin
[94] Rogers

In reserve, a budding interest in the removable appliances seems to be discernible in the New World.

In this manner the work towards the elimination of dental occlusal anomalies and jaw deformities has developed in the course of the last hundred years from an initial endeavor to serve purely cosmetic purposes to a scientifically founded branch of dentistry which is predominantly oriented around function. While it appears that a certain stagnation has set in in the other specialties of dentistry at this time, that is not to be perceived in orthodontics, where a great deal of development is still going on. Surely, the goal is clearly recognized: a biological treatment of malocclusion through mechanical and functional means. The optimal path, however, is not yet ascertained.

For the indispensable specialist's advice provided for this chapter, the author thanks his wife, Dr. Irmtraut Hoffmann-Axthelm. He also thanks Dr. Thomas Rakosi, professor of Orthodontics at the University of Freiburg im Breisgau, for revising the English edition.

References

Ainsworth, George C(ook)
Some thoughts regarding methods, and a new appliance for moving dislocated teeth into position. Int. Dent. J. 25 (1904) 481—495

Andresen, Viggo
a) The Norwegian system of functional gnatho-orthopedics. Acta gnatholog. 1 (1936) 5—36
b) Über das sogenannte "Norwegische System der Funktions-Kiefer-Orthopädie". Dtsch. zahnärztl. Wschr. 39 (1936) 235—238; 283—286

Angell, E(merson) H.(error; recte Colon)
Treatment of irregularity of the permanent or adult teeth. Dent. Cosmos 1 (1860) 540—544; 599—600

Angle, Erdward H(artley)
a) Notes on orthodontia, with a new system of regulation and retention. Dent. Cosmos 29 (1887) 757—763
b) The angle system of regulation and retention of the teeth, . . . 4th ed., Philadelphia 1895
c) Classification of malocclusion. Dent. Cosmos 41 (1899) 248—264; 350—357
d) Further steps in the progress of orthodontia. Dent. Cosmos 55 (1913) 1—13
e) The ribbon arch mechanism and some new auxiliary instruments. Dent. Cosmos 62 (1920) 1158—1167; 1279—1294
f) The latest and best in orthodontic mechanism. Dent. Cosmos 70 (1928) 1143—1158; 71 (1929) 164—174; 260—270; 409—421

Artzney Buchlein/wider allerlei kranckeyten und gebrechen der tzeen . . . Leyptzigk 1530

Baume, Robert
Lehrbuch der Zahnheilkunde. Leipzig 1890

Bell, Thomas
The anatomy, physiology, and diseases of the teeth. London 1828

Bonwill, W. G(ibson) A(rlington)
Apparate und Methoden zur Regulierung von Unregelmäßigkeiten. Korresp. bl. Zahnärzte 18 (1889) 209—232

Brewster, C(hristopher) S(tarr)
Développement anormal de la portion antérieure du maxillaire supérieur avec rétraction de la lèvre supérieure. Gaz. hôp., Paris 15 (1840) 538—539

Broadbent, B(irdsall) Holly
a) Investigations on the orbital plane. Dent. Cosmos 69 (1927) 797—805
b) The orthod. value of cephalometric studies . . .: The use of X-ray silhouettes in tracing facial growth. J. Dent. Res. 13 (1933) 151—154

Carabelli, Georg von
Systematisches Handbuch der Zahnheilkunde. Vol. II (Anatomie des Mundes), With: Kupfertafeln zu v. Carabelli's Anatomie des Mundes. Wien 1842

Case, Calvin S(uveril)
a) Principles of force and anchorage in the movement of teeth. Dent. Cosmos 39 (1897) 1011—1024
b) The question of extraction in orthodontia. Dent. Cosmos 54 (1912) 137—157; 276—284
c) The bodily movement of the teeth in orthodontia. Dent. Cosmos 58 (1916) 877—893

Casto, Frank M.
A historical sketch of orthodontia. Dent. Cosmos 76 (1934) 110—135

Civen, O. I.
A historical review of the progress of orthodontics from 1840 to 1940. Amer. J. Orthod. Oral Surg. 31 (1945) 203—213

Cohen, R. A.
The Talma family. Brit. Dent. J. 126 (1969) 319—326

Coleman, Alfred
On certain points in the treatment of dental irregularity. Transact. Odont. Soc. G. B. N. S. 10 (1877/78) 111—112

Crozat, George B.
Possibilities and use of removable labio-lingual appliances. Int. J. Orthod. 6 (1920) 1—6

Delabarre, C(hristophe) F(rançois)
a) Odontologie, ou observation sur les dents humaines. Paris 1815
b) Traité de la seconde dentition, et méthode naturelle de la diriger. Paris 1819

Farrar, John Nutting
a) Inquiry into the physiologic and pathologic changes in animal tissues in regulation teeth. Dent. Cosmos 18 (1876) 13—24
b) Mechanical appliances for regulating teeth. Dent. Cosmos 28 (1886) 153—169
c) A treatise on the irregulations of the teeth and their correction. Vol. I, New York City 1888; II, 1889/97

Fitch, Samuel Sheldon
A system of dental surgery. Philadelphia 1829

Fox, Joseph
a) The natural history of the human teeth . . . London 1803
b) The history and treatment of the disease of the teeth, the gums and the alveolar processes, . . . London 1806

Herbst, Wilhelm
Methoden und Neuerungen auf dem Gebiet der Zahnheilkunde. Berlin (1895)

Hofrath, Herbert
Die Bedeutung der Röntgenfern- und Abstandsaufnahme für die Diagnostik der Kieferanomalien. Fortschr. Orthod. 1 (1931) 232—258

Iszlai, Josef
Einige Worte zur Nomenklatur der sog. "Bißarten". Österr.-ung. Vjschr. Zahnheilk. 7 (1891) 263—272

Jackson, Victor H(ugo)
a) Regulating appliance. Dent. Cosmos 29 (1887) 373—379
b) Correcting irregularities of the teeth. Dent. Cosmos 32 (1890) 874—882
c) Correction of irregularities by "Crib" appliance. Dent. Cosmos 35 (1893) 784—791

Jessen, Ernst
On the dental inspection and treatment of the children in the communal schools of Strassburg. (Ash's) Quart. Circ. (1902) 145—148

Ketcham, Albert H.
A preliminary report of an investigation of apical root resorption of permanent teeth. Int. J. Orthod. 13 (1927) 97—127

Kingsley, Norman W(illiam)
A treatise on oral deformities as a branch of mechanical surgery. New York 1880

Kneisel, (Friedrich Christoph)
Der Schiefstand der Zähne, . . . Berlin/Posen/Bromberg 1837

Koecker, Leonard
Principles of dental surgery, . . . London 1826

Körbitz, Alfred
Eine einfache Art der frühzeitigen Zahnbogendehnung. Zschr. zahnärztl. Orthop. 4 (1910) 355—364

Lefoulon, J(oachim)
Nouveau traité théorique et pratique de l'art du dentiste. Paris 1841

Linderer, C(allman) J(acob)
Lehre von den gesammten Zahnoperationen . . . Berlin 1834

Linderer, Joseph
a) Handbuch der Zahnheilkunde. 2nd ed., Berlin 1842
b) Handbuch der Zahnheilkunde. Vol. II, Berlin 1848
c) Die Zahnhk. nach ihrem neuesten Standpunkte. Erlangen 1851

Lomnitz, Carl Berthold Alexander
Die Lehre vom Schiefstand der Zähne. Berlin 1840

van Loon, J. A. W.
Neue Methoden zur Feststellung normaler und anormaler Beziehungen der Zähne zu den Gesichtslinien. Zschr. zahnärztl. Orthop. 10 (1916) 1—11; 22—29; 42—55; 61—69

Lourie, Lloyd S(teele)
The concealed labial arch wire with spring extensions. Int. J. Orthod. 4 (1918) 24—35

Lundström, Axel F(redrik)
Malocclusion of the teeth regarded as a problem in connection with the apical base. Med. Diss. Stockholm 1923. Also in: Int. J. Orthod. 11 (1925) 591—602; 724—731; 793—812; 933—941; 1022—1042; 1109—1133

Maclean, Samuel
a) On the removal of the four permanent first molars, in certain cases, at an early period of life. Transact. Odont. Soc. Gr. Britain 1 (1856/7) 49—66
b) Obituary Maclean. Brit. J. Dent. Sci. 7 (1864) 526—527

Magitot, Emile
Traité des anomalies du système dentaire chez l'homme et les mammifères. Paris 1877

Marjolin, (Jean Nicolas René)
Catch-word "Dent (pathologie)" in: Dictionnaire de Médecine. 2nd. ed., Paris 1832—1845. Vol. VI, pp. 447—474

Maury, F.
a) Vollständiges Handbuch der Zahnheilkunde. Weimar 1830
b) Traité complet de l'art du dentiste. Nouv. éd., Paris 1833

Mershon, John V(alentine)
a) Band and lingual arch technic. Int. J. Orthod. 3 (1917) 195—203
b) The removable lingual arch as an appliance for the treatment of malocclusion of the teeth. Int. J. Orthod. 4 (1918) 578—587

Nessel, Franz
Handbuch der Zahnheilkunde. Prag (1840)

Nord, Ch(arles) F(rederick) L(eopold)
Loose appliances of orthodontia. Dent. Cosmos 70 (1928) 681—687

Oppenheim, Albin
a) Tissue changes, particularly of the bone, incident to tooth movement. Transact. Europ. Orthod. Soc. 8, pp. 303—359. In: Österr.-ung. Vjschr. Zahnheilk. 27 (1911)
b) Wurzelresorption bei orthodont. Maßnahmen. (Öst.) Zschr. Stomat. 27 (1929) 605—653

Parmly, Levy Spear
Lectures on the natural history of the teeth. London 1820

Pfaff, Wilhelm
Lehrbuch der Orthodontie . . . mit Einschluß der Geschichte der Orthodontie. Dresden 1906

Pont, A(lbéric)
Der Zahnindex in der Orthodontie. Zschr. zahnärztl. Orthop. 3 (1909) 306—321

Quinby, Henry C(lay)
Notes on dental practice. London 1883

Robertson, William
A practical treatise on the human teeth. London 1835

Robin, Pierre
a) Observation sur un nouvel appareil de redressement. Revue Stomat., Paris 9 (1902) 423—432
b) Démonstration pratique . . . d'un nouvel appareil de redressement. Revue Stomat., Paris 9 (1902) 561—590

Rogers, Alfred Paul
a) The correction of facial inharmonies. Dent. Cosmos 49 (1907) 850—852
b) Muscle training and its relation to the orthodontia. Int. J. Orthod. 4 (1918) 555—577

Rogers, William
L'encyclopédie du dentiste . . . 2nd ed., Paris 1845

Saunders, Edwin
Lectures on the diseases and operations of the teeth, VII. The Forceps 2 (1845) 25—27

Schange, J. M. A(lexis)
Précis sur le redressement des dents . . . Paris 1841

Schwarz, A(rthur) Martin
Gebißregelung mit Platten. Berlin/Wien 1938

Schwarz, A(rthur) Martin; Max Gratzinger
Removable orthodontic appliances. Philadelphia 1966

Simon, Paul W(ilhelm)
a) Gnathostatik. Neue Wege der orthodontischen Diagnostik. Dtsch. Mschr. Zahnheilk. 37 (1919) 33—70
b) On the gnathostatic diagnosis in orthodontics. Int. J. Orthod. 10 (1924) 755—785
c) Über neuere und bewährte Apparaturen in der Orthodontie. Berlin 1928
d) The spring-beam apparatus. Int. J. Orthod. 16 (1930) 658—664

Talma, A(madée)-F(rançois)
a) Mémoire sur la conversation des dents. Bruxelles 1843. Extract in: Der Zahnarzt, Berlin 6 (1851) 167—178; 211—223
b) Mémoires sur . . . la médecine dentaire . . . Bruxelles 1852

Tomes, John
A system of dental surgery. Philadelphia 1859

Wedl, C(arl)
Pathologie der Zähne. Leipzig 1870

Weinberger, Bernhard Wolf
Orthodontics. 2 vols., St. Louis 1926

Welcker, Hermann
Untersuchungen über Wachsthum und Bau des menschlichen Schädels. Leipzig 1862

Chapter 15

Research and Teaching

The fundamentals of the development of odontological science in the 19th century were provided in the second half of the preceding century by an outsider, John Hunter, a surgeon, with his first book entitled "The Natural History of the Teeth."[1] For his part, he was able to draw on the totality of odontological scientific knowledge that had been summarized first in the western culture by Aristotle[2]. Enriched by the knowledge supplied by the Alexandrian school, specifics were noted by Celsus and Galen[3] which remained valid until Vesalius initiated the great overthrow in anatomy[4]. His followers, in turn, Falloppia and Eustachi—to the latter of whom we owe the first specialized anatomy—were especially interested in explaining tooth formation, a subject to which Rau also devoted his dissertation in Leyden in 1694[5]. Bunon, in Paris in the 18th century, studied the genesis of enamel erosion, also quoted by Fauchard, while Ludwig and Kemme, Berdmore, Hunter and Plenck dealt with dental enamel[6]. Schaeffer's investigations in 1757 finally freed the profession of its erroneous belief in the toothworm[7].

Speculative remnants, based in the final analysis on Plato's natural philosophy, were finally eliminated from medical research in the 19th century by Berlin's great physiologist, Johannes Müller. His student, Rudolf Virchow, founded a new phase of normal and pathological anatomy through his study of the cell. The clinical experience of Ignaz Semmelweis (contact infection) and Joseph Lister (antisepsis), and the researches of Louis Pasteur and Robert Koch provided the new subject of microbiology, and the trailblazing invention of Wilhelm Conrad Röntgen opened the way for new diagnostic and therapeutic developments.

Anatomy of the Tooth

The advances in the subject of anatomy of the tooth were achieved through the aid of the microscope, a device that had been used chiefly by its earlier developer Leeuwenhoek and by the great Malpighi to study this difficult material, while de la Hire and Winslow examined it probably with magnifying glasses only[8].

In addition to the long differentiated enamel and dentin, the third hard tissue component, cementum, was described in 1767 by Jacques René Tenon, a Frenchman, as *cortical osseux.* His work was brought to light only in a lecture in 1797. Cementum was described by John Corse and Everard Home in 1780 and was designated as "crusta petrosa" by Robert Blake[9] who made his studies with animal teeth. The same is true for the founder of paleontology, George Cuvier, who in his 1805 "Leçons d'anatomie comparée" (Lectures in Comparative Anatomy) determined in the section dealing with "cement" that this *appears to be like calculus that has become crystallized on the tooth ... I am convinced that this is deposited by the same membrane and* (on) *the same surface as enamel*[10]. Probably Cuvier was the first (from Retzius) to speak of "cement." In 1835 the candidate for a doctor's degree of Purkinje, Fraenkel, described it for the human tooth as "substantia osteoidea" (Fig. 495), while his colleague Raschkow already speaks of "caementum."[11]

Two anatomical works devoted to the anatomy of teeth, from Paris, brought no significant advances. The 1817 "Essai" of the anatomist Augustin Serres includes the first description of the "glands" later to be named after him on the alveolar processes of the newborn. These were said to secrete calculus later, but in fact contain epithelial inclusions from the root

[1] See pp. 219 f.
[2] See p. 65
[3] See pp. 72 and 76
[4] See pp. 136 f.
[5] See pp. 140 f. and 223
[6] See pp. 214 f. and 198
[7] See p. 214 f.
[8] See pp. 171 f., 174, and 193
[9] Cohen
[10] Cuvier (a) pp 109 f., (b) pp. 103 f.
[11] Retzius p. 543; Fraenkel Fig. 1—2; Raschkow p. 10. Magitot (see pp. 346 f.) regrettet again in 1857 that "the prestige of Cuvier rules in our schools and delays our progress so much in this question (of tooth development), while Germany and England make further progress" (Magitot (a) p. 37 f.).

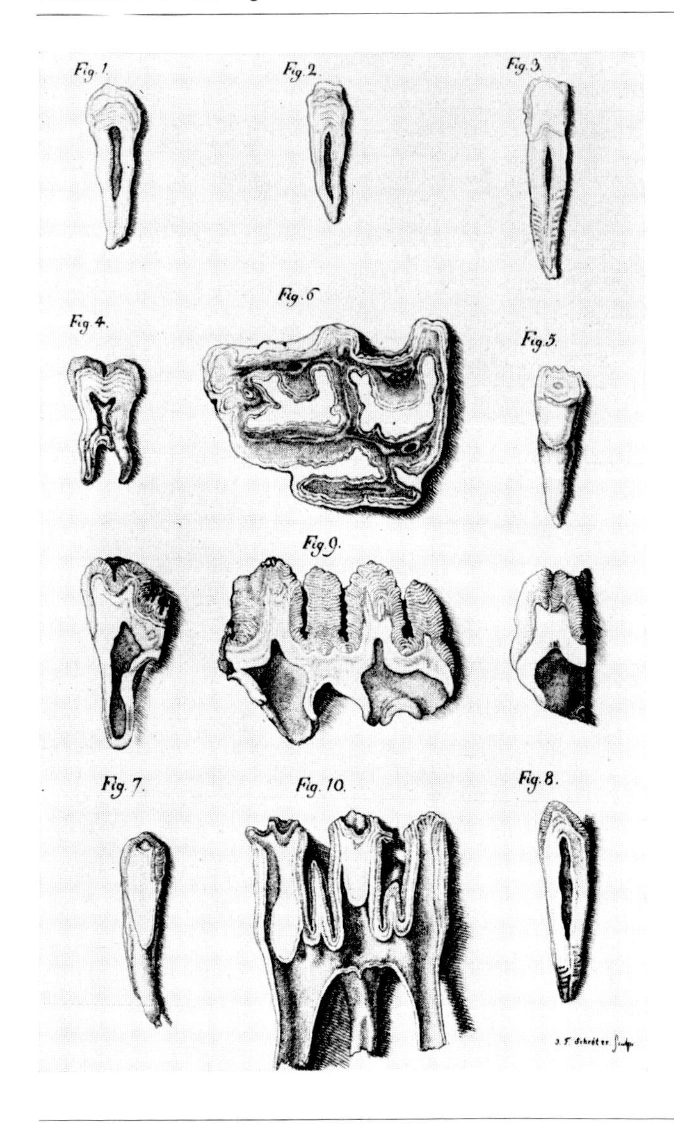

Fig. 494 *Schreger: Hunter-Schreger bands in the enamel of animal and human teeth, 1800*

sheath[12]. Even less productive is the "Anatomie du système dentaire" of Philippe Frédéric Blandin, anatomist and surgeon, who did not even mention the cementum in 1836. The hard tissue called "ostéide dentaire" consisted for him only of dentin (ivoire) and enamel (émail). For the London dentist Thomas Bell this third hard tissue of the tooth was also unknown in the second edition of his book in 1835[13].

In 1800, Christian Heinrich Theodor Schreger, then in training with his elder brother in Erlangen, and later to be professor of the healing arts of the university in Halle, described the bands later to be named after him and Hunter.

These bands in the enamel, visible in magnifications attainable by a magnifying glass, had already been observed by Malpighi (1661), Clopton Havers (1689), de la Hire (1699, see Fig. 135), Winslow (1733), Berdmore (1768), Hunter (1771, see Fig. 181), and the Dublin dentist Robert Blake (1798, in fibres of the Cortex striatus)[14]. Schreger provided the following description:

[12] Serres pp. 28 f. See also pp. 348 f.
[13] Blandin pp. 57 f.; Bell pp. 4 f.
[14] Blake (a) p. 16; (b) p. 80; Boyde

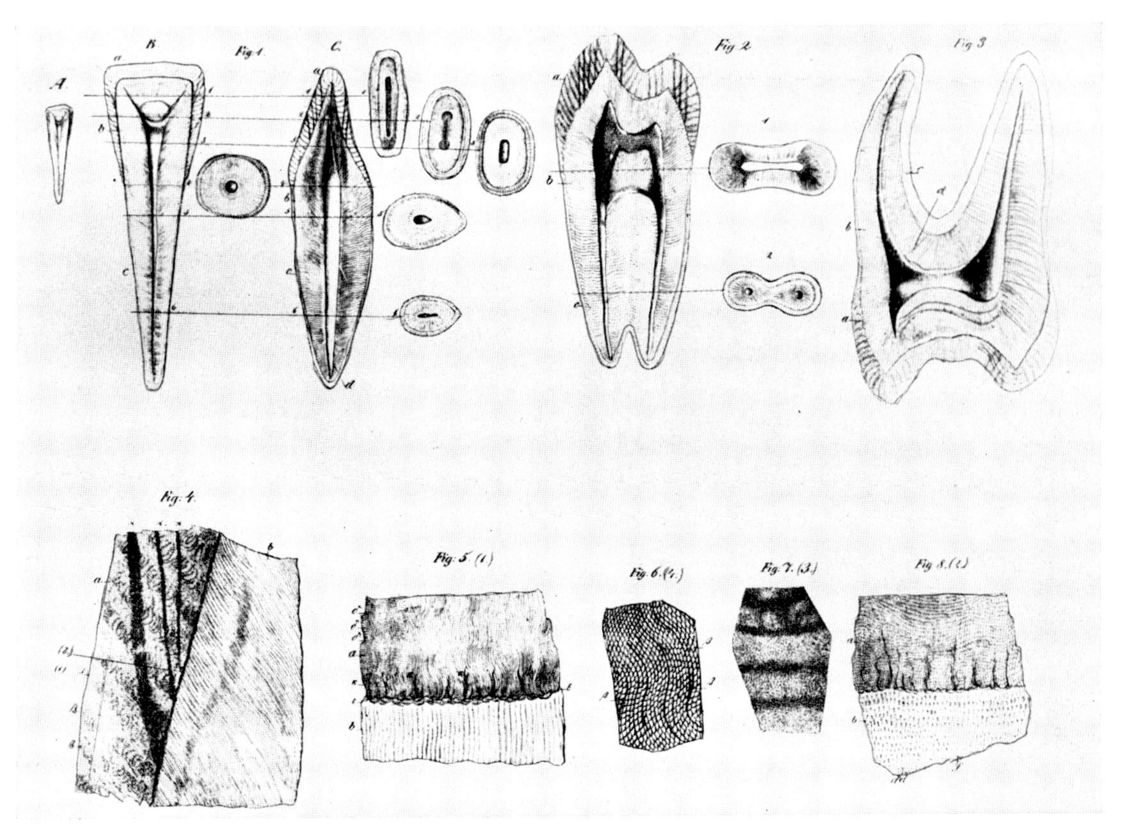

Fig. 495 *Meyer Fraenkel: Tooth sections showing Hunter-Schreger bands (e. g., Fig. 2 a), striae of Retzius (Fig. 4 a), and cement (Figs. 1 c and 2 c), 1835*

All the bands actually run in arch shapes in human enamel, not—as Hunter says and illustrates—in straight rays. (They course) *so that their concave surfaces are directed toward the crown and the convex toward the root of the tooth* (Fig. 494). The *horny substance of the root* (*substantia cornea*), incidentally, is described by Schreger as *the product of diseased bone tissue substance,* a description true only of hypercementosis[15]. Almost simultaneously around 1835, three researchers took up the study of fine structure in dental tissue: at first the physiologist Johann Evangelista Purkinje, then in Breslau and later to work in Prague, then, in 1833 guided by Purkinje, the Swedish anatomist Adolph Retzius, who published in 1836 and 1837 in Stockholm and Berlin; and finally, stimulated by Johannes Müller and Theodor Schwann, the Berlin dentist Joseph Linderer[16].

Purkinje, who developed the technique of preparation of slice preparations and decalcified sections and later arranged for the construction of the first microtome, caused the problem to be discussed in two dissertations in 1835. These were "De penitiori dentium humanorum structura observationes" (Observations concerning the Internal Structure of Human Teeth, Fig. 495) by Meyer Fraenkel, and Isaak Raschkow's "Meletemata circa mammalium dentium evolutionem" (Studies of the Development of the Teeth of Mammals).

The Hunter-Schreger bands were described by Retzius in 1835 as *parallel shadows of the cross-striations of the enamel fibers*[17]. In the same year, Fraenkel came closer to the truth with the assumption that they arose through

[15] Schreger
[16] See pp. 272 ff.
[17] Retzius p. 540

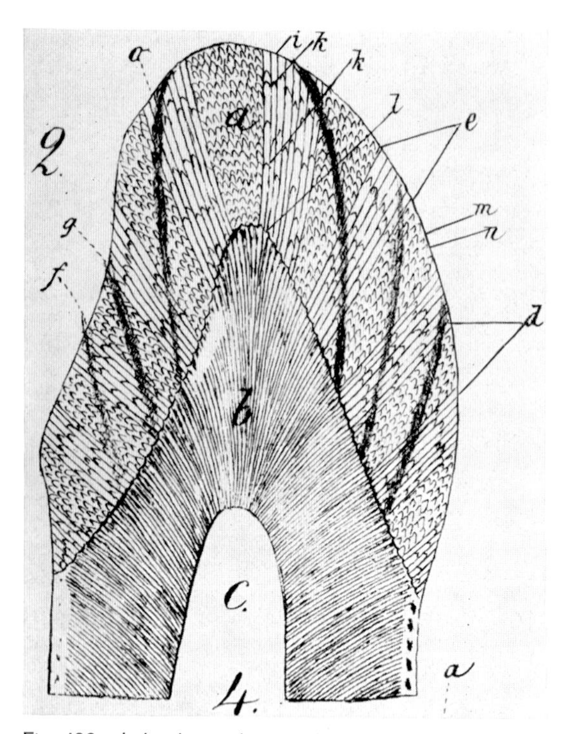

Fig. 496 *J. Linderer: Longitudinal section through an incisor (f, g, o = layer bands), 1837*

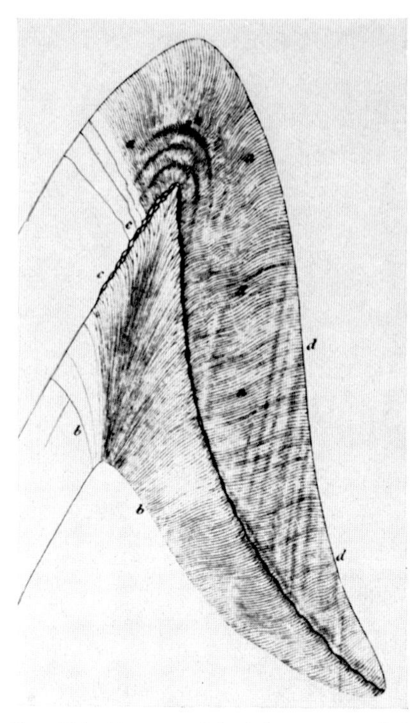

Fig. 497 *Retzius: "d d brown parallel lines," 1837*

the refraction of light by the naturally alternating course of the columns[18]. Joseph Linderer, who himself noted that he had made his observations before Fraenkel *in the presence of Professor Müller* (Fig. 496) wrote in 1837 in his "Handbuch der Zahnheilkunde" (Handbook of Dentistry) that these band-forming light and dark lines arise through enamel prisms which are hit lengthwise or cross-wise in section.[19] The anatomist of Würzburg, Albert Koelliker[20] and the Danish histologist Adolph Hannover[21] came to the same conclusion in 1852 and 1855, respectively, a conclusion still valid today, while the anatomist Wilhelm Waldeyer, in Königsberg and Breslau in 1864/1865 and later in Strassburg and Berlin, wrote that he *would ascribe a good part of these cross-lines* (striations) *to* (the effects of) *enamel prism crossing*[22]. In 1895, Gustav Preiswerk in Basel called this type of enamel bands *Zonien* (zones), whereby he differentiated between the light (*Parazonien*) and the dark (*Diazonien*), vertical sections and cross-sections[23]. Preiswerk later (from 1895) provided the first dental instruction at the University of Basel, from 1902 on as lecturer.

The other bands recognizable in the enamel, the brownish parallel striae, bear the name of Retzius (Fig. 497). Like Meyer Fraenkel before him[24], and like Joseph Linderer in 1837[25] (layer bands, Fig. 496) and Koelliker[26] and Hannover[27] later, in 1837 Retzius determined that this phenomenon arose from the changing rhythm of intensity

[18] Fraenkel p. 16: "Haec enim strata lucis radiis varie reflexis originem debent, eodem, modo, quo versicolores dentalis subst. propriae striae, ut supra fusius explicavimus." But here the wording is (p. 13): "Quas strias nos quoque in dente polito perspeximus, at opticum tantum phaenomenon esse invenimus, hac reortum, quod lucis radii in diversis fibrarum curvationibus refringuntur."
[19] Linderer (a) pp. 166 and 176 f.
[20] Koelliker (a) p. 375; (b) p. 53
[21] Hannover p. 91
[22] Waldeyer p. 269
[23] Preiswerk pp. 94 f.
[24] Fraenkel pp. 19 f.
[25] Linderer (a) p. 182
[26] Koelliker (a) p. 375; (b) p. 53
[27] Hannover p. 902 f.

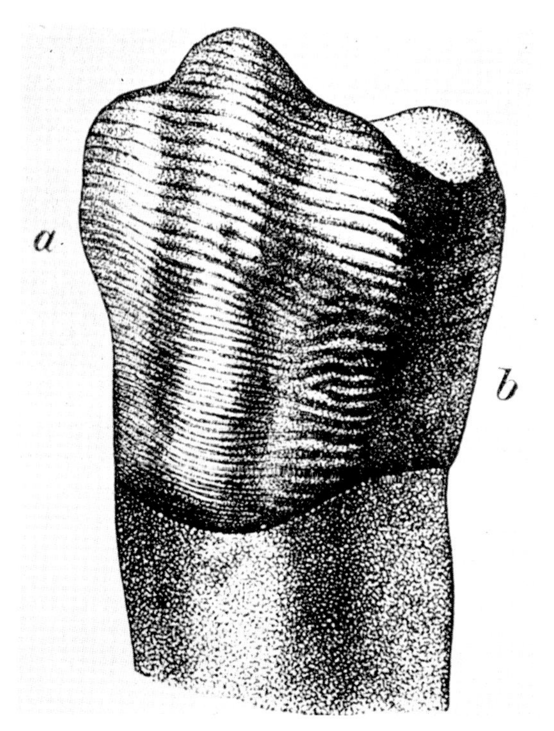

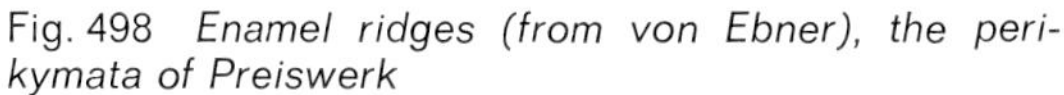
Fig. 498 *Enamel ridges (from von Ebner), the perikymata of Preiswerk*

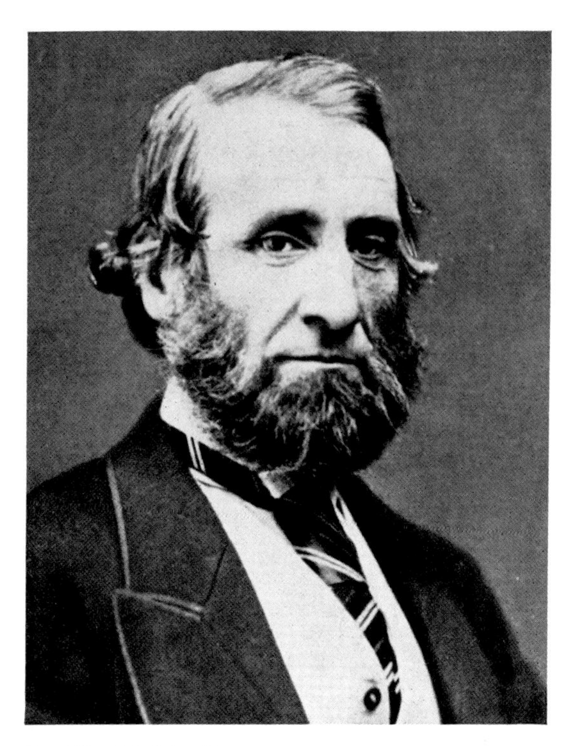
Fig. 499 *Sir John Tomes*

of calcification of enamel formation. They appeared to be the traces of different periods of enamel formation, like the lines running around the pulp cavity in the tooth substance (i.e., the Owen's contour lines)[28]. *I cannot determine whether they arise from brown discoloration of the tooth substance itself, from the coming together of parallel shadows of the cross-bands of the enamel fibers, or through both of these effects jointly*[29]. In Vienna in 1890, von Ebner saw this as an optical phenomenon: *The brownish parallel stripes of Retzius rest on the appearance of air between rows of enamel prisms on dry teeth*[30]. In 1895, Gustav Preiswerk called the striae of Retzius contour lines, a designation which has become less accepted than his term "perikymata" for the small transverse ridges on the exposed surface of enamel (Fig. 498) and "zones" for the Schreger bands[31]. In the 1848 edition of his handbook, Linderer describes the tuft fibers (*Büschelfasern*) of the enamel for the first time[32]. Today these regions of low calcification near the amelodentinal junction are called enamel tufts, as they do not contain true fibers.

Stimulated by lectures of Owen, the anatomist, and without being aware of the publications of the Breslau and Berlin schools, John Tomes at the age of 23 presented "On the Structure of the Teeth" to the Royal Society in 1838. Here, left entirely to his own devices, he attained the level of his predecessors.

The advancement of British dentistry is inseparably connected scientifically, practically, and from the point of view of professionalism with the name of Sir John Tomes (Fig. 499). He was born on March 21, 1815 in Weston on Avon, the son of a farmer. Following his schooling he was apprenticed to an apothecary and from 1836 on studied medicine in London at King's College and then in the Medical School of the Middlesex Hospital. As early as 1837, Tomes

28 See p. 394
29 Retzius p. 539
30 von Ebner (a) p. 100
31 Preiswerk p. 89 f.
32 Linderer (b) pp. 24 f.

devoted himself to the study of tooth structure and in 1840 he decided to give up the study of medicine and to become a dentist. As such, he entered King's College and simultaneously opened an office, devoting himself untiringly to his histological research. Berlin's great pathologist, Rudolf Virchow, called his 1848 effort a *classical work*[33]. The high point was the publication in 1856 of the work quoted below about dentinal fibrils, the Tomes' fibres. In 1859, "A System of Dentistry" was published, *a strictly practical work*, of which a German translation was published in 1861, a French one in 1873 and an American edition in 1887. His interest also extended to amalgams[34]. In addition, he invented numerous instruments and devices for the dental office[35]. The last 30 years of his efforts were devoted with success to the elevation and organization of dentistry as a profession. In 1856 jointly with Samuel Cartwright and others he founded the "Odontological Society." This group attained recognition as a profession through an examination in the College of Surgeons in 1858. The examination attained legal status with the passage of the "Dentists Act" in 1878. Tomes participated in the founding of an educational institution, the "Dental Hospital of London," as well in a leading role[36]. To crown his efforts, he was elected in 1880 as the first president of the newly founded "British Dental Association" and was elevated to the peerage in 1886.

Full of honors, the initiator of British dentistry died in London on July 29, 1895.—His son Charles Sismore followed in the footsteps of the father, being elected president of the "British Dental Association" in 1894, and being awarded the Association's prize named for his father for scientific merit[37].

In the previously noted publication, "On the Presence of Fibrils of Soft Tissue in the Dentinal Tubes," Tomes described and drew the fibrils now named after him in 1856. These had been seen by other researchers but—with a single exception—not precisely recognized or showed[38]. He writes: *With proper care in manipulating, nothing is more easy than to demonstrate the existence of the dentinal fibrils, in any tooth which has been recently extracted. If a thin section be made in the plane of the direction of the tubes, and then placed in dilute hydrochloric acid until the whole or a greater part of the lime is removed, and the section be afterwards torn in a direction transverse to that of the tubes, many of the fibrils will be seen projecting from the torn edges* (Fig. 500). *It is desirable, in repeating the experiment, to place the decalcified section upon a slide before tearing, as in moving it from the surface upon which it has been torn, some of the longer fibrils may be folded back upon the body of the specimen and thus become obscured. Where the separation between the torn surfaces has been but slight, we may often see a fibril, unbroken, stretching across from the separated orifices of the tube to which it belongs. It is not necessary, however, to decalcify dentine in order to show the fibrils. If a similar section to that already described be divided with the edge of a knife, many of these delicate organs will be seen, but they are usually broken off much shorter, many of them scarcely projecting beyond the orifices of the tubes*[39].

Twenty years earlier, Johannes Müller, the founder of precise medicine based on natural science in Germany and teacher of Rudolf Virchow, von Helmholtz, Henle, Schwann, and others, had provided a quite similar description in 1836. As it is largely unknown, it is quoted here: *In breaking fine tooth sections in a vertical direction to the fibres, I saw these frequently sticking out for a short distance from the edge from the dental hard tissue. Under these conditions, they are quite straight and do not appear to be bendable. If, however, calcium salts have been removed with acid from the fine sections, and the remaining cartilaginous sections are torn against the fibres, the fibres at the edge of the tear appear to be quite bendable and transparent and frequently extend for quite a distance. From this it may be concluded that the tubes have an animal matrix, membrane, and that this is rigid and fragile in the solid tooth which is still penetrated with calcium salt, but soft in the tooth that has lost its calcium salts . . .*[40]. Especially on the basis of this example, one can see how difficult it is to assign priority; even the situations described here need not be assumed to describe the definitive events, for fibre struc-

33 Virchow p. 300
34 See pp. 292 f.
35 See pp. 263 and 328 f.
36 See p. 410
37 Cope p. 95
38 Tomes (b); (c) pp. 327 f.; see Cope pp. 41 f.
39 Tomes (a)
40 Müller p. 336

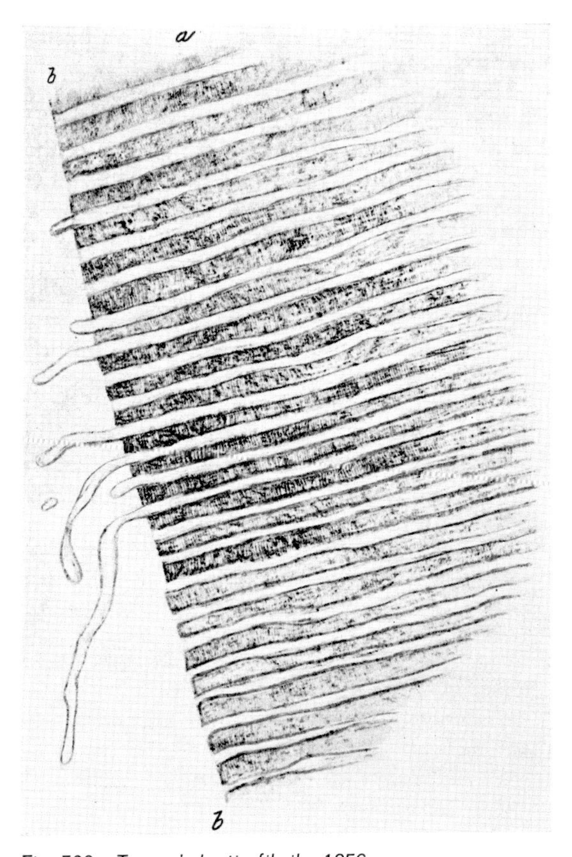

Fig. 500 *Tomes' dentin fibrils, 1856*

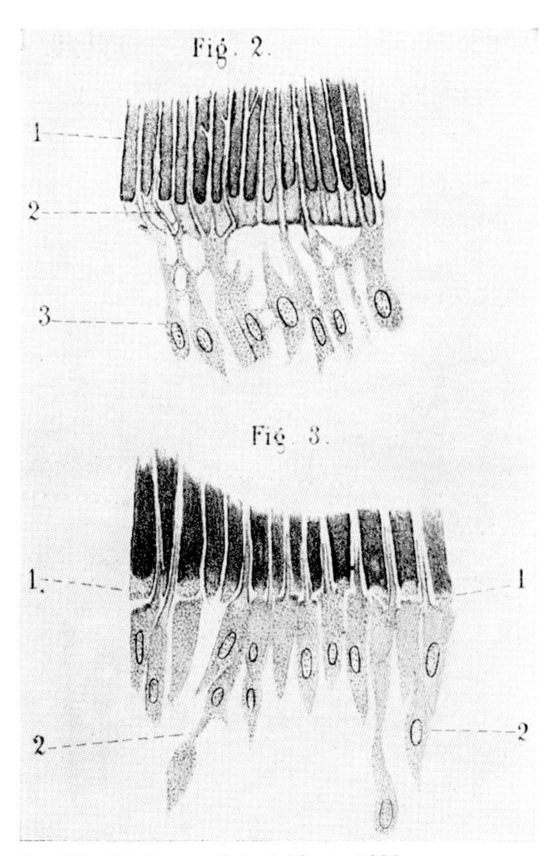

Fig. 501 *Waldeyer: Odontoblasts, 1865*

ture of dentin was already known to the other Purkinje-student, Raschkow, in 1835: *Substantiae dentalis structura in omnis fibrosa est* (The structure of the dental substance (dentin) is completely fibrous [p. 10]).

In 1839, Müller's student, the anatomist Schwann, later in Louvain and Liège, described the dentinal fibres quite similarly as his teacher. He had already recognized also what these structures really represented because he says *that each of the cylindrical cells of the surface of the pulp extend toward the tooth substance as a short, fine fibre and that these fibres extend beyond the surface of the pulp approximately as the dentinal tubules. I believed earlier that they extended into the tubules and that they were extensions of the cells in the interstitial substance between the tubules and that they were exposed intercellular substances.* [41] Schwann is thus the discoverer of the odontoblasts, the dentin-forming cells.

A long accepted version of the development of dentin was provided by Wilhelm Waldeyer, in 1865: *The formation of dentin consists in a transformation of a portion of the protoplosm of the ivory cell into a glue-like substance with subsequent calcification of the latter, whereby the other portion of the cell protoplasm remains unchanged in the hardening mass in the form of soft fibres* [42] (Fig. 501). Only in the last quarter of the century the older secretion theory prevailed, at first indicated by Rau, then mentioned by Raschkow and established by Koelliker, a concept still accepted today [43].

[41] Schwann p. 106
[42] Waldeyer (b) p. 189
[43] See p. 223 and the Waldeyer quotation p. 394

The other student of Purkinje, Isaak Raschkow of Breslau, introduced the still valid concept of an "enamel organ" in his dissertation, similarly written in Latin: *This spherical nucleus we have now called the enamel organ (organon adamantinae) because ... it is fated to form the enamel substance in that it will be transformed into the membrane which brings forth the enamel substance*[44]. A membrane seen by Raschkow between the pulp and the enamel organ was described by him as "Membran(ul)a praeformativa"[45], of which Waldeyer in 1864 believes *without fear of contradiction to be able to claim that no histologist has seen it properly, let alone that he has been able to make a proper preparation of it or that he has been able ... to make of Raschkow's description precisely what its discoverer meant by it*[46]. Nonetheless, the concept will appear frequently because there is hardly an investigator in this field around the middle of the 19th century who did not base his own investigations on these two Latin dissertations from the school of Purkinje from 1835.

We find an especially clear description of the enamel organ in Linderer's Handbook of 1837: *The enamel organ has the shape of the earlier enamel ... and at its summit it has a more smooth surface, not the points and the fissures of enamel. The inner surface, however, which lies on the top of the dental pulp has as many points and fissures as the latter, but of course in the reverse relationship. The external surface of the enamel organ touches the inner surface of the dental follicle; the inner surface of the enamel organ touches the external surface of the dental pulp*[47] (Fig. 502). The dental pulp, here still the dentin-forming organ, *is surrounded, as it were, by a skin ... Raschkow calls this skin the membranula praeformativa*[48].

Schwann believed, in 1839, *that the prismatic cells of the enamel membrane separate from it and grow into the already formed enamel, while their cavities either fill with calcium salts simultaneously or while they ossify in their entire thickness after their cavities are filled with an organic substance*[49]. Later this was also the view of Tomes[50], and Waldeyer also agreed in 1864. The latter differentiated between external and internal epithelium in the enamel organ and called the latter the *enamel membrane*. Cylindrical cells grow from this, which provide the enamel *in that they calcify themselves directly*[51]. Today one recognizes, analogously to dentin, the enamel prisms as excretion products of these cells, the ameloblasts.

Richard Owen, already mentioned as a teacher of Tomes, was a London anatomist and director of the Hunter collections of the Royal College of Surgeons. In his publication of 1840/1842 entitled "Odontography," a work devoted to comparative anatomy, he already used the current terms *dentine, enamel* and *cement* without any further explanation. The designation *dentine* (usually "dentin" in the American and the non-British European literature) probably should be ascribed to him[52]. He had previously already described the *contour lines* later named after him in the dentin; these correspond to the striae of Retzius in the enamel, that is, they similarly arise through the layer-like deposits of the substance.

Alexander Nasmyth (Fig. 503), dentist and member of the Royal College of Surgeons of London, who was acquainted with the work of the Purkinje school and of Müller and Retzius[53], in 1839 described to the Royal Society a tissue he called *Capsular Investment of the Enamel*[54], one known to us today through Koelliker as "Schmelzoberhäutchen" (enamel cuticle) or through Waldeyer as "Cuticula dentis." Nasmyth placed this structure (erroneously) in an analogous position to the "crusta petrosa" of Blake, i.e., root cementum, and in his posthumously published "Researches" he interpreted this *persistant dental capsule* more clearly as analogous to coronal cement of certain mammals as a rudiment of the enamel-covering portion of cementum[55] (Fig. 504).

This assumption was rejected as early as 1841 by William Lintott, a surgeon and surgical and mechanical dentist of London, who believed that *this membranous apparatus ... is the rudiment of the enamel organ of the embryo, in the structure of which the crystalline substance was originally deposited*[56]. The designation "Nasmyth's membrane" for the enamel

[44] Raschkow p. 2
[45] Raschkow p. 5 f.
[46] Waldeyer (b) p. 177
[47] Linderer (a) p. 85
[48] Ibid. p. 89
[49] Schwann p. 101
[50] Tomes (c) pp. 313 f.
[51] Waldeyer (a) p. 275
[52] Owen pp. 302 f.; Cohen
[53] Pindborg
[54] Nasmyth (a); (b) pp. 113 f.
[55] Ibid. (b) pp. 79 f.
[56] Lintott p. 8

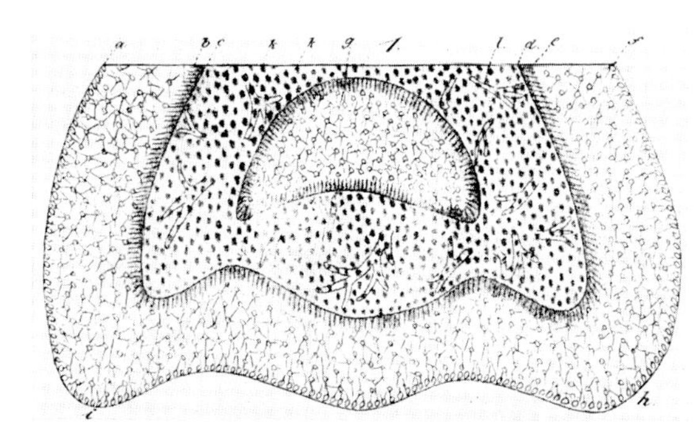

Fig. 502 *J. Linderer: Enamel organ of a calf tooth, 1837*

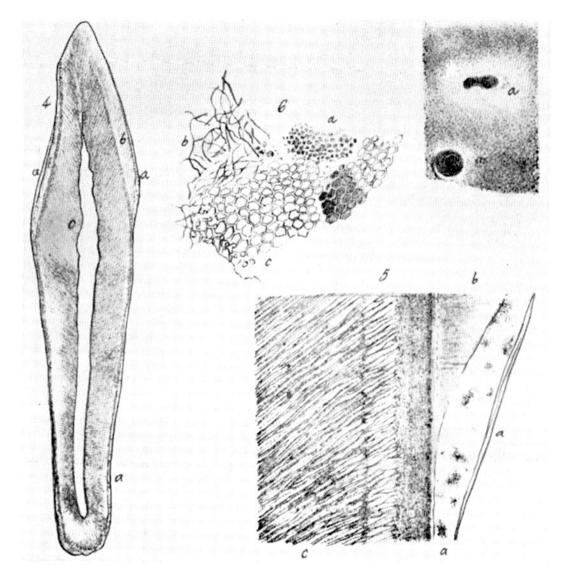

Fig. 504 *Nasmyth: "Capsular investment" (4 a and 5 a), 1849*

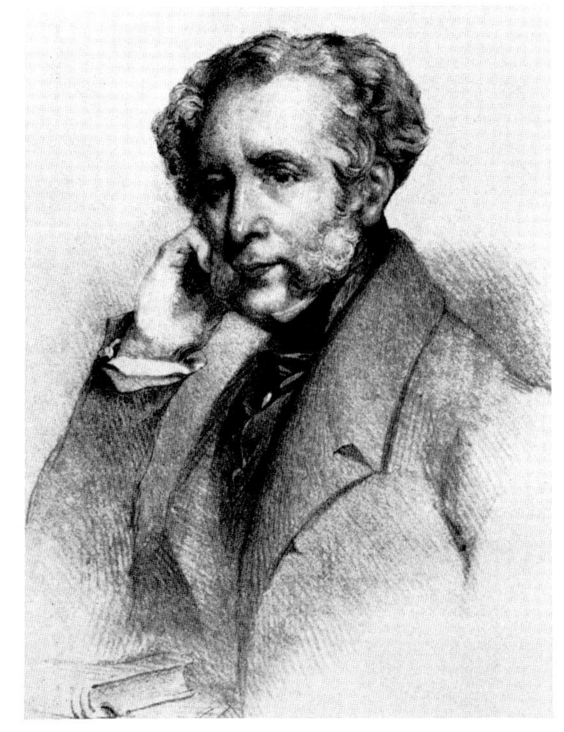

Fig. 503 *Alexander Nasmyth*

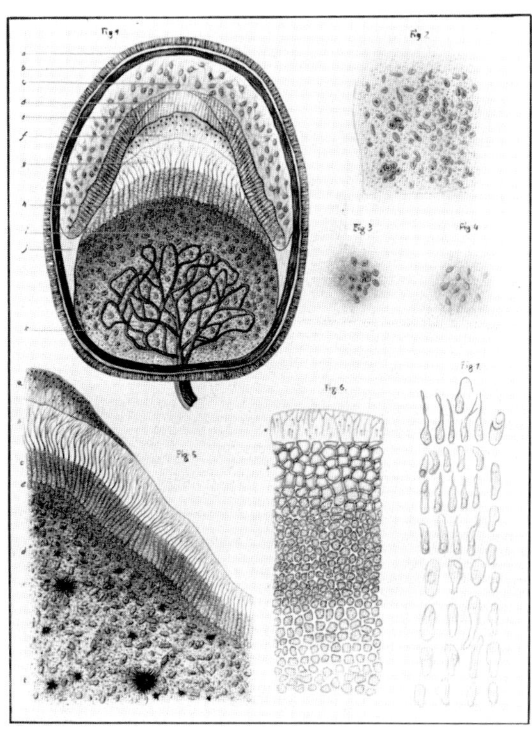

Fig. 505 *Magitot: "Follicule dentaire" (Enamel organ), 1857*

cuticle owes its existence to the famed London biologist and comparative anatomist Thomas Henry Huxley who supported the experimental results of Nasmyth in 1853 but drew conclusions different, in part from them. Teeth and hair, he alleged, were *in all respects homologous, and true dermal organs.* He provided an exact description of the toothforming epithelial sheath, which therefore occasionally bears his name but which is also frequently identified by the name of the Berlin anatomist, Oscar Hertwig. The latter, in 1874, recognized the epithelial character first, in comparative anatomical studies of the shark [57]. Raschkow's *"enamel organ,"* always cited in quotation marks by Huxley, was not admitted to have enamel-forming capacity at all, a conclusion through which Huxley also put himself in opposition to Tomes and Koelliker [58]. According to him, the enamel cuticle developed from Raschkow's legendary membrana praeformativa, which he named *basement membrane* in accordance with his colleague William Bowman. This membrane, according to Huxley's wrong interpretation, produces all three tooth tissues: *Neither the capsule nor the "Enamel-organ" take any direct share in the development of the dental tissues, all three of which—viz. enamel, dentine and cement—are formed beneath the membrana preformativa, or basement membrane of the pulp* [59].

Magitot of Paris, who, unlike Raschkow, did not believe in the formative role of the membrane, assumed that dentin cells formed beneath it but that it then *disappeared through atrophy* [60] (Fig. 505). John Tomes joined the coronal cement theory of Nasmyth in his evaluation of the significance of the enamel cuticle [61]. Magitot, too, in his, regarding literature, unusually careful prepared dissertation [63], Wedl in 1870 [64], and Baume in his textbook in 1875 and 1877 [65] followed this false path. Linderer, on the contrary, *had never noted this in human teeth* in 1851 [66].

Koelliker finally brought this coronal cementum hypothesis ad absurdum when he claimed to be able to demonstrate a *Schmelzoberhäutchen* (enamel cuticle) between the enamel and coronal cementum of guinea pigs in 1852 [67]. He believed it to be the last layer secreted by the enamel organ [68], while Waldeyer recognized a remnant of the external enamel epithelium [69]. For a long time, an interpretation of von Ebner remained valid; the latter, like Koelliker, described the enamel cuticle as an end product of the enamel-forming cells, the ameloblasts [70]. Despite the efforts of Gottlieb in Vienna (1921) and other researchers of the time, the type and origin of this substance remains controversial [71].

The physiologist Johann Czermak, whose work was done chiefly in Leipzig, described the *interglobular spaces* (Fig. 506) especially noticeable in youths in regions adjacent to the enamel and cementum, in his dissertation of 1850 entitled "Beiträge zur mikroskopischen Anatomie der menschlichen Zähne" (Contributions to the Microscopic Anatomy of Human Teeth) as a student of Koelliker in Würzburg. For a long time, those spaces bore his name, although they had been seen previously within the "granular layer" by Tomes. As Tomes and Czermak already assumed, these are uncalcified spaces between ball-shaped calcification centers, the dentinal globules of Koelliker [72]. Owen perceived dentinal cells in them, a belief that was still shared halfway by Hannover in 1859 [73]. Magitot [74], on the other hand, followed Czermak's lead, and this teaching was sustained by von Ebner and others up to our own days. Probably as the first, Czermak assumed the presence of some sort of adhesive substance (Kittsubstanz) between the single enamel prisms [75]. He was the first—and for a long time the only—one who indicated the size relations in illustrations of his sections.

Joseph Linderer's odontological collection, but also his intellectual succession was assumed in Berlin by the previously noted Robert Baume, who provided worthwhile contributions to pathological and comparative

[57] Huxley p. 164; Hertwig
[58] Huxley pp. 153 and 164
[59] Ibid. pp. 157 f.
[60] Magitot (a) p. 22. See p. 346
[61] Tomes (c) pp. 315 f.
[63] Magitot (a) pp. 76 f.
[64] Wedl p. 46
[65] R. Baume (a); (b) p. 61
[66] Linderer (c) p. 50
[67] Koelliker (a) p. 373; (b) p. 49; v. Ebner (c) pp. 335 f.
[68] Koelliker (a) p. 387; (b) p. 70
[69] Waldeyer (a) p. 294
[70] von Ebner (c) p. 287
[71] Lenz
[72] Czermak pp. 16 f.; Tomes (b) pp. 315 f.; Koelliker (a) p. 372; (b) p. 47
[73] Owen pp. 861 f.
[74] Magitot (a) pp. 34 f.
[75] Czermak p. 6

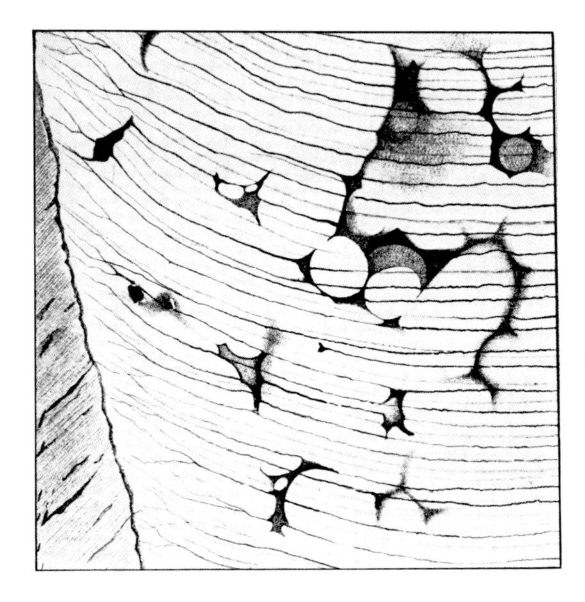

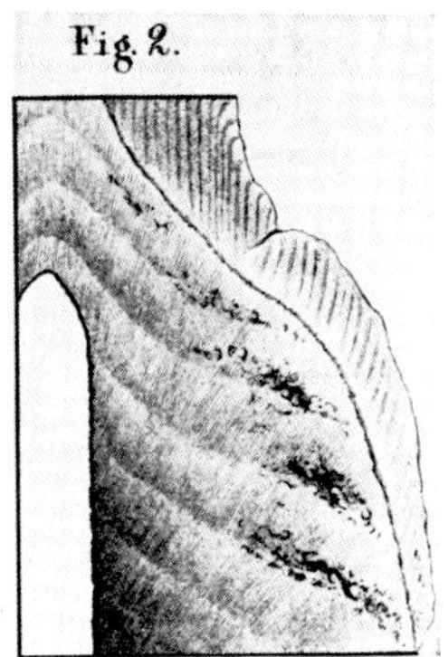

Fig. 506 *Czermak: "Interglobularräume" (Interglobular spaces), 1850*

anatomy in the several editions of his "Lehrbuch der Zahnheilkunde" (Textbook of Dentistry) of 1877, 1886 and 1900, and in his "Odontologische Forschungen" (Odontological Researches, 1882)[76]. In 1874 he provided a clear and histologically founded description of a "tooth within a tooth" but, like the dental surgeon of Guy's Hospital in London, Samuel James Augustus Salter, who described the condition first and called it "warty tooth" in 1855, like Quincy, a dentist in Illinois, who gave it the English name in 1856, and Tomes in 1859, he did not recognize the etiology as invagination of a tooth germ. The popular Latin expression, "dens in dente," was coined by the first director of the Berlin University Dental Institute, Friedrich Busch, in 1897, the earlier eponymic "Salter's tooth" may be found only in older English literature. They all believed the deformity to be a kind of gemination[77]. In 1953 these terms were proposed to be replaced by "dens invaginatus[78]."

The Viennese stomatological school, without doubt under the influence of the outstanding pathologist Karl von Rokitansky, devoted itself to the study of macroscopic normal and pathological anatomy of the organs of mastication, under the leadership of Carabelli. Georg Carabelli (Fig. 507) was a true son of the Austrian mixture of nations. Of Italian origin through his father, he was born of a Hungarian mother on December 11, 1787 in Budapest, and spent his life working in Vienna. He studied medicine at that city's university and was trained as a surgeon at its military medical academy, the Josephinum. As its pupil he took part in the Napoleonic wars of 1809 and 1813. In 1815 he was awarded the doctorate in surgery and turned to dentistry. When peace was declared, he completed his special education in Paris and, as the first at Vienna's university, was appointed professor of dentistry. Through untiring scientific effort and an extensive private practice, Carabelli made a superb position for himself, one which was enhanced in 1831 by the bestowal of a Hungarian hereditary title—he was now Edler von (nobleman of) Lunkaszprie—and stabilized in 1833 by his appointment as court dentist to emperor Franz. In 1831, the first volume of a planned comprehensive "Systematisches Handbuch der Zahnheilkunde" (Systematic Handbook of Dentistry) was published containing an "Historical Survey of Dentistry." This first extensive documented chronicle of the profession later met with some criticism. Nevertheless, one must surely agree

[76] Guttmann
[77] R. Baume (a); Salter; "Socrates;" Tomes (c) pp. 266 f.; Busch; see Kitchin, who provides an extensive historical review
[78] Hallet

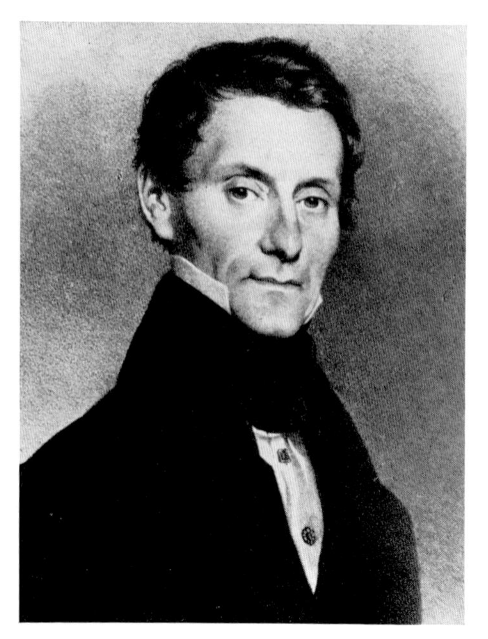

Fig. 507 *Georg Carabelli, Lithograph by Josef Kriehuber, 1835*

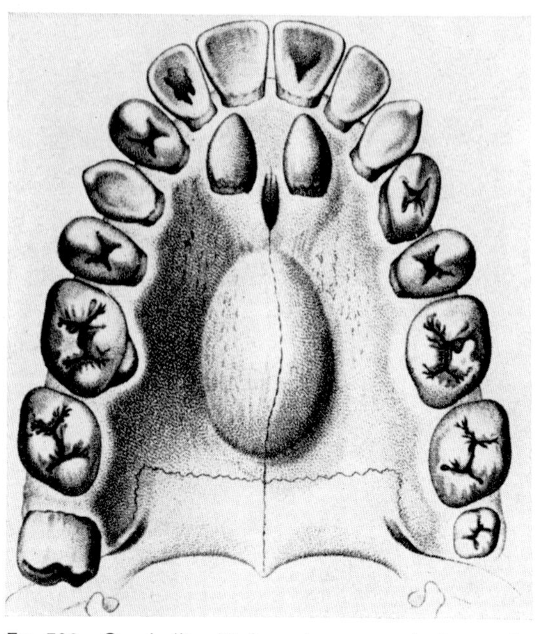

Fig. 508 *Carabelli: "Tuberculus anomalus" at the upper right first molar, 1842*

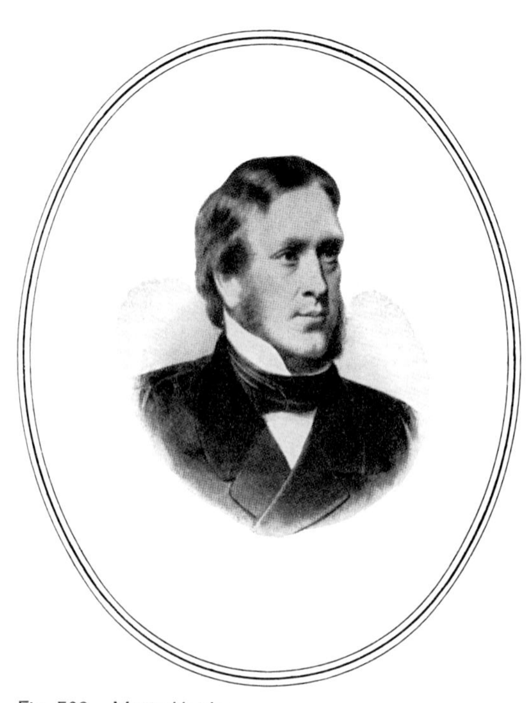

Fig. 509 *Moriz Heider*

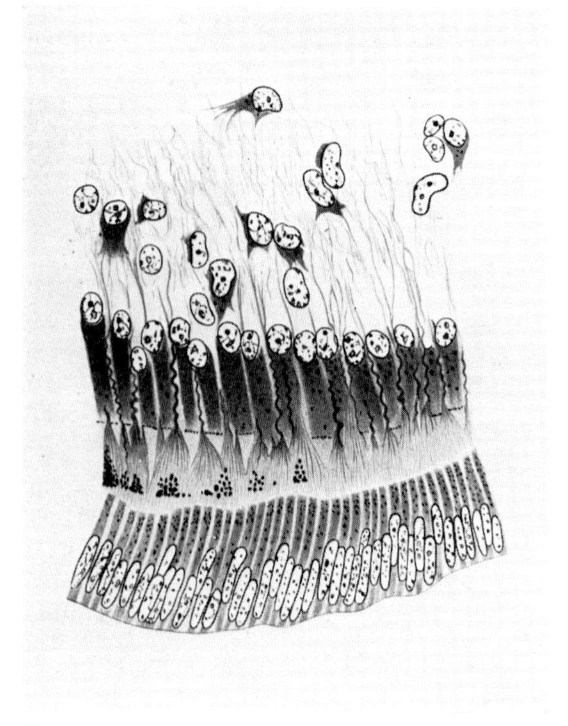

Fig. 510 *von Korff: Intercellular collagenous fibres, 1906*

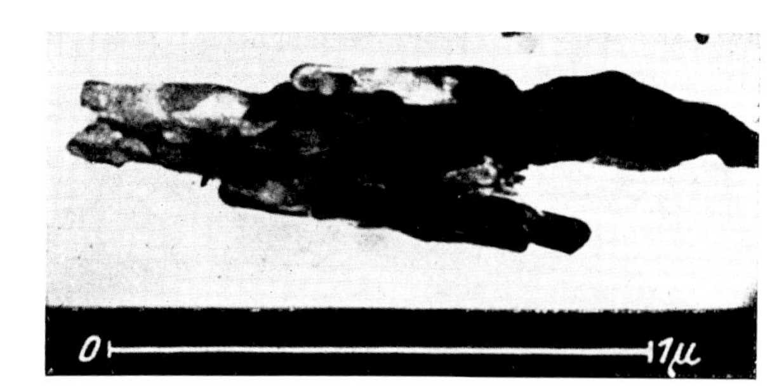

Fig. 511 *First electron microscopic photograph of enamel crystals by Keck and Helmcke, 1944*

with J. Linderer, who spoke in 1851 of *inevitable errors and omissions*[79]. In 1842, the year of Carabelli's death, volume II, the "Anatomie des Mundes" (Anatomy of the Mouth) followed, with a special volume of illustrations[80]. The latter contained a description of the abnormal tuberculum which has taken his name, Carabelli's tubercle (*tuberculus anomalus;* Fig. 508)[81]. Two years after his death on October 24, 1842, both volumes by this founder of the important Viennese odontological research tradition were published in a second edition.
Carabelli, who died at age 55, lived on through his students, of whom Prague's professor Franz Nessel previously has been quoted several times. Another, Adolf Fröhlich, founded a private dental institute in Graz, and Friedrich Turnovsky another one in Budapest. The most important among them, however, was Heider.
Moriz Heider (Fig. 509), born in Vienna on June 21, 1816, studied medicine there until 1841 but was also interested in astronomy as a sideline. The offer of Carabelli, to make Heider his assistant, was rejected with the frequently quoted phrase that *an honourable young man who has studied, too, can't become a dentist*[82]. But because he could not find a position as an assistant either in a physical laboratory or in a clinic, in 1842 he became Carabelli's assistant for the six months still left to him. Then was made heir to Carabelli's practice and collections; in 1843 he became a lecturer and in 1859 professor at the University of Vienna. In the same year the first 23 members of the "Central-Verein deutscher Zahnärzte," the predecessor of today's "Deutsche Gesellschaft für Zahn-, Mund- und Kieferheilkunde," elected him president at their inaugural meeting in Berlin. He founded the publication of that society, the *Deutsche Vierteljahrsschrift für Zahnheilkunde* in 1861 and served as its editor until his untimely death on July 29, 1866. His greatest goal, however, to establish a university dental institute in Vienna, which would be a *model charitable institution for all of Germany* was not fulfilled because of the lack of insight of the authorities. This was achieved by Julius Scheff only in 1890[83].
Heider introduced gold foil restorations to Austria; in 1845 he constructed what may have been the first electrocautery, with which he cauterized pulp. Most importantly, however, was his "Atlas to the Pathology of the Teeth" with Carl Wedl, the histopathologist which was published in 1869, three years after Heider's death. It was republished in 1889 in German and in 1872 and 1893 in German and English. In 1870, this beautifully made, richly illustrated work was followed by Wedl's "Pathologie der Zähne" (Pathology of the Teeth), so that these fortunate cooperative efforts produced not only the first, but also an excellent textbook of the special pathology of the subject[84]. The same year saw the publication of the purely macroscopic "Anatomie des menschlichen Gebisses" (Anatomy of the Human Dentition) by Eduard Mühlreiter, a Salzburg dentist and student of Heider. This is a work whose subsequent editions have continued into our own times. Adolph Zsigmondy, also a student of Heider whose

[79] Linderer (c) p. 373
[80] Carabelli I. See p. 368
[81] Carabelli II p. 107. That this cusp, enlarging approximately 67 % of all upper first molars, had been noted by the anatomist Samuel Thomas von Sömmering as early as 1791 could not be verified by the author in the editions of 1791 and 1839, at least not expressis verbis: "Its crown has four, five, or even more cusps, usually three labial and two lingual . . ." Sömmering I p. 201
[82] Steinberger
[83] Heider; Lesky
[84] Heider; Wedl

entire working life was spent in Vienna, in 1861 proposed the tooth designation system characterized by angular notations; the system became particularly accepted in Europe. In 1887, the Danish dentist Viktor Haderup devised the tooth identification scheme which is characterized by the use of plus and minus signs [85]. The Viennese tradition of anatomy was continued successfully by Victor von Ebner, the histologist. Collagenous dentinal fibrils bear his name, as does a type of serous glands of the retrolingual region of the tongue [86]. He was succeeded by Fleischmann and Gottlieb in the 20th century [87]. The latter transfered this Viennese tradition of research to the USA.

One of the first to apply photographic illustrations to the depiction of dental tissue was Otto Walkhoff, a dentist then working in Braunschweig in 1894 and 1897 in the two volumes of his splendidly produced, trilingual microphotographic atlas of the normal and the pathological histology of the teeth. In his dissertation of 1899 he denied the adhesive substance between enamel prisms first proposed by Czermak. Also in 1894, a "Sammlung von Mikrophotographien ... der mikroscopischen Struktur der Zähne" (Collection of Microphotographs ... of the Microscopic Structure of the Teeth), an atlas with 12 great plates, was published by Gysi and Röse in Zürich [88].

Walkhoff, appointed professor in Munich in 1902, and later, from 1922 to 1927, in Würzburg, resolutely filled the gap in German dentistry left by the departure of Miller in 1906 [89], in that he became the chairman (1906—1925) of the "Centralverein" as well as the president of the Vth International Dental Congress in Berlin in 1909. He was a pugnacious leader of the profession and a strong protagonist for the introduction of the doctor's degree for dentists, a proposal legalized in Germany in 1919.

In 1906, Karl von Korff described the fibers noted by him (and named after him) in odontogenesis (Fig. 510). This work was done at the University of Kiel; later, and until his death, he worked at the University of Rosario, in Argentina. He depicted the fibers as fibrils arising in the tooth germ, later to be the pulp, and saw in them, and not in the odontoblasts, the true dentin forming structures. Von Ebner strongly opposed this point of view and called the fibrils illusions. For this reason, von Korff left his country. At present the structures are usually held to be collagenous fibrils which have been raised from the other fibrous substance through a bundling process [90].

The established British tradition of anatomical-odontological research led Henry Percy Pikkerill to far-off New Zealand where he founded the first dental educational institution in 1907. His "The Structure of the Enamel", in which he concentrated largely on the course of prisms and the amelodentinal junction, appeared in 1912. He also dealt with caries research, but under the influence of World War I he turned completely to maxillary and facial surgery [91].

Thus we have reached a point of connection with the present. The construction of the electron microscope in 1927 by Ernst Ruska in Berlin initiated a new epoch in the study of dental tissue, too, especially as these tissues served as most suitable ones for examination. The first investigations of this material were made in 1944 by the Berlin biologist Johann-Gerhard Helmcke together with J. Keck, a dentist (Fig. 511). As Leeuwenhoek had opened a new world for himself with the lenticular microscope three centuries earlier, so today's scientists made progress at the viewers of these new, constantly improving devices. Later generations will make the efforts to understand the now visible microstructures and to place them in their proper arrangement.

Caries Research

The great caries researcher Willoughby Dayton Miller provided a historical classification of earlier caries theories in 1889 [92]. He introduced these theories with *depraved juices accumulated in the teeth,* the final end of Hippocratic beliefs in dentistry [93] as were still mentioned by Fauchard and Bourdet [94].

According to Galen and his successors, the blame was to be put on nutritional disturb-

[85] Zsigmondy; Haderup
[86] von Ebner (b) p. 343
[87] See p. 318
[88] Walkhoff (a and b); (c) p. 8; Gysi/Röse
[89] See p. 407
[90] von Korff; von Ebner (d); L. J. Baume pp. 106 f.
[91] Pickerill; Schmid. See pp. 320 f.
[92] Miller (c) p. 92; (d) p. 120
[93] See p. 62
[94] See pp. 198 f. and 211

ances. Thus his admirer Eustachi attributed disturbances of nutrition to his theory of decay: *The excesses cause a disease like that of inflammation of the fleshy organs, despite the hard, even stony hardness of the teeth*[95]. The inflammation theory was especially accepted in England. Hunter still avoided a clear definition in 1778. He spoke of *mortification* of the tooth substance but believed that this was not the sole cause because the teeth did not decay after death[96]. Fox, in 1806, ascribed caries ("decay") largely to inflammation of dentin, which, in turn, was said to be the consequence of inflammation of the periodontal membrane. Other causes were said to be related to constitutional or nutritional nature, and infection alco appeared in crowding[97]. In 1826 Koecker took up the inflammation theory, and in 1829, Thomas Bell took up the cudgels clearly when he noted that caries, which he called *gangrene of the teeth,* arose through inflammation. Dentin had a propensity for caries because it had only *a small degree of vital power* and could hardly resist injuries such as those from cold. The periodontal membrane theory of caries, propounded by Fox, was strictly rejected by Bell, however[98].

The millenia-old worm theory, definitely disproved by Schaeffer[99] in 1757, still vegetated in the medical literature up to the 19th century. In 1790 the surgeon and later professor at the University of Berlin, Johann Gottlieb Bernstein suggested that winter cherries with yellow wax be placed in teeth afflicted *with toothache from worms in teeth with cavities,* and that henbane fumigation be used. This prescription is still to be found in the fifth edition of his handbook of 1819[100].—Even in the respected *Magazin für die gesamte Heilkunde,* its editor, the surgeon Rust, reviewed the report of a Silesian local physician who had reported the elimination of toothache in two patients by the withdrawal of 20 toothworms, as follows: *Because after one has coated the surrounding region with the gastric juice of a pig, the sick persons noted how these worms bored through the teeth and reached the oral cavity*[101]. —The German translator and commentator of Laforgue's "Dental Arts," the Saxon court surgeon and municipal dentist of Leipzig, Carl Friedrich Angermann, showed toothworms *in natural look* in 1803 (Fig. 512). Although he made an effort to establish a sensible reason for the appearance of both types of toothworm, he tends to view *worms that live in carious teeth as the cause of toothache*[102]. The belief in toothworms remained among the peoples of central Europe well into the 20th century[103].—Pfaff's putrefaction theory of 1756, however, lived (after Miller) only in the concept of "tooth-rot."

The chemical theory of caries dominated the 19th century. Based on the acid experiments of Ludwig and Kemme[104], especially the Germans, but later the British and American authors agreed with it. Thus the North American dentist Levi Spear Parmly in his textbook of 1819, while otherwise completely following the footprints of Fox, saw, *comprising a discovery of the origin of the caries,* the primary cause *in relics of the food and beverage, which, from heat and stagnation, undergoing a putrefactive fermentation, acquire a sufficient solvent power to produce a disease*[105]. While the previously mentioned hypotheses were built exclusively on speculation, experimental science now assumed its proper place again. Karl Joseph Ringelmann, the first instructor of dentistry (from 1824?) at the University of Würzburg whose reputation is dubious dissolved enamel in sulfuric acid. Note, however, that this "professor's " opponent, the dentist Johann Franz Gallette of Mainz, proved his opus was plagiarism from A to Z, taken from several contemporaneous books[106].

Joseph Linderer in the middle of the '30s was probably the first to subject carious tissue to microscopic examination. As seen in figure 513, he consistently found in enamel as well as in dentin processes that became pointed as they ran inwards, brown in color and surrounded in the dentin by lighter lines caused by the continuing spread. These discolorations led him to distinguish between the state of decay (decomposition), in which *the calcified fibers dissolve* to form *a friable mass,* and the subsequent *softening,* characterized by complete

95 Eustachius p. 94
96 Hunter II pp. 1 f.
97 Fox p. 12 f.
98 Bell pp. 123 f.
99 See pp. 241 f.
100 Bernstein p. 159
101 Rust
102 Laforgue and Angermann p. 75 Note; p. 335 f.
103 Kobusch
104 See p. 241
105 Parmly p. 81
106 Ringelmann (a) pp. 77 f.; Gallette (b)

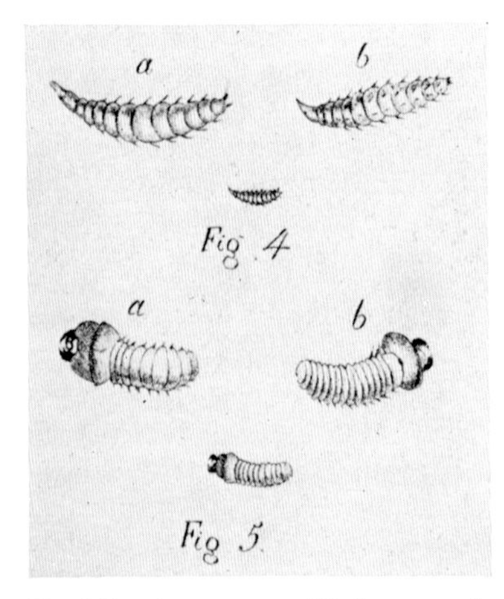

Fig. 512 *Angermann: "Zahnwürmer" (Toothworms), 1803*

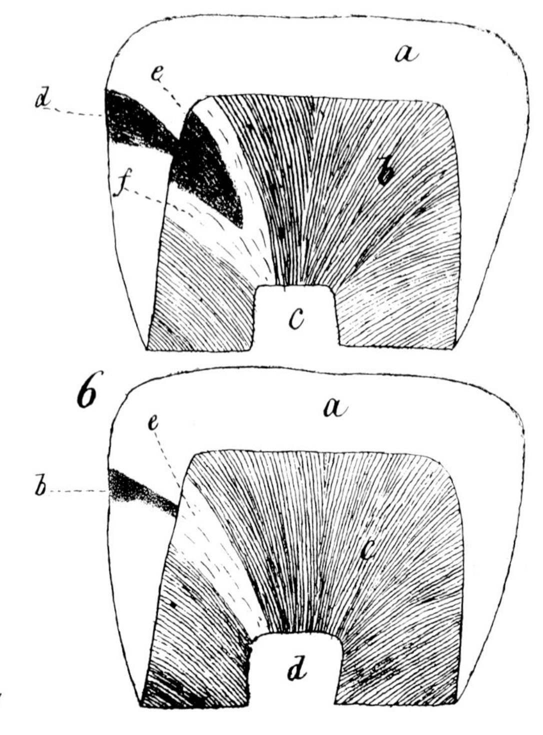

Fig. 513 *J. Linderer: Microscopic depiction of caries, 1837*

loss of structural organization [107]. In the edition of 1848 of the "Handbook" this was elaborated as the author took a position on the causes of caries, which he perceived as *acid oral fluids;* i.e., he adopted the chemical theory [108].

The first Anglo-Saxon exponent of this theory was probably William Robertson, a dentist practicing in Birmingham (England). He noted clearly in his "Practical Treatise" that, contrary to Hunter, Fox and Bell, the decay is *entirely the result of external agencies,* that this in turn consists in *a chemical action of the food lodging in that situation,* i.e., in the fissures, especially of the grinders [109].

John Tomes, who properly complained that Robertson ignored more recent histological findings, joined the chemical and inflammation theories in the decade of the '50s. Like Linderer, he too assumed that the eliciting factor was a pathological excess of acids in the oral fluids. Acids elicit an inflammatory process in the dentin which, because of the particular anatomic conditions, does not run with the classical characteristics. Following destruction of the vitality of the tissue the chemical reaction begins to affect the enamel secondarily [110].

Like Linderer, Tomes recognized by microscopic examination a conical shape of the carious process in the dentin, caused by the course of the fibers. These he found broken within the canals (Fig. 514).

The New York dentist Amos Westcott (Fig. 515) extended in 1843 the well-known acid experiments to organic acids, including acetic, citric, malic, and other acids, and noted that these attack the teeth equally. *Sugar has no effect until it is transformed to acetic acid, but then the effect is the same as when the acid is applied directly* [111]. A similar result was obtained by Paolo Mantegazza in 1864, then working in Pavia. He placed teeth into solutions of sugar; traces of calcium were found in these solutions only after it had become acid in reaction [112].

With his characteristic meticulousness Magitot of Paris repeated these acid experiments and published the results in 1867. He placed

107 Linderer (a) pp. 189 f.
108 Linderer (b) pp. 85 f.
109 Robertson pp. 37 f.; vita see Cohen (b)
110 Tomes (b); (c) pp. 353 f.
111 Cf. Harris p. 299
112 Mantegazza

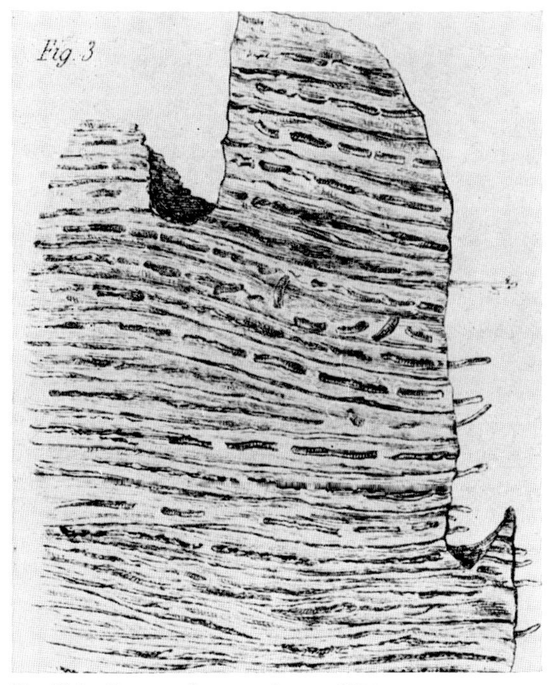

Fig. 514 *Tomes: Carious dentin, 1856*

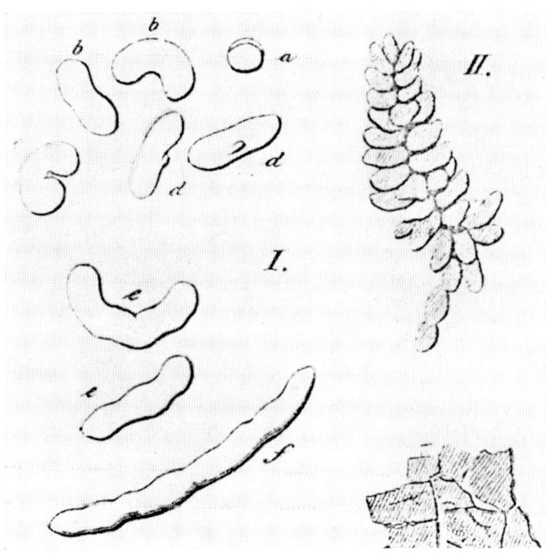

Fig. 516 *Ficinus: "Denticola" (I), 1847*

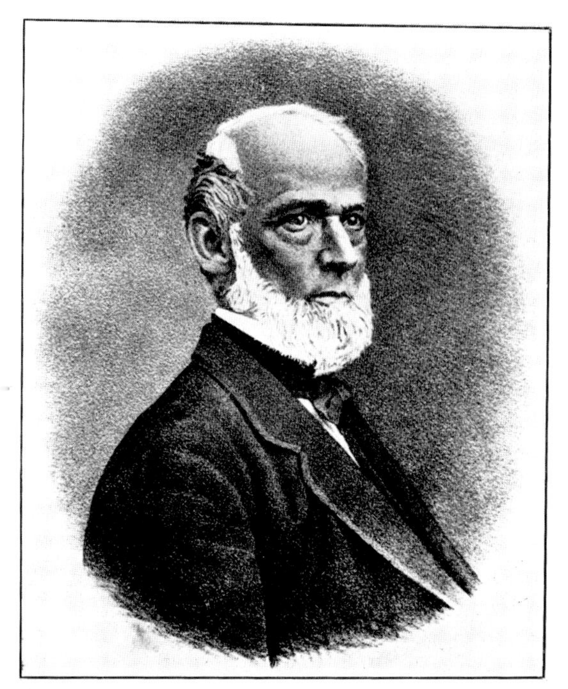

Fig. 515 *Amos Westcott*

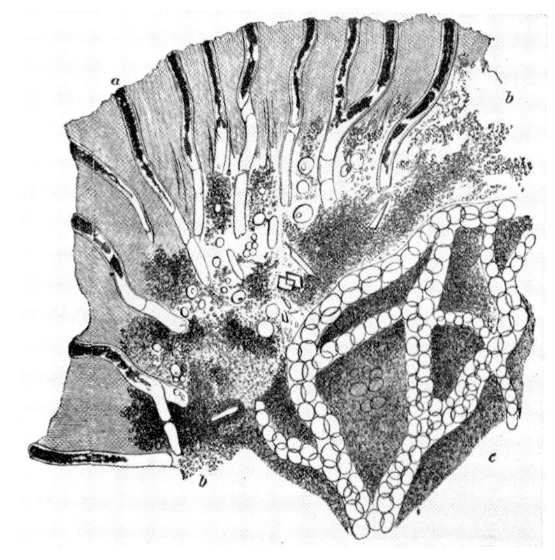

Fig. 517 *Klencke: "Centrale Zahnverderbnis" (Central tooth corruption), allegedly caries arising from the pulp, 1850*

teeth which had been protected on some surfaces with wax into a sugar solution for two years, and then found a softening at the unprotected areas [113]. He believed, properly, that caries was a complex process but in principle adopted the chemical theory [114]. The surest protection against caries was, he believed, an intact enamel cuticle. He was the first to describe the formation of secondary dentin by the pulp [115].

Carl Wedl of Vienna was also an adherent of the chemical theory (1870). He recognized caries as a process *which owes its existence to abnormal secretions of the gingiva, then of the remaining oral mucosa and the salivary glands* [116].

The parasitic theory, of which, strictly speaking, the ancient toothworm belief is a part, was taken up again by Michael Erdl, the Munich anatomist. He perceived the carious substance in 1843 as a parasitic vegetable which he tried to kill with a mixture of creosote and saltpeter (potassium nitrate), a rather impractical proposal for treatment [117].

Two further physicians and adherents to this theory, Ficinus and Klencke, met through a competition intended to clarify the causes of caries in 1844. The event was sponsored by the "Deutscher Verein für Heilwissenschaft zu Berlin" (German Society for Healing Science of Berlin). Robert Ficinus, a general physician in Dresden, proposed the name "Denticola" in 1847 for the "Animalcula" discovered by Leeuwenhoek (Fig. 516). Initial caries, he believed, was the brown deposit of such *tooth animals and decomposed organic matter* on the enamel cuticle, i.e., that which we call dental plaque today. This material decomposes, and the decay thus transfers to the enamel. *Without transfer of the decay process from the enamel cuticle, incidentally, neither the enamel or the dentin substance is affected by caries* [118]. He found masses of infusoria in decomposed dentin. Acids and sugar were strictly rejected as causative agents.

The winning prize essay about "Die Verderbnis der Zähne" (The corruption of teeth) by Hermann Klencke of Hannover, physician, professor, man of letters and prolific author, was published in 1850. In this work, marked by several errors, we are presented with a *central tooth corruption*, i.e., caries that arises in the inflamed pulp (Fig. 517). Klencke (like Ficinus) ascribed peripheral caries to the enamel cuticle as a matrix: *This enamel cuticle is the matrix on which Caries humida of the tooth germinates,* (it) *begins with cell deformation and then gives the tooth the brownish color which precedes caries* [119]. This cariogenic cell is Protococcus dentalis, which acts destructively in a manner similar to that of dry rot. Even the old fairy tale of worms and fumigation was built into his hypothesis [120]. He also found the "Denticola" of Ficinus and made this and other infusoria responsible for the third, the putrid, form of caries. The chronic form, caries sicca, was described as a *disintegration process* caused by lactic acid formed in the oral cavity. Here, finally, we find Klencke on the right track.

We read in the booklet of 1867 "Dental Caries and its Causes" by Theodor Leber and Jean Baptist Rottenstein, two Berlin physicians, about the first attempts to coordinate the chemical theory with the parasitic one. They too found, on the basis of their microscopic and chemical experiments, that the acids formed in the mouth initiated caries. Into this initial caries, however, they believed that the Leptothrix fungus (Leptotrichia today), now known as harmless and involved in calculus formation moves in and *produces by their extension, especially in the dentine, an effect of softening and destruction much more rapid than the action of acids alone is able to accomplish* [121]. The paper was widely distributed: after the Berlin edition it appeared in 1868 and in 1878 in Paris, in 1873 in Philadelphia, and in 1878 in London in appropriate translations.

Quite differently these two theories were combined as the "chemo-parasitic theory", not quite renounced today, by Miller. Willoughby Dayton Miller came from a North American farmer family whose founder, his great-grandfather, had been an immigrant from Germany. Born on August 1, 1853 on his father's farm near Alexandria, Ohio, he grew up on the farm, went to school in Newark, and studied mathematics and physics from 1871 to 1875 at the University of Michigan in Ann Arbor, from

113 Magitot (b) pp. 107 f.
114 Ibid. (b) p. 135
115 Ibid. (b) pp. 141 f.
116 Wedl pp. 343 f.
117 Erdl
118 Ficinus p. 31
119 Klencke p. 47
120 Ibid. p. 61
121 Leber and Rottenstein p. 98

which he graduated with a B. A. with honors. To round out his education, he took himself to Edinburgh, where he was stranded as a result of the failure of his bank. He managed to survive by tutoring, but proceeded in tenacious pursuit of his scientific goals to Berlin in the same year, 1876, and here audited especially the lectures of Hermann von Helmholtz, the physician and physicist. Soon Miller had reached the end of his financial—and thus his physical—means. In search of help, he sought out his countryman, Francis Peabody Abbot[122], who had been practicing dentistry in Berlin since 1851. Abbot recognized the character of this man at first glimpse and took him under his wing by obtaining a translator's position for him and having him give instruction in natural science to his wife and daughter. The direct result of these lessons was the engagement of Miller to Miss Caroline Abbot, as a consequence of which Miller, the natural scientist, decided to study dentistry.

With the support of his future father-in-law, Miller began to study at the Pennsylvania Dental College in 1877, and returned to Berlin in the Spring of 1879 as a graduated Doctor of Dental Surgery, having won the prize for the best essays on "The Conservative Treatment of the Dental Pulp." In Berlin he became the assistant and the son-in-law of Dr. Abbot, continuing nevertheless to audit lectures in medicine and natural sciences at the University. On August 30, 1880, Miller appeared in public for the first time at the annual meeting of the "American Dental Society of Europe" in Lucerne with a presentation entitled "Chemical versus Electrical Theory of Caries." This work, based on experiments and the first of 164 contributions to be published by 1907, refuted the "electrical theory" proposed in 1863 by William Kencely Bridgman and extended in 1879 by the American, Henry Seymour Chase, who saw caries as an electrolytic process[123]. Bridgman's was the "Prize Essay on the Pathology of Dental Caries" of the Odontological Society in London.

Already in the following year, Miller attracted attention with a study of "The Effect of Micro-organisms on Caries of the Human Teeth," an excursion into the still unstudied subject of the microflora of the oral cavity. Thorough studies in the school of Robert Koch, the pathfinder of microbiology who had been working in Berlin since 1880, preceded the attention given by Miller to his topic. His experiments were done with rare skill and tenacious persistence, frequently extending over periods of years. It is Miller's unquestioned merit that he introduced precise investigative methods of natural science to dental research.

Further publications, including some from other areas of dentistry, followed, some in German, others in British, and still others in American journals, so that the attention of Prussian authorities were directed to Miller when in the fall of 1884 it was necessary to find a lecturer for the University Dental Institute to be opened in Berlin. Initially he was attached to the chief of the department of conservative dentistry as assistant department head; in 1892 the department came under his direction (Fig. 518).

Above all, Miller's name had become known to the entire profession through the publication of "The Micro-Organisms of the Human Mouth," a summarization of the results of his bacteriological investigations published in German in 1889 and in English in 1890. The book was published with the sub-title "The Local and General Diseases which are Caused by them." There followed in 1896 the "Lehrbuch der konservierenden Zahnheilkunde" (Textbook of Conservative Dentistry), and now Miller the practicing dentist came to the foreground, to present his rich experience in restorative dentistry but also to present here the results of experimental investigations into the methods described and to provide support for the materials recommended.

Thus, Miller soon was recognized internationally as the leading personality in dentistry, but he also took a decisive role in the development of the profession in Germany. The membership of the "Central-Verein deutscher Zahnärzte" tripled in the six years of his leadership, and we are told that he had written for it 1300 letters in a single year. He was presiding officer of the Docent's Association and of the

[122] Varying information is available about the year of Abbot's settling in Berlin, ranging from 1851 to 1854. The Prussian diplomat Kurd von Schlözer wrote in his "Jugendbriefe" of January 23, 1852: "For some months an American dentist has been here (in Berlin), Mr. Abbot, who understands the filling of teeth like no German dentist! He takes out the nerve and then fills, not like the German dentists with lead and other things, but rather with pure gold. . . Removal of the nerve costs 7 Taler, simple filling 4 Taler for the tooth. Despite the bad times, I have decided to undertake this expense." Abbot is the inventor of the combined gold and tinfoil restoration.

[123] Miller (a); Bridgmann; Chase

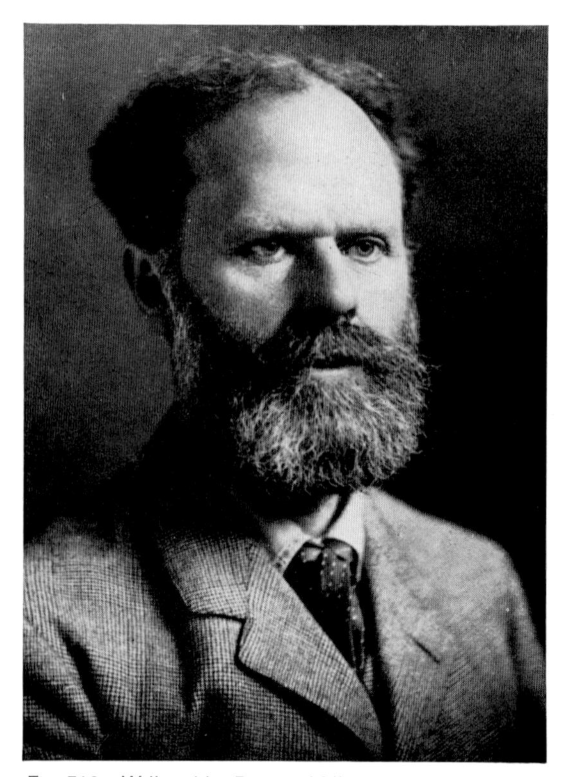

Fig. 518 *Willoughby Dayton Miller*

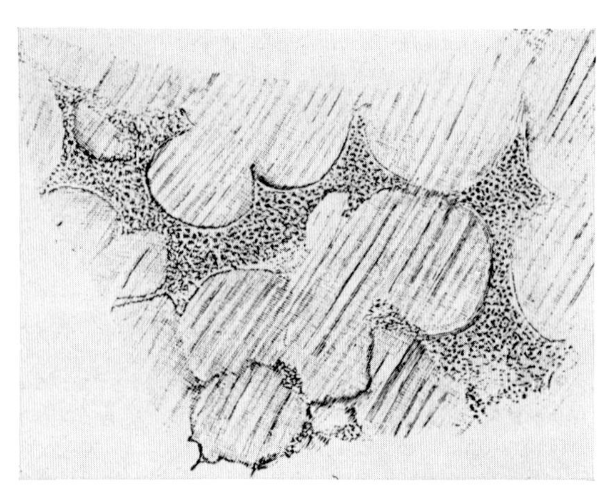

Fig. 520 *Miller: "Interglobular spaces filled with micrococci"*

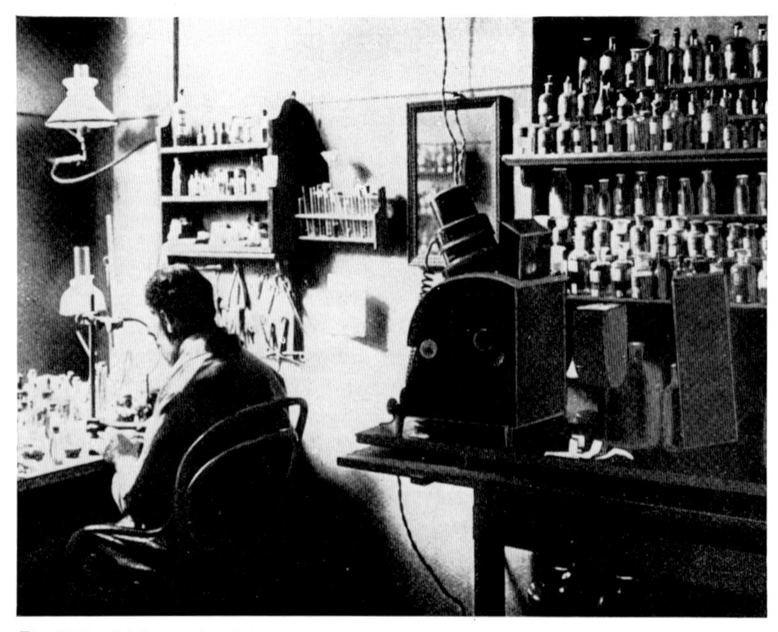

Fig. 519 *Miller in his laboratory*

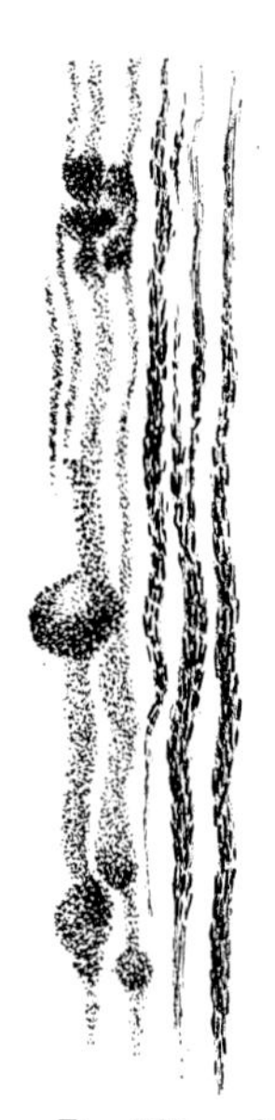

Fig. 521 *Miller: "Decayed dentine showing a mixed infection with cocci and bacilli"*

fund to support German Dentists. He organized continuing education of his Prussian colleagues and was named honorary member of 39 professional societies; he was awarded honorary doctorates by numerous universities. In 1904 he became president of the Fédération Dentaire Internationale, founded in Paris by Charles Godon in 1900, and was elected, unanimously, president of the Vth International Dental Congress, which was to be held in Berlin in 1909.

Despite all his success, Miller remained personally a modest man, a benevolent and patient leader for his colleagues. He was the central personality in Berlin's American colony and served as treasurer of its church. He never forgot his own time of need and *not infrequently visited attics to see the poverty and need for himself*[124]. He found harmonious balance and peaceful happiness in his marriage, blessed with three children, but also found time to defend his title as German champion on the grounds of the Berlin Golfklub.

His working conditions, however, in the dilapidated Dental Institute of the University of Berlin were unsurpassed for wretchedness. The clinic area was constantly crowded and students were prohibited from applause in the lecture hall because of the danger of collapse. Miller's research space, a laboratory of about 30 square feet, became a topic of discussion in the Prussian Landtag (legislature)—without success (Fig. 519)[125]. In recognition of these conditions, well equipped American universities had for years made various efforts to bring their countryman back to his native land and it is understandable that Miller accepted the call from the University of Michigan at Ann Arbor in 1906, the site of his first education in science.

Now the authorities tried everything to retain the great man in Berlin. His family and his friends from the American Club, however, pressed him to accept the call and to be able to represent his profession without worries about budget and other restrictions imposed by Prussian bureaucracy. Miller was greatly troubled with this decision, and it was made difficult for him. Finally, in October 1906, he resigned from his official positions; his resignation was accepted while he was designated a Medical Privy Counselor. Still he delayed his departure; on May 8, 1907, he gave the keynote lecture at the meeting of the Central-Verein in Hamburg. A few days before he left Berlin, he accepted the charter of a Miller Foundation from the hands of organized German dentistry; the foundation continues today to honor scientific efforts of dental students.

Miller left Germany during the first days of June, after twenty years of activity of seminal importance for dental science. He was received with enthusiasm by his American colleagues. Before beginning his work in Ann Arbor, he went to visit his sister on the home farm near Alexandria. A tragic fate destined him to become ill here of appendicitis, to which he succumbed on July 27, 1907 after an appendectomy performed in the Newark, Ohio, hospital.

Miller had taken up the problem of the microbiology of the oral cavity with the thoroughness of a biological researcher. He had grown pure cultures of the fungi found in the normal and in pathological milieus, and had studied their effects on carbohydrates, fatty acids, etc. in numerous series of experiments. In the first publication of his results in 1883, he formulated a new contention: *I am not an advocate of the pure acid theory of caries nor of the pure germ theory; I believe rather that both acids and fungi are concerned in producing caries, that the tendency of late has been to underestimate the former and over-estimate the latter, and that both together cannot furnish a satisfactory solution of all cases of caries*[126] (Figs. 520 and 521). Following further investigation and consideration of all the requirements, he offered the following valid definition in 1889: *Dental decay is a chemico-parasitical process consisting of two distinctly marked stages: decalcification, or softening of the tissue, and a dissolution of the softened residue. In the case of enamel, however, the second stage is practically wanting, the decalcification of the enamel practically signifying its total destruction.* This second stage, the dissolution of decalcified dentin, proceeds by *the bacterium-ferment, as albumen by the pepsine of the gastric juice*[127]. Thus we have here the same classification in two stages taken by Linderer 50 years earlier through microscopic studies[128].

Miller's chemico-parasitic theory remains unshaken today, although it is not necessarily

124 Dieck (Wilhelm Dieck was Miller's chief assistant and became his successor at the University of Berlin in 1907)
125 Hoffmann-Axthelm pp. 43 f.
126 Miller (b)
127 Miller (c) p. 163; (d) p. 205
128 See pp. 401 f.

the definitive solution of this complex process. The theory has been expanded and supplemented with other theories, but no one has been able to refute it. We can agree with him less when, entirely the prisoner of the bacteriological era, he proposes the chemical desinfection of the oral cavity as a prophylactic measure. *Under all conditions, however, the chief thing is the thorough mechanical cleansing of the teeth* [129]. Because of this position, too, he showed little understanding for Röse's stimulus of caries prevention through nutrition [129].

Miller's life-work has found acceptance throughout the world. As its highest honor for scientific achievement, the Federation Dentaire Internationale awards the International Miller Prize, founded in 1908, at five-year intervals. A memorial statue was erected to Miller in 1915, today placed in the courtyard of Postle Hall in the Ohio State University College of Dentistry, side by side the bust of John R. Callahan. In 1912, the new building of the Berlin Dental Institute included a window with his likeness; unfortunately it was destroyed in 1945. More importantly, however, wherever in the world caries is discussed at present, Miller's theories remain the starting point and doubtless will continue to do so for a long time.

Dental Education

As in so many other things, the United States was the site of ground-laying efforts for dental education in institutions especially intended for the purpose. This fact may be attributed to the joint efforts of two dentists working in Baltimore, Hayden and Harris, the first of whom took the lead scientifically while Harris provided the driving organizational strength.

Horace H. Hayden (Fig. 522), born October 13, 1769 on the farm of his ancestors in Connecticut, was at first active in the profession of his father, architecture, and in his hobby, geology, but was not entirely satisfied with either. Thus he turned to dentistry in 1793. In New York as a patient of John Greenwood, he studied in his library (of which we know that it contained a copy of Hunter's work [130]) and then went to Baltimore in 1800, where he practiced with success. As a sideline, he studied anatomy and medicine, served in the war in 1814 against England, and soon became a teacher of his profession. He did research in the subject of glandular function, gaining high personal and scientific respect, and was invited in 1819 to teach dentistry at the University of Maryland, the first such invitation extended in the United States. He and Harris were unsuccessful in organizing a dental school there, however. As a consequence, they jointly founded the Baltimore College of Dental Surgery (Fig. 523) in 1839, the first such specialized institution in the world. Hayden was president until his death, always supported by the true organizational force, Harris, who was his successor in the presidency. Here in 1841, the title "Doctor of Dental Surgery" (D. D. S.) was awarded for the first time to two graduates. Hayden died three years later, on January 25, 1844, this *father of American Dental Science* having reached the age of 75 years, after a full life in Baltimore, the city of his long and effective efforts on behalf of his profession.

At the advanced age of 71, Hayden had founded the American Society of Dental Surgeons in New York in 1840, a group which, apart from a brief-lived local New York association founded in 1834, is the world's oldest dental society. Here, too, Harris bore the burden of work as secretary. The unfortunate position taken by this group in the amalgam war of 1843, a position rescinded in 1859, lowered its prestige to such an extent that it dissolved in 1856. The American Dental Association, founded thereafter in 1859, was maintained up to our days, only the period between 1897 and 1926 was characterized by problems and internal struggles. In 1926 48 regional associations of the separate states joined in this national organization.

Chapin Aaron Harris (Fig. 524), born May 6, 1806 in New York State, at first studied medicine but turned to dentistry in 1827, probably under the influence of his brother, Dr. John Harris, who, a physician, had been providing would-be dentists medical and odontological fundamentals in Bainbridge, Ohio since 1825. Harris was educated by his brother in dentistry [131]. He worked successfully at numerous places, studied the writings of Hunter, Fox and Delabarre intensively, and finally settled in Baltimore in 1835. His first book, entitled "The Dental Art, a Practical Treatise on Dental Surgery," was published in 1839. It was en-

[129] Miller (c) p. 109; (d) p. 237; (f) pp. 294 f. See p. 320
[130] See p. 258
[131] Mills.—John Allen and James Taylor were among the students of John Harris.

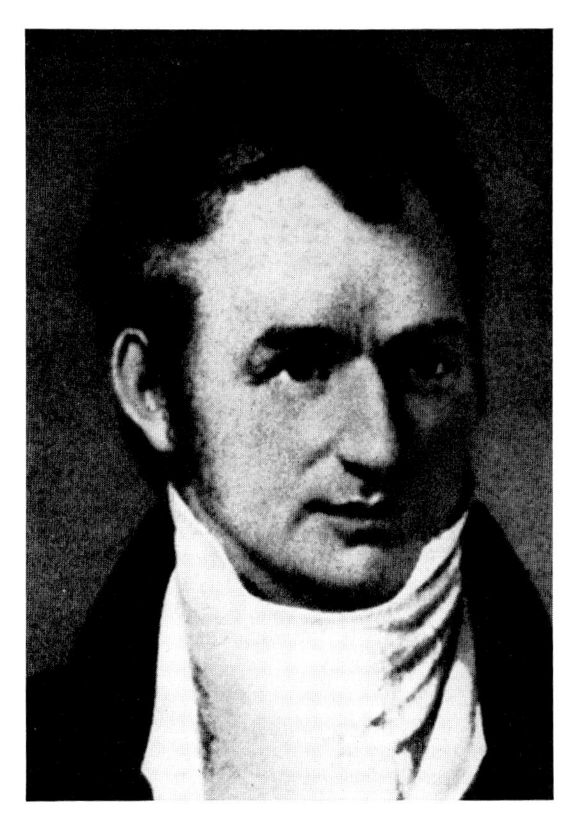

Fig. 522 *Horace H. Hayden*

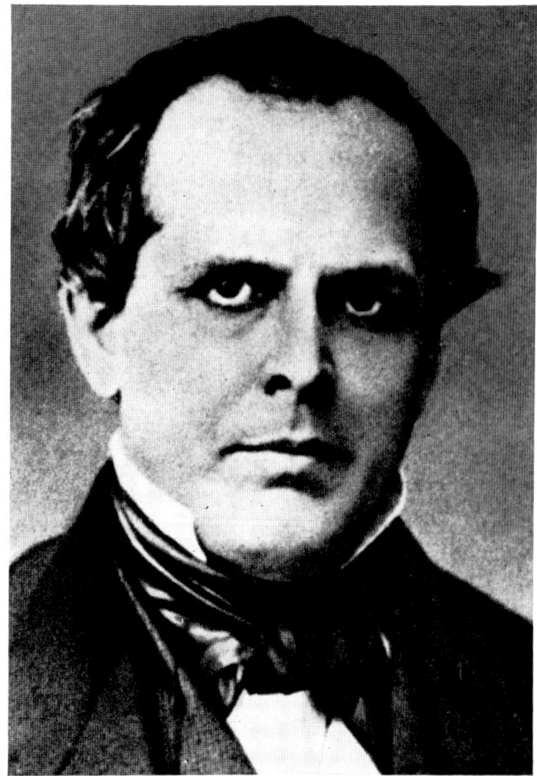

Fig. 524 *Chapin Aaron Harris*

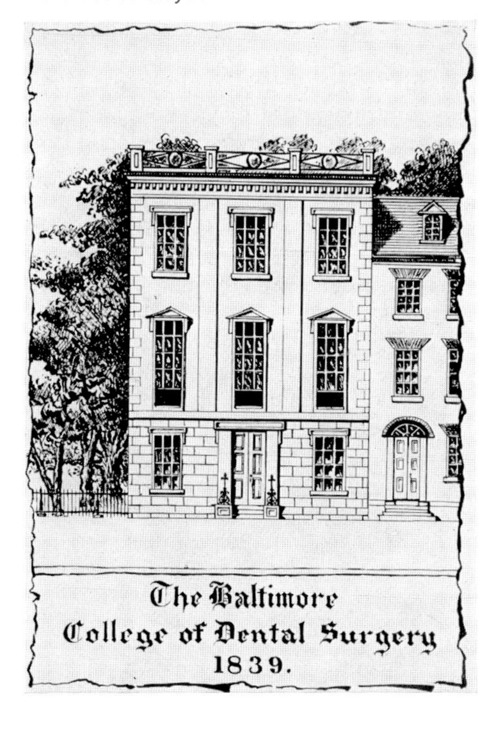

Figure 523

larged to twice the original size and published again in 1845 as "The Principles and Practice of Dental Surgery." One new edition followed another until 1899, with many translations, so that it became one of the most popular text-books ever. He published numerous other works dealing with the entire field, but also translations of the works of the French dentists Duval, Delabarre, Lefoulon and Désirabode. In 1839, together with the prominent New York dentist Eleazar Parmly (see Fig. 312), he founded *The American Journal of Dental Science,* which was taken over in the following year by the newly organized American Society of Dental Surgeons and jointly edited with Solyman Brown, Amos Westcott, and others until Harris' death.

This dynamic personality exhausted himself in the service of his profession. Harris died at the age of 55 on September 29, 1860, leaving his family destitute. A collection taken up by American dentistry came to $85 after deduction of expenses; his widow rejected this *beggarly gift* and she died in indigent circumstances [132].

Another student of John Harris and friend of Chapin, James Taylor founded the "Ohio College of Dental Surgery" in 1845 as the second educational institution of its kind in the world. In 1852 the New York College followed in Syracuse, with Amos Westcott as the founder (see Fig. 515) and approximately at the same time the Philadelphia College was organized. Soon similar new institutions turned up almost every year, good ones and bad ones, until the founding of the National Association of Dental Faculties in 1884 brought gradually an element of order into the educational system of the nation [133].

Complete independence had been attained in dental education in the United States in these important years of 1839 and 1840, a status which was largely to be continued even though there was a gradual contact with universities. The start in this direction was made in 1867 with the Dental School of Harvard University; by the turn of the century, *32 of the 52 schools which were members of the National Association of Dental Faculties were, in fact, departments of universities or of medical schools* [134].

In Europe in the second half of the century a certain reflux to general medicine came about. As late as 1845, Jena's Professor Heinrich Haeser, after listing the most important dentists from Fauchard to Carabelli, wrote in his "Geschichte der Medizin" (History of medicine) that these men had caused the surgical component of dentistry to be elevated to a high level of education: *Nonetheless, this specialty is still too much neglected by the physicians and in consequence finds itself in the hands of the semi-educated, whose appearance too often recalls that of market-criers of earlier centuries* [135]. In the same year, for example, there were not more than 96 dentists in the Kingdom of Prussia, of whom 37 were in Berlin alone [136].

The first independent educational institution in Germany was founded by Eduard Albrecht (Fig. 525), a physician and son of a dentist, induced thereto by the famous ophthalmologist Albrecht von Graefe. He opened the school as the "Öffentliche Klinik für Mundkrankheiten" (Public clinic for oral diseases) in Graefe's private clinic in Berlin in 1855. Attendance there was made obligatory for students of dentistry by the Prussian minister of culture in 1866. From 1868, it received subventions from the state and it was absorbed into the medical faculty as the "Zahnärztliches Universitätsinstitut" (University Dental Institute; Fig. 526) in 1884, a year after the tragic death of Albrecht, who died of an infection through his work shortly before attainment of his life's goal [137].

The first specialized lectures in London were held approximately by the Surgeon-Dentist to the King, William Rae, a pupil of John Hunter, in 1872. Rae's manuscripts were published for of their historical interest in 1859 at the request of John Tomes in the first volume of the *British Journal of Dental Science,* predecessor of today's still flourishing *British Dental Journal* [138]. Rae's student, Joseph Fox, continued the line of lecturers in dentistry in Guy's Hospital of London; he was followed in turn by Thomas Bell. In 1858, through the initiative of the Odontological Society, the "Dental Hospital of London" (Fig. 527) opened its doors, in the following year to devote itself to education as the "London School of Dentistry." In 1859 the "Metropolitan School of Dental

132 Thorpe pp. 66 f.
133 Miller (e)
134 Miller (e)
135 Haeser pp. 769 f.
136 Schmedicke
137 Hoffmann-Axthelm pp. 12 f.
138 Rae

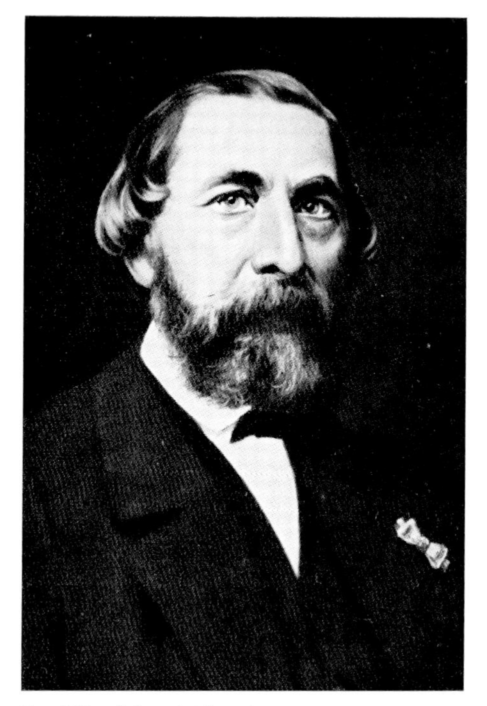

Fig. 525 *Eduard Albrecht*

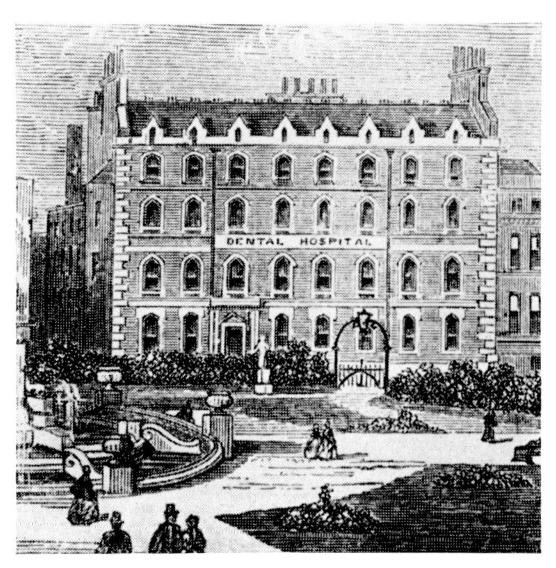

Fig. 527 *Dental Hospital of London, in Soho Square, 1858*

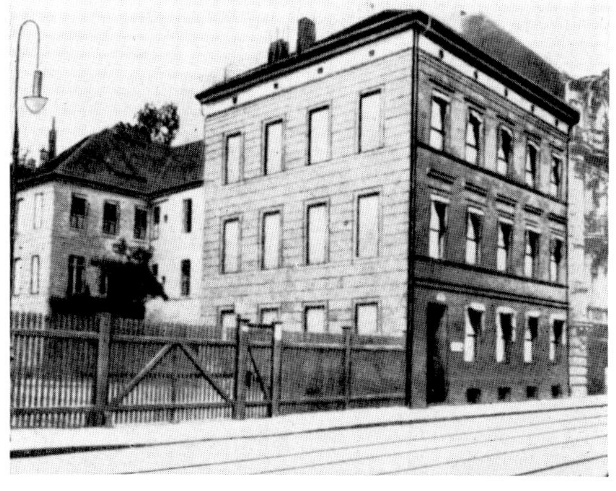

Fig. 526 *University Dental Institute in Berlin, 1884*

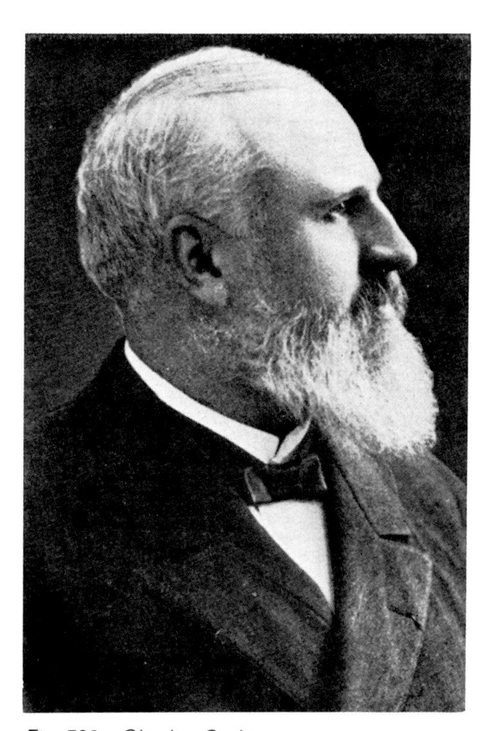

Fig. 528 *Charles Godon*

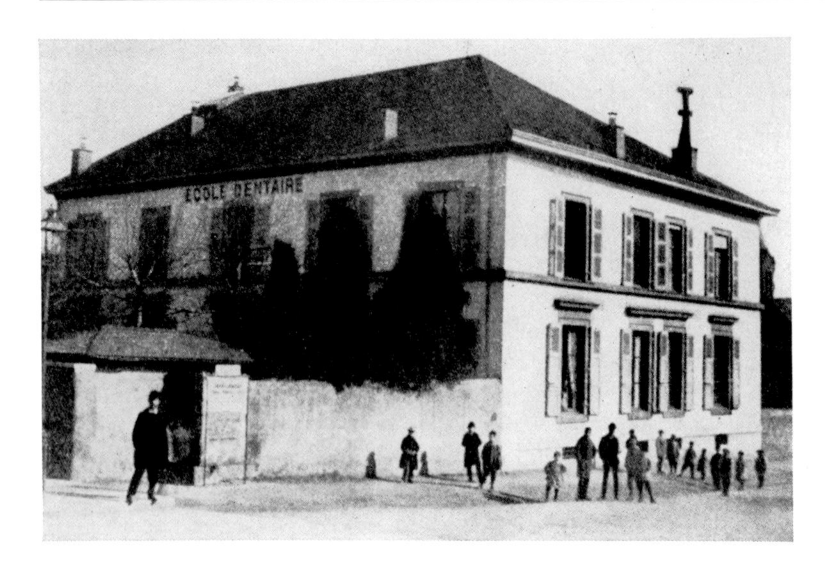

Fig. 529 *École dentaire, Geneva, 1881*

Science" opened as a kind of competing association, but it lasted only until 1863.
Activity in Paris began relatively late. Here an "Ecole dentaire" privately sponsored by the "dentistes" was opened under the leadership of Charles Godon (Fig. 528) in 1880. An "Institut odontotechnique de France" followed for reasons similar to those in London in 1884 and another "Ecole dentaire pratique" in 1892. The latter joined with the first of these institutions four years later. Both schools, whose examinations for "Chirugien-Dentiste" achieved state recognition in 1892, continue to exist up to the present day[139]. The first educational institution within the framework of the medical faculty specially intended for the education of stomatologists in the sense proposed by Magitot was founded in Paris in 1909 as the "Institut de Stomatologie de la Faculté de Médecine."
The "Ecole dentaire de Genève" was founded in 1881 in Geneva as the first state institution of the world. Operative dentistry was represented by the previously noted Camille Redard[140] (Fig. 529). In 1888 Göteborg followed, with Victor Bensow and Hjalmar Carlson as initiators[141], as did Copenhagen and, as noted above, Vienna with Julius Scheff in 1890[142].
Up to our own times dental education has existed as either of two extremes: the American type of dental college completely independent of the medical faculty, and the specialized training following completion of the medical curriculum as proposed initially by Heider in Vienna and Magitot in Paris, and in the extreme demonstrated by exclusion of dentists from a meeting of "stomatologists" by Arkövy in Budapest in 1909[143], who was not a student but a spiritual adherent of Magitot in each relation. This practice continues to be followed in certain successor states of the Danubian monarchy with the inevitable result that these nations have a large contingent of persons who was founded in Paris in 1909 as the "Institut de education.
Similar conditions exist in the Soviet Union, in which nowadays two separate groups of persons are active: the physician specialists in stomatology who are trained in oral and maxillofacial surgery as well as dentistry during their five-year professional curriculum, and the dentists of so-called "mid-level medical personnel" who have three years of practical training[144]. These conditions exist, it should be noted, only since the October Revolution of 1917. Before that time, training in the *healing art of dentistry* was provided by apprenticeship appoint-

139 Godon pp. 139 f.
140 Levay. See p. 338
141 Löfgren
142 Lesky. See p. 399
143 Trebitsch; Huszár. See pp. 315 and 346
144 Müller-Dietz. The author thanks the director of the Section of medicine of the Osteuropa Institut at the Free University of Berlin, Prof. Dr. Heinz Müller-Dietz, for the friendly advice and for the translation of Russian texts.

ments and in private dental institutions, of which the first was founded in 1881 by the dentist Fom Ignatjevič Važinskij in Petersburg [145]. Despite the unflagging efforts of the Petersburg physician Alexander Karlovič Limberg, previously a dentist, it was impossible to establish a dental training program on a university-level in czarist Russia because of the disapproval of official agencies and the disinterest of medical faculties [146].
A middle course is generally followed in the rest of Europe: education in special institutions integrated with the medical faculty. Only most recently have there been movements in the direction of formation of separate faculties, so that it appears that here, too, there will be an approach of the organizational forms.
Each of these systems has advantages and disadvantages which have largely become balanced. While the training of the North American dentist was characterized at first by the purely mechanical aspects, his European-trained colleague had better education in the medical sciences than in techniques. This afforded American dentists a certain degree of practical superiority until approximately the turn of the century. Today the scientific training provided by the American dental colleges does not take second place in any way to the European schools, while the latter have directed increased attention to manual skills in the twentieth century. The goal of preparing a scientifically and technically trained dentist able to meet all the demands expected of him, a *dentiste habile et experimenté (skillfull and experienced),* as he was called by Fauchard in 1728, has been reached through sometimes serious differences of opinions and in a variety of ways.
This achievement has assured the position of dentistry within medicine. In the future, too, the position may be changed by mutual give and take as we experience today, for example, in the specialty of maxillofacial surgery and in materials science. Together the dentists of the entire world today build on those foundations developed over the millenia and strengthened by events within the young profession in the 19th and 20th centuries in the cultures of Europe and North America.

[145] Michalowski; for professional designations in the USSR, see p. 244
[146] Kowarski pp. 16 f.; Bassalyk

References

Albrecht, Eduard
Klinik der Mundkrankheiten. Berlin 1862

Bassalyk, A.
Zur Geschichte der zahnärztlichen Ausbildung im vorrevolutionären Rußland. Transl. from "Stomatologija" 1 (1961) 82 f. by Dieter Nünchert in: Zahnärztl. Mitt. 52 (1962) 1199—1201

Baume, Louis J(ean)
The biology of pulp and dentine. Basel, etc. 1980

Baume, Robert
a) Zahnmißbildungen. I. Ein Zahn im Zahne. Dtsch. Vjschr. Zahnk. 14 (1874) 25—29. Engl. transl. in: Monthly Rev. Dent. Surg. 2 (1874) 399 f.
b) Bemerkungen über die Entwicklungen und den Bau des Säugetierzahnes. Dtsch. Vjschr. Zahnhk. 15 (1875) 125—142, 265—285
c) Lehrbuch der Zahnheilkunde. Leipzig 1877
d) Versuch einer Entwicklungsgeschichte des Gebisses. Odontolog. Forschungen I, 1882

Bell, Thomas
The anatomy, physiology and diseases of the teeth. London 1829

Bernstein, Johann Gottlob
Prakt. Handbuch für Wundärzte und Geburtshelfer. Part II, 2nd ed. Leipzig 1790

Blake, Robert
a) An essay on the structure and formation of the teeth in man and various animals. (Med. Diss. Edinburgh 1798). Dublin 1801
b) Idem. Americ. rev. ed. Cyreneus O. Cone, Baltimore 1848

Blandin, Ph(ilippe) F(rédéric)
Anatomie du système dentaire. Paris 1836

Boyde, A(lan)
The history of 'enamel fibres'. Brit. Dent. J. 121 (1966) 85—89

Bridgman, W(illiam) K(encely)
The prize essay on the pathology of dental caries. Trans. Odont. Soc. G. B. 3 (1861—63) 369—425

Busch, (Friedrich)
Über Verschmelzung und Verwachsung der Zähne. Dtsch. Mschr. Zahnhk. 15 (1897) 469—486

Carabelli, Georg von
Systematisches Handbuch der Zahnheilkunde. Vol. I (Geschichtl. Übersicht der Zahnheilkunde) (2nd ed.) Wien 1844. Vol. II (Anatomie des Mundes) Wien 1842. Kupfertafeln (copper engravings) zu v. Carabelli's Anatomie des Mundes. Wien 1842

Chase, Henry S(eymour)
Oral electricity. Dent. Cosmos 21 (1879) 205—207

Cohen, R. A.
a) The development of dental histology in Britain. Brit. Dent. J. 121 (1966) 59—71
b) William Robertson of Birmingham. Brit. Dent. J. 142 (1977) 64—69, 99—102

Cope, Zachary
Sir John Tomes. London 1961

Cuvier, G(eorge)
a) Leçons d'anatomie comparée. Vol. III, Paris 1805
b) Vorlesungen über vergl. Anatomie. Part III, transl. I. F. Meckel. Leipzig 1810

Czermák, Johann
Beiträge zur mikroskop. Anatomie der menschlichen Zähne. Med. Diss. Würzburg 1850

Dieck, W(ilhelm)
W. D. Miller. Korresp. bl. Zahnärzte 37 (1908) 1—23

Duval, Jacques René
Recherches historiques sur l'art du dentiste chez les anciens. Paris 1808

Ebner, Victor von
a) Strittige Fragen über den Bau des Zahnschmelzes. Sitzg.-Ber. K. Akad. Wiss. Wiener Math.-Naturw. Kl., III 99 (1890) 57—104
b) A. Koelliker's Handbuch der Gewebelehre. Vol. III, Leipzig 1902
c) Histologie der Zähne mit Einschluß der Histogenese. Scheff's Handbuch der Zahnhk., 3rd ed., vol. I., Wien, Leipzig 1909
d) Über scheinbare und wirkliche Radiärfasern des Zahnbeines. Anat. Anz. 34 (1909) 289—309

Erdl, Michael
Chemische Analyse der Cariesmaterie der menschlichen Zähne. Allg. Ztg. Chir. 4 (1843) 159—160

Eustachius, Bartholomaeus
Libellus de dentibus. Venetiis 1563

Ficinus, Robert
Über das Ausfallen der Zähne und das Wesen der Zahnkaries. J. Chir. Augenhk., Berlin 6 (1847) 1—43

Fox, Joseph
The history and treatment of the diseases of the teeth, . . . London 1806

Fraenkel, Meyerus
De penitiori dentium humanorum structura observationes. Diss. anat.-physiol. Vratislaviae 1835

Gallette, J(ean) Fr(ançois)
a) Einige Betrachtungen über den Schmelz der Zähne. . ., Mainz 1824
b) Abgeforderter Beweis, daß der Titular-Professor Dr. Ringelmann zu Würzburg ein Plagiarius sei. Mainz 1828

Godon, Charles
L'école dentaire. Paris 1901

Gottlieb, Bernhard
Der Epithelansatz am Zahne. Dtsch. Mschr. Zahnhk. 39 (1921) 142—147

Guttmann, Curt
Ein Pionier der wissenschaftlichen Zahnheilkunde. Zahnärztl. Mitt. 53 (1963) 861—865

Gysi, A(lfred); C(arl) Röse
Sammlung von Mikrophotographien zur Veranschaulichung der mikroskopischen Struktur der Zähne des Menschen. Zürich 1894

Haderup, V(iktor)
Vorschlag zu einer internationalen Bezeichnung der Zähne. Korresp. bl. Zahnärzte 16 (1887) 314—315

Haeser, H(einrich)
Lehrbuch der Geschichte der Medicin . . . Jena 1845

Hallet, G. E. M.
The incidence, nature, and clinical significance of palatal invaginations in the maxillary incisor teeth. Proc. roy. Soc. Med. 46 (1953) 491—499

Hannover, Adolph
Über die Entwicklung und den Bau des Säugethierzahns. Verh. Leopold. Carolin. Akad. Naturforscher 25/II (1855) 807—936. Engl. transl. in: Brit. J. Dent. Sc. 1 (1857) 324—325, 353—360, 382—384

Harris, Chapin A(aron)
The principles and practice of dental surgery. 5th ed., Philadelphia 1853

Heider, Moriz
Über die Verhältnisse der zahnärztlichen Bildung und Praxis in Österreich. Wien 1858

Heider, M(oriz), C(arl) Wedl
Atlas zur Pathologie der Zähne. 2nd ed., Leipzig, London, New York 1893

Helmcke, J(ohann)-G(erhard)
Bau und Struktur der Zahnhartsubstanzen. Dtsch. zahnärztl. Zschr. 15 (1960) 155—168

Hertwig, Oscar
Über Bau und Entwicklung der Placoidschuppen und Zähne der Selachier. Jena. Zschr. Naturw. 8 (NF 1) (1874) 330—402

Hoffmann-Axthelm, Walter
Vorgeschichte und Geschichte des Berliner Zahnärztlichen Universitäts-Institutes. Köln 1965

Hunter, John
A practical treatise on the diseases of the teeth. London 1778

Huszár, Gy(örgy)
The role of Hungarian dentists in the history of odontology. Int. Dent. J. 19 (1969) 502—510

Huxley, Thomas H(enry)
On the development of the teeth, and on the nature and import of Nasmyth's "Persistant Capsule". Quart. J. microsc. Sc. 1 (1853) 149—164

Kitchin, Paul C.
Dens in dente. Oral. Surg. Med. Path. 2 (1949) 1181—1193

Klencke, H(ermann)
Die Verderbnis der Zähne. Leipzig 1850

Koelliker, Albert
a) Handbuch der Gewebelehre des Menschen. Leipzig 1852
b) Manual of human histology. Transl. and ed. George Busk, Thomas Huxley, vol. II, London 1854

Korff, K(arl) von
Die Entwicklung der Zahnbeingrundsubstanz der Säugetiere. Arch. Mikrosk. Anat. 67 (1906) 1—17

Kowarski, M. O.
Die Zahnheilkunde in Rußland im 18. und 19. Jahrhundert. Greifswald 1933

Laforgue, L(ouis)
Die Zahnarzneikunst . . . Übers. C. F. Angermann, Leipzig 1803

Leber, Th(eodor), J(ean) B(aptist) Rottenstein
Dental caries and its causes. Transl. Thomas H. Chandler, Philadelphia 1873

Lenz, Hans
Elektronische Untersuchungen am Schmelzoberhäutchen. Dtsch. Zahnärztl. Zschr. 21 (1966) 1056—1062; 22 (1967) 1466—1482; J. dent. Res. 46 (1967) 1246—1247

Lesky, Erna
150 Jahre zahnärztlicher Unterricht in Wien. Österr. Ärzteztg. 26 (1971) 1015—1020

Levay, Etienne
Die "Ecole dentaire" in Genf. Österr.-Ung. Vjschr. Zahnhk. 1 (1885), Nr. 2, 71—72

Linderer, Joseph
a) Handbuch der Zahnheilkunde, . . . Berlin 1837 (with J. C. Linderer)
b) Handbuch der Zahnheilkunde. Vol. II, Berlin 1848
c) Die Zahnheilkunde nach ihrem neuesten Standpunkte. Erlangen 1851

Lintott, William
On the structure, economy and pathology of the human teeth. London 1841

Löfgren, Åke B.
Göteborgs Tandläkareinstitut. In: Göteborgs Tandläkare-Sällskaps, Årsbok 1967, pp. XLI—LX

Magitot, Emile
a) Etude sur le développement des dents humaines. Thèse méd. Paris 1857
b) Traité de la carie dentaire. Paris 1867
c) Traité des anomalies du système dentaire chez l'homme et les mammifères. Paris 1877

Mantegazza, Paolo
An experimental inquiry into the action of sugar and of certain acids upon the teeth. Brit. J. Dent. Sc. 7 (1864) 49—54

Michalowski, J.
Die ersten 5 Jahre des Bestehens der ersten russischen zahnärztlichen Schule. Korresp. bl. Zahnärzte 16 (1887) 261—265

Miller, W(illoughby) D(ayton)

a) Chemical versus the electrical theory of caries. Dent. Cosmos 23 (1881) 91—98

b) The agency of acids in the production of caries of the human teeth . . . Dent. Cosmos 25 (1883) 337—344

c) Die Mikroorganismen der Mundhöhle. Leipzig 1889

d) The micro-organisms of the human mouth. Philadelphia 1890

e) Das zahnärztliche Unterrichtswesen in Amerika. Dtsch. zahnärztl. Wschr. 4 (1900) 369—382

f) Lehrbuch der Conservirenden Zahnheilkunde. Leipzig 1896

g) Obituary. Dent. Cosmos 49 (1907) 1009—1014

Mills, Edward C.
Bainbridge, Ross County, Ohio, the cradle of dental education. J. Am. Dent. Ass. 19 (1932) 361—389

Mühlreiter, E(duard)
Anatomie des menschlichen Gebisses. Leipzig 1870

Müller, J(ohannes)
Über die Structur und die chemischen Eigenschaften der thierischen Bestandtheile der Knorpel und Knochen. Ann. Phys. Chem. (Poggendorf) 38 II (1836) 295—253

Müller-Dietz, H(einz)
Die zahnärztliche Versorgung in der Sowjetunion. Zahnärztl. Rdsch. 71 (1962) 345—347

Nasmyth, Alexander

a) Report on a paper on the cellular structure of the ivory, enamel, and pulp of the teeth, . . . London (1839) Reprint in Brit. Ass. Adv. Sc., Vol. 3

b) Researches on the development, structure, and diseases of the teeth. London 1849

Nedden, A(dolf) zur
Die Verderbnis der Zähne. Erlangen 1858

Owen, Richard
Odontography; or a treatise on the comparative anatomy of the teeth, . . . Vol. I, London 1840—1845

Parmly, L(evi) S(pear)
A practical guide to the management of the teeth, . . . Philadelphia 1819

Pickerill, H(enry) P(ercy)
The structure of the enamel. Dent. Cosmos 55 (1912) 959—988

Pindborg, Jens J.
Anders Adolf Retzius and Alexander Nasmyth: a Correspondence . . . J. Hist. Med. 17 (1962) 388—392

Preiswerk, Gustav
Beiträge zur Kenntnis der Schmelzstructur bei Säugethieren. Basel 1895

Rae, (William)
Lectures on the teeth. Brit. J. Dent. Sc. 1 (1857) 386—387, 429—430, 457—465

Raschkow, Isacus
Meletemata circa mammalium dentium evolutionem. Med. Diss. Vratislaviae (Breslau) 1835

Retzius, A(dolph)
Bemerkungen über den inneren Bau der Zähne, . . . (Müllers) Arch. Anat. Phys., Berlin (1837) 486—566

Ringelmann, K(arl) J(oseph)

a) Der Organismus des Mundes, besonders der Zähne, . . . Nürnberg 1824

b) Gedanken über die Pflege des Mundes, besonders der Zähne. 2nd ed., Nürnberg

Robertson, William
A practical treatise on the human teeth: . . . London 1835

R(ust, Johann Nepomuk)
Miscellen. (Rusts) Magazin für die ges. Heilkunde, Berlin 18 (1825) 186—187

Salter, James
Warty tooth. Trans. pathol. Soc., London 6 (1855) 173—177

Schmedicke, C(arl) W(ilhelm)
Statistische Notizen über die Zahl der Zahnärzte im Preußischen Staate. Der Zahnarzt, Berlin 1 (1846) 56—59

Schmid, Hans
Henry Percy Pickerill (1879—1956). Med. Diss. Zürich 1960

Schreger, (Bernhard Gottlob)
Beitrag zur Geschichte der Zähne. Beitr. Zergliederungskunst 1 (1800) 1—7

Schwann, Th(eodor)
Microscopische Untersuchungen über die Übereinstimmung in der Struktur und dem Wachstume der Thiere und Pflanzen. Berlin 1839 (Reprint Leipzig 1910)

Serres, A(ugustin)
Essai sur l'anatomie et la physiologie des dents, ou nouvelle théorie sur la dentition. Paris 1817

"Socrates" (pseudonym of Quincy)
Tooth within a tooth. Dent. Reg., Cincinnati 10 (1856) 355—356

Sömmering, S(amuel) Th(omas)
Vom Baue des menschlichen Körpers. Part I, Knochenlehre. Frankfurt am Main 1791; Vol. II, Leipzig 1839

Steinberger, (Philipp)
Nekrolog (Heider). Dtsch. Vjschr. Zahnhk. 6 (1866) 245—252

Thorpe, Burton Lee
History of dental surgery. Ed. Charles R. E. Koch. Vol. III, Chicago 1909

Tomes, John

a) On the structure of the dental tissues of marsupial animals, and more specially of the enamels. Phil. Trans. Roy. Soc. (1849) 403—412

b) On the presence of fibrils of soft tissue in dentinal tubes. Phil. Trans. Roy. Soc. (1856) 515—526

c) A system of dental surgery. Philadelphia 1859

Trebitsch, Hugo
Odontologen und Stomatologen. Zahnärztl. Rdsch. 18 (1909) 195—197, 231—232

Virchow, Rudolf
Über parenchymatöse Entzündung. Virchows Arch. path. Anat. 4 (1852) 261—324

Waldeyer, Wilhelm
Untersuchungen über die Entwicklung der Zähne.

a) 1. Abt. Königsberger med. Jahrbücher 4 (1864) 236—299

b) 2. Abt. Zschr. ration. Med. 3/24 (1865) 169—212

Walkhoff, Otto

a) Mikrophotographischer Atlas der normalen Histologie menschlicher Zähne. Stuttgart 1894

b) Mikrophot. Atlas der patholog. Histologie menschl. Zähne. Stuttgart 1897

c) Beiträge zum feineren Bau des Schmelzes und zur Entwicklung des Zahnbeins. Phil. Diss. Erlangen 1897; idem. in: Dtsch. Mschr. Zahnhk. 16 (1898) 1—16, 64—79, 119—133

Wedl, C(arl)
Pathologie der Zähne . . . Leipzig 1870

Zsigmondy, Adolph
Grundzüge einer praktischen Methode zur . . . Vormerkung . . . Dtsch. Vjschr. Zahnhk. 1 (1861) 209—211

General Works of Reference and Bibliographies

Asbell, Milton B.
A bibliography of dentistry in America 1790—1840. New Jersey 1973

Biographisches Lexikon der hervorr. Ärzte, see Hirsch et al.

Boissier, Raymond
L'évolution de l'art dentaire. Paris 1927

Bremner, M. D. K.
The story of dentistry. Rev. 3rd ed., Brooklyn, London 1964

Burgess, Renate
Portraits of doctors and scientists in the Wellcome Institut of the history of medicine. London 1973

Callisen, Adolph Carl Peter
Medicinisches Schriftsteller-Lexicon der jetzt lebenden Ärzte . . . Vols. I—XXXIII, Copenhagen 1830—1845

Campbell, J(ohn) Menzies
Dentistry then and now. Glasgow 1963

Cecconi, L. J.
Notes et mémoires pour servir à l'histoire dentaire . . . Paris 1959

Crowley, C. Geo.
Dental Bibliography: . . . Philadelphia 1885

Dagen, Georges
Documents pour servir à l'histoire dentaire en France . . . Paris (1926)

David, Th.
Bibliographie française de l'art dentaire. Paris 1889

Dechaume, Michel; Pierre Huard
Histoire illustrée de l'art dentaire. Paris 1977

Diepgen, Paul
Geschichte der Medizin. Vol. I, Berlin 1949; vol. II/1, 2nd ed., Berlin 1959; Vol. II/2, 2nd ed., Berlin 1965

Geist-Jacobi, G(eorge) P(ierce)
a) Geschichte der Zahnheilkunde . . . Tübingen 1896
b) Geschichte der Zahnheilkunde. In: Handbuch der Geschichte der Medizin von Max Neuburger and Julius Pagel. Vol. III, Jena 1905, pp. 355—392

Guerini, Vincenzo
A history of dentistry. Philadelphia, New York 1909

Gurlt, Ernst
Geschichte der Chirurgie. Vols. I—III, Berlin 1898

Hirsch, August, E(rnst) Gurlt and A(lbrecht) Wernich
Biographisches Lexikon der hervorragenden Ärzte . . . 3rd ed., München 1962

Hoffmann-Axthelm, Walter
a) The writing of dental history: a commentary. J. Am. Dental. Ass. 88 (1974) 1355—1357
b) Die Geschichte der Zahnheilkunde, Berlin 1973
c) Lexikon der Zahnmedizin. 2nd ed., Berlin 1978

Koch, Charles R. E.
History of dental surgery. Vol. I, 1910; vol. II, 1909; vol. III (Burton Lee Thorpe) Chicago 1909

Linderer, Joseph
a) Geschichte der Zahnheilkunde. In: Handbuch der Zahnheilkunde. Vol. II, Berlin 1848, pp. 398—483
b) Geschichte und Litteratur. In: Die Zahnheilkunde nach ihrem neuesten Standpunkte. Berlin 1851, pp. 343—480

Lindsay, Lilian
A short history of dentistry. London 1933

Lufkin, Arthur Ward
A history of dentistry. 2nd ed., London 1948

Maretzky, Kurt; Robert Venter
Geschichte des deutschen Zahnärzte-Standes. Köln 1974

Mettler, Cecilia C.
History of medicine. Ed. Fred A. Mettler, Philadelphia, Toronto 1947

Morton, Leslie T.
A medical bibliography. 3rd. ed., London 1970

Poletti, Johannes Baptista
De re dentaria apud veteres. 2nd ed., Mediolani 1951

Prinz, Hermann
A historical review of the therapeutic concept during the last hundred years. Dent. Cosmos 76 (1934) 91—109

Proskauer, Curt
Iconographia odontologica. Berlin (1926)

Proskauer, Curt; Fritz H(einz) Witt
Bildgeschichte der Zahnheilkunde. Köln 1962

Sarton, George A. L.
Introduction to the history of science. Vols. I—III, Washington 1927

Sigerist, Henry E.
A history of medicine. Vol. I, New York 1951/1955; vol. II, New York 1961

Strömgren, Hedvig Lidforss
a) Die Zahnheilkunde im 18. Jahrhundert. Kopenhagen 1935
b) Die Zahnheilkunde im 19. Jahrhundert. Kopenhagen 1945
c) Index of dental and adjacent topics in medical works before 1800. Copenhagen 1955

Sudhoff, Karl
Geschichte der Zahnheilkunde. 1st and 2nd ed., Leipzig 1921 and 1926

Thorpe, Burton Lee
History of dental surgery. Ed. Charles R. E. Koch, vol. III, Chicago 1909

Waller, Erik
Bibliotheca Walleriana. Vols. I and II, Stockholm 1950

Weinberger, Bernhard Wolf
a) Orthodontics. Vols. I and II, St. Louis 1926
b) An introduction to the history of dentistry. Vols. I and II, St. Louis 1948
c) Dental Bibliography. 2 parts, New York 1929 (2nd ed.) and 1932

Index of Persons

A

B

C

D

E

F

H

M

N

O

P

Q

R

Richter, August Gottlieb (1742—1812) *235*, 236, 237
Riethe, Peter (b. 1921) 157
Riggs, John Mankey (1811—1885) *317*, 318, 332, 333
Ringelmann, Karl Joseph (1776—1854) 401
Ritter, Frank (1852—1915) 308
Rivière, Lazare (Lazarus Riverus; 1589—1655) *189*
Rivius see Ryff
Robert, Alphonse (1801—1862) 351, 355
Robertson, William (1794—1870) 370, 402
Robin, Charles Philippe (1821—1885) 346
Robin, Pierre (1867—1950) 384
Robinson, James Esq., (1816—1862) *263*, 290, 312, 334, 335, 369, 370
Robicsek, Salomon (1845—1928) 294
Röntgen, Wilhelm Conrad (1845—1923) 344, 387
Röse, Carl (1864—1947) 320, 400, 408
Roger II, King of Sicily (1095—1154) 110
Roger Baron (circa 1214—1292) 124
Roger (Frugardi) of Salerno (fl. 1170) *113*, 115, 123, 124, 129
Rogers, Alfred Paul (1873—1959) 384
Rogers, William (fl. 1845) 264, 373
Roggensack, Bruno (b. 1901) 57, 58
Rokitansky, Karl von (1804—1878) 397
Roland of Parma (fl. 1st h. of the 13th cent.) *113*, 115, 129
Rombouts, Theodor (1597—1637) 171
Romero, Javier (fl. 1951/64) 51
Rostaing, A. (fl. 1858) 294
Rostaing, Charles Sylvester (fl. 1858) 294
Rottenstein, Jean Baptiste (fl. circa 1867) 404
Rousseau, Jean Jacques (1712—1778) 163
Routledge, W. G. (d. 1907) 308
Roux, Albert (1850—1924) 384
Rowlandson, Thomas (1756—1827) 222, 255
Rümelin, Johannes (Remmelinus, Ioannes; 1583—1632) 170
Rütenick (d. 1825?) 350, 353
Ruffer, Sir Marc Armand (1859—1917) 23
Rufus of Ephesos (fl. 115) *74*, 75, 92, 95, 110
Ruiz de Alarcón, Hernando (fl. 1629) 51
Runge, Ludolf Heinrich (1688—1760) 229, 346
Rush, Benjamin (1745—1813) 274
Ruska, Ernst (b. 1906) 400
Ruspini, Bartholomew (1728—1813) 215, *218*, 258
Rust, Johann Nepomuk (1775—1840) 401
Ruysch, Frederik (1638—1731) 223
Ryff, Walther Hermann (Rivius; d. 1562) 163, *165* 167, 180, 350
Rynd, Francis (1803—1861) 339

S

Sachs, Hans (1494—1576) 160
Sahagún, Bernardino de (1499—1590) 47, 50, 57
Salter, Samuel James Augustus (1825—1897) 397
Sarābiyūn: Yūḥannā ibn Sarābiyūn, Serapion (fl. 873) *92*, 130
Sargon I. (circa 2334—2279 B. C.) 27
Sauer, Carl (1835—1892) *266*, 356, 358
Saunders, Sir Edwin (1814—1901) 370
Sauvages, François Boissier Sauvages de Lacroix (1706—1767) 194
Saville, Marshall Howard (1867—1935) 58
Savonarola, Giovanni Michele (1384?—1440?) *131*, 132
Schaeffer, Jacob Christian (1718—1790) 145, 237, *241*, 387, 401
Schalit, Albert (circa 1928) 281
Schange, J. M. Alexis (b. 1807) 279, 366, 368, 373
Scheff, Julius (1846—1922) 399, 412
Schenck von Grafenberg, Johann (1531—1598) *169*, 170, 177
Scheref ed-Din Sabuncuoğlu (fl. 15th cent.) 106
Schiller, Friedrich von (1759—1805) 326
Schiltsky, Otto (d. circa 1907) 279
Schleich, Carl Ludwig (1859—1922) 341
Schlözer, Kurd von (1822—1894) 405
Schneider, Friedrich (1844—1899) 308
Schreger, Christian Heinrich Theodor (1768—1833) *388*, 391
Schreier, Emil (1862—1944) 315
Schreiter, Richard (1846—1925) 315
Schröder, Hermann (1876—1942) 271
Schrott, Johann Joseph (1822—1899) *269*, 279
Schultheiss, Johannes see Scultetus
Schwann, Theodor (1810—1882) 389, 392, 393, 394
Schwarz, Arthur Martin (1887—1963) 383
Scribonius Largus (fl. 47) *73*, 83, 97, 145, 231
Scultetus, Johannes (Schultheiss; 1595—1645) 143, *180*, 181, 187, 199, 240, 346
Sebizius, Melchior (Sebiz; 1578—1671) 174
Šem'ōn de Ṭaibūṭā (End of the 18th cent.) *92*, 93
Semmelweis, Ignaz, (1818—1865) 387
Serapion see Sarābiyūn
Sercombe, Edwin (1826—1875) 302, 305, 307
Serre, Johann Jacob Joseph (1759—1830) 234, *239*, 240, 241, 299, 326, 362
Serres, Etienne Reynaud Augustin (1786—1868) 387
Sethos I (reigned 305—290 B. C.) 19
Shepard, Luther Dimmick (1837—1911) 374

T

U

V

W

Y

Z

U

V

W

Y

Z

Subject Index

Subject Index

A

B

C

D

E

F

G

H

I

J

K

L

M

N

O

P

Q

R

S

T

U

V

W

X

Z

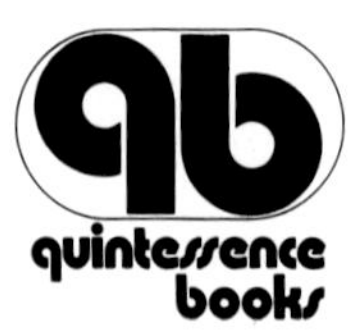

Samuel Fastlicht

Tooth Mutilations and Dentistry in Pre-Columbian Mexico

Recognized as the world's leading authority on pre-Columbian dentistry, Dr. Samuel Fastlicht of Mexico City, has made numerous major contributions to the literature in this field.
He was graduated in Dentistry from the National University of Mexico in 1932. Dr. Alfonso Caso, considered the greatest Mexican archeologist, inspired him to investigate pre-Columbian arts, medicine and dentistry. Fastlicht has published three books:
The Art of Tooth Mutilation (1951)
Mexican Dental Bibliography (1954)
Dentistry in pre-Hispanic Mexico (1971)
According to Dr. Caso, "Fastlicht is one of three Mexican researchers who have dedicated themselves to the subject of 'tooth mutilations and dentistry in pre-Columbian Mexico,' and has carefully studied the very rich collection of our Department of Physical Anthropology of the National Museum of Mexico."
This book contains a report of the investigation, proving that the mutilations of the teeth, as well as the pre-Columbian inlays, were made during the life of the individuals. This has been clearly shown by the use of Xrays.
Also the contribution of Mexico to the Western World, with foodstuffs, industrial and pharmacological products, revolutionized the economy, medicine and nutrition in the Old World.
The author studied the cement used in the fixation of the inlays, and analyzed it in several laboratories in the United States and Europe (London). The inlays in which this cement was used, are still in place, after probably more than a thousand years.
The fascinating chapter on jade in America proves that Chinese jade is a nephrite, and was not used in America, while in Meso-America all of the masterpieces made by the Olmecs, as well as other fabulous archeological pieces, many of them belonging to Museums and private collections, were jadeite.
In addition, the "appendix" contains information about migrations of the peoples, who after thousands of years settled the American continent. Mongolian heredity is clearly indicated in the shovel-shaped-teeth of the ancient Mexicans.

164 pages, 125 illustrations (40 multi-colored). Size: 17.5 x 24.5 cm, linen-bound with gold stamping and protective cover, slip-case.
Order FTM $ 46.– plus handling and 6 % sales tax in Illinois/USA.
ISBN 3 87652 611 6
Quintessence Publishing Co., Inc., 10 South La Salle Street, Suite 1338, Chicago, Illinois 60603